An Atlas of Gynecologic Oncology

An Atlas of Gynecologic Oncology Investigation and Surgery

Third Edition

Edited by

J. Richard Smith MBChB MD FRCOG
Consultant Gynaecological Surgeon and Honorary Senior Lecturer in Gynaecology,
West London Gynaecological Cancer Centre,
Queen Charlotte's and Chelsea Hospitals,
Imperial College NHS Trust,
London, UK

Giuseppe Del Priore MD MPH
Mary Fendrich Hulman Professor and Director of Gynecologic Oncology,
Indiana University School of Medicine, Simon Cancer Center,
Indianapolis, Indiana, USA

Robert L. Coleman MD
Professor & Vice Chair, Clinical Research, Ann Rife Cox Chair for Gynecology,
Department of Gynecologic Oncology, MD Anderson Cancer Center,
University of Texas, Houston, Texas, USA

John M. Monaghan MB ChB FRCS (Ed) FRCOG
Retired Consultant Gynaecological Oncologist,
Senior Lecturer in Gynaecological Oncology,
University of Newcastle Upon Tyne, UK

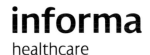

informa
healthcare

First published in 2005 by Taylor & Francis, an imprint of the Taylor & Francis Group.

This edition published in 2011 by Informa Healthcare, Telephone House, 69-77 Paul Street, London EC2A 4LQ, UK.

Simultaneously published in the USA by Informa Healthcare, 52 Vanderbilt Avenue, 7th Floor, New York, NY 10017, USA.

Informa Healthcare is a trading division of Informa UK Ltd. Registered Office: 37–41 Mortimer Street, London W1T 3JH, UK. Registered in England and Wales number 1072954.

A CIP record for this book is available from the British Library.

ISBN-13: 9780415450591

Library of Congress Cataloging-in-Publication Data

An atlas of gynecologic oncology: investigation and surgery/edited by J. Richard Smith ... [et al.]. -- 3rd ed.
    p. ; cm.
  Includes bibliographical references and index.
  ISBN 978-0-415-45059-1 (hb : alk. paper) 1. Generative organs, Female--Cancer--Surgery--Atlases. I. Smith, J. Richard.
  [DNLM: 1. Genital Neoplasms, Female--Surgery--Atlases. WP 17]
  RC280.G5.A85 2011
  616.99'465--dc22
                                                                                    2011008292

Orders may be sent to: Informa Healthcare, Sheepen Place, Colchester, Essex CO3 3LP, UK
Telephone: +44 (0)20 7017 5540
Email: CSDhealthcarebooks@informa.com
Website: http://informahealthcarebooks.com/

For corporate sales please contact: CorporateBooksIHC@informa.com
For foreign rights please contact: RightsIHC@informa.com
For reprint permissions please contact: PermissionsIHC@informa.com

Typeset by Exeter Premedia Services Private Ltd., Chennai, India
Printed and bound in the United Kingdom
Transferred to Digital Print 2011

Dedication

To Mr. Tom Lewis and Dr. Bruce A. Baron, whose friendship was responsible for bringing the editors together. Also to my wife Deborah and my four children for their patience, support, and tolerance of this and many other projects.

JRS

To my family—from the smallest latest joyous addition, to the oldest and wisest, some departed, and in the center of them all, my wife, Men-Jean Lee.

GDP

To my extraordinary wife, Fay, for her unwavering support and understanding, mentorship, love and friendship and to our six blessing children, of whom I could not be prouder. And, to my Parents, who through their years of sacrifice and guidance enabled me to pursue my dreams.

RLC

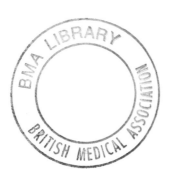

Contents

CONTENTS

Contributors

James Aikins
Division of Gynecologic Oncology, Cooper University Hospital, Voorhees, and Robert Wood Johnson Medical School at Camden, Camden, New Jersey, USA

Thanos Athanasiou
Department of Cardiothoracic Surgery, National Heart and Lung Institute, Imperial College London, Hammersmith Hospital, London, UK

Syed Babar Ajaz
Consultant Radiologist, Hammersmith Hospital, London, UK

Richard R. Barakat
Gynecology Service, Department of Surgery, Memorial Sloan-Kettering Cancer Center, New York, New York, USA

John F. Boggess
University of North Carolina, Chapel Hill, North Carolina, USA

Mark Bower
Consultant Medical Oncologist, Chelsea & Westminster Hospital, London, UK

Deborah C. M. Boyle
Consultant Gynaecologist, The Royal Free Hampstead NHS Trust, London, UK

Gary Bradley
London, UK

Jane Bridges
Unit of Gynaecologic Oncology, Royal Marsden Hospital, London, UK

Erkan Buyuk
Department of Obstetrics and Gynecology, Division of Reproductive Endocrinology and Infertility, Albert Einstein College of Medicine of Yeshiva University, Bronx, New York and Montefiore's Institute for Reproductive Medicine and Health, Hartsdale, New York, USA

Jayanta Chatterjee
Department of Obstetrics and Gynaecology, Queen Charlotte's & Chelsea Hospitals, London, UK

Carmel Cohen
Division of Gynecologic Oncology, Mount Sinai Medical Center, New York, New York, USA

Robert L. Coleman
Department of Gynecologic Oncology, MD Anderson Cancer Center, University of Texas, Houston, Texas, USA

Kathleen Connell
Urogynecology, Yale University Medical School, New Haven, Connecticut, USA

Peter G. Cordeiro
Plastic and Reconstructive Surgery Service, Memorial Sloan-Kettering Cancer Center, New York, New York, USA

David J. Corless
Department of Surgery, Leighton Hospital, Crewe, UK

Jonathan A. Cosin
Gynecologic Oncology, Washington Hospital Center, Washington, DC, USA

Sarah Cox
Palliative Medicine, Chelsea & Westminster Hospital Foundation Trust, London, UK

Daniel Dargent†
Gynécologie Obstétrique, Hôpital Edouard Herriot, Lyon, France

Peter A. Davis
Department of Surgery, The James Cook University Hospital, South Tees Hospitals NHS Trust, Mar on Road, Middlesbrough, UK

Giuseppe Del Priore
Indiana University School of Medicine, Simon Cancer Center, Indianapolis, Indiana, USA

Scott M. Eisenkop
Gynecological Oncologist, Northridge, California, USA

Paul Farquhar-Smith
Department of Anaesthetics, Royal Marsden Hospital, London, UK

Jeffrey M. Fowler
Division of Gynecologic Oncology, The Ohio State University Medical Center, Columbus, Ohio, USA

Michael Frumovitz
Gynecologic Oncology, MD Anderson Cancer Center, University of Texas, Houston, Texas, USA

Ektoras Georgiou
Department of Biosurgery & Surgical Technology, Imperial College Healthcare NHS Trust, Hammersmith Hospital, Imperial College London, London, UK

Sadaf Ghaem-Maghami
Department of Obstetrics and Gynaecology, Imperial College London, Hammersmith Hospital NHS Trust, London, UK

Catherine Gillespie
Lead Cancer and Palliative Care Nurse and Cancer Services Manager, Chelsea & Westminster Hospital Foundation Trust, London, UK

Gary L. Goldberg
Department of Obstetrics and Gynecology and Women's Health, Albert Einstein College of Medicine, and Montefiore Medical Center, Bronx, New York, USA

Rabbie K. Hanna
Department of Obstetrics and Gynecology, Division of Gynecologic Oncology, University of North Carolina, Chapel Hill, North Carolina, USA

Paul Hilton
Directorate of Women's Services, Royal Victoria Infirmary, Newcastle upon Tyne, UK

Sean Hislop
University of Rochester Medical Center, Rochester, New York, USA

Michael Höckel
Department of Obstetrics and Gynaecology, University of Leipzig, Leipzig, Germany

Simon A. Hurst
Charing Cross Hospital, Imperial College, London, UK

Karl A. Illig
Division of Vascular Surgery, University of Rochester Medical Center, Rochester, New York, USA

---

†Deceased.

Thomas Ind
Unit of Gynaecologic Oncology, Royal Marsden Hospital, London, UK

Ian Jacobs
Department of Gynaecological Oncology, EGA Institute for Women's Health, University College London, London, UK

Christina L. Kushnir
Women's Cancer Center of Nevada, Las Vegas, Nevada, USA

Andrew Lawson
Department of Anaesthetics, Royal Berkshire Hospital, Reading, UK

Charles M. Levenback
Gynecologic Oncology, MD Anderson Cancer Center, University of Texas, Houston, Texas, USA

Werner Lichtenegger
Klinik für Frauenheilkunde und Geburtshilfe, Charité/Universitätsmedizin Berlin, Berlin, Germany

Ranjit Manchanda
Department of Gynaecological Oncology, EGA Institute for Women's Health, University College London, London, UK

Angus McIndoe
West London Gynaecological Cancer Centre, Hammersmith & Queen Charlotte's and Chelsea Hospitals, Imperial College Healthcare NHS Trust, London, UK

Usha Menon
Department of Gynaecological Oncology, EGA Institute for Women's Health, University College London, London, UK

John M. Monaghan
Whitton Grange, Whitton, Northumberland, UK

Nimesh P. Nagarsheth
Division of Gynecologic Oncology, Mount Sinai Medical Center, New York, and Englewood Hospital and Medical Center, Englewood, New Jersey, USA

Farr Nezhat
Department of Clinical Obstetrics and Gynecology, Columbia University, College of Physicians and Surgeons; Minimally Invasive Gynecologic & Robotic Surgery, and Division of Gynecologic Oncology, Department of Obstetrics and Gynecology, St. Luke's and Roosevelt Hospitals, New York; Department of Obstetrics, Gynecology & Reproductive Medicine, State University of New York at Stony Brook, School of Medicine; and Minimally Invasive Surgery in Gynecologic Oncology, Department of Obstetrics and Gynecology, Winthrop University Hospital, Mineola, New York, USA

Katherine A. O'Hanlan
Laparoscopic Institute for Gynecologic Oncology, Portola Valley, California, USA

Kutluk H. Oktay
Department of Obstetrics & Gynecology, Medicine, and Cell Biology & Anatomy, Division of Reproductive Medicine & Infertility, and Institute for Fertility Preservation; Laboratory of Molecular Reproduction and Fertility Preservation, Department of Obstetrics & Gynecology, New York Medical College, Valhalla, New York, USA

David Oram
Department of Gynaecology, Barts and the London NHS Trust, The Royal London Hospital, Whitechapel, London, UK

Kenneth Ouriel
Columbia University, New York, New York, USA

Laszlo Palfalvi
Department of Obstetrics and Gynecology, St Stephen Hospital, Budapest, Hungary

Isabel Pigem
Chelsea & Westminster Hospital, London, UK

Marie Plante
Gynecologic Oncology Division, L'Hôtel-Dieu de Québec, Laval University, Quebec, Canada

Andrea L. Pusic
St Paul's Hospital, Vancouver, Canada

Michel Roy
Gynecologic Oncology, CHUQ-Hôtel-Dieu, Quebec, Canada

Srdjan Saso
Department of Obstetrics and Gynaecology, Hammersmith Hospital, Imperial College London, London, UK

Jeanne M. Schilder
Indiana University School of Medicine, Simon Cancer Center, Indianapolis, Indiana, USA

Michael J. Seckl
Director of the Charing Cross Gestational Trophoblastic Disease Centre, Head of Section of Molecular Oncology, Division of SORA CR-UK Laboratories, Hammersmith Hospital Campus of Imperial College London, London, UK

Eileen M. Segreti
Department of Obstetrics and Gynecology, Division of Gynecologic Oncology, Western Pennsylvania Hospital, Pittsburgh, Pennsylvania, USA

Jalid Sehouli
Universitätsklinikum Charité Medizinische Fakultät der Humboldt-Universität, Berlin, Berlin, Germany

Krishen Sieunarine
Consultant in Obstetrics & Gynaecology, Kettering General Hospital NHS Foundation Trust, Northants, UK

J. Richard Smith
West London Gynaecological Cancer Centre, Queen Charlotte's and Chelsea Hospitals, Imperial College NHS Trust, London, UK

Nick M. Spirtos
Women's Cancer Center of Nevada, Las Vegas, Nevada, USA

Paniti Sukumvanich
Department of Obstetrics, Gynecology & Reproductive Sciences, Magee-Womens Hospital of the University of Pittsburgh Medical Center, Pittsburgh, Pennsylvania, USA

Jessica Thomes-Pepin
Department of Obstetrics and Gynecology, Indiana University School of Medicine, Indianapolis, Indiana, USA

Laszlo Ungar
Department of Obstetrics and Gynecology, St Stephen Hospital, Budapest, Hungary

Louis J. Vitone
Department of Surgery, Mid Cheshire Hospital NHS Trust, Crewe, UK

David Warshal
Division of Gynecologic Oncology, Cooper University Hospital, Voorhees, and Robert Wood Johnson Medical School at Camden, Camden, New Jersey, USA

Ruth Williamson
Clinical Radiology, Hammersmith Hospital, London, UK

Preface

We, the editors, are pleased to introduce you to an updated third edition. We believe that in the mould of the previous editions we have included the standard repertoire of the gynecologic oncologist plus all that is new and leading edge. All chapters have been reviewed by both the editors and their authors, some chapters have been replaced, and we have added some new chapters, including preoperative work-up, robotic surgery, uterine transplantation, and the impact of organ retrieval on training. In addition to this, we have included a new chapter on removal of upper abdominal ovarian cancer. New sections have been added to the chapter on anatomy and these tie in with a new chapter on total mesometrial resection. The superb artwork of Dee McLean and Joanna Cameron is continued and we believe allows easy step-by-step breakdown of each procedure. This book follows the "cookbook" formula of the previous editions, that is, nobody is telling you which operation to do, but rather telling you how to do the operation you have decided upon. Many of our contributors have developed/improved the operations they describe and we believe it is a sign of the success of the book that innovative surgeons are keen to take part. It has once again been a privilege and a pleasure to collect together and edit this selection of contributions which we hope covers all the mainline procedures currently in use in gynecologic oncology, not to say a few which we believe may become important.

J. Richard Smith
Giuseppe Del Priore
Robert L. Coleman
John M. Monaghan

Acknowledgments

Mr. Smith would like to thank Miss Rodena Kelman, Dr. Charles J. Lockwood, Chief of Obstetrics and Gynaecology at Yale University, and Professor P. J. Steer, Professor of Obstetrics, Imperial College School of Medicine, at Chelsea and Westminster Hospital. He would also like to thank Dr. J. A. Davis, Stobhill Hospital, Glasgow, and Mr. B. V. Lewis of Watford General Hospital, for their surgical teaching and stimulus "to go and see new things." In addition, he would like to express his gratitude to his new colleagues, Mr. Angus McIndoe, Mr. Peter Mason, Mr. Alan Farthing, Ms. Sadaf Ghaem-Maghami, and Professor Hani Gabra for their warm welcome to the West London Gynaecological Cancer Centre, a truly inspirational environment in which to work. Dr. Del Priore wishes to thank his family for indulging his passion for his work and patients. He also thanks his trainees for constant inspiration to learn and teach more. He thanks his colleagues for their continued guidance and constructive feedback and especially Drs. Smith and Lee.

1 Introduction

J. Richard Smith, Giuseppe Del Priore, and Simon A. Hurst

INTRODUCTION

This chapter reviews three specific areas relevant to virtually all surgical procedures and surgeons, namely infection prophylaxis, deep venous thrombosis prophylaxis, and universal precautions: the latter facilitate the protection both of surgeons and their assistants, both medical and nursing, and of patients. Preoperative and postoperative check lists now form a vital part of risk reduction. James Reason CBE formulated the "Swiss cheese theory" of risk. This is based on a piece of Swiss cheese with holes in it and the more slices one puts in the cheese the less likely it is that an arrow could fly through the holes, the holes are less likely to tally with each other. Thus the more layers of checking that one puts in pre- and postoperatively the less likely it is that the antibiotic prophylaxis will be forgotten or the postoperative DVT prophylaxis will not be given. A simple check list is shown below.

CHECK LIST FOR SURGERY ON ADMISSION Date :-	

NAME :   DATE OF BIRTH :

OPERATION PLANNED :

RISKS	
Infection	
Anaesthetic	
Haemorrhage	
Deep Venous Thrombosis	
Uterine Perforation	
Other Organ Damage	
Others	

PAST GYNAECOLOGICAL HISTORY	
Last Menstrual Period	
Contraception	
x/y	
Pregnancy Test	

PERTINENT MEDICAL/ANAESTHETIC PROBLEMS	

Signed _____

POSTOPERATIVE CHECK LIST	
Low molecular weight heparin or other measures prescribed	
Antibiotics prescribed	
Photographs taken and collected	

Signed _____

INFECTION PROPHYLAXIS

Most gynecology units now routinely use antibiotic prophylaxis prior to both minor and major surgery. In the absence of such prophylaxis, abdominal hysterectomy is complicated by infection in up to 14% of patients, and following vaginal hysterectomy, infection rates of up to 38% have been reported (Sweet and Gibbs 1990). This results in much morbidity, increased length of hospital stay, increased prescribing of antibiotics, and a large financial burden. The risk factors for postoperative infection are shown in Table 1. By its very nature, oncological surgery carries greater risks of infection than routine gynecological surgery, owing to the length of the procedures and increased blood loss.

It is difficult to compare many of the studies on prophylaxis, as diagnosis and antibiotic regimens are not standardized. However, there seems to be general agreement that approximately 50% of infections are prevented in this way and that the potential dangers of increased microbial resistance do not justify withholding prophylaxis. Prophylaxis is thought to work by reducing, but not eradicating, vaginal flora. The antibiotic used, its dose, and the duration of therapy do not appear to influence results. It is therefore suggested that short courses of antibiotics should be used, involving a maximum of three doses. First-generation cephalosporins, broad-spectrum penicillins, and/or metronidazole are all reasonable choices on grounds of efficacy and cost. Antibiotic prophylaxis should not detract from good surgical technique, with an emphasis on strict asepsis, limitation of trauma, and good hemostasis. This should be coupled with adequate drainage of body cavities, where particularly blood and also lymph are likely to pool postoperatively.

PREVENTION AND TREATMENT
OF THROMBOEMBOLIC DISEASE

Thromboembolic disease (TED) is a significant cause of morbidity and mortality in gynecologic oncology patients. If sensitive methods of detection are employed and no preventive measures are taken, at least 20% and as many as 70% of gynecologic cancer patients may have some evidence of thrombosis. In certain situations, such as with a long-term indwelling venous catheter of the upper extremity, nearly all patients will have some degree of TED, though it may not be clinically significant. On the other hand, lower extremity TED has a much more certain and clinically significant natural history. Venous thromboses below the knee may spread to the upper leg in approximately 10% to 30% of cases or resolve spontaneously in approximately 30%. Once the disease has reached the proximal leg, the risk of pulmonary embolism (PE)

increases from less than 5% for isolated below-the-knee TED, to up to 50% for proximal TED. The mortality rate for an undiagnosed PE is high. Up to two-thirds of patients who die from PE do so in the first 30 minutes after diagnosis. Early recognition and effective treatment can reduce this mortality; however, postoperative TED is still a leading cause of death in gynecologic oncology patients. In the past, it was clear that only one-third of hospitalized high-risk patients received appropriate prophylaxis and this figure has now much improved particularly with the use of check lists.

PREVENTION AND RISK ASSESSMENT

Patients may be considered for prevention of TED based on their clinical risk category. Laboratory tests such as euglobulin lysis time do correlate with the risk of TED but are no more helpful than clinical risk assessment in selecting patients for prophylaxis. Low-risk patients are young (less than 40 years old), undergoing short operative procedures (less than one hour) and do not have coexisting morbid conditions such as malignancy or obesity that would elevate the risk of TED. Moderate-risk patients include those undergoing longer procedures, older or obese patients, and patients having pelvic surgery. High-risk patients include otherwise moderate-risk patients who have cancer and those with a previous history of TED. Positioning for vaginal surgery lowers the risk of TED when compared with the abdominal approach.

All patients should have some form of TED prevention. Low-risk patients, with an incidence of approximately 3% for TED, may be adequately protected with early ambulation, elevation of the foot of the bed, and graduated compression stockings. 'Early ambulation' has been defined by some investigators as walking around the nursing station at least three times within the first 24 hours. Graduated compression stockings are readily available; however, ensuring their proper application and size can be difficult. Obese patients may suffer from a "tourniquet" effect if the stocking rolls off the thigh; this may actually increase the risk of TED, not prevent it.

Moderate-risk patients include the majority of general gynecology patients and have approximately 10% to 40% chance of developing TED. These patients should receive the same measures as low-risk patients with the addition of low-dose unfractionated low molecular weight heparin (LMWH), 5000 units subcutaneously twice a day. An alternative to the administration of heparin is the application of pneumatic compression devices to the lower extremities. High-risk category patients require even more measures owing to the estimated 40% to 70% risk of TED.

The vast majority of gynecologic oncology cases will fall into the high-risk category. Standard unfractionated heparin (UH) is ineffective in these cases in low doses, such as 5000 units twice daily. If given three times daily, UH is effective but no better than pneumatic calf compression. Unfortunately, more frequent dosing is associated with significantly more wound hematoma formation and blood transfusions. It also requires additional nursing and pharmacy personnel time, and is more uncomfortable for the patient. These may be some of the reasons why only a minority of surgeons regularly use UH prophylaxis. Unfortunately, although compression devices are effective in gynecologic oncology patients, the

---

Table 1 Risk Factors for Postoperative Infection

1	Hospital stay for more than 72 hours before surgery
2	Prior exposure to antimicrobial agents in the immediate preoperative period
3	Morbid obesity
4	Chronic illness, e.g., hypertension, diabetes
5	History of repeated infection
6	Prolonged operative procedure (>3 hr)
7	Blood loss in excess of 1500 ml

devices are somewhat cumbersome, and are disliked by patients and nursing staff. In fact, improper application of the devices occurs in approximately 50% of patients on routine inpatient nursing stations. Compression devices are also contraindicated in patients with significant peripheral vascular disease.

The LMWHs have many potential advantages over the previously cited alternatives. These include excellent bioavailability, allowing for single daily dosing. This reduces nursing effort and therefore cost, and may be better accepted by the patient. This form of prophylaxis is also associated with less thrombocytopenia and postoperative bleeding. Patients with UH-associated thrombocytopenia will usually tolerate LMWH without difficulty. In summary, in extremely high-risk patients such as gynecologic patients, LMWH may be more efficacious, more cost-effective and less toxic than the alternatives.

Many other agents have been tried in an attempt to overcome the imperfections of existing options. All have limitations and are not used routinely; however, all are effective to some degree and may be appropriate in highly selected patients. Some of these agents include aspirin, warfarin and high molecular weight dextran. The most promising are direct thrombin inhibitors and oral factor Xa inhibitors. In comparison with LMWH, aspirin results in more bleeding complications and is less effective than heparin in preventing TED. Warfarin has a prophylactic effect similar to aspirin, but again is less effective than heparin and is associated with a higher risk of complications and requires more intensive monitoring. Dextrans are effective but have been associated with rare cases of allergic reactions. Other complications reported include fluid overload and nephrotoxicity. Further research to avoid some of these limitations may improve the therapeutic value of these alternatives.

PREVENTION AND TREATMENT OF THROMBOEMBOLIC DISEASE

The duration of prophylaxis has traditionally been limited to the duration of hospital stay. In many older studies, when health care was less cost-conscious, this may have been several days to weeks. Lengths of stay are now much shorter and as a result, so is the duration of TED preventive measures. Even before this forced change in clinical practice, it was recognized that a significant minority of TED either developed or was diagnosed long after discharge from the hospital. The optimal duration of prophylaxis is still not known and depends on the method used. For instance, patients should be instructed to walk every day once discharged from the hospital. Similarly, graduated compression stockings may be worn after surgery until discharge with little risk and possibly some benefit. Some authors also advocate compression stockings to be worn at home following discharge. However, pharmacologic therapies have side effects, may require some training (e.g., self or nurse injections) and are associated with considerable cost in both monitoring and potential toxicity. For these reasons, the optimal method and duration of TED prophylaxis following discharge have not been determined. General guidance has been to use prophylaxis until the patient is fully mobile. However, one patient's fully mobile is another's complete stasis. Clear exercise parameters are probably the only definers of full mobility.

The agents discussed above are all designed to prevent TED and thereby reduce the risk of developing a clinically significant PE. When these methods are used properly, most patients will not develop TED and therefore will be at low risk for a PE. However, it is not uncommon for a gynecologic oncology patient to present with TED as the first manifestation of disease; for instance, it is the presenting symptom in up to 10% of ovarian cancer patients. In these patients, and in those who develop TED despite appropriate prophylaxis, something must be done to prevent the progression to a potentially fatal PE. This becomes especially difficult if the patient requires surgical treatment for the malignancy. One common management technique for these difficult situations is mechanical obstruction of the inferior vena cava. This can be accomplished preoperatively via peripheral venous access and interventional radiologic techniques. Care must be taken to delineate the extent of the clot so that no attempt is made to pass the filtering device through an occluded vein. If peripheral caval interruption is not possible, a vena caval clip may be applied intraoperatively. However, large pelvic masses, not uncommon in gynecologic cancer patients, may prevent access. Additional problems with vena caval interruption include migration of the device, complete occlusion of the cava, perforation and infection. In preoperative cases where the patient cannot have a filter or clip placed, one option is the discontinuation of intravenous UH one hour before the perioperative period, with resumption approximately six hours after completion of the surgery. Most patients will do well with this technique, but they are still vulnerable to intraoperative PEs. Another pharmacologic option may include the preoperative lysis of the thrombus with thrombolytic agents such as urokinase followed by resumption of standard prophylactic measures. Oral anticoagulation is used after caval interruption, if not contraindicated, to prevent post-thrombotic venous stasis of the lower extremity. Therefore, mechanical devices, while reducing perioperative pulmonary emboli, do not obviate the need for long-term anticoagulation. It is vitally important if one is operating on patients who have traveled on long haul flights that major surgery should be avoided within 48 hours of this flight. NICE guidance on venous thromboembolism in patients undergoing surgery (NICE 2007) states that "immobility associated with continuous travel of more than three hours in the four weeks before or after surgery may increase the risk of VTE". For those patients traveling by plane postoperatively, the relatively new oral preparations of Dabigatran and rivaroxaban, licensed for the prevention of VTE after hip and knee replacement surgery may be prescribed (Gomez et al. 2009).

DIAGNOSIS

Given the imperfection of prophylaxis and the high risk of TED in gynecologic oncology patients, all physicians caring for these women should be familiar with the treatment and diagnosis of TED including PE. Fewer than one-third of patients with TED of the lower extremity will present with the classic symptoms of unilateral edema, pain and venous distension. A positive Homan's sign, calf pain with dorsiflexion of the foot, is also unreliable and is seen in less than half of patients with TED. Calf TED occurs bilaterally in approximately 40% of cases and is more common on the left (40%)

than on the right (20%). Only a high index of suspicion and objective testing can correctly identify patients with TED.

In high-risk patients with a high baseline prevalence of TED, sensitive but nonspecific tests are useful owing to their high positive predictive value. To exclude disease in these same high-risk patients, repeat testing on subsequent days or more sensitive techniques are needed. Noninvasive diagnostic testing should always be considered before interventional techniques including venography and arteriography. Lower extremity Doppler and real-time two-dimensional ultrasonography scans are fairly sensitive (85%) and specific (>95%) for TED. If results are positive in high-risk patients, including those with symptoms suggestive of PE, no further testing is indicated and therapy may be initiated. Ventilation–perfusion scans and spiral CT thoracic scanning may be used similarly in patients in whom PE is suspected. If the scan indicates an intermediate or high probability of PE, treatment is usually advisable. In patients at higher risk for hemorrhagic complications, such as during the immediate postoperative period where there is residual tumor, confirmatory tests may be indicated before therapy. Pulmonary arteriography may be indicated in this setting, although magnetic resonance arteriography or venography is rapidly becoming the test of choice.

TREATMENT

If there is no contraindication to anticoagulation, therapy should be started as soon as the diagnosis of TED is made. Outcomes are correlated with the time it takes to achieve therapeutic anticoagulation, so the fastest means available should be employed. Low molecular weight heparin has an advantage over UH in that a single daily dose of approximately 175 units/kg subcutaneously will be therapeutic almost immediately. Unfractionated heparin may require approximately 24 hours and repeated blood testing before becoming therapeutic. Treatment with warfarin can be started once the anti-coagulation effect of either heparin is confirmed. With UH, this may be as early as day 1, although two to three days of therapy may be needed before anticoagulation is achieved. With LMWH, warfarin can be started within a few hours, and definitely on the same day. Either heparin should be continued until the warfarin has achieved an international normalized ratio of 2 to 3. Anti-coagulation with warfarin should continue for at least three months. Patients with recurrent TED or persistent precipitating events, e.g., vessel compression by tumor, may need indefinite anticoagulation.

Disseminated cancer and chemotherapy will unavoidably increase the risk of complications from anticoagulation. Cancer patients who have nutritional deficits, organ damage, and unknown metastatic sites are particularly vulnerable. Chemotherapeutic agents alter the metabolism of anticoagulants through their effect on liver and renal function, making dosing more difficult. Chemotherapeutic drugs may also share similar toxicities with anticoagulants and thereby worsen hemorrhagic complications from thrombocytopenia and anemia. For these reasons, treatment of TED may not be desired by the patient nor recommended by her physician in all situations. Thrombosis restricted to the calf may be followed with frequent ultrasonograms in such situations, although the decision to treat or not is controversial and thus a matter for clinical judgment.

INFECTION CONTROL[a]

There is increasing awareness of the risks of transmission of blood-borne pathogens from surgeon to patient and vice versa during surgical practice. These risks have been highlighted by the publicity surrounding human immunodeficiency virus (HIV), but are generally greater from other pathogens including hepatitis B virus (HBV). Infection with hepatitis C virus (HCV) also poses a risk of transmission from patient to surgeon. The prevalence of these viral infections varies widely with different populations, and this exerts an influence on the surgeon's risk, as does the number of needlestick (or sharps) injuries sustained and the surgeon's immune status. The risks of transmission of these viruses and their subsequent pathogenicity are discussed below. The necessity for universal precautions in surgical practice need not affect overmuch operator acceptability or cost.

Antenatal anonymous surveys have shown a seroprevalence of HIV in metropolitan areas of the United Kingdom to be as high as 0.26% (Goldberg et al. 1992, Evans et al. 2009). HIV prevalence has increased in the United Kingdom over the last decade, with an estimated 73,000 individuals living with HIV by 2006. Seroprevalence data of women undergoing gynecological or general surgical procedures are not currently available, but an unlinked anonymous survey of 32,796 London hospital inpatients aged 16 to 49 years from specialties not usually dealing with illness related to HIV infection has found a seroprevalence of 0.2% (Newton and Hall 1993).

The risk of acquiring HIV from a single-needlestick injury from an infected patient is in the region of 0.10% to 0.36% (Shanson 1992, Ippolito et al. 1993, Cardo et al. 1997a, b). Pooled data from several prospective studies of health-care personnel suggest that the average risk of HIV transmission is approximately 0.3% (95% confidence interval, 0.2 to 0.5) after a percutaneous exposure to HIV-infected blood and approximately 0.09% (95% confidence interval, 0.006 to 0.5) after a mucous-membrane exposure (Gerberding 2003). However, using mathematical models to predict lifetime risks of acquiring the infection in a population with a low HIV seroprevalence (0.35%), it has been suggested that 0.26% of surgeons would seroconvert during their working lives (Howard 1990). Needlestick injuries pose a significant occupational risk for surgical trainees. A study by Markay et al. (2007) in *The New England Journal of Medicine* found that virtually all surgical residents (99%) had had a needlestick injury by their final year of training, and concluded that needlestick injuries are common among surgeons in training and are often not reported. Improved prevention and reporting strategies are needed to increase occupational safety for surgical providers (Markay et al. 2007). If the seroprevalence of HIV infection in surgical patients were as high as 5%, then the estimated 30-year risk of HIV seroconversion for the surgeon might be as high as 6%, depending on the number and type of injuries sustained (Lowenfels et al. 1989). In December 2001, 57 health-care workers in the United States had seroconverted to HIV as a result of occupational exposure. Of the adults reported with acquired immune deficiency syndrome (AIDS) in the United

---

[a]This section is adapted and updated from *Br J Gynaecol Obstet* (1995) **102**: 439–41.

States through December 31, 2002, 24,844 had a history of employment in healthcare. These cases represented 5.1% of the 486,826 AIDS cases reported to the Centers for Disease Control and Prevention for whom occupational information was known (www.cdc.gov). This website is a valuable resource particularly with respect to new and ever changing drug regimens currently in use in the management of blood-borne pathogens.

Intact skin and mucous membranes are thought to be effective barriers against HIV. Only a very few cases of transmission via skin contamination are known to have occurred, and these health-care workers had severe dermatitis and did not observe barrier precautions when exposed to HIV-infected blood (Centers for Disease Control 1987) Aerosol transmission of HIV is not known to occur, and the principal risks are related to injuries sustained from hollow-bore needles, suture needles, and lacerations from other sharp instruments. Infectivity is determined by the volume of the inoculum and the viral load within it: thus a hollow-bore needlestick injury carries greater risk than injury from a suture needle. Prior to highly active antiretroviral therapy, infection with HIV results in the AIDS in 50% of patients over a 12-year period and had a long-term mortality approaching 100%. The situation is now radically different. For HIV seropositive surgeons, further operative practice involving insertion of the fingers into the body cavity is precluded owing to the potential risk of doctor-to-patient transmission: for gynecologic surgeons, this encompasses virtually their entire surgical practice, with the exception of laparoscopic and hysteroscopic procedures. There is a whole classification related to exposure-prone procedures (EPP) which is categorised into non-exposure prone (category 0) and exposure (1-3). Category 3 encompasses all open procedures. This classification is available from the UK Dept of Health website related to UKAP (United Kingdom Advisory Panel for Health Care Workers infected with blood-borne pathogens). At present there is no vaccine available to prevent infection with HIV. Should needlestick injury occur, the injured area should be squeezed in an attempt to expel any inoculum, and the hands should be thoroughly washed. There is good evidence that after exposure prophylactic zidovudine (azidothymidine, AZT) reduces transmission by 79%. Most occupational health departments now advise their health-care workers to commence treatment within one hour of injury with multiple therapy which depending on the risk of HIV exposure should either be two drug regimen for four weeks or for those at higher risk a three drug regimen. These usually include zidovudine (AZT), lamivudine (3TC), although these may be modified in the event of known drug resistance in the index case. This type of regimen may well reduce the risks of seroconversion further. A further study suggested a reduced risk from multiple therapy of 81% (95% CI 43% to 94%) (Cardo et al. 1997a, b). In some countries surgeons with a persistently undetectable viral load (less than 50 copies) may be allowed to return to performing EPPs under occupational health supervision.

Intraoperative transmission of HBV occurs more readily than with HIV, and exposure of skin or mucous membrane to blood from a hepatitis B e antigen (HBeAg) carrier involves a highly significant risk of transmission for those who are not immune. The risk of seroconversion following an accidental inoculation with blood from an HBeAg carrier, in the absence of immunity, is up to 30% for susceptible HCWs without post-exposure prophylaxis (PEP) or sufficient hepatitis B vaccination (Wicker et al. 2008). Hepatitis B surface antigen (HBsAg) is found in 0.5% to 1% of patients in inner cities and in 0.1% of patients in rural areas and blood donors. Given a needlestick rate of 5% per operation, the risk of acquiring the virus in a surgical lifetime is potentially high. Prior to the introduction of HBV vaccination an estimated 40% of American surgeons became infected at some point in their careers, with 4% becoming carriers. Acute infection with HBV is associated with the development of fulminant hepatitis in approximately 1% of individuals. Carriers may go on to develop chronic liver damage, cirrhosis, or hepatocellular carcinoma, carrying an overall mortality of approximately 40%.

Transmission of HBV from infected health-care workers to patients is rare but well documented. Welch et al. (1989) reported a case of an infected gynecologist who transmitted HBV to 20 of his patients; the operations carrying greatest risk of infection were hysterectomy (10/42) and caesarean section (10/51). In view of this risk government guidelines in most countries stipulate that surgeons should be immune to HBV, either through natural immunity or vaccination, the exceptions being staff who fail to respond to the vaccine (5% to 10%) and those who are found to be HBsAg positive in the absence of "e" antigenemia [(United Kingdom) Advisory Group on Hepatitis 1993]. In the United Kingdom, the United States, and other countries this is a statutory obligation. Those who fail to respond to vaccination should receive hepatitis B immunoglobulin following needlestick injury where the patient is HBV positive.

Hepatitis C virus, the commonest cause of non-A non-B hepatitis in the developed world, is also known to be spread by blood contamination. Routine screening for antibodies amongst blood donors in the United Kingdom has shown that 0.05% were seropositive in 1991; many of these were seemingly healthy asymptomatic carriers. However, as many as 85% of injecting drug users may be seropositive. Antibodies to HCV were detected in 4.3% of 599 pregnant women screened anonymously in a North American inner city (Silverman et al. 1993). In the United Kingdom, infection with HCV is second only to alcohol as a cause of cirrhosis, chronic liver disease and hepatocellular carcinoma, although the clinical course in seemingly healthy individuals is unclear.

A recent anonymous seroprevalence study of staff at an inner London teaching hospital reported that infection with HCV was no higher than that previously seen in blood donors. The seroprevalence was no different for workers involved with direct clinical exposure (medical and nursing staff) compared with those at risk of indirect clinical exposure (laboratory and ancillary staff) (Zuckerman et al. 1994). However, these findings should not lead to complacency. From epidemiological data, it would appear that HCV infection is less contagious than HBV, but more so than HIV. The risk of a HCV infection is estimated at between 3 and 10%; it increased 10-fold if the source patient has high levels of virus load (Wicker et al. 2008). It would however appear that transmission is very rare with solid bore needles, i.e., almost exclusively follows inoculation with hollow bore needles. Transmission has rarely followed mucous membrane exposure and never via non-intact or intact skin. The possibility of HCV infection should be considered in the event of needlestick injury.

Immunization and PEP are not available for those exposed to HCV. In the United Kingdom recently for those health-care workers infected with hepatitis C, the same restrictions with respect to HIV, i.e., preclusion from performing exposure prone procedures has been introduced; this is not the case in any other country.

PREVENTION OF BLOOD-BORNE INFECTION

Some surgeons have advocated preoperative screening of patients for HIV infection. They argue that patients shown to be infected should be treated as high-risk, while the remaining patients would be labeled as low-risk, with the consequent development of a two-tier infection control policy. However, such an approach is fraught with political, ethical, logistical, and financial implications and, furthermore, wrongly assumes that infected patients can always be identified by serological testing. The universal precautions suggested below are practicable, and effectively minimize the intraoperative infection risk of both surgeon and patient. These precautions are based on the procedure rather than the perceived risk status of the patient. As discussed above, the greatest risk of contracting a blood-borne pathogen is from needlestick injury. Vaginal hysterectomy has been shown to have the highest rate (10%) of needlestick injury of any surgical procedure (Tokars et al. 1991). Glove puncture has been used as a measure of skin contamination and a reflection of needlestick injury; the highest rate of glove puncture reported in any surgical procedure was 55% at caesarean section (Smith and Grant 1990). Double gloving has shown a six-fold diminution in inner glove puncture rate, and anecdotally appears to result in a reduction in needlestick injury, but it is uncomfortable, particularly during protracted procedures, making it unsuitable for many gynecologic oncological operations. Blunt-tipped needles, such as the Protec Point (Davis & Geck, Gosport, United Kingdom) and Ethiguard (Ethicon, Edinburgh, United Kingdom), appear to reduce the rate of glove puncture, and one of the authors (J.R.S.) has never sustained a needlestick injury in eight years of continuously using these needles. The newer needles are capable of penetrating the majority of tissues including uterine muscle, vaginal vault, cervix, peritoneum, and rectus sheath. They are unsuitable for bowel and bladder surgery and do not penetrate skin, but they have been used subcutaneously for abdominal wound closure. Abdominal skin closure can also be safely undertaken with the use of staples. This is particularly important since it has been shown that 5% of glove punctures occurred during this stage of the procedure (Smith and Grant 1990). Just under half of punctures occur in the right hand (Smith and Grant 1990)—a surprising finding considering that most surgeons are right-handed and therefore grasp the needleholder with the dominant hand. Injury appears to occur during knot tying, and a safety needleholder with provision for guarding the needle tip at this stage and when returning the needle to the scrub nurse is now available (Thomas et al. 1995) (Fig. 1). The use of a kidney dish for passing scalpels between staff should also be encouraged, as should safe needle and blade disposal in hands-free surgical sharps boxes. Blades or needles that have fallen on the floor should be retrieved with a magnet prior to disposal. Blunt towel clips are also available to prevent injury while draping. Reusable self-adhesive drapes are available, as are disposable

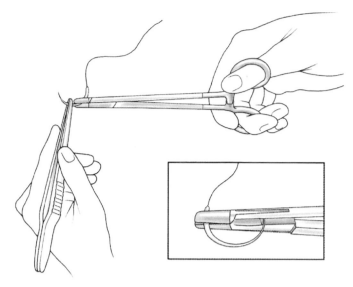

Figure 1 Safety needle holder.

Table 2 Risk Factors for Transmission of Blood-Borne Pathogens During Surgical Practice

1	Prolonged surgical procedure
2	Heavy blood loss
3	Operating within a confined space, e.g., pelvis or vagina
4	Poor lighting
5	Guiding the needle by feel

Table 3 Simple Precautions Available to Reduce Needlestick Injury

1	Blunt-tipped needles: available from Davis & Geck (Protec Point) and Ethicon (Ethiguard needle)
2	Staple guns for skin closure: available from Autosuture and Ethicon Endosurgery
3	Staples for bowel anastomosis: available from Autosuture and Ethicon Endosurgery
4	Spectacles/protective eyewear: blood-borne pathogens have however only been shown to be transmitted very rarely and usually only in the presence of gross ocular contamination
5	Magnet for picking up sharps
6	Hands-free disposable sharps boxes for needles and blades
7	Blunt towel clips
8	Self-adhesive drapes

self-adhesive drapes with a surrounding bag to prevent gross contamination.

Skin and mucous membrane contamination should be avoided by the use of masks and waterproof gowns. Spectacles or other protective eyewear should be worn to prevent contamination by facial splashes of blood and other body fluids.

The risks and safety measures discussed above are summarized in Tables 2 and 3. Table 2 demonstrates that oncological surgery carries the greatest risk. However, the simple and relatively cheap procedures and precautions suggested in Table 3 can reduce the risk for both surgeon and patient to extremely low levels.

REFERENCES

Advisory Group on Hepatitis (1993) *Protecting Health Care Workers and Patients from Hepatitis B.* London: HMSO.

Cardo DM, Culver DH, Ciesielski CA, et al. (1997a) A case-control study of HIV seroconversion in health care workers after percutaneous exposure. *N Engl J Med* **337**:1542–3.

Cardo DM, Culver DH, Ciesielski CA, et al. (1997b) A case control study of HIV seroconversion in health care workers after percutaneous exposure. *N Engl J Med* **337**:1485–90.

Centers for Disease Control (1987) Update: human immuno deficiency virus infection in health care workers exposed to blood of infected patients. *MMWR* **36**:285–9.

Evans HE, Mercer CH, Rait G, et al. Trends in HIV testing and recording of HIV status in the UK primary care setting: a retrospective cohort study 1995–2005. *Sex Transm Infect* 2009; **85**: 520–6.

Gerberding JL (2003) Occupational exposure to HIV in health care settings. *N Engl J Med* **348**:826–33.

Goldberg DJ, MacKinnon H, Smith R, et al. (1992) Prevalence of HIV among childbearing women and women having termination of pregnancy: multi-disciplinary steering group study. *Br Med J* **304**:1082–5.

Gomez-Outes A, Lecumberri R, Pozo C, Rocha E. New anticoagulants: focus on venous thromboembolism. *Curr Vasc Pharmacol* 2009; **7**: 309–29.

Howard RJ (1990) Human immunodeficiency virus testing and the risk to the surgeon of acquiring HIV. *Surg Gynaecol Obstet* **171**:22–6.

Ippolito G, Puro V, De Carli G (1993) The risk of occupational human immunodeficiency virus infection in health care workers: The Italian Study Group on occupational risk of HIV infection. *Arch Intern Med* **153**:1451–8.

Lowenfels AB, Worsmer GP, Jain R (1989) Frequency of puncture injuries in surgeons and estimated risk of HIV infection. *Arch Surg* **124**:1284–6.

Makary MA, Al-Attar A, Holzmueller CG, et al. Needlestick injuries among surgeons in training. *N Engl J Med* 2007; **356**: 2693–9.

Newton L, Hall SM (1993) Unlinked anonymous monitoring of HIV prevalence in England and Wales: 1990–1992. *Common Dis Rep* **3**:1–16.

NICE (2007) Guidance on venous thromboembolism in patients undergoing surgery (April 2007) states that 'immobility associated with continuous travel of more than 3 hours in the 4 weeks before or after surgery may increase the risk of VTE'.

Shanson DC (1992) Risk to surgeons and patients from HIV and hepatitis: guidelines on precautions and management of exposure to blood or body fluids. (Joint Working Party of the Hospital Infection Society and the Surgical Infection Study Group). *Br Med J* **305**:1337–43.

Silverman NS, Jenkin BK, Wu C, et al. (1993) Hepatitis C virus in pregnancy: seroprevalence and risk factors for infection. *Am J Obstet Gynecol* **169**:583–7.

Smith JR, Grant JM (1990) The incidence of glove puncture during caesarean section. *J Obstet Gynaecol* **10**:317–18.

Sweet RL, Gibbs RS (1990) *Infectious Diseases of the Female Genital Tract*, 2nd edn. Baltimore: Williams & Wilkins.

Thomas PB, Falder S, Jolly M, et al. (1995) The role of blunt-tipped needles and a new needle-holder in reducing needlestick injury. *J Obstet Gynaecol* **15**:336–8.

Tokars J, Bell D, Marcus R, et al. (1991) Percutaneous injuries during surgical procedures (Abstract). VII International Conference on AIDS, Florence, Italy.

Wicker S, Cinatl J, Berger A, et al. Determination of risk of infection with blood-borne pathogens following a needlestick injury in hospital workers. *Ann Occup Hyg* 2008; **52**: 615–22.

Welch J, Webster M, Tilzey AJ, et al. Hepatitis B infections after gynaecological surgery. *Lancet* 1989; **1**: 205–7.

West DJ. The risk of hepatitis B infection among health professionals in the United States: a review. *Am J Med Sci* 1984; **287**: 26–33.

Zuckerman J, Clewley G, Griffiths P, Cockroft A (1994) Prevalence of hepatitis C antibodies in clinical health-care workers. *Lancet* **343**:1618–20.

2 Preoperative work up

Jessica Thomes-Pepin and Jeanne M. Schilder

ASSESSMENT OF PERIOPERATIVE CARDIAC RISK

The current leading cause of all female mortality is coronary artery disease. Perioperative cardiovascular complications remain the most treatable causes of morbidity and mortality associated with noncardiac surgery. The 2007 ACC/AHA perioperative cardiac risk guidelines can be implemented to determine a patient's cardiovascular risk and decrease perioperative morbidity and mortality (Fleisher et al. 2007). Perioperative deaths related to noncardiac procedures are most commonly the result of cardiovascular stress (Mangano 1990), and nearly one-third of all patients undergoing major elective surgery have at least one cardiac risk factor. Acute myocardial infarction (MI) comprises 50% of all perioperative cardiovascular complications, most commonly occurring within the first three days after surgery (Asthon et al. 1993). Following perioperative MI, patients carry a 28-fold increase in cardiovascular complications during the subsequent six months (Mangano 1990). A postoperative MI markedly increases the risk of death (40–70%) (Shah et al. 1993). Preoperative cardiac assessment and management allows the physician to minimize adverse cardiac events in the post-operative period, and to identify those with a poor long-term prognosis. Improvements in perioperative assessment and management have allowed for a decrease in re-infarction rates in the patients who undergo surgery within three months following MI. A postoperative re-infarction is inversely related to the time interval between the initial myocardial infarction and the surgical procedure. At less than three months the associated risk is 30% and at four to six months, the risk is 14%. At greater than six months, the associated risk is 4% (Eagle et al. 1997).

2007 ACC/AHA PERIOPERATIVE CARDIAC RISK GUIDELINES

Step 1: Determine the Urgent or Emergent Nature of the Procedure

A procedure that has been determined to be emergent or urgent will require a history and physical, but no additional testing will be necessary. However, the surgeon must acknowledge there is a two- to five-fold increase in the risk of cardiovascular complications in comparison to elective procedures (Goldman et al. 1977). This suggests the operative medical team employ more aggressive perioperative surveillance. Additionally, risk stratification and risk factor management in the postoperative period can help ensure improved patient outcomes. If a procedure will be performed on an elective basis, active cardiac conditions may be evaluated and treated, further clarifying the perioperative risks and needs for management.

Step 2: Determine the Presence of Active Cardiac Disease or Active Clinical Risk Factors of Cardiac Disease

There remains a persistent underestimation of cardiac disease in women when evaluating cardiac risk preoperatively (Table 1). In patients with established cardiovascular disease, preoperative assessment must include any recent change in symptoms including shortness of breath, palpitations, fatigue, or chest pain. Any history of unstable angina, MI, significant arrhythmias, or severe cardiac valvular disease all increase risk of a perioperative cardiac event. In the Goldman series, although only 12 patients were included, MI within four weeks prior to a surgical procedure conferred a 33% increase in perioperative MI and mortality rate. Patients who had experienced an MI between six weeks and six months prior to surgery had a 20% increase in perioperative cardiovascular events (Goldman et al. 1977, Charlson et al. 1994). Smoking, hyperlipidemia, and diabetes mellitus are important historical factors that encourage further investigation for cardiac disease and could lead to the discovery of subclinical disease. In the original ACC/AHA guidelines, the committee separated clinical risk factors into major, intermediate and minor risk factors (Eagle et al. 2002) (Table 1). The presence of one or more active cardiac conditions with major clinical risk warrants further investigation prior to proceeding with surgery. The intermediate risk category from the Revised Cardiac Index includes clinical risk factors including a history of heart disease, compensated or prior heart failure, cerebrovascular disease, diabetes mellitus, and renal insufficiency (Lee et al. 1999). Patients within the intermediate risk category should have their functional capacity measured, and the degree of risk associated with the planned procedure should be determined to assess for the need for further testing or intra-operative monitoring (Table 1). Advanced age (>70 years), abnormal ECG (LV hypertrophy, left bundle branch block (LBBB), ST-T abnormalities), rhythm other than sinus, and uncontrolled hypertension represent minor predictors, which are considered markers for cardiovascular disease but have not been proven to independently increase perioperative risk (Lee et al. 1999).

Step 3: Determine the Patient's Functional Capacity, or their Ability to Perform Common Daily Tasks

Functional capacity is measured in METS (metabolic equivalents), which correlate with oxygen demands in stress testing (Table 2) (Hlatky et al. 1989). If a patient has not had a recent exercise test, their functional status can be estimated from the ability to perform activities of daily living (Reilly et al. 1999). A patient's functional capacity can be assessed by questioning their ability to perform activities of daily living. Functional capacity is classified from excellent (10), moderate (4–6) to poor (4 or less) or unknown. If a patient can achieve a level of four or greater without symptoms of a stressed myocardium, then it is acceptable to proceed with surgery (Class I, LOE B). In patients with poor or unknown functional capacity the number of active clinical risk factors should guide the need for further testing.

Step 4: In Patients with Poor Functional Capacity, the Presence of Active Clinical Risk Factors will Determine the Need for Future Invasive Testing

In patients with poor functional capacity, refer to the presence of active clinical risk factors, which will determine the need for future evaluation prior to surgery. Caution should be taken in patients with low performance scores (<4). In patients with no clinical risk factors, proceeding with surgery is appropriate (Class I, LOE B) Patients with one to two clinical risk factors may proceed to surgery with perioperative beta blocker therapy (Class IIA, LOE B) or preoperative non-invasive testing if it will change clinical management (Class IIB, LOE B). In patients with more than three clinical risk factors, the level of risk associated with the surgical procedure should be used as a tool for guidance to determine the need for further non-invasive cardiac assessment. If the procedure is vascular, further cardiac testing should be considered if it will change management. If the procedure is intermediate risk, the patient may proceed to surgery with intra-operative heart rate control. (Class IIA, LOE B). Cardiac risk increases with a history of a positive treadmill test, recent use of nitroglycerin, or chest complaints consistent with coronary ischemia. Patients with pulmonary edema, paroxysmal nocturnal dyspnea, peripheral edema, bilateral rales, S3, pulmonary re-distribution on chest x-ray, cerebrovascular disease, transient ischemic attack, or stroke warrant further evaluation (Fleisher et al. 2007).

Step 5: Determine the Procedural Based Cardiac Risk (Table 3)

Determining the procedural based cardiac risk is particularly important in those patients with poor functional capacity and 3 or more clinical risk factors. Fleischer et al. determined the procedure specific combined incidence of cardiac death and nonfatal MI and whether further preoperative cardiac testing would be indicated in patients undergoing each type of procedure (Table 3). High-risk procedures carry a risk of a postoperative nonfatal MI or cardiac death of ≥5% (Fleisher et al. 2007). It is imperative to determine those patients with baseline cardiac disease in order to identify those with a higher risk for associated perioperative morbidity and mortality. Patients undergoing procedures determined to be highest risk (vascular procedures) who also have a high risk of cardiac perioperative risk, further cardiac testing should be considered if it would change preoperative management. Intermediate procedural risk is 1% to 4% (Fleisher et al. 2007). There is insufficient data to determine whether perioperative beta blockade or further cardiovascular testing will change management or decrease perioperative morbidity associated with those procedures. Low risk procedures, not requiring any further testing carry an operative risk of <1% (Fleisher et al. 2007).

DISEASE-SPECIFIC APPROACHES

A patient's perioperative risk may also be determined in a disease-specific approach. For example, according to the 2007 ACC/AHA guidelines, in a patient with coronary artery disease, it may be important to determine how much cardiac tissue will be at jeopardy or how much procedural stress will produce an ischemic event. In a patient with known abnormal ventricular function, the key to ensuring prevention of further disease lies in optimization of medication and determining the extent of disease. Despite this, assessment of left ventricular function has not been found to be a consistent predictor of perioperative ischemic events. A patient with stage 3 hypertension (>180/110) should have the benefits and risks of delaying the procedure and optimizing therapy weighed against proceeding with an intravenous antihypertensive (Weskler et al. 2003). Patients on angiotensin converting enzyme inhibitor or

Table 1

Major cardiac risk factors	Unstable coronary syndromes
	  Unstable or severe angina
	  Recent myocardial ischemia
	    History of MI—Q waves on EKG
	    Acute MI—acute event 7 days or prior
	    Recent MI—>7 days or ≤1 mo prior
	Decompensated heart failure
	Significant arrhythmias
	Severe valvular disease

Intermediate cardiac risk factors	History of heart failure History of compensated heart disease or prior heart failure History of cerebrovascular disease Diabetes mellitus Renal insufficiency
Minor cardiac risk factors	Abnormal EKG—LBBB, LVH, ST abnormality Rhythm other than sinus Uncontrolled systemic hypertension

Abbreviations: MI, myocardial infarction; EKG, electrocardiogram; LBBB, Left Bundle Branch Block; LVH, Left ventricular hypertrophy.
Source: Reproduced from Freeman WK, Gibbons RJ (2009), Adapted from Fleisher et al. (2007), Eagle et al. (2002).

Table 2

#MET	
1	Ability to eat, dress, use the toilet
2	Walk indoors and around the house
3	Walk a block or two on level ground at 2–3 mph
4	Ability to perform light work around the house including dusting or washing dishes Climb a flight of stairs or walk up a hill. Walk on level ground at 4 mph
5+ to 10	Run a short distance Heavy house work including scrubbing floor or lifting or moving heavy furniture Moderate recreational activity participation including golf, bowling, dancing, doubles tennis or throwing a baseball or football Strenuous sport activity like running, swimming, singles tennis, football, basketball, and skiing

Modified from Hlatky et al, 1989; Fletcher et al 1995; Fleisher et al 2007

Table 3 Procedural-based Risk

High risk (5%)	Aortic and other major vascular procedures Peripheral vascular procedures
Intermediate risk (1–5%)	Intraperitoneal and intrathoracic surgery Carotid endarterectomy Head and neck surgery Orthopedic surgery Prostate surgery
Low risk (<1%)	Endoscopic procedures Superficial procedures Cataract surgery Breast surgery Ambulatory surgery

Reproduced from Fleisher et al. 2007.

Preoperative cardiac evaluation algorithm. Based on ACC/AHA 2007 guidelines

Without known active cardiac condition	Low-risk procedure	Proceed with planned procedure regardless of cardiac risks
	Intermediate- or high-risk procedure	Determine functional capacity, proceed with planned procedure if ≥4 METs without symptoms
Low or unknown functional capacity	Intermediate- or high-risk procedure	Consider cardiac testing if it will change management Proceed with heart rate control or consider noninvasive testing if it will change management

Adapted from Fleisher LA et al. ACC/AHA 2007 guidelines on perioperative cardiovascular evaluation and care for noncardiac surgery. J Am Coll Cardiol 2007;50:1707–32

aldosterone receptor blocker antihypertensives should have these medications withheld, particularly in procedures where large fluid shifts can be anticipated, lessening the risk of perioperative renal failure (Bertrand et al. 2001, Coriat et al. 1994, Comfere et al. 2005). Patients with symptomatic aortic stenosis or mitral valve stenosis should undergo preoperative cardiac assessment prior to elective surgery (Raymer and Yang 1998, Torsher et al. 1998). Patients with mechanical prosthetic valves should receive prophylactic antibiotics to reduce the risk of subacute bacterial endocarditis (ACC/AHA Guidelines 1998).

PERIOPERATIVE MEDICAL MANAGEMENT
Several randomized control trials have suggested there is a benefit to perioperative beta blockade during noncardiac procedures in high-risk patients conferring reduced risk of perioperative ischemia. This theoretically reduces the risk of perioperative MI and death in patients with known coronary artery disease, with best outcomes acheived by titrating the patient's heart rate to <70 beats/min. Recent studies suggest no benefit to the use of perioperative beta blockade creating controversy for current practice. (Yang et al. 2005, Juul et al. 2006, Feringa et al. 2006, Goldman 1981, Shammash et al. 2001, Hoeks et al. 2007).

Similar studies of perioperative medical therapy have recently been investigated. A meta analysis by Hindler and colleagues suggests a 44% reduction in mortality in patents with perioperative statin use. LeManch et al. found that perioperative statin withdrawal was an independent predictor of myonecrosis (Hindler et al. 2006, Le Manach et al. 2007). Other studies have suggested that alpha 2 agonists reduce mortality and MI in vascular procedures and perioperative calcium channel blockers may also reduce perioperative ischemia and SVT with trends towards reduced MI and death (Wijeysundera et al. 2003, Wallace et al. 2004, Wijeysundera and Beattie 2003).

SURVEILLANCE PERIOPERATIVE MI
In patients with perioperative signs and symptoms of cardiovascular complications, serial ECGs and cardiac specific biomarkers including troponin T and I may be obtained to assess for the need of intervention. Routine troponin measurements and postoperative ECGs are not recommended in clinically low risk patients and low risk procedures (Landesberg et al. 2004). Peri-operative MI treatment includes peri-reperfusion anticoagulation and antiplatelet therapy, emploring the treating physician to weigh the benefits of a reperfusion procedure with the risks of postoperative bleeding. Intraoperative nonfatal MI carries a significantly elevated risk for postoperative cardiac events, the greatest concern being cardiovascular death. The occurence of a perioperative MI mandates left ventricular (LV) function be evaluated prior to discharge (Mangano and Goldman 1995, Berger et al. 2001, Mangano et al. 1992).

SUPPLEMENTAL PERIOPERATIVE ASSESSMENT
Assessment of left ventricular function by echocardiography at rest has not been found to be a consistent predictor of perioperative ischemic events prior to noncardiac surgery. Echocardiography can be used to predict postoperative congestive heart failure (CHF) in patients with an ejection fraction (EF) <35%, but does not accurately predict ischemia. Echocardiography can be useful in the evaluation of valvular diseases and patients with known left ventricular dysfunction. No research study has determined when to obtain an electrocardiogram (ECG) in the preoperative period; however, it is generally accepted that an ECG within 30 days of surgery is adequate for those with stable disease in whom a preoperative ECG is indicated (Beattie et al. 2006). Exercise stress testing can be an accessory in determining functional capacity, and identifying preoperative myocardial ischemia or cardiac arrhythmias. Perioperative cardiac risk is directly linked to the extent of jeopardized viable myocardium identified by stress cardiac imaging (Beattie et al. 2006). Noninvasive stress testing utilizing pharmacologic stress linked with cardiac imaging has been shown to predict perioperative cardiac events. Patients requiring a high risk procedure with unstable myocardiac ischemia should proceed directly to coronary angiography.

ASSESSMENT OF HEMATOLOGIC RISK
Thromboembolic Disease
Gynecologic cancer alone significantly increases a patient's risk of venous thromboembolic complications with an incidence of 11% to 18% (Geerts et al. 2008). Additionally, a great majority of gynecologic oncology patients have more than one

Table 4

Risk	Factors
Low	Minor surgery in patients <40 yrs without an additional risk factor[a]
Moderate	Minor surgery in patients with additional risk factor[a]
	Minor surgery in patients 40–60 yrs
	Major surgery in patients <40 yrs without an additional risk factor[a]
High	Minor surgery in patients >60 yrs or with an additional risk factor[a]
	Major surgery in patients older than 40 yrs or an additional risk factor[a]
Highest	Major surgery in patients >60 yrs of age with a history of venous thromboembolism, cancer or a molecular hypercoagulable state

[a]Cancer, obesity, lower extremity edema, non-white race, varicose veins, history of radiation therapy, history of deep venous thrombosis or pulmonary embolism, current estrogen use, tamoxifen, oral contraceptive use, thrombophilia, acute medical conditions.
Adapted from ACOG Practice Bulletin 84. American College of Obstetricians and Gynecologists. Obstet Gynecol. 2007;110:429–40.

Table 5

Incision location—thoracic > midline abdomen > low abdomen
Duration of anesthetic—2 hrs or greater
Nasogastric tube—use increases risk
Analgesic modality—parenteral > epidural
Smoking history—increased with positive history
Other factors—increased with a history of dyspnea, COPD, pneumonia and sleep apnea

Adapted from Smetana GW, Lawrence VA, Cornell JE. Preoperative pulmonary risk stratification for noncardiothoracic surgery: systematic review for the American College of Physicians. Ann Intern Med. 2005; 144:581–95.

risk factor, further increasing the risk of venous thromboembolism at some point during their disease span. Perioperatively, the patient with cancer has a 38% risk of developing a venous thromboembolism (Geerts et al. 2008). Contributing to this elevated risk includes intra-operative risk factors including longer operative duration, time under anesthesia, increased operative blood loss and need for intraoperative blood transfusion. Thromboembolic disease is the most frequent cause of postoperative death in patients with uterine or cervical carcinoma. Forty percent of all postoperative gynecologic deaths are directly related to pulmonary emboli. Other significant risk factors for venous thromboembolism are listed in Table 4. Chemotherapy, radiation therapy and hormonal treatment place the cancer patient at additional risk for venous thromboembolism.

Pharmacologic and mechanical methods are both used for prophylaxis against thromboembolic disease by reducing the hypercoagulable state and reducing stasis, respectively. The incidence of venous thromboembolism is decreased to a risk of 2% to 6% with the standard using those preventive measures including sequential compression devices (SCDs), unfractionated heparin (UFH), and low molecular weight heparin (LMWH) (Prevention of deep vein thrombosis and pulmonary embolism (2007)). The ENOXACAN II study found that four weeks of postoperative anticoagulation decreased the incidence of VTE from 12% to 4.8% in cancer patients undergoing abdominal, gynecological, or urological surgery (Bergqvist et al. 2002). Current American College of Chest Physicians and American College of Gynecologists suggest extended prophylaxis in the highest risk patients for four weeks (Level C evidence) (Geerts et al. 2008).

Comparisons of LMWH to UFH have shown equal efficacy in the prophylaxis of VTE. LMWH may be associated with decreased risk of bleeding complications and greater ease of use with once daily dosing. Patients with a low preoperative risk do not need prophylaxis; however, the patient should be encouraged to begin early ambulation. Those patients determined to be at moderate risk should have at least one type of preventative measure (mechanical or pharmacologic). Those deemed to be high risk should receive both mechanical and pharmacologic prevention with SCDs and LMWH or UFH (Douketis et al. 2005). High risk patients who have undergone a major cancer procedure are currently recommended to receive thromboprophylaxis after hospital discharge for up to 28 days postoperatively (Geerts et al. 2008).

Duplex ultrasonography is ordered when there is suspicion for the presence of deep venous thromboembolism (DVT), and treatment is with heparinization to 1.5 times control prothrombin time or with therapeutic doses of LMWH. Increasing sensitivity of dynamic contrast-enhanced computerized tomography has confirmed the replacement of the prior gold standard of pulmonary arteriogram in the diagnosis of pulmonary embolism. Upon diagnosis, the patient is anticoagulated with intravenous heparin or LMWH. Long-term anticoagulation should last for three months in the case of DVT and six months in the case of pulmonary embolism with coumadin therapy converted from heparin or LMWH.

ASSESSMENT OF PULMONARY RISK
Pulmonologic associated procedural based risk may be either specific to the patient, the procedure, or both. Approximately 25% of early postoperative mortality in the early postoperative period is pulmonary related, including atelectasis, pneumonia, respiratory failure, and exacerbation of underlying chronic lung disease. Commonly performed gynecologic oncology procedures, high risk procedures, place each patient at a 20% to 30% overall risk of a pulmonary complication (Ferguson (1999)). Laparotomy is associated with 45% decrease in vital capacity and a 20% reduction in functional residual capacity (Qaseem et al. 2006). Atelectasis, a complication of dorsal lithotomy, results as the functional residual capacity is reduced below the alveolar closing volume. Several intraoperative factors increase the risk of perioperative pulmonary complications. (see Table 5). Procedural based pulmonary risk factors include duration of surgery, choice of anesthetic, the emergent nature of the procedure, and the location of incision. Risk factors specific to the patient include increasing age, chronic lung disease, cigarette use, functional status, obesity, congestive heart failure, asthma, obstructive sleep apnea, poor mental status, alcohol use, and neurologic impairment (Ametana et al. 2006, Doyle (1999)).

Several multivariable studies have demonstrated age to be the most commonly associated risk factor for perioperative pulmonary complications. Patients >60 years of age are subject to increasing perioperative pulmonary morbidity even after adjusting for co-morbid conditions. Congestive obstructive pulmonary disease, COPD, remains the most common risk factor for the postoperative period. Patients with COPD retain carbon dioxide, have poor gas exchange, and an increased residual volume. Smoking increases the risk of postoperative complications even in the absence of chronic lung disease. Perioperative pulmonary risk is particularly increased in those who have been smoking more than 20 years and is highest in patients still smoking within two months of surgery. Good evidence exists that perioperative complications are decreased in those patients who stop smoking more than six months prior to surgery. Obstructive sleep apnea increases risk for airway management difficulties in the immediate perioperative period, however, associated complications have not been studied. Patients with a history of asthma or other restrictive lung diseases are at a minimal risk for postoperative complications.

There is no associated predictive value in obtaining a chest x-ray in a well, normal adult and should therefore not be included in the preoperative evaluation. Alternatively, patients at increased risk for perioperative pulmonary complications including those older than 50 years of age and those with diagnosed lung disease may benefit from a baseline chest x-ray (Qaseem et al. 2006). Pulmonary function testing may be supportive for the assessment of the extent of disease and predictive of the risk for postoperative complications. However, few clinical trials actually support pulmonary function testing in diseases other than restrictive lung disease, which, from an anesthesiologists perspective, tend not to produce acute exacerbations and do not require specific anesthetic agents. (Qaseem et al. 2006.) Patients with long standing restrictive lung disease are at a significantly elevated risk for pulmonary hypertension. Preoperative functional status in addition to recommendations from the patient's pulmonologist help to guide the surgeon and anesthesiologist for perioperative pulmonologic care. Spirometry may be helpful in diagnosing obstructive lung disease; however, it has not been proven to be predictive of postoperative pulmonary complications. Pulmonary function tests may be particularly helpful in patients unable to detect a difference in their disease status and whether a patient responds to therapy. In the setting of unacceptably poor preoperative PFTs, a procedure should be cancelled and preoperative pulmonary rehabilitation considered. One study found that an FEV1 of <50% and a FEV1/FVC ratio of <70% was a predictor of six deaths and seven major pulmonary complications following 107 surgical procedures (National Emphysema Treatment Trial Research Group. 2001). Preoperative arterial blood gases are not considered an acceptable routine test; however, in the work up for a patient with an obstructive lung disease they are indicated. Patients with elevated $PaCO_2$ above 45 mmHg have been proven to have increased complications and in those patients with hypoxemia ($PO_2 < 50$ mmHg), surgery is contraindicated.

Prevention of postoperative pulmonary complications is derived from careful preoperative assessment and maximization of the patient's current medication regimen. Risk reduction strategies in the postoperative period include pulmonary expansion by means of incentive spirometry, chest wall expansion, deep breathing and cough, none of which has been proven to be superior to the other. The best outcomes by anecdotal data support counseling in all modalities. Available evidence suggests that for all patients undergoing abdominal surgery, any type of lung expansion is better than no prophylaxis at all. Any recent increased use of bronchodilators, steroids, recent exacerbations, or smoking are risk factors for perioperative bronchospasm. Prophylaxis in reactive airway disease is supported by the use of perioperative inhaled beta agonists whether by inhaler or nebulizer therapy. Steroid therapy should be reserved for those patients already using them as a part of their current regimen, however, they may be helpful in decreasing inflammation preoperatively and minimization of bronchospasm postoperatively. Prophylactic antibiotics have no place in perioperative therapy to prevent pulmonary complications. Patients on oral steroids for prolonged periods of time should be considered for a preoperative stress dose steroid (see below; adrenal suppression). Preoperative consultation with an anesthesiologist is imperative in this patient population for planning medication use, optimization of therapy, and communication.

ASSESSMENT OF ENDOCRINOLOGIC RISK
Diabetes Mellitus

Diabetes continues to pose significant issue for postoperative outcomes as 15% to 20% of all surgical procedures are performed on diabetics, and as the incidence of disease continues to increase, the postoperative complication rate is sure to increase as well. Diabetes places the patient at an elevated risk for wound complications including infection and impaired healing and significantly increases a patient's risk for cardiovascular and renal complications. More than 90% of all diabetics are type II, included all patients treated by diet alone, oral hypoglycemic agents, or with insulin (Schiff and Welsh 2003).

Diabetes associated perioperative risk can be uncovered by determining the extent of the disease. Microvascular disease associated with diabetes causes complications such as retinopathy, neuropathy, nephropathy, and cardiovascular disease. The risk of which, is even more elevated in those who have had the disease for 10 years or greater (Schiff and Welsh 2003). Preoperative assessment including a thorough history and physical evaluates for the presence of end organ dysfunction by identifying the presence of cardiac disease, nephropathy, peripheral neuropathy, and retinopathy. A hemoglobin A1C in addition to fasting and postprandial blood glucose levels can reveal the extent of glucose control, thereby suggesting a patient's likelihood of associated comorbidities.

Operative physiologic stress induces a hyperglycemic state in the diabetic patient. This is caused by the adrenal stress response releasing epinephrine, norepinephrine, cortisol, and growth hormone, which all suppress insulin function, directing the patient to utilize an increased pool of intravascular glucose for the fight or flight response. Gluconeogenesis and lipolysis support the stress response by mobilizing glucose precursors inducing a net protein catabolism. Intraoperative glucose assessment is necessary in procedures lasting longer than two hours to rule out the presence of ketosis or acidosis from the hyperglycemia stress response (Hoogwerf (2006)). Diabetic patients have an increased risk for postoperative cardiac complications including ischemia and infarction. Preoperative prevention of acute renal failure in diabetic patients can be acheived by recognizing the potential for large fluid shifts, increased peritoneal evaporative loss, perioperative respiratory loss and decreased intravascular volume effects of anesthetic agents.

Wound complications and postoperative infections are a significant risk for the diabetic patient in the postoperative period. Hyperglycemia significantly impairs phagocytes, granulocytes, and collagen synthesis at glucose levels >200 mg/dl, placing the uncontrolled diabetic patient at a significantly elevated risk for wound and fascial dehiscence. The associated microvascular changes of diabetes impair oxygen delivery to tissues, compounding the already poor ability to ward off infection within the wound. Several retrospective studies have found a lower incidence of postoperative wound complications, including reduced infectious morbidity, is associated with tighter glycemic control (Marks 2003).

Patients on oral antihyperglycemics should cease their medications on the morning of their procedure. Oral antihyperglycemic agents metformin or chloropropramide should be stopped 24 to 48 hours prior secondary to their longer half life. Insulin dependent diabetics should take one-third to two-thirds of their insulin dose on the morning of minor procedures and should be monitored closely with i.v. insulin therapy intraoperatively in major procedures. A diabetic controlled by diet alone does not require additional antihyperglycemic therapy preoperatively or intraoperatively. A diabetic on oral hypoglycemics should have a preoperative glucose reading in addition to every two hour intraoperative glucose reading with insulin therapy as needed per recommendations as above. A type II diabetic on insulin therapy should also have preoperative and frequent intraoperative glucose measurements with intravenous insulin therapy as needed.

Thyroid Dysfunction

Thyroid dysfunction, in particular hypothyroidism, increases the risk of perioperative complications associated with cardiac, vascular, metabolic, and central nervous systems. Thyroid stimulating hormone and thyroxine (T4) levels should be obtained preoperatively to rule out laboratory abnormalities preoperatively, particularly in patients with a history of fatigue and new-onset depression. Avoidance of rare but serious complications including myxedema coma and thyroid storm can be accomplished by appropriate preoperative assessment.

Hypothyroidism influences many physiologic functions including cardiac, respiration, gastrointestinal, hemostasis, and free water balance. The severity of the underlying hypothyroidism determines the nature by which a surgeon should proceed to the operating room. Retrospective studies have demonstrated that euthyroid, to mild or even moderate hypothyroidism should not be denied necessary surgery in order to correct the underlying disorder. Perioperative risks associated with hypothyroidism include intraoperative hypotension, gastrointestinal complications including ileus, postoperative neuropsychiatric complications, and inability to mount fever. Patients with severe hypothyroidism, identified by those suffering from myxedema coma, decreased mentation, pericardial effusions, heart failure or very low levels of thyroxine, who are in need of an urgent/emergent procedure, should

receive intravenous thyroxine and stress dose glucocorticoids administered in the perioperative period. Hypothyroid patients with concern for development of myxedema coma include those who develop perioperative seizures, coma, unexplained heart failure, hypothermia, prolonged ileus, or postoperative delirium, and should be promptly treated for such a complication. (Stathatos and Wartofsky (2003)).

Hyperthyroidism poses significant perioperative cardiac risk, as thyroxine (T4) and triiodothyronine (T3) impose both inotropic and chronotropic effects on cardiac function. The greatest perioperative risk to an untreated hyperthyroid patient is the development of thyroid storm and should be investigated in any patient suffering postoperative fever, tachycardia, confusion, cardiovascular collapse, or death. Mild hyperthyroids may proceed with surgery with the support of perioperative beta blockade. Moderate to severe (thyrotoxic) patients should have surgery delayed unless the procedure is emergent or urgent. Premedication for these patients is necessary with antithyroid agents, beta blockade, and corticosteroids. Treatment of a thyroid storm includes beta blockade, thionamides, iodine, and corticosteroids in addition to admittance to an intensive care unit for appropriate monitoring.

Adrenal Suppression

Exogenous corticosteroid use over a prolonged period of time poses a potential risk for hypothalamic pituitary axis (HPA) suppression. In preoperative evaluation, the surgeon must determine the type of steroid used, the duration of treatment, and whether a taper was used if the medication was discontinued. Preoperative stress dose steroids are used for the prevention of HPA suppression and its life-threatening sequelae. Administering stress–dose glucocorticosteroids must be weighed against the potential side effects of the medication including possible poor wound healing, fluid retention, and increased risk for infection.

Doses seldom resulting in HPA suppression and not requiring stress-dose corticosteroids include steroid equivalents to 5 mg of prednisone as a single daily dose, alternate day steroids given as a morning dose and any steroid used for less than three weeks. Alternatively, patients taking 20 mg equivalents of prednisone daily for more than three weeks or those who appear clinically cushingoid require stress-dose steroids in the perioperative period (Salem et al. (1994)).

ASSESSMENT OF RENAL RISK

As the incidence of diabetes, hypertension and obesity increases alongside an aging population, the prevalence of impaired renal disease continues to rise in surgical patients. Additionally, advancements in dialysis allows many patients to live with end stage renal disease (ESRD), who are subject to increased risks of perioperative morbidity and mortality. Patients with ESRD also tend to have other co-morbid conditions such as coronary artery disease and peripheral vascular disease. Postoperatively, these patients tend to have difficulty with fluid balance, anemia, electrolyte, acid-base abnormalities and postoperative wound complications secondary to an immuno-compromised state.

Preoperative evaluation of ESRD patients includes a cardiac evaluation, electrolyte and fluid management, assessing for anemia or bleeding diatheses, and optimizing glycemic control.

Cardiac disease is the leading cause of death amongst peri-operative ESRD patients and tends to be asymptomatic. Consultation with the patient's nephrologist to ensure coordination of the procedure with the patient's dialysis schedule can help ensure euvolemia, pre-procedure electrolyte replacement within 24 hours and postoperative fluid shift management. Erythropoetin is a common medication administered to ESRD patients to maintain hemoglobin levels. Transfusions may be required in the immediate preoperative period to increase hemoglobin levels. Uremic patients may have dysfunctional platelets resulting in bleeding. If a patient has a history of bleeding secondary to a uremic platelet dysfunction, they can be treated with 1-deamino-8-D-arginine vasopressin (dDAVP) intravenously, intranasally with cryoprecipitate, or with intravenous conjugated estrogens, which may be given four to five days prior to surgery at a dose of 0.6 mg/kg, to prevent intra-operative bleeding.

ASSESSMENT OF HEPATIC RISK
Routine testing of liver function rarely yields an abnormality-and rarely tends to change perioperative management in the routine surgical patient. However, liver disorders can impact perioperative risk enough to significantly confer unnecessary morbidity and mortality. Decompensated liver disease increases the perioperative risks of acute hepatic failure, sepsis, bleeding and renal dysfunction. A patient presenting with a history of jaundice, blood transfusions, the use of alcohol or recreational drugs, hepatitis or physical findings of icterus, hepatosplenomegaly, palmar erythema, or spider nevi should be tested to rule out occult or active liver disease.

The extent of liver dysfunction and type of surgery play key roles in determining perioperative risk. Liver disease easily affects many other organ systems in the body including the cardiorespiratory and circulatory systems, the brain, the kidney and the immune system. Patients with chronic hepatitis without cirrhosis have very minimal perioperative morbidity; however, those patients with acute hepatitis have an associated mortality rate of up to 50% and should hold on nonemergent/urgent procedures until the acute phase has resolved. Patients with cirrhotic disease have significantly increased perioperative surgical risk.

REFERENCES
ACC/AHA guidelines for the management of patients with valvular heart disease: report of the American College of Cardiology/American Heart Association Task Force on Practice Guidelines (Committee on Management of Patients with Valvular Heart Disease) (1998). J Am Coll Cardiol 32:1486–588.

Ametana GW, Lawrence VA, Cornell JE (2006) Preoperative pulmonary risk stratification for noncardiothoracic surgery: systematic review for the American College of Physicians. Ann Intern Med 144:581–95.

Asthon CM, Petersen NJ, Wray NP, et al. (1993) The incidence of perioperative myocardial infarction in men undergoing noncardiac surgery. Ann Intern Med 118:504–10.

Beattie WS, Abdelnaem E, Wijeysundera DN, Buckley DN (2006) A meta-analytic comparison of preoperative stress echocardiography and nuclear scintigrapy imaging. Anesth Analg 102:8–16.

Berger PB, Bellot V, Bell MR, et al. (2001) An immediate invasive strategy for the treatment of acute myocardial infarction early after noncardiac surgery. Am J Cardiol 87:1100–2.

Bergqvist D, Agnelli G, Cohen AT, et al.; Dietrich- Neto F (ENOXAXAN II Investigators) (2002) Duration of prophylaxis against venous thromboembolism with enoxaparin after surgery for cancer. N Engl J Med 346(13):975–80.

Bertrand M, Godet G, Meerschaert K, et al. (2001) Should the angiotensin II antagonists be discontinued prior to surgery? Anesth Analg 92:26–30.

Charlson M, Peterson J, Szarowski TP, et al. (1994) Long-term prognosis after peri-operative cardiac complications. J Clin Epidemiol 47:1389–400.

Comfere T, Sprung J, Kumar MM, et al. (2005) Angiotensin system inhibitors in a general surgical population. Anesth Analg 100:636–44.

Coriat P, Richer C, Douraki T, et al. (1994) Influence of chronic angiotensin-converting enzyme inhibition on anesthetic induction. Anesthesiology 81:299–307.

Douketis JD, Johnson JA, Turpie AG (2005) Low-molecular-weight-heparins as periprocedural anticoagulation for patients on long-term warfarin therapy: a standardized bridging therapy protocol. J Thromb Thrombolysis 20:11–16.

Doyle RL (1999) Assessing and modifying the risk of postoperative pulmonary complications. Chest 115:77–81.

Eagle KA, Berger PB, Calkins K, et al. (2002) ACC/AHA guideline update for perioperative cardiovascular evaluation for noncardiac surgery-executive summary: a report of the American College of Cardiology/American Heart Association Task Force on Practice Guideline (Committee to Update the 1996 Guidelines on Perioperative Cardiovascular Evaluation for Noncardiac Surgery). J Am Coll Cardiol 39:542–53.

Eagle KA, Rihal CS, Mickel MC, et al. (1997) Cardiac risk of non-cardiac surgery: influence of coronary disease and type of surgery in 3368 operations. Circulation. 96:1882–7.

Ferguson MK (1999) Preoperative assessment of pulmonary risk. Chest 115:58–63.

Feringa HH, Bax JJ, Boersma E, et al. (2006) High-dose beta-blockers and right heart rate control reduce myocardial ischemia and troponin T release in vascular surgery patients. Circulation 114:1344–9.

Fleisher LA, Beckman JA, Brown KA, et al. (2007) ACC/AHA 2007 Guidelines on perioperative cardiovascular evaluations and care for noncardiac surgery: executive summary: a report of the American College of Cardiology/American Heart Association Task Force on Practice Guidelines (Writing committee to revise the 2002 guidelines on perioperative cardiovascular evaluation for noncardiac surgery). Circulation 116:1971–96.

Fletcher GF, Balady G, Froelicher VF, et al. (1995) Exercise standards: a statement for healthcare professionals from the American Heart Association. Circulation 91:580–615.

Freeman WK, Gibbons RJ (2009) Perioperative Cardiovascular Assessment of Patients Undergoing Noncardiac Surgery. May Clin Proc 84(1):79–90

Geerts WH, Bergqvist D, Pineo GF, et al. (2008) Prevention of venous thromboembolism: American College of Chest Physicians Evidence-Based Clinical Practice Guidelines, 8th edn. Chest 133:381S–453S.

Goldman L, Caldera DL, Nussbaum SR, et al. (1977) Multifactorial index of cardiac index of cardiac risk in noncardiac surgical procedures. N Engl J Med 297:845–50.

Goldman L (1981) Noncardiac surgery in patients receiving propranolol. Case reports and recommended approach. Arch Intern Med 141:193–6.

Hindler K, Schaw AD, Samuels J, et al. (2006) Improved postoperative outcomes associated with preoperative statin therapy. Anesthesiology 105:1260–72.

Hlatky MA, Boineau RE, Kigginbotham MB, et al. (1989) A brief self-administered questionnaire to determine functional capacity (the Duke Activity Status Index). Am J Cardiol 64:651–4.

Hoeks SE, Scholte Op, Reimer WJ, et al. (2007) Increase of 1-year mortality after perioperative beta-blocker withdrawal in endovascular and vascular surgery patients. Eur J Vasc Endovasc Surg 33:13–19.

Hoogwerf BJ (2006) Perioepartive management of diabetes mellitus: how should we act on the limited evidence? Cleve Clin J Med 73(Suppl 1):S95–9.

Juul AB, Wetterslev J, Gluud C, et al. (2006) Effect of perioperative beta blockade in patients with diabetes undergoing major non-cardiac surgery: randomized placebo controlled, blinded multicentre trial. BMJ 332:1482.

Landesberg G, Mosseri M, Shatz V, et al. (2004) Cardiac troponin after major vascular surgery: the role of perioperative ischemia, preoperative thallium scanning and coronary revascularization. J Am Coll Cardiol 44:569–75.

Lawrence VA, Cornell JE, Smetana GW. Strategies to reduce postoperative pulmonary complications after noncardiothoracic surgery: systematic review for the American College of Physicians. Ann Intern Med 2005;144:596–608.

Le Manach Y, Godet G, Coriat P, et al. (2007) The impact of postoperative discontinuation or continuation of chronic statin therapy on cardiac outcome after major vascular surgery. Anesth Analg 104:1326–33.

Lee TH, Marcantonio ER, Mangione CM, et al. (1999) Derivation and pro-spective validation of a simple index for prediction of cardiac risk of major noncardiac surgery. *Circulation* **100**:1043–9.

Mangano D (1990) Perioperative cardiac morbidity. *Anesthesiology* **72**:153–84.

Mangano DT, Browner WS, Hollenberg M, Li J, Tateo IM (1992) Long-term cardiac prognosis following noncardiac surgery. The Study of Perioperative Ischemia Research Group. *JAMA* **268**:233–9.

Mangano DT, Goldman L (1995) Preoperative assessment of patients with known or suspected coronary disease. *N Engl J Med* **333**:1750–6.

Marks JB (2003) Perioperative management of diabetes. *Am Fam Physician* **67**:93–100.

National Emphysema Treatment Trial Research Group. (2001) Patients at high risk of death after lung volume-reduction surgery. *New Eng J of Med* **345**:1075–83.

Nelson CL, Herndon JE, Mark DB, et al. (1991) Relation of clinical and angio-graphic factors to functional capacity as measured by the Duke Activity Status Index. *Am J Cardiol* **68**:973–5.

Prevention of deep vein thrombosis and pulmonary embolism (2007) ACOG practice Bulletin No. 84. American College of Obstetricians and Gynecolo-gists. *Obstet Gynecol* **110**:429–40.

Qaseem A, Snow V, Fitterman N, et al. (2006) Clinical Efficacy Assessment Subcommittee of the American College of Physicians. *Ann Intern Med* **144**(8):575–80.

Raymer K, Yang H (1998) Patients with aortic stenosis: cardiac complications in non-cardiac surgery. *Can J Anaesth* **45**:855–9.

Reilly DF, McNeely MJ, Doerner D, et al. (1999) Self-reported exercise toler-ance and the risk of serious perioperative complications. *Arch Intern Med* **159**:2185–92.

Salem M, Tanish RE Jr, Bromber J, Loriaux DL, Chernow B (1994) Periopera-tive glucocorticoid coverage. A reassessment 42 years after emergence of the problem. *Ann Surg* **219**:416–25.

Schiff RL, Welsh GA (2003) Perioperative evaluation and management of the patient with endocrine dysfunction. *Med Clin North Am* **87**:175–92.

Shah KB, Kleinman BS, Sami H, et al. (1993) Reevaluation of perioperative myocardial infarction in men undergoing noncardiac surgery. *Ann Intern Med* **118**:504–10.

Shammash JB, Trost JC, Gold JM, et al. (2001) Perioperative beta-blocker withdrawal and mortality in vascular surgical patents. *Am Heart J* **141**: 148–53.

Smetana GW, Lawrence VA, Cornell JE. Preoperative pulmonary risk stratifi-cation for noncardiothoracic surgery: systematic review for the American College of Physicians. *Ann Intern Med* 2005;**144**:581–95.

Stathatos N, Wartofsky L (2003) Perioperative management of patients with hypothyroidism. *Endocrinol Metab Clin North Am* **32**:503–18.

Torsher LC, Shub C, Rettke SR, Brown DL (1998) Risk of patients with severe aortic stenosis undergoing noncardiac surgery. *Am J Cardiol* **81**:448–52.

Wallace AW, Galindez S, Salahieh A, et al. (2004) Effect of clonidine on cardio-vascular morbidity and mortality after noncardiac surgery. *Anesthesiology* **101**:284–93.

Weskler N, Klein M, Szendro G, et al. (2003) The dilemma of immediate pre-operative hypertension: to treat and operate, or to postpone surgery? *J Clin Anesth* **15**:179–83.

Wijeysundera DN, Beattie WS (2003) Calcium channel blockers for reducing cardiac morbidity after noncarac surgery: a metaanalysis. *Anesth Analg* **97**:634–41.

Wijeysundera DN, Naik JS, Beattie WS (2003) Alpha-2 antagonists to prevent perioperative cardiovascular complications: a meta-analysis. *Am J Med* **114**:742–52.

Yang H, Raymer K, Butler R, Parlow J, Roberts R (2005) The effects of perioperative beta-blockade: results of the metoprolol after vascular surgery (MaVS) study, a randomized controlled trial. *Am Heart J* **152**: 983–90.

3 Complications
David Warshal and James Aikins

INTRODUCTION

Complications are an inevitable consequence of surgery. A clear understanding of surgical principles and technique is essential but is not always sufficient to prevent complications, particularly when normal anatomical relationships have been altered by the presence of a malignancy. Furthermore, some complications are beyond the control of the surgeon. The judicious surgeon must always be cognizant of the potential complications associated with each step of a particular surgical procedure and actively work to minimize these risks. The prompt detection and management of perioperative complications is of paramount importance in order to minimize adverse sequelae.

For this chapter, we have chosen to address what we believe are the most relevant issues in regard to complications associated with gynecologic surgery. Urinary tract complications have not been included in this section since they are discussed in Chapter 26.

BOWEL COMPLICATIONS

Preoperative bowel preparation had been considered to be an essential factor in preventing complications associated with colorectal surgery for over a century. However, over the past several years, a series of studies have challenged this belief. A 2009 Cochrane review examining this issue concluded, based on over 4000 subjects participating in 13 randomized trials and one non-randomized trial, that there was no benefit conferred by preoperative bowel preparation. In fact, they discovered a trend toward increased postoperative infectious complications with bowel preparation. It has been suggested that this association may be due to leakage of liquid stool from inadequately prepped bowel or from local structural and inflammatory changes of the bowel wall that can result from a mechanical bowel prep. Intravenous antibiotics with both aerobic and anaerobic coverage, such as a second generation cephalosporin with metronidazole or amoxicillin/clavulanic acid, should be administered preoperatively. Ciprofloxicin or clindamycin may be substituted for the cephalosporin in the penicillin allergic cases. If bulky stool is encountered intraoperatively, it should be gently milked away from the area of resection or washed out from the anus to facilitate reanastomosis.

Historically, injury to the colon, particularly with gross contamination of the peritoneal cavity, was managed by colostomy formation. Recent prospective randomized studies examining the management of traumatic colon injuries have demonstrated either equal or improved outcomes with primary repair. Though the risk for intra-abdominal sepsis is increased with multiple associated abdominal injuries, massive blood transfusion, and severe peritoneal contamination, the method of management of the colon injury does not affect the incidence of sepsis. In addition, the repair technique, hand sewn versus stapled, also does not influence the complication rate. In the face of a colon injury with peritoneal contamination, broad spectrum antibiotic prophylaxis should be continued for 24 hours.

Intraoperative bowel injuries are most likely to occur during entry into the abdominal cavity and during lysis of adhesions. If entering the abdomen through an old scar, the risk of injury is reduced if entry is gained just beyond the limit of the old scar. Sharp entry is preferred over use of an electrocoagulation device due to the clean, defined nature of a sharp injury. Thermal injuries are more difficult to detect and evaluate due to the potential for delayed tissue necrosis up to a few centimeters beyond the point of visible damage. When a significant thermal injury to the bowel occurs, a wide resection up to 3 to 5 cm from the edges of the injury with primary reanastomosis is recommended. Thin filmy intra-abdominal adhesions can be safely lysed using blunt dissection and the electrocautery devise. Thicker, less yielding adhesions require sharp dissection to avoid injury to the bowel.

Following difficult bowel dissections, direct visual inspection of all bowel surfaces is important. Of note, the risk of compromise of the distal sigmoid colon is increased in cases of ovarian cancer with extensive pelvic disease and with endometriosis where the cul de sac may be obliterated. Injury in this area may be particularly difficult to visualize. When concern is raised, a large gauge foley catheter should be inserted into the rectum and the balloon inflated. With the pelvis filled with saline and the proximal sigmoid occluded with gentle pressure, air is injected into the foley to inflate the bowel. Air will bubble to the surface if a laceration is present.

Small bowel lacerations involving less than half of the circumference of the bowel are repaired without resection. A single layer of full thickness delayed absorbable 3-0 sutures are placed 3 mm apart. The closure is oriented perpendicular to the path of the bowel to limit narrowing of the lumen. A second seromuscular layer imbricating the first layer is sometimes placed provided that it does not compromise the bowel lumen. The closure should be water-tight and is tested by gently milking bowel contents and intraluminal gas past the repair site. Pinching the bowel lumen at the anastomotic site should confirm a luminal diameter of at least 1 cm. If a larger laceration occurs, the edges are devascularized, or multiple small enterotomies involve a short segment of bowel, resection of the injured area with primary reanastomosis is warranted.

Repair of large bowel lacerations is similar to that for the small bowel with a few exceptions. Lacerations of up to 30% of the circumference of the bowel are closed primarily with larger injuries requiring bowel resection. Two layer closures as described above are the standard. There is generally no concern regarding narrowing of the large bowel lumen by repair.

Routine use of a nasogastric tube following extensive gynecologic procedures or bowel resection has recently been re-examined. Nasogastric tube suctioning does not reduce the duration of ileus and may actually delay return of normal bowel function. Following bowel resection, the presence of a tube did not affect the incidence of anastomotic leakage or incisional hernia development. In addition to the substantial discomfort associated with nasogastric tubes, they are also a major risk factor for postoperative pulmonary complications. Two recent meta-analyses suggested that only up to 10% of patients undergoing bowel resection and managed without nasogastric decompression would warrant insertion later in their postoperative course.

Several studies have recently evaluated the feasibility of early feeding of patients who have undergone bowel resection and other types of intraabdominal surgery. Early feeding was found to be safe and not associated with the development of a prolonged ileus or anastomotic leakage. A reduced length of stay and a reduction in the postoperative infection rate have also been reported. Conversely, many of these studies have also shown that those fed early have an increased risk for nausea, vomiting, and abdominal distention.

Following laparotomy, a *postoperative* ileus occurs routinely. Small bowel motility and absorption generally returns within a few hours of surgery followed by stomach emptying which begins after 24 hours. The colon remains inactive for approximately from 48 to 72 hours. This process is controlled by the autonomic nervous system. Occasionally a paralytic ileus may develop that can last from days to weeks. A *paralytic* ileus is associated with bowel mucosal injury secondary to bowel manipulation, hypoxia, endotoxins, and/or hypoperfusion, and all bowel segments are affected. Pain and opioid use can prolong both postoperative and paralytic ileuses. Techniques to reduce the risk of ileus include gentle handling of tissue, appropriate intraoperative fluid management, minimizing opioid use, epidural infusion of local anesthetics for pain management, and use of peripherally acting gastrointestinal opioid receptor antagonist. Alvimopan, approved by the FDA for postoperative use, has been found to shorten the time to return of bowel function without compromising pain control in patients undergoing bowel resection and radical hysterectomy.

Patients with a paralytic ileus develop abdominal bloating, anorexia, nausea, and vomiting if early feeding is initiated. Abdominal cramping and pain in excess of that anticipated by the patient's postoperative state are usually absent. Physical exam reveals a distended, tympanitic abdomen without bowel sounds. Obstruction series imaging will show a nonspecific bowel gas pattern with dilated loops of small and often large bowel. It can often be difficult radiographically to distinguish an ileus from an early obstruction. It is important to rule out infectious and metabolic causes such as peritonitis, abscess, and electrolyte abnormalities such as hypokalemia and hypomagnesemia. Patients are kept nil per orum (NPO) and observed with supportive measures instituted. For patients with persistent nausea and vomiting, a nasogastric tube should be inserted. However, nasogastric tubes have not been shown to shorten the duration of an ileus. If possible, narcotic use should be minimized. No currently available medications have been demonstrated to relieve a postoperative ileus once it is established. Watchful waiting with periodic obstruction series imaging to exclude an obstruction and blood work to exclude infection and metabolic derangement are recommended. For a prolonged ileus lasting more than one week, hyperalimentation should be considered. We have anecdotally found that hunger develops shortly before flatus and that diarrhea is common during the first 24 hours following the onset of bowel movements.

Bowel obstructions, characterized as partial or complete, prevent passage of bowel contents through the intestines. Obstruction most commonly involves the small bowel with adhesions followed by hernias accounting for the majority of postoperative causes. Symptoms associated with bowel obstructions include colicky abdominal pain that comes in waves, bloating, and rapid onset of nausea, often with forceful emesis that temporarily relieves these symptoms. Auscultation reveals high pitched, rushing bowel sounds, and borborygmi. An obstruction series imaging will show distended loops of bowel with air-fluid levels arranged in a stepladder fashion. Conservative management with placement of a nasogastric tube is appropriate if evidence of bowel strangulation, such as fever, tachycardia, abdominal guarding, rebound tenderness, and leukocytosis are absent. A spontaneous resolution rate of approximately 80% is seen, with partial obstructions responding better than complete blockages. If improvement is not evident within the first one to two days of conservative management, or if signs and symptoms of bowel compromise develop, surgical exploration should be performed.

Patients who have undergone extensive enterolysis or bowel resection either due to injury or to disease are at risk for perforation or leakage at the anastomotic site with the subsequent development of peritonitis, an abscess, or an enterocutaneous fistula. Leakage from small bowel anastomoses occurs in up to 3% cases whereas the risk rises to up to 20% for colorectal anastomoses. Patients with perforation or free anastomotic leaks allowing soiling throughout the peritoneum present with fever, tachycardia, increasing abdominal pain, and acute abdominal signs such as guarding and rebound tenderness. In the immediate postoperative period, intra-abdominal free air detected by X-ray will not be diagnostic. Septic shock with hypotension and end-organ dysfunction can rapidly ensue. A high level of suspicion must be maintained when evaluating such patients since the use of postoperative narcotics can minimize these signs and symptoms. If significant concern for peritonitis is present, medical stabilization should be promptly initiated, including the use of broad spectrum antibiotics, and the patient returned to the operating room for re-exploration. Intraoperative management must be individualized based on the condition of the patient and the complexity of the complication. Often a simple perforation or a small bowel anastomotic leak can be repaired primarily. Distal colonic and rectal anastomotic leaks will usually necessitate colostomy formation.

Postoperative abscess formation following contamination of the peritoneal cavity during gynecologic surgery has become much less frequent due to the use of preoperative prophylactic antibiotics. Simple vaginal cuff abscesses can often be opened and allowed to drain through the vagina. Deeper pelvic or abdominal abscesses can occur spontaneously or in association with a contained leakage from the bowel. Intravenous antibiotics and drainage are usually required. Percutaneous placement of a drainage catheter is favored if a safe approach that avoids bowel and major blood vessels is available. Small collections that cannot be drained percutaneously can be managed with antibiotics and observed for resolution.

Bowel injury or anastomotic leakage can also lead to the development of enterocutaneous or enterovaginal fistulas. A fistula can extend directly from the involved bowel to the abdominal wall or vagina or it can drain from deep within the abdomen through a complex abscess channel. An additional infrequent cause of enterovaginal fistulas is inclusion of a portion of the rectosigmoid wall in stitches used to close the vaginal cuff at the time of hysterectomy. Patients with scarring in the cul de sac from tumor or endometriosis are at increased risk for this. Small bowel fistulas drain copious amounts of caustic effluent that irritates the surrounding skin. Colonic fistulas, particularly those that are more distal, leak stool. A step-wise management plan is used in which fluid resuscitation and measures to protect the skin surrounding the fistula are initiated first. The patient is made NPO, and hyperalimentation is started. Somatostatin is often used to further reduce the output from a small bowel fistula. Radiographic imaging including CT scanning, upper GI with small bowel follow-through, barium enema, and fistulagram are helpful in determining the anatomy of the fistula and whether an abscess is associated with it. When healthy bowel in close proximity to the skin surface is involved, expectant management with an approximately 70% likelihood of spontaneous closure is appropriate. Surgical management is required for more complex fistulas and for those that do not close within two months.

INTRAOPERATIVE BLEEDING

It is essential for the gynecologic surgeon to have an "emergency" plan of action in the event of intraoperative hemorrhage. Under most circumstances, the routine steps of applying pressure to the site of bleeding and obtaining good visualization of the area will maximize the likelihood of a quick resolution. Arterial bleeders need to be identified and either coagulated, ligated, or repaired as outlined in Chapter 28. It has been our experience that several minutes of direct pressure to the site of venous bleeding, even from the inferior vena cava, is enough to control hemorrhage in many cases. Electrocoagulation must be used judiciously around veins due to their thin walls. If these maneuvers are insufficient and the injury is limited in size, Debakey forceps can be used to carefully stabilize the vessel and surgical clips applied. Care must be taken to not inadvertently enlarge the vascular defect. The next step in our approach has been to use one of several hemostatic agents that are now available. A general understanding of the similarities and differences between these products and their availability will aid the surgeon in the choosing the appropriate agent.

The first and simplest group of agents includes Gelfoam® (Pfizer NY, NY), Surgicel® (Ethicon, Somerville, NJ), Avitene® (Bard Warwick, RI), Arista® (Medafor, Minneapolis, MN), [Vitasure® (Orthovita, Malvern, PA)], and others. These work early in the intrinsic clotting cascade to accelerate hemostasis and require adequate concentrations of clotting factors. Gelfoam® and Surgicel® should be applied to dry surfaces and held in place with moderate pressure until bleeding stops. It is recommended that Surgicel® be removed when hemostasis is achieved, but both of these products are absorbable and may be left in place. The other products in this group can be used

on bloody surfaces and are left in situ. The second group of agents uses topical thrombin either alone or in conjunction with a collagen or gelatin matrix. FloSeal® (Baxter, Deerfield, IL) combines topical thrombin and a gelatin matrix. Some surgeons will saturate Gelfoam® with thrombin for a similar effect. These are applied to areas with active bleeding and rely on the conversion of the patient's fibrinogen to fibrin to complete hemostasis. Products using bovine thrombin carry a black box warning from the FDA regarding the potential development of antibodies to bovine thrombin and/or factor V that can cross react against human factor V, causing a factor V deficiency. This can lead to hematologic abnormalities that affect the prothrombin (PT) and the partial thromboplastin (PTT) times and can cause severe bleeding or thrombosis. The last of these groups, the fibrin sealants, include Tisseal® (Baxter Dearfield, IL), Evicel® (Ethicon Somerville, NJ), and Vitagel® (Orthovita Malvern, PA), and contain thrombin and fibrinogen. Vitagel® is unique in that it uses plasma obtained from the patient to supply concentrated autologous fibrinogen, platelets, and other coagulation factors. However, the thrombin in this product is bovine-derived.

There are few studies directly comparing these agents. A rat neurosurgical model was recently used to compare the safety and efficacy of Surgicel®, FloSeal®, Arista®, and Avitene® against a negative control. A standardized defect was made in the rats' brain and the agents were then applied to the area. Time to hemostasis was recorded. The rats were sacrificed according to a predetermined schedule and their brains were examined for inflammation and residual hemostatic agent. In this relatively small study, all the hemostatic agents performed better than the negative control with hemostasis at one minute achieved in approximately 65% to 95% of active cases. Avitene® and FloSeal® showed a propensity to promote granuloma formation and residual material remained for all of the agents but Arista®. Clearly these latter two attributes are less critical in abdominal/pelvic surgery.

If the above steps are unsuccessful, suturing of a venous defect in a large vessel such as the vena cava is performed using a 5-0 monofilament suture. Proximal and distal occlusion of the vessel around the site of injury using sponge sticks will facilitate the ease of repair. Alternatively, a finger may be placed over the vascular defect and slowly moved down the length of the vessel as successive stitches are placed. For bleeding deep in the pelvis, a bilateral hypogastric artery ligation will reduce the pulse pressure in the more distal vessels and control bleeding in up to 50% of cases.

Recent reports including a meta-analysis have shown that intravenous infusion of recombinant activated factor VIIa has an approximately 75% likelihood of reducing or stopping major abdominal bleeding. Thromboembolic complications occurred in 16% of cases. If all else fails, a base of hemostatic agents are applied to the area of bleeding and packing is placed in an effort to apply pressure to this area when the abdominal wall is closed. A variety of techniques have been described including a "parachute" packing that comes out through the vagina and is placed on traction to apply pressure to the deep pelvis. The patient remains intubated and sedated while medical stabilization is achieved. Prophylactic antibiotics are given and the patient is returned to the operating room for pack removal in 24 to 72 hours.

In situations of excessive hemorrhage, the surgeon must remain aware of the extent of blood loss. If this loss is rapid or extreme, it may be necessary to stop active efforts to identify and repair bleeding sites, which often allows ongoing loss of blood, in favor of controlling the bleeding with pressure and allowing the anesthesiologist to stabilize the patient with crystalloid and blood products. Additional assistants and specialists should be summoned as needed. As blood loss mounts, monitoring of the patient's coagulation profile with replacement using fresh frozen plasma, platelets, and cryoprecipitate as indicated becomes essential.

WOUND COMPLICATIONS

The incidence of postoperative wound complications is associated with patient-related factors such as obesity, older age, poor nutritional status, and intercurrent medical conditions such as diabetes and pulmonary disease. Intraoperative factors adversely affecting wound healing include extended duration of surgery, inadequate wound hemostasis, and poor surgical technique. Wound infections occur in up to 12% of cases while fascial dehiscences are discovered in up to 3% of wounds. Superficial wound separations affect up to 20% of cases.

The choice of abdominal incisions is dependent primarily on issues related to access to the pelvis and upper abdomen. Transverse incisions provide excellent exposure to the pelvis while minimizing the cosmetic side effects of pelvic surgery when laparoscopy is not feasible. In addition, many studies including a recent Cochrane review have found that, when compared to vertical incisions, transverse incisions are associated with less pain, less compromise of pulmonary function, and lower rates of dehiscence and hernia formation. Despite the increased operative time, greater blood loss, and increased risk for nerve damage with transverse incisions, they are the default surgical route when access to the upper abdomen is not needed or large masses do not require intact removal. Entrapment of the ilioinguinal or iliohypogastric nerve within the fascial closure of a transverse incision can occur when the fascial incisions have extended beyond the lateral border of the rectus muscles. Patients present with sharp, moderate to severe pain localized to the lower quadrant. Relief of the pain following injection of local anesthetic helps to establish the diagnosis. Under extreme circumstances, the fascial stitch may need to be modified.

When pelvic exposure is limited with a Pfannenstiel incision, we recommend conversion to a Cherney incision in which the tendinous insertions of the rectus muscles onto the symphysis pubis are divided. A portion of the tendon is left on both the muscle and the insertion site to facilitate reapproximation with permanent suture at the completion of the procedure. The inferior epigastric vessels are isolated along the lateral edge of each muscle and divided. Partially or fully cutting the rectus muscles under these circumstances is discouraged since the attachment of the muscles to the fascia was taken down as part of the Pfannenstiel incision and closure of the fascia at the completion of the procedure will not reapproximate the cut portion of muscle.

The obese patient presents a special challenge in regard to incision location. The inclination to make a suprapubic incision below the pannus must be resisted due to the high rate of wound breakdown and infection associated with this location. The lone exception to this rule is when a panniculectomy is performed which facilitates the intra-abdominal portion of the procedure and reduced postoperative complications. Gallup has described a technique in which the pannus is retracted caudally and a vertical incision is made either periumbilically or, for those with a very large pannus, entirely supraumbilically. Care must be taken to not extend the incision on to the pannus and inadvertently go through it and on to the mons. The fascial incision is taken down to the symphysis pubis. Issues in regard to closure are discussed below.

Epithelialization begins within hours following wound closure with a watertight seal established within 48 hours. Wounds should be covered with a clean, dry dressing for 24 to 48 hours. The wound's tensile strength increases rapidly during the initial six weeks following surgery. Staples may be removed from low tension, transverse incisions in seven days. For vertical incisions that are under increased tension, particularly in the obese, staples should remain in place for up to 14 days despite the increased scarring that can develop at the staple sites when they remain in place beyond 7 to 10 days. Tapes such as Steri-strips are placed across the wound following removal of staples to reduce tension on the skin edges. Alternatives to standard staples for large wounds or those under mild tension are subcuticular stitches or use of co-polymer subcutaneous staples that are absorbed over several months and therefore do not need to be removed. For smaller incisions, dermal glues provide fast closure with good cosmeses.

The role of surgical preparation and technique in the development of wound complications has been extensively studied. There is no clear evidence that bathing preoperatively with chlorhexidine reduces the risk for skin infections. Furthermore, scrubbing and painting the abdomen holds no advantage over an iodine-based paint only skin prep, and using a second scalpel after opening the skin also does not reduce the incidence of wound infections. Clipping rather than shaving pubic hair that might interfere with skin closure has been shown to be beneficial. Incising the subcutaneous fat with either a scalpel or with electrocautery using cutting current also does not appear to affect wound outcome. Coagulation current should not be used for general opening of the subcutaneous tissue or fascia due to the wider path of thermal injury caused by this mode.

Closure of the peritoneum is associated with adhesion formation, infection, and delayed return of bowel function. A running mass closure of the abdominal wall using either delayed-absorbable or permanent monofilament suture with stitches placed 1.5 to 2 cm from the fascial edge and 1 cm apart has a dehiscence rate of less than 0.5%. It is important when closing the fascia to reapproximate the tissue but to not strangulate it by pulling too tightly on the sutures which can predispose to dehiscence.

Management of the subcutaneous tissue in overweight and obese women remains controversial. A meta-analysis from 2004 examined suture closure of subcutaneous fat greater than 2 cm in thickness during Cesarean, section. Though only one of the studies independently showed benefit, the analysis concluded that closure decreased the risk of wound disruption by 34%. However, a prospective, randomized study involving 222 evaluable subjects compared a control group to subcutaneous closure or closed suction drainage of the subcutaneous space in gynecologic patients with vertical incisions and 3 cm or more of subcutaneous fat. The overall wound complication rates and wound disruption rates were similar for all groups. Of additional interest is an obstetrical study that showed no difference between suture closure with or without closed suction drainage.

Superficial wound separations occur when excessive tension is placed on the skin edges. Often the subcutaneous tissue has not reapproximated and an infection, seroma, or hematoma may be present. Loculated subcutaneous fluid will usually begin to seep through the wound within three to seven days following surgery, heralding an impending wound separation. If the drainage is copious and persistent, fascial dehiscence must be considered and gentle probing of the fascia with a long Q-tip or a gloved finger should be performed. Purulent drainage due to infection needs to be cultured and drained by opening the incision. Debridement of the wound as described below is usually sufficient. If cellulitis of the skin is present, characterized by erythema, warmth, tenderness, and swelling, antibiotic therapy using a first generation cephalosporin or a quinolone is prescribed for 10 days.

When a superficial wound separation is apparent, the extent of the defect in the subcutaneous tissue is assessed. If a significant portion of the defect tunnels under an intact area of the wound, particularly if access for debridement and packing is limited, the overlying skin is opened. In the occasional case where the wound surfaces are clean, immediate closure with permanent monofilament suture is performed. Mattress stitches are placed approximately 2 cm apart and tied tight enough to reapproximate but not necrose the tissue. Steri-strips can be placed between sutures to further approximate the wound edges. It is important to close the deep subcutaneous space to avoid seroma development. We have successfully utilized a modification of the figure-of-eight closure described by Dodson et al. for patients with particularly deep wounds. Sutures are removed in 10 to 14 days. Antibiotics are used only when infection is present.

If necrotic or infected tissue is present, debridement is performed. Studies evaluating various means of wound debridement including sharp dissection, mechanical debridement using wet-to-dry normal saline dressing changes, and enzymatic or autolytic agents have failed to identify significant outcome differences between these methods. Once the wound is free of necrotic or infected debris and granulation tissue is present, the wound may be closed using the techniques noted above. Secondary closure significantly reduces recovery time versus healing by secondary intention and is successful in approximately 90% of cases. An additional option to speed healing is a vacuum-assisted closure (VAC) devise which cyclically applies negative pressure to the wound bed, facilitating the removal of interstitial fluid, formation of granulation tissue and reduces bacterial colonization. A 2004 study from M.D. Anderson showed that this devise could be used for a variety of complex gynecologic oncology wounds.

Fascial dehiscence (separation of the fascial closure) and evisceration (dehiscence with protrusion of the bowel through the wound) are surgical emergencies that historically had been associated with a mortality rate of up to 35%. Recent series have demonstrated much lower mortality rates, possibly due to earlier recognition and better supportive care. Fascial dehiscence usually occurs one to two weeks following surgery. When suspected, the incision must be thoroughly inspected, preferably using a gloved finger on the fascia. When a dehiscence is discovered, broad spectrum antibiotics are started, and the patient is immediately moved to the operating room. Under most circumstances, the point of failure will be the fascia rather the breakage or untying of the suture. The wound should be opened entirely and cleaned of any necrotic or infected tissue. The bowel should be inspected for injury, and copious irrigation of the abdominal cavity performed. A nasogastric tube is placed to help decompress the bowel. A continuous mass closure technique as described above is used to close the abdominal wall. In addition, many surgeons continue to place retention sutures using large permanent sutures place through the entire thickness of the abdominal wall, spaced approximately 3 cm apart, and secured using skin bridges that allow for adjustment of the tension of the suture. The skin is usually closed secondarily.

BIBLIOGRAPHY

Chelmow D, Rodriguez EJ, Sabatini MM (2004) Suture closure of subcutaneous fat and wound disruption after cesarean delivery: a meta-analysis. *Obstet Gynecol* **103**:974–80.

Guenaga KKFG, Matos D, Wille-Jorgensen P (2009) Mechanical bowel preparation for elective colorectal surgery. *Cochrane Database Syst Rev* (1).

Pursifull NF, Morey AF (2007) Tissue glues and nonsuturing techniques. *Curr Opin Urol* **17**:396–401.

Stany MP, Farley JH (2008) Complications of gynecologic surgery. *Surg Clin N Am* **88**:343–59.

Sweeney KJ, Joyce M, Geraghty JG (2002) Management of intraoperative bowel injuries. *CME J Gynecol Oncol* **7**:178–82.

Tanguy M, Seguin P, Malledant Y (2007) Bench-to-bedside review: routine postoperative use of the nasogastric tube—utility of futility? *Crit Care* **11**:201–7.

Von Heymann C, Jonas S, Spies C, et al. (2008) Recombinant activated factor VIIa for the treatment of bleeding in major vascular and urological surgery: a review and meta-analysis of published data. *Crit Care* **12**:R14.

Wydra D, Emerich J, Ciach K, et al. (2004) Surgical pelvic packing as a means of controlling massive intraoperative bleeding during pelvic posterior exenteration—a case report and review of the literature. *Int J Gynecol Cancer* **14**:1050–4.

4   Anatomy
Werner Lichtenegger, Jalid Sehouli, and Giuseppe Del Priore

INTRODUCTION

Surgical anatomy is the synthesis of topographic and functional anatomy and surgical techniques. Surgical anatomy presents much more than the systematic description of organs and anatomic structures with particular emphasis on the relationships of the parts to each other. The tumor biology and tumor spread will also be taken into account with the different surgical techniques. To achieve the primary goal of cancer treatment to extirpate the tumor masses completely and to preserve important relevant anatomic structures, a detailed knowledge of the anatomy of the pelvis and abdomen is essential. This skill will also influence the complication rate (morbidity) and the optimal debulking rates (survival) of patients with gynecologic tumors directly. Studies have shown that the strongest clinician-driven predictor of survival is the optimal surgical outcome (Nguyen et al. 1993, Lichtenegger et al. 1998). In a national survey on 12,316 patients with ovarian carcinoma from 904 American hospitals, Nguyen and coworkers have demonstrated that gynecologic oncologists frequently performed more hysterectomies, oophorectomies, omentectomies, lymph node, and peritoneal biopsies and yielded higher debulking rates than other specialists. With the exception of patients with Stage I disease, patients treated by general surgeons had significantly reduced survival than those treated by gynecologic oncologists ($p < 0.004$). To optimize clinical management, systematic and continual teaching in anatomy is required for all physicians who are involved in the surgical treatment of patients with gynecologic malignancies.

PELVIC FASCIA AND PELVIC SPACES

Within the space lined by the pelvic fascia lies a mass of subserous tissue which as a whole is termed the *tela urogenitalis* (Fig. 1). The tissue has various functions. It forms the fascia of the pelvic viscera as well as denser tissues conducting blood vessels and nerves from the pelvic wall. Between the pelvic wall, the uterus, and the denser tissue, lie spaces filled with loose connective tissues. These spaces can be easily opened during surgery. The anatomic nomenclature includes many different interpretations and synonyms of the connective tissue structures in the pelvis. These terms include endopelvic fascia, intrapelvic fascia and connective tissue body, neurovascular plate, corpus intrapelvinum, paratissue (Stoeckel) parametrium, parangium hypogastricum (Pernkopf), transverse ligament of the collum (Mackenrodt), cardinal ligament (Kocks), web (Meigs), broad ligament, and hypogastric sheets. The mass of the connective tissue body originates at the pelvic wall and runs in a transverse direction to the uterus and the vagina. Before reaching it, it provides one connective tissue sheet to the rectum and one to the bladder. These structures can be distinguished as the uterovaginal pillar, the bladder pillar, and the rectal pillar. In a transverse section of the pelvis, it resembles a horizontal letter Y, the base of which originates at the pelvic wall and which follows the pelvic axis. The body of the corpus intrapelvinum can originate only from the posterior ascending field of the arcus. Pernkopf took this into account in describing what he called the *frontal dissepiment* as meaning the pelvic wall at the posterior part of the arcus (Fig. 2).

A confluence of this connective tissue from the sidewall to the uterus is called the *cardinal ligament* (Fig. 3). This is the strongest thickening of the pelvic fascia between the pelvic wall and the uterus. It emits the rectal pillar and the bladder pillar. Only the parametrium actually reaches the supravaginal part of the cervix and therefore the uterus. The paracolpium, the part of the uterovaginal pillar below the level of the ureter, reaches the vagina and the cervix at the level of the vaginal fornix.

The bladder pillar from the abdominal view stretches from the body of the corpus intrapelvinum to the bladder. Viewed from the vagina, the distal pillar, which also lies in a sagittal plane, rises to the bladder. The sagittal bladder pillar is also called the *vesicouterine ligament*. The part of the ligament covering the ureter (the ureteral roof) forms the upper limit of the paracystium. Loose connective tissue lies between the uterus and the wall of the canal of the ureter. This tissue contains the blood supply for the ureter and has been called the *mesoureter*.

The rectal pillar (uterosacral) spans the distance from the dorsal of the cardinal ligament to the sacrum. The upper portion represents the sagittal rectal pillar. The sagittal rectal pillar does not lie in a sagittal plane, but deviates far laterally to accommodate the pouch of Douglas. This brings it very close to the pelvic wall. The rectouterine ligament splits into an anterior leaf that emits the rectal fascia and a posterior leaf, which reaches the sacrum at the level of anterior sacral foramina II to IV. The insertion at the sacrum can extend upward beyond the sacral promontory (Figs. 3 and 4).

The paravesical space is limited medially by the vesical fascia and the bladder pillar that enters it. Laterally, it reaches the parietal pelvic fascia and medially and anteriorly, it merges into the prevesical space. The major pelvic vessels lie in the lateral margin. Posteriorly, it is limited by the body of the corpus intrapelvinum and the uterine artery in the cardinal ligament. The roof of the paravesical and prevesical space is formed by the vesicoumbilical fascia, which forms a vertical plane at the anterior abdominal wall and horizontal plane in the pelvis.

The pararectal space is limited medially by the rectal fascia and the rectal pillar and laterally by the parietal pelvic fascia. After being opened from the abdomen, the pararectal space is narrow, because the rectal pillar lies close to the pelvic wall. The space is best demonstrated by pulling the uterus anteriorly so that the rectal pillar is lifted off the pelvic wall. The retrorectal/presacral space lies behind the rectum and is

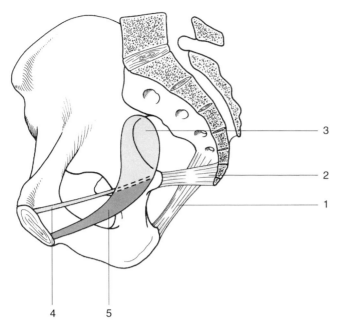

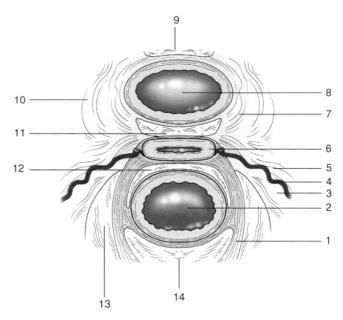

Figure 1 1 Ischiosacral ligament; 2 Sacrospinous ligament; 3 Origin of corpus intrapelvicum at lateral pelvic sidewall; 4 Arcus tendineus levatoris ani; 5 Arcus tendineus fasciae pelvis.

Figure 3 1 Uterosacral ligament; 2 Rectum; 3 Adventitia; 4 Vessels; 5 Cardinal ligament; 6 Vagina; 7 Bladder pillar; 8 Urinary bladder; 9 Prevesical space; 10 Paravesical space; 11 Vesicovaginal space; 12 Rectovaginal space; 13 Pararectal space; 14 Retrorectal space.

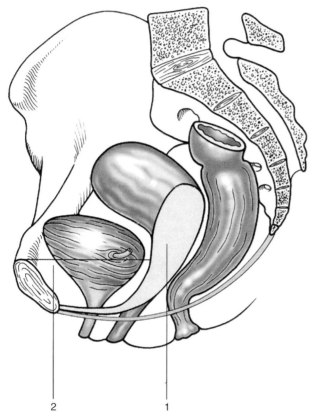

Figure 2 1 Corpus intrapelvicum; 2 Arcus tendineus levatoris ani.

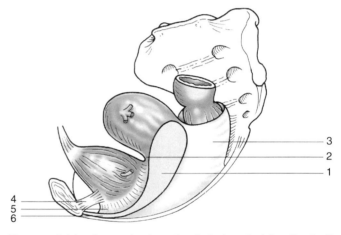

Figure 4 1 Origin of connective tissue, detached at lateral pelvic wall; 2 Cardinal ligament; 3 Uterosacral ligament; 4 Pubovesical ligament; 5 Laterovesical ligament; 6 Arcus tendineus fasciae pelvis.

The vesicocervical and vaginal spaces are limited by the vesical fascia and the cervix. They reach the peritoneum and are inferiorly separated by the supravaginal septum. The vesicovaginal space reaches caudally the origin of the urethra and lies between the bladder pillars.

UPPER PART OF THE ABDOMEN

Although in most patients with primary gynecologic cancers the highest tumor mass is concentrated in the pelvis, the upper quadrants of the abdomen are predominantly involved by metastasis in patients with recurrence ("change of level").

The omental bursa is limited ventrally by: stomach, lesser omentum, and gastrocolic ligament; dorsally by: peritoneum (ceiling), pancreas, duodenum (middle), and greater omentum; posterior lamina (bottom) cranially by: caudate lobe of liver, left diaphragmatic vault; caudally by: transverse colon, transverse mesocolon, greater omentum (with inferior recession). To the

limited by rectal fascia and the parietal pelvic fascia. The retrorectal space is separated from the pararectal spaces by the part of the rectal pillar that joins the pelvic sacral foramina II to IV.

Between the vaginal and rectal fascia lies the rectovaginal space. It reaches caudally to the centrum tendinum. Superiorly, it is limited by the peritoneum of the pouch of Douglas. Laterally, the space is limited by the rectal pillars.

left this space is limited by the following structures and organs: spleen, gastrophrenic ligament, gastrolienal ligament, splenorenal ligament, phrenico-splenal ligament, and splenocolic ligament (Fig. 5). The omental bursa communicates with the peritoneal cavity via the epiploic foramen (foramen of Winslow). This foramen is located below the free right margin of the hepaticoduodenal ligament and is limited cranially by the caudate lobe of the liver and distally by the superior duodenal flexure. The best way to explore the omental bursa is to prepare the space between the gastrocolic ligament and the transverse colon. During primary surgery of ovarian cancer the greater omentum is often resected incompletely. As a consequence, residuals of the omentum will be detected during surgery in relapse, frequently. In the case of an acute pancreatitis, necrosis or effusion can also affect this pouch.

Peritonectomy is often applied in diffuse peritoneal carcinomatosis. This can also be performed in the case of involvement of the right diaphragm. Therefore, the falciform ligament of the liver should be cut in order to inspect the diaphragm completely. The falciform ligament is a wide, sickle-shaped fold of the peritoneum and attached to the lower surface of the diaphragm, internal surface of the right rectus abdominis muscle, and the surface of the liver.

The duodenum is about 25-cm long, C-shaped and begins at the pyloric sphincter. It is entirely retroperitoneal and is the most fixed part of the small intestine. The duodenum has four parts: (1) superior, (2) descending, (3) horizontal, and (4) ascending.

The fourth part of the duodenum terminates at the duodenojejunal flexure with the jejunum. The ligament of Treitz is a musculofibrous band (suspensory muscle) that extends from the upper aspect of the ascending part of the duodenum to the right crus of the diaphragm and tissue around the celiac artery.

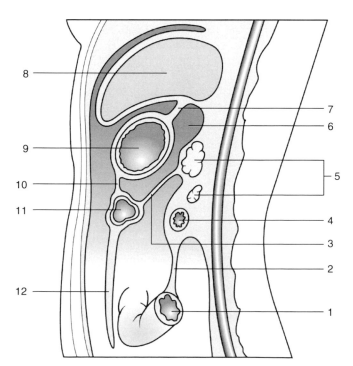

Figure 5 1 Small intestine; 2 Mesentery; 3 Transverse mesocolon; 4 Duodenum; 5 Pancreas; 6 Omental bursa; 7 Lesser omentum; 8 Liver; 9 Stomach; 10 Gastrocolic ligament; 11 Transverse colon; 12 Greater omentum.

VASCULAR SUPPLY

Most vessels encountered during oncologic procedures can be interrupted without ill effect because of the rich collateral circulation (Figs. 6–8). These anastomoses prevent ischemia unless more than one of the major vessels is occluded. However, patchy ischemia, especially induced by atherosclerosis, fibrosis or irradiation, can occur since the small vessels that enter the gut wall are essentially terminal arteries. Obstruction of these vessels results in segmental ischemia. However, whenever possible, vessels should be spared in order to promote healing and optimize chemotherapy and radiotherapy. Certain vessels, such as the superior mesenteric artery, can never be interrupted without reanastomosis. Care must be exercised around these structures, as blood vessels are not entirely consistent in their course or points of origin.

Some helpful guidelines for locating these vessels include the bony, cutaneous, and muscle relationships. For instance, the aortic bifurcation often occurs over the fourth lumbar vertebra which, in thin individuals, is at the level of the umbilicus. The renal vessels originate around the second lumbar vertebra. The ovary arteries arise just inferiorly to these at the third lumbar vertebra, around the level of the third part of the duodenum. The duodenum is also helpful in identifying the superior mesenteric artery, which leaves the aorta immediately cephalad to the third part, and the inferior mesenteric artery, which leaves the aorta just caudad to this same duodenal section. The ovary veins, on the other hand, are asymmetric, with the left vein emptying into the left renal vein, and are accompanied by many lymph vessels.

The umbilical artery originates where the uterine artery originates, at the termination of the internal iliac vessel. The distal region of this artery runs as the obliterated medial umbilical ligament and the proximal region is the origin of the superior vesical artery. The identification of the umbilical ligament is very helpful by the preparation of the parametrium; during radical hysterectomy, in the case of cervical cancer.

The external iliac artery and vein are additional important anatomic landmarks of the pelvis and can be easily palpated during surgery. The external iliac artery has two branches to the pelvic region: the deep circumflex iliac artery and the inferior epigastric artery.

The external iliac artery continues as the femoral artery after crossing under the inguinal ligament through the lacuna vasorum. The lacuna vasorum is the anatomic space for the passage of the femoral vessels to the thigh. The femoralis vein, the femoral ramus of the genitofemoral nerve, and the superior lymph node ("node of Rosenmüller") of the deep inguinal nodes are also located in the lacuna vasorum. The femoral nerve (L1–L2) is located between the psoas muscle and iliac muscle and passes laterally from the femoral artery with the lateral cutaneous femoral nerve and the lacuna musculorum.

In advanced cancer, regions of the intestinum are frequently involved. Knowledge of the blood supply of the mesenteric arteries is required to determine the area of intestinal resection in order to obtain maximal debulking. The superior mesenteric artery has branches to the stomach, inferior part of the duodenum, jejunum, ileum, cecum, ascending and transverse colon, ending at the left flexura. The inferior mesenteric artery

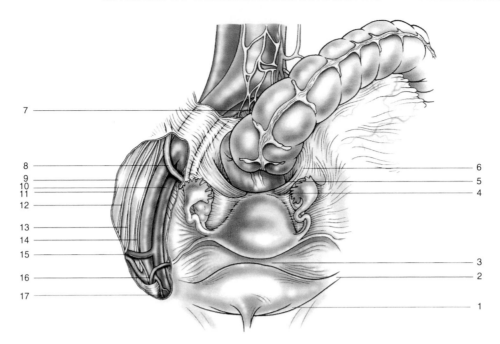

Figure 6 1 Paravesical fossa; 2 Transverse vesical fold; 3 Uterovesical pouch; 4 Rectovesical pouch; 5 Sacrogenital fold of uterosacral ligament; 6 Pararectal fossa; 7 Superior hypogastric plexus; 8 Ureter; 9 Psoas muscle; 10 Internal iliac artery; 11 Iliohypogastric nerve; 12 Ilioinguinal nerve; 13 Lateral femoral cutaneous nerve; 14 Genitofemoral nerve; 15 Circumflex iliac artery; 16 Round ligament inserting into internal inguinal ring; 17 Inferior epigastric artery.

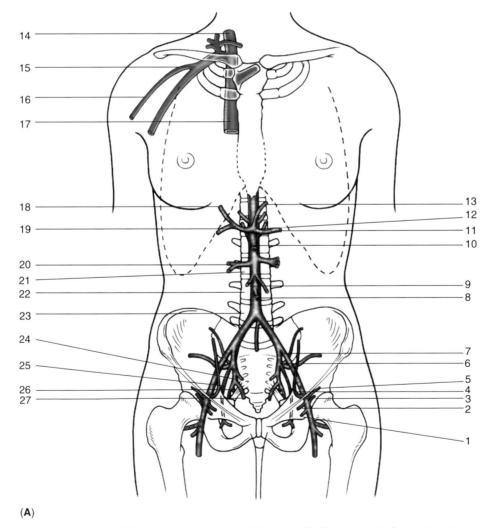

(A)

Figure 7 (**A**) 1 External pudendal artery; 2 Superficial epigastric artery; 3 Superficial circumflex iliac artery; 4 Inferior epigastric artery; 5 Deep circumflex iliac artery; 6 Internal iliac artery; 7 External iliac artery; 8 Inferior mesenteric artery; 9 Gonadal artery; 10 Superior mesenteric artery; 11 Splenic artery; 12 Celiac trunk; 13 Left gastric artery; 14 Internal jugular vein; 15 Subclavian vein; 16 Cephalic vein; 17 SVC; 18 Hepatic artery; 19 Gastroduodenal artery; 20 Renal artery; 21 L2; 22 L3; 23 L4; 24 Inferior rectal artery; 25 Obturator artery; 26 Internal pudendal artery; 27 Uterine artery. (*Continued*)

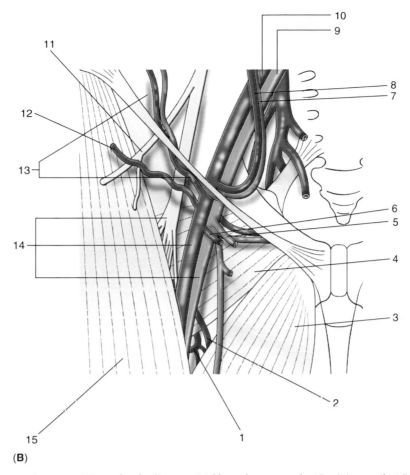

(B)

Figure 7 *(Continued)* (**B**) 1 1st perforating artery; 2 Femoral pudendis artery; 3 Adductor longus muscle; 4 Pectinius muscle; 5 External pudendal vein; 6 External pudendal artery; 7 Inferior epigastric vein; 8 Inferior epigastric artery; 9 External iliac vein; 10 External iliac artery; 11 Lateral femoral cutaneous nerve; 12 Superficial circumflex iliac artery; 13 Deep circumflex iliac artery + vein; 14 Femoral nerve, artery + vein; 15 Sartorius.

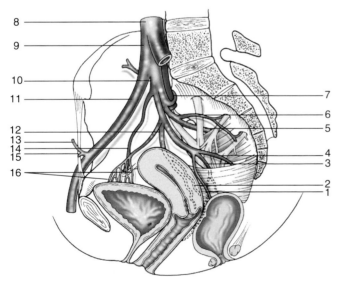

Figure 8 1 Middle rectal artery; 2 Descending cervical of uterine artery; 3 Internal pudendal artery; 4 Inferior gluteal artery; 5 Superior gluteal artery; 6 Lateral sacral artery; 7 Iliolumbar artery; 8 Aorta; 9 Common iliac artery; 10 Internal iliac artery; 11 External iliac artery; 12 Uterine artery; 13 Circumflex iliac artery; 14 Obturator artery; 15 Inferior epigastric artery; 16 Superior vesical.

gives branches to the descending and sigmoid colon and the rectum. The lower mesenteric vein carries blood from the descending colon, sigmoid colon, and rectal vein plexus into the portal vein. The superior mesenteric vein takes blood from the jejunum, ileum, cecum, ascending colon, and the transverse colon into the portal vein and receives additional blood from veins of the duodenum and the pancreas.

The celiac artery is the first branch of the abdominal aorta and supplies the stomach, liver, spleen, duodenum, and pancreas. There are also various anastomoses between the superior mesenteric artery and celiac trunk (pancreaticoduodenal artery) and the superior mesenteric artery and inferior mesenteric artery. The so-called Riolan's arch is an inconstant artery which is parallel to a portion of the middle colic artery and can be identified in the area of the left flexura of the colon. When Riolan's arch is not developed—narrowed by irradiation or artherosclerosis—a ligation of the inferior mesenteric artery can induce necrosis of the descending colon because arterial perfusion by the medial colic artery is interrupted.

Lymphatic drainage parallels the course of venous blood supply. However, drainage is not always as straightforward as the blood supply. Lymph node metastases can obstruct flow and lead to retrograde metastases, which appear to skip regional chains. For instance, some endometrial and ovarian cancers can have isolated para-aortic lymph node spread through the lymph vessels of the infundibulopelvic ligament and show a retrograde lymphatic spread (Fig. 9).

For performing a systematic pelvic lymphadenectomy and for extraperitoneal preparation in the case of bulky disease, it is advisable to distinguish the different anatomic spaces

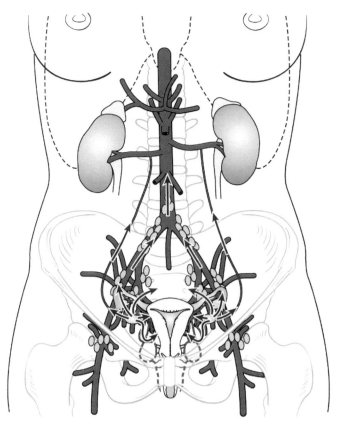

Figure 9 Lymphatic spread in ovarian cancer.

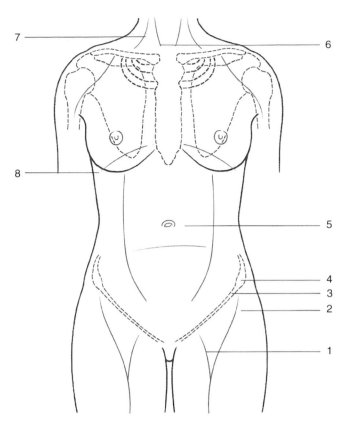

Figure 10 1 Adductor longus groove; 2 Sartorius muscle groove; 3 Inguinal ligament; 4 Anterior superior iliac spine; 5 Level of L4/L5 vertebral bodies; 6 Sternal head; 7 Clavicular head (6 and 7 sternocleidomastoid muscle); 8 Seventh rib.

around the pelvic vessels and structures. For simplification, it is helpful to visualize four associated spaces.

1. *Lateral pelvic wall.* Entrance between the medial part of the psoas muscle and laterally from the external iliac artery,
2. *Paravesical fossa.* Entrance between the posterior wall of the urinary bladder and the external pelvic vein,
3. *Obturator fossa.* Entrance between external iliac vein and medial umbilical artery,
4. *Prevesical (retropubical) space (space of Retzius).* Entrance between the lower portion of the abdomen (pubic bones) and urinary bladder.

NERVES

There are few procedures that require a complete dissection of nerves in gynecologic oncology. In particular, the nerves of the pelvis and abdomen show a wide spectrum of variation in topographic anatomy.

Nevertheless, the general course and function of many nerves should be known in order to avoid their injury and minimize surgical complications (Fig. 10). The larger nerves are sometimes used as landmarks during surgical dissections, for instance, the obturator (L1–L4) nerve may serve as the near-to-inferior border of the pelvic lymphadenectomy (obturator fossa) and the phrenic nerve as the posterior border of the scalene node dissection.

To avoid injury, at the very beginning of a surgical procedure, the anatomy of the nervous system should be kept in mind when positioning the patient. For instance, because laparoscopy requires the surgeon to be further cephalad than

during the same procedure done by laparotomy, both arms should be tucked at the patient's side to avoid excessive superior traction on the brachial plexus by the surgeon leaning on the extended arm. During vaginal procedures, an assistant unfamiliar with the course of the femoral nerve might rest an arm on the patient's medial anterior thigh and compress the femoral nerve. This nerve may also be injured by an abdominal retractor placed too deeply over the psoas muscle. Finally, some of the smaller nerves, such as the genital femoral nerve, may be transected during the removal of suspicious lymph nodes.

Femoral nerve injury results in decreased hip flexion and leg extension due to the loss of the iliacus, rectus femoris, vastus lateralis, intermedius and medialis, and sartorius muscle function. Injury to the obturator nerve results in loss of leg adduction and pronation from loss of the adductor brevis, longus and magnus, as well as obturator externus, and gracilis muscle innervation.

The obturator nerve is surrounded by soft tissue consisting of lymph nodes and vessels and can be easily seen at the lateral pelvic wall medially from the lumbosacral trunk and the obturator fossa. In 30% of cases, an accessory obturator vein runs across the fossa. The obturator nerve leaves the pelvic wall by traversing through the obturator canal of the hip bone and crossing the paravesical fossa. The obturator canal is an opening in the obturator membrane and located a distance of 2 to 4 cm directly under the upper part of the symphysis.

The sciatic nerve is located laterally to the internal iliac artery and is not usually injured during surgical procedures.

The sciatic nerve leaves the pelvis together with the inferior gluteal vein through the sciatic foramen. The sciatic nerve can be compromised by inadequate positioning during surgery and by advanced cancer (e.g., cervical cancer) spread to the lateral pelvic wall. Pain, secondary to cancer or postoperatively, can be controlled in the pelvis by regional anesthetic blockade of the dorsal nerve roots of T10, T11, and T12 to the uterus tubes and ovary, and S2, S3, and S4 to the remaining genital structures (see chapter 35).

The sympathetic trunk and the hypogastric nerves are responsible for the sympathetic innervation of the pelvis. Both lumbar trunks run across the medial origin of the iliopsoas muscle and ventrally to the lumbar veins. Injury to the sympathetic trunk can cause homolateral vasodilatation postoperatively: a feeling of hyperthermia in the lower extremity. The splanchnic nerves take the parasympathetic innervation of the pelvis and control micturition and defecation.

MUSCLES

Many of the cutaneous landmarks used in planning gynecologic surgery comprise borders of the superficial muscles (Figs. 10 and 11). In some of the reconstructive techniques discussed in this book, the muscles are the primary focus of the procedure. For the most part, however, they are structures to be retracted or transected. Nevertheless, they are helpful in identifying related anatomical structures, and therefore should be familiar to the operating surgeon.

One useful relationship is that between the rectus abdominis muscle and the epigastric vessels. When performing laparoscopy, it is best to place the lateral trocars completely laterally to these muscles to ensure avoidance of epigastric vessels. This procedure facilitates surgery also by keeping the surgical instruments as far apart as possible. It is this relationship with the epigastrics that makes the rectus abdominis muscle an ideal vascular pedicle flap for reconstructive

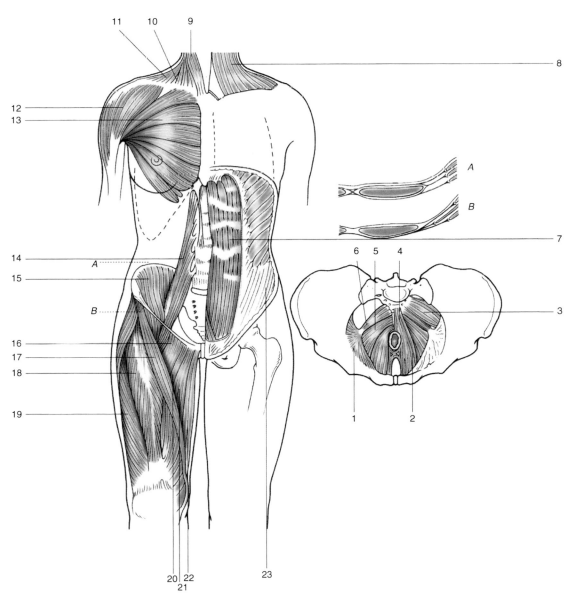

Figure 11 A Transverse level, umbilicus; B Transverse level, arcuate line; 1 Obturator internus; 2 Puborectalis; 3 Piriformis; 4 Pubococcygeal muscle; 5 Iliococcygeal muscle; 6 Coccygeus; 7 Rectus abdominis; 8 Platysmus; 9 Sternocleidomastoid muscle; 10 Anterior scalene muscle; 11 Trapezius; 12 Deltoid; 13 Pectoralis major; 14 Psoas; 15 Iliacus; 16 Pectineus; 17 Sartorius; 18 Rectus femoris; 19 Adductor brevis; 20 Adductor longus; 21 Vastus lateralis; 22 Gracilis; 23 Anterior superior iliac spine.

procedures. The gracilis muscle is also a suitable pedicle flap, but because it is more variable, the rectus is preferred for perineal reconstruction.

The muscles of the abdominal cavity are sometimes involved in either the disease process or surgical procedures in gynecologic oncology. However, they do serve as borders for lymph node dissections. For example, the middle of the psoas muscle marks the lateral extent of the pelvic lymphadenectomy and the internal obturator muscle does the same for the obturator space lymphadenectomy. The muscles of the proximal lower extremity are similarly used as landmarks in inguinofemoral dissection. During a scalene node biopsy, dissection is carried to the surface of the scalenus anterior muscle between the sternocleidomastoid and the trapezius muscles (Fig. 11).

BONY AND CUTANEOUS LANDMARKS

Bony and cutaneous landmarks are sometimes overlooked by junior surgeons in their eagerness to enter the abdomen (Fig. 11). However, more experienced surgical oncologists will recognize their value in planning successful gynecologic oncology procedures. For instance, gaining central venous access always begins with determination of the location of the distal third of the clavicle or the heads of the sternocleidomastoid muscle. Vascular access may also be achieved through a cephalic vein cut-down. This vein is identified by the cutaneous border of the deltoid and pectoralis major muscles (Mohrenheim's space).

These same landmarks are also useful in initiating a scalene node biopsy. An inguinal node dissection may be performed through different incisions provided that the operator recognizes the relationship of the nodes to the inguinal ligament. Tube thoracotomy and thoracocentesis require recognition of the location of the inferior scapula at the seventh and eighth rib. Finally, although the patient's soft tissue dimensions are important, the truly limiting factor for most is the bony confine of the operative field. For instance, a large patient may have a wide and shallow pelvis, making the patient an acceptable candidate for a radical hysterectomy. This may be determined before the incision by noting the distance between the anterior iliac crests in relation to the distance from the crest to the ischial tubercle. Similarly, for vaginal procedures, emphasis should be placed on the distance between the ischial tubercles and the angle of the pubic arch. The best way to assess the patient preoperatively is by recognizing the significance of the bony and cutaneous landmarks of the operative field.

REFERENCES

Lichtenegger W, Sehouli J, Buchmann E, et al. (1998) Operative results after primary and secondary debulking operations in advanced ovarian cancer (AOC). *J Obstet Gynaecol Res* **24**(6):447–51.

Nguyen HN, Averette HE, Hoskins W, et al. (1993) National Survey of Ovarian Carcinoma: V. The impact of physician's specialty on patient's survival. *Cancer* **72**:3663–70.

BIBLIOGRAPHY

Amreich I (1958) Zusammenhänge zwischen normaler und chirurgischer Anatomie des Beckenbindegewebes der Frau. *Klin Med* **13**:443.

Bristow RE, Tomacruz RS, Armstrong DK, et al. (2002) Survival effect of maximal cytoreductive surgery for advanced ovarian carcinoma during the platinum era: a meta-analysis. *J Clin Oncol* **20**(5):1248–59.

Burghardt E, Girardi F, Lahoussen M, et al. (1991) Patterns of pelvic and para-aortic lymph node involvement in ovarian cancer. *Gynecol Oncol* **40**(2):103–6.

Lee Anne MR, Agur AMR (1999) *Grant's Atlas of Anatomy*. Philadelphia: Lippincott Williams & Wilkins.

Netter FH (2003) *Atlas of Human Anatomy*. Whitehead, UK: Icon Learning Systems.

Pernkopf E (1943) *Topographische Anatomie des Menschen*, 2nd edn. Berlin: Urban & Schwarzenberg.

Possover M, Krause N, Drahonovsky J (1998) Left-sided suprarenal retrocrural para-aortic lymphadenectomy in advanced cervical cancer by laparoscopy. *Gynecol Oncol* **71**(2):219–22.

Richter K (1985) Spezielle Gynäkologie 1. In: Ober KG, Thomsen K, eds. *Gynäkologie und Gerburtshilfe*, Vol. III/1, 2nd edn. Stuttgart: Thieme.

Richter K, Frick H (1985) Die Anatomie des Fascia pelvis visceralis aus didaktischer Sicht. *Geburtshilfe Frauenheilkd* **45**:275.

5 Cross-sectional imaging

Syed Babar Ajaz and Ruth Williamson

INTRODUCTION

Pelvic imaging has seen a revolution in the recent times with increasing availability and utilization at almost all levels from initial assessment of tumors to role in management and disease response evaluation. Various classification systems are in use for staging gynecological malignancies but International Federation of Gynaecology and Obstetrics (FIGO) is currently widely used in this regard. Although FIGO does not take into account the role of cross-sectional imaging for staging of gynecological malignancies, computed tomography (CT) and magnetic resonance imaging (MRI) have become the mainstay for assessment and staging in developed countries; however, FIGO manual and surgico-pathological staging is vital for full international comparison of incidence and results of treatment. The role of imaging is valuable in the initial assessment of indeterminate adnexal masses and endometrial assessment but not in diagnosing cervical and endometrial cancers. These tumors are diagnosed by clinical examination supplemented by examination under anesthesia (EUA), biopsy, and hysteroscopy. The gold standard for staging of endometrial cancer remains histopathological. CT and MRI also have a vital role in radiotherapy treatment planning. Following treatment, cross-sectional imaging plays an important role in assessing response to treatment and also for evaluating for any recurrence. 2-(F-18) Fluor-2-deoxy-D-glucose positron emission tomography (18 FGD PET) is also now part of the mainstay of imaging when it comes to response assessment, disease recurrence and prior to pelvic exenteration.

CARCINOMA OF THE ENDOMETRIUM

Endometrial cancer is one of the commonest cancers of the female genital tract with almost 42,160 new cases diagnosed in 2009 in USA with 7780 deaths as per the figures released by the American Cancer Society. This is a disease of elderly females with 95% of endometrial cancers occurring in women aged 40 and above. The cancer is also related to un-apposed estrogen exposure such as in early menarche, late menopause, infertility, exposure to Tamoxifen (an anti breast cancer drug) and hormone replacement therapy (HRT). The disease predominantly affects post-menopausal women who present with vaginal bleeding. Because of this most of the women are diagnosed early with 75% presenting with disease confined to the endometrium. The majority of endometrial tumors arise from the glandular epithelium and hence are adenocarcinomas of the endometriod type (75%). The other less common type of tumors are serous papillary, adenosquamous and the clear cell type, all of which have a worse prognosis. Sarcomas including the mixed malignant mullerian tumors (MMMT) and leiomyosarcomas are also relatively rare.

The diagnosis of the endometrial cancers is by hysteroscopy and curettage with histological confirmation. Carcinoma of the endometrium is staged using either the TNM classification or the FIGO staging system, which is surgico-pathological (Table 1).

It is important to add here that the FIGO staging system has been recently revised (Pecorelli 2009) and the new staging system has been changed for stage I disease to stage IA where the endometrial tumor either does not or invades less than half of the depth of the myometrium. Previously stage IA was disease confined to the endometrium with no myometrial invasion. Stage IB now replaces the previous 1C disease in which the tumor invades equal to or more than half of the depth of the myometrium. Similarly, cervical glandular epithelium now is staged as stage I instead of stage IIA as per the old staging system.

Role of Imaging

Imaging has a role in early detection of abnormality of the endometrium, which may warrant further assessment by hysteroscopy and dilatation and curettage. This may be in the form of abnormal thickening of the endometrial lining on ultrasound, which would then by assessed by a hysteroscopy and once the diagnosis of endometrial cancer is made on biopsy, imaging evaluation by MRI would be required. Imaging would also be able to assess for advanced disease, which might affect the choice of treatment or the surgical approach. If it is demonstrated on imaging that the disease is quite advanced with peritoneal and nodal disease then adjuvant therapy may be indicated. Some patients may require lymph node sampling. These are patients with high-grade tumor, lymphovascular spread, cervical and deep myometrial involvement and adeno-squamous histology. Of these factors imaging is able to assess the depth of myometrial invasion, nodal enlargement and also invasion of the cervix.

Ultrasound

Ultrasound is usually the first imaging modality of choice for assessment of the endometrium in patients who present with vaginal bleeding. Trans-vaginal ultrasound is more accurate and allows precise measurement of the endometrial thickening compared to the trans-abdominal ultrasound. In addition, in obese patients and in patients with retro-verted uterus, it may be difficult to assess the endometrial lining on a trans-abdominal ultrasound.

Normal endometrial thickness and appearances vary not only with the age of the patient but also with the phase of the menstrual cycle. In the early part of the menstrual cycle, the endometrium is visualized as a thin reflective line (Fig. 1). During the proliferative phase, the endometrium is thickened and is seen as a triple line (Fig. 2) and lastly during the secretory phase the endometrial lining is at its maximum thickness with homogenously increased reflectivity and through transmission (Fig. 3).

Table 1 Endometrial Cancer-FIGO Staging 2009

Stage IA	No or less than half of myometrial invasion Endocervical glandular invasion is also stage IA
Stage IB	Invasion of half or more than half of myometrium
Stage II	Tumor invades cervical stroma but does not extend beyond the uterus
Stage IIIA	Tumor invades uterine serosa and or adnexa
Stage IIIB	Vagina and or parametrial spread
Stage IIIC	Metastases to pelvic and para-aortic nodes
Stage IVA	Invasion of bladder and or rectal mucosa
Stage IVB	Distant metastases and or inguinal node involvement

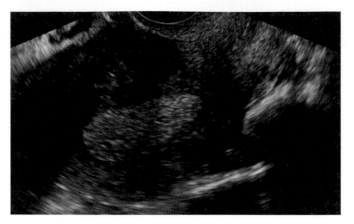

Figure 3 Trans-vaginal ultrasound during the secretory phase of the menstrual cycle shows thickened hyper-reflective endometrial echoes with through transmission.

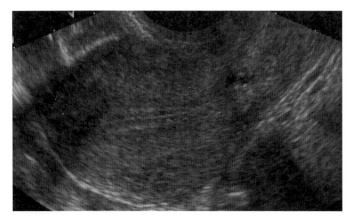

Figure 1 Trans-vaginal ultrasound during the early phase of the menstrual cycle shows a thin reflective endometrial lining.

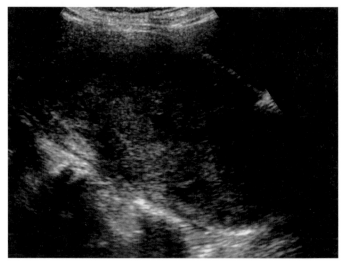

Figure 4 Trans-abdominal ultrasound shows a large uterus with complete replacement of the normal endometrial lining by a heterogeneous mass which shows ill-defined margins. Histology confirmed this to be endometroid adenocarcinoma of the uterus.

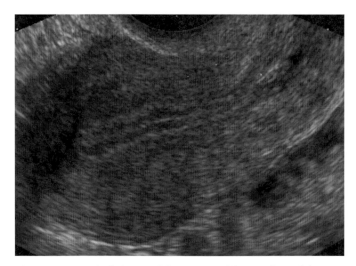

Figure 2 Trans-vaginal ultrasound during the proliferative phase of the menstrual cycle shows a triple line appearance of the endometrial echoes.

In post-menopausal women, the endometrium lining is thin and generally measures <4 mm unless the patient is on HRT or Tamoxifen for breast cancer. If the patient is on sequential HRT and is asymptomatic then the endometrial thickness can be up to 8 mm. Endometrial thickness between 5 and 8 mm will require a biopsy if the patient is symptomatic and presents with vaginal bleeding. Thickness >8 mm would require a follow-up ultrasound in asymptomatic patients and a biopsy in symptomatic ones (Levine et al. 1995).

Endometrial cancer is characterized by increased endometrial thickness often associated with heterogeneous reflectivity

and irregular and ill-defined margins (Fig. 4). There, however, remains an overlap between endometrial cancer, polyps, and hyperplasia. Trans-vaginal ultrasound appears to have a sensitivity of about 94.3% for detecting endometrial cancer but has a low specificity of 52.4%. In a recent analysis the diagnostic accuracy, sensitivity, specificity, positive, and negative predictive value of trans-vaginal ultrasound have been reported as 69%, 66%, 72%, 60%, and 75% (Kanat-Pektas et al. 2008) respectively.

Computed Tomography
CT has a major role in assessing for distant spread when it comes to staging endometrial carcinoma. MRI, however, best stages the tumor locally. The staging investigation generally includes a contrast enhanced scan of the chest, abdomen, and pelvis. Although contrast enhanced CT can detect endometrial thickness and the primary tumor as a hypodense lesion, it is difficult to assess for the depth of myometrial invasion on CT (Fig. 5). The depth of myometrial infiltration can be assessed as can the cervical involvement but generally CT is considered

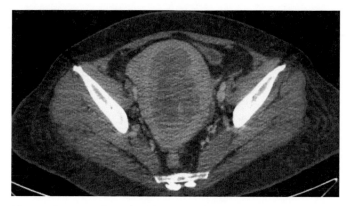

Figure 5 Contrast-enhanced axial CT scan shows an enlarged uterus with a large mass filling the endometrial cavity. There is irregular interface between the mass and the left myometrium suggesting inner myometrial invasion.

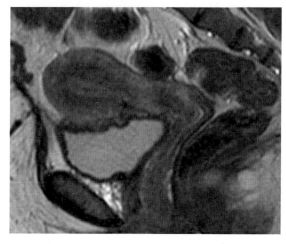

Figure 6 Sagittal T2-weighted MR scan demonstrates the normal zonal anatomy of uterus. The endometrial cavity is hyperintense on the T2W sequences. This is surrounded by a hypointense thin layer of junctional zone and the intermediate signal intensity outer myometrium.

inferior to MRI in this regard. In locally advanced disease, CT may show the involvement of parametrial structures and pelvic sidewalls. In addition, CT is useful in detecting enlarged pelvic as well as para-aortic lymph nodes, peritoneal, and omental disease in the abdomen and distant metastases in the liver, lung, bones, and brain. CT can detect enlarged lymph nodes generally based on the size criterion and this may help plan management pre-operatively, if the surgeons are contemplating doing lymph node dissection. Alternatively, CT may also provide useful information regarding the nodal map for radiotherapy planning.

Contrast enhanced CT has an accuracy of about 58% to 76% or staging of endometrial carcinoma (Kim et al. 1995). Other studies have demonstrated a slightly better accuracy of 84% to 88% for staging of endometrial cancers (Ascher and Reinhold 2002).

Magnetic Resonance Imaging

MRI is the modality of choice for local staging of the endometrial cancer once the diagnosis has been confirmed on histology. MRI is not appropriate for diagnosing endometrial cancer, as there is an overlap between the MRI appearances of endometrial cancer, hyperplasia, endometritis, and polyps. Hence, the role of MRI is in local staging of the disease after its diagnosis.

MRI exquisitely assesses normal uterine anatomy. The uterus is best assessed on the T2-weighted scans for its zonal anatomy. A normal uterus demonstrates three separate zones on the T2-weighted sequence (Fig. 6). The endometrial cavity is seen as a bright linear hyperintensity because of the presence of endometrial glands and their secretions. The thickness of the endometrial cavity can vary with the phase of the menstrual cycle. It is thickest in the mid-secretory phase and thinnest after menstruation. This is surrounded by the junctional zone, which is part of the myometrium and appears as a low signal intensity rim bordering the endometrium. This is low signal because of the low water content and the tight arrangement of the cells with paucity of the extra-cellular matrix. This is surrounded by the intermediate signal intensity outer myometrium, which can also vary in its signal intensity and reaching maximum intensity in the mid-secretory phase. The myometrial appearances can also vary with use of oral contraceptives and can be high signal on the T2W sequences.

On post-contrast dynamic scans the endometrial cavity and the outer myometrium show intense enhancement whilst the low signal intensity junctional zone remains as it is. However, there is a sub-endometrial zone, which enhances earlier than the rest of the myometrium and corresponds to the junctional zone.

The standard protocol varies from department to department but generally includes a T1W-weighted scan in the axial or coronal planes, Sagittal and axial T2W sequences through the pelvis, axial-oblique T2W small field of view perpendicular to the long axis of the endometrial cavity, a coronal or axial STIR (Short Tau Inversion sequence), and finally a T1W fat saturated dynamic contrast enhanced scan in the sagittal or axial oblique plane. In addition diffusion-weighted sequences using a B value of 1000 sec/mm^2 along with apparent diffusion coefficient (ADC) map is now part of the routine imaging.

On the T2-weighted sequences the tumor is seen as a mass or thickening of the endometrial cavity, which is of intermediate signal abnormality in comparison to the high signal of the endometrial cavity (Fig. 7). This demonstrates a good contrast between the tumor and the endometrial cavity as well as between the intermediate signal intensity tumor and the low signal intensity junctional zone. This spread into the surrounding myometrium is best assessed on the axial oblique small field of view T2W sequences. The tumor also appears heterogeneous and can have ill-defined margins and demonstrate less or no enhancement compared to the rest of the endometrium and the myometrium on the post-contrast enhanced dynamic scans. The depth of the myometrial infiltration is closely associated with lymph node involvement as well as patient survival. The FIGO staging of the endometrium has recently been revised as described above with stage IA being involvement of the inner half of the myometrium and stage IB with extension into the outer myometrium (Fig. 8). The tumor can invade the cervical lumen as well as the surrounding stroma and the parametrial tissues (Fig. 9). This is also best depicted on the sagittal and axial oblique T2W small field of view sequences. The endocervical lumen is bright because of the secretions of the endocervical glands whilst the surrounding cervical stroma is of low signal intensity. Hence,

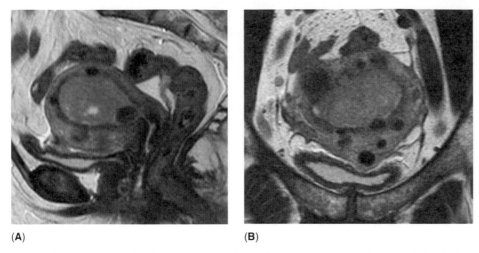

(A)   (B)

Figure 7 (**A, B**) Sagittal and axial-oblique T2-weighted MR scans show complete replacement of the normal endometrial cavity by a large intermediate signal intensity mass in keeping with an endometrial carcinoma. The tumor is confined to the endometrial cavity with no invasion into the adjacent myometrium on both planes in keeping with FIGO stage IA. Incidental small low signal intensity fibroids are noted.

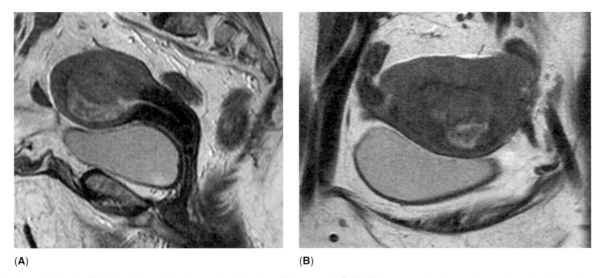

(A)   (B)

Figure 8 (**A, B**) Sagittal and axial-oblique T2-weighted scans show invasion of the posterior half of the myometrium by an intermediate signal intensity endometrial carcinoma. The tumor is seen to invade into the outer half of the myometrium in keeping with FIGO stage IB.

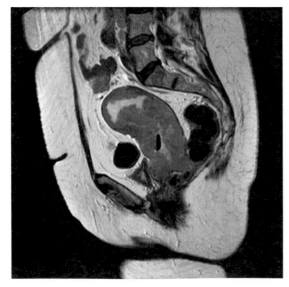

Figure 9 Sagittal T2-weighted MR shows a large endometrial tumor with invasion of both the endocervical canal as well as the surrounding cervical stroma. The low signal intensity centrally with the cervix represents gas secondary to necrotic breakdown of the tumor.

there is a good contrast between the tumor and the cervix. MR is also excellent in demonstrating involvement of the adjacent structures like the bladder and the rectum (Fig. 10). Diffusion-weighted imaging (DWI) has been shown to differentiate normal from diseased endometrium especially using high-B values (Fujii et al. 2008). Tumors are generally higher signal intensity than the surrounding myometrium on the DWI sequences and are of low signal intensity on the ADC map (Fig. 11). Uterine sarcomas including MMMT and leiomyosarcoma can have a similar appearance to endometrial cancer and may be indistinguishable on MRI. However, sometimes these tumors are seen as large intermediate to high signal intensity mass completely replacing the normal uterine architecture (Fig. 12).

The overall sensitivity and staging accuracy of MRI in assessing for myometrial invasion is 87% and 90% (Ortashi et al. 2008). The depth of myometrial invasion can be improved by using a dynamic contrast enhanced technique compared to the T2W sequence (Hricak et al. 1991). The staging may also be affected by the atrophy of the myometrium and other factors like the presence of fibroids and adenomyosis, which

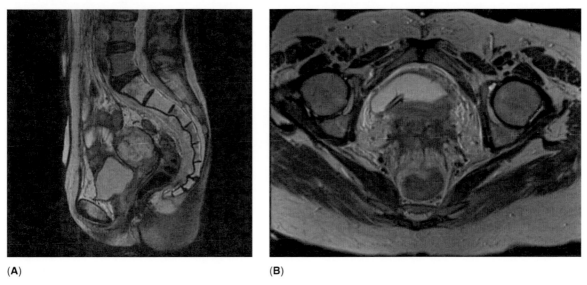

(A)   (B)

Figure 10 (**A, B**) Sagittal and axial T2-weighted sequences show a large endometrial carcinoma invading the bladder and the rectum on the right side in keeping with stage IV disease.

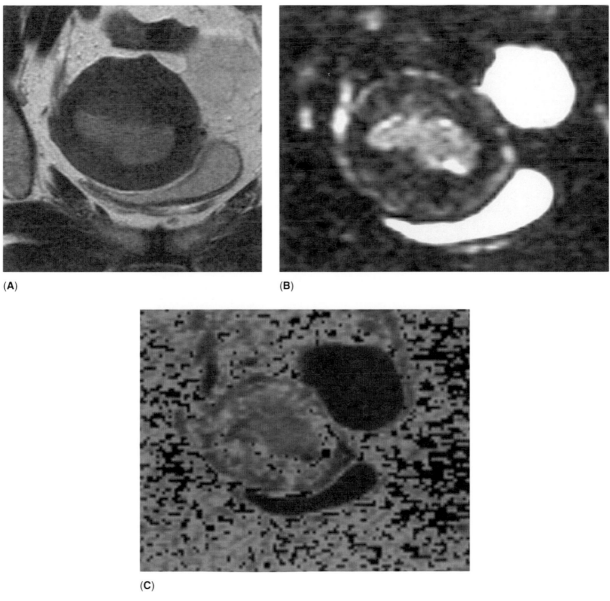

(A)   (B)

(C)

Figure 11 (**A–C**) A large endometrial adenocarcinoma with myometrial invasion on T2 weighted, diffusion-weighted imaging and the corresponding ADC map.

may distort the anatomy. MRI accuracy reduces slightly when assessing for the invasion of the outer myometrium and the cervix. In a recent study MRI differentiation of deep myometrial invasion from superficial disease agreed with

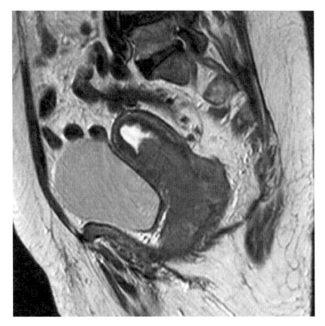

Figure 12 Sagittal T2-weighted MR scan in a 56-year-old patient with mixed malignant mullerian tumor (MMMT) presenting as a large intermediate signal intensity mass completely involving the lower uterine segment extending into the cervix and vagina.

pathological findings in 77% of cases, with a sensitivity of 83%, specificity of 72%, and a diagnostic accuracy of 77%. In regards to cervical invasion, MRI had a sensitivity, specificity, and diagnostic accuracy of 42%, 92%, and 81%, respectively. In assessing lymph node invasion, MRI presented a sensitivity of just 17%, a specificity of 99%, and a diagnostic accuracy of 89% (Cabrita et al. 2008).

Positron Emission Tomography-CT (PET-CT)
PET-CT also has an evolving role in patients with gynecological cancer in general and endometrial cancer in particular. FDG PET-CT is used for detecting nodal metastases and also has a useful role in assessing patients prior to exenterative surgery (Fig. 13). The presence of lymph nodes in patients with endometrial cancer has important implications in terms of prognosis, patient survival and surgical management. CT and MRI use size criteria to detect lymph node metastases. However, it is well known that the sensitivity and specificity of both techniques in detecting nodal metastases is low as enlarged nodes may be reactive and small nodes may harbor metastases. In a recent study the overall node-based sensitivity, specificity, PPV, NPV and accuracy of PET-CT for detecting nodal metastases in patients with endometrial cancer has been reported as 51.1%, 99.8%, 85.2%, 98.9%, and 98.7% respectively (Kitajima et al. 2009).

CERVICAL CANCER
Cervical cancer is the third most common cancer among women after breast and colorectal cancer. According to the

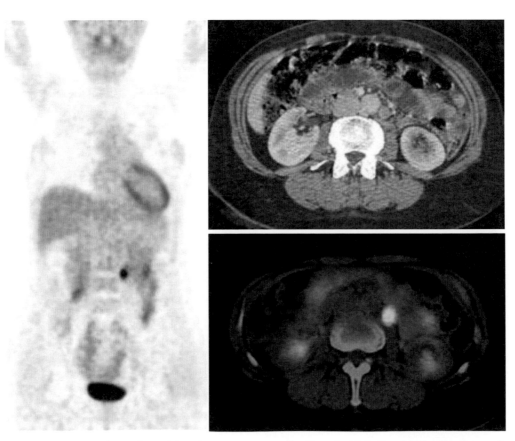

Figure 13 Fifty-eight-year-old stage IIIA grade 2 endometrial carcinoma two years earlier. Treated with TAH and BSO with adjuvant chemoradiotherapy. On follow-up small left para-aortic node on contrast enhanced CT (*top right*) not enlarged by CT criteria. PET-CT confirms metabolically active and solitary site of relapse therefore suitable for radiotherapy.

statistics of the American Cancer Society there were 11,270 new cases of cervical cancer diagnosed in 2009 with 4070 cervical cancer-related deaths. Cervical cancer is a disease of a younger age group with peak incidence between 35 and 50 years. There is also a greater incidence in developing countries and is seen in patients in the lower socio-economic class. Risk factors for cervical cancer include early sex and multiple sexual partners, smoking and long-term use of oral contraceptives has also been implicated. It is now accepted that the Human Papilloma virus is causative. Approximately 80% of cervical cancers are squamous cell in origin and the remainder being primarily adeno and adeno-squamous carcinomas.

Role of Imaging

The FIGO staging system for cervical cancer is clinical (Table 2). This involves EUA. Hence, there are inherent weaknesses in this staging. EUA may misinterpret inflammation in the parametrial tissues as local invasion. Although cross-sectional imaging is not officially included in the staging, CT and MRI are almost universally used for assessment and staging of cervical cancers. In developed countries, cross-sectional imaging is used to provide information about the size and volume of the tumor, involvement of the parametrium and adjacent structures and also to assess for nodal and metastatic disease. Tumor volume and parametrial involvement are critical factors for decisions regarding operability versus radiotherapy.

Ultrasound

Ultrasound both trans-abdominal and trans-vaginal have very limited role in staging and assessing cervical cancer. Trans-rectal ultrasound has also been used in assessing cervical tumors. The tumor is seen as a hypoechoic mass in majority of the patients (Fig. 14). Parametrial extension is inferred when there is soft tissue stranding from the lateral margin of the tumor. In early staging, ultrasound has been reported to have an accuracy of about 75% (Yang et al. 1996).

Computed Tomography

CT has a useful role in staging advanced disease, i.e., stages III and IV but has a limited role in staging early stage cervical cancer. The primary tumor may be seen as a hypodense lesion in an otherwise dense looking cervix after a post-contrast enhanced scans (Fig. 15). However, it is not possible to accurately assess the tumor volume because of lack of soft tissue contrast between the tumor and the cervical stroma. In addition, it is very difficult to assess for parametrial extension on CT as surrounding inflammation may be over-estimated as parametrial extension. An eccentric mass extending into

Table 2 Cervical Cancer-FIGO Staging

Stage 0	Carcinoma in situ
Stage I	Invasive carcinoma confined to the cervix
Stage IA	Diagnosed only by microscopy
Stage IA1	Micro-invasive carcinoma with stromal invasion <3 mm in depth and <7 mm wide
Stage IA2	Micro-invasive carcinoma not exceeding 5 mm in depth or 7 mm in width
Stage IB	Clinically visible or microscopic lesion >IA2
Stage IB1	Clinical lesions not exceeding 4 cm in diameter
Stage IB2	Clinical lesions larger than 4 cm
Stage II	Extension beyond the cervix but not to the pelvic wall
Stage IIA	Involvement of the vagina but not the lower third
Stage IIB	Parametrial involvement not reaching the pelvic side wall
Stage III	Extension to the pelvic wall or lower third of the vagina. Hydronephrosis or non-functioning kidney, unless due to a cause other than obstruction by tumor
Stage IIIA	Involves the lower third of the vagina
Stage IIIB	Extension to the pelvic wall (includes hydronephrosis)
Stage IV	Extension beyond the true pelvis or involving bladder or rectum
Stage IVA	Involvement of the bladder or rectal mucosa
Stage IVB	Spread outside the true pelvis or metastases to distant organs

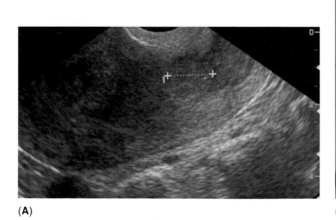

(A)

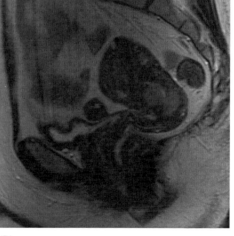

(B)

Figure 14 (**A, B**) Trans-vaginal ultrasound shows a small hypoechoic lesion at the level of the cervix in keeping with a cervical carcinoma. Corresponding sagittal T2-weighted MR images confirms the presence of an intermediate signal intensity tumor.

the surrounding soft tissues is considered an important sign of parametrial extension. Involvement of the pelvic sidewall may be seen as tumor extending to involve the obturator internus and piriformis muscle. CT has been reported to

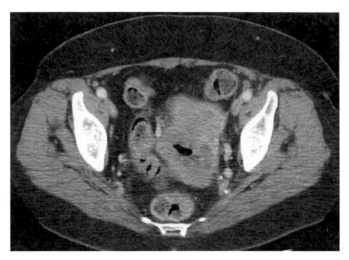

Figure 15 Axial post contrast enhanced CT scan shows a large cervical squamous cell carcinoma presenting as a mixed density mass in the cervix with central gas lucency suggestive of necrosis.

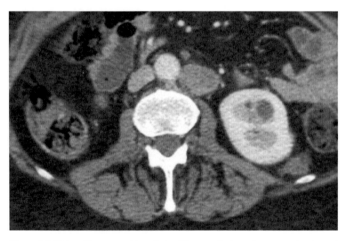

Figure 16 Thirty-five-year-old patient with a cervical carcinoma and enlarged left para-aortic lymph node.

have an accuracy of over 90% for pelvic sidewall involvement (Walsh and Jones 1992). CT is also useful in detecting nodal enlargement and distant metastases (Fig. 16). CT has a role in detection of recurrent disease at the vaginal vault and also in the pelvic and para-aortic nodes. There are however limitations in differentiating radiation fibrosis from recurrent tumor and in assessing vesico-vaginal and recto-vaginal fistulas on CT.

Magnetic Resonance Imaging

MRI is the imaging modality of choice for local staging of cervical cancer. MR provides information about the tumor volume, parametrial spread, bladder, and rectal involvement as well as assessment of local nodes.

The cervix shows a bi-zonal anatomy on the T2-weighted sequence in contrast to the three zones visible in the uterus (Fig. 17). The endocervical cavity is hyperintense because of the presence of endocervical glands and mucus. The surrounding stroma is low signal on the T2-weighted sequence because of the presence of fibrous tissue and the compact arrangement of the cells with reduced extra-cellular matrix.

The MR protocol for the assessment of cervical cancer is the same as that of endometrium with the exception that there is no additional benefit in the staging accuracy by the use of intravenous contrast. Hence, contrast is not normally given in staging of cervical tumor. The small field of view axial oblique T2W scan is performed perpendicular to the long axis of the cervix.

Invasive cervical carcinoma less than stage IB is not visualized on MR. It is important to remember that the patients will have their MR after they have had a biopsy and diagnosis made on histology. Hence, the cervix may demonstrate edema and hemorrhage at the site of the biopsy, which generally appears as an area of diffuse hyperintensity on the T2W sequences. The tumor is of intermediate signal intensity on the T2-weighted scans, which contrasts nicely with the hyperintense cervical lumen and low signal intensity fibrous stroma (Fig. 18). The tumor volume is calculated in three dimensions using the formula of antero-posterior dimension × transverse diameter × cranio-caudal height × 0.5. In many centers, tumor volume of more than 12 cc is generally considered a cut-off between surgical treatment versus radiotherapy. Extension of

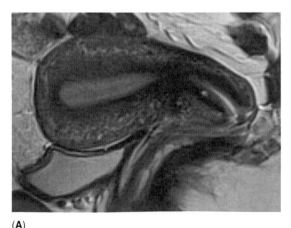

(A)

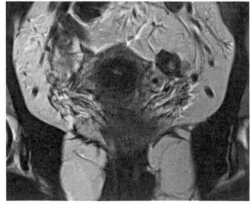

(B)

Figure 17 (**A, B**) Sagittal and axial oblique T2-weighted MR scan demonstrating the normal zonal anatomy of the cervix. The central endocervical gland shows high signal surrounded by a low signal intensity fibrous stroma.

the tumor into the parametrial tissues is another important parameter, which defines surgical versus non-surgical treatment. The presence of a well-defined low signal intensity fibrotic rim around the circumference of the cervical tumor is a good sign that there is no parametrial extension (Fig. 19). This sign has been shown to have a high negative predictive value of almost 97%.

MRI is also excellent in detection of disease outside the cervix. The involvement of the ureter can be seen on both sagittal and axial T2W scans as a dilated tubular structures. Similarly, MRI can assess involvement of bladder and rectum in stage IV disease (Fig. 20). However, MRI can over stage disease by false positive identification of disease in the bladder or rectum as mucosal edema may be interpreted a local invasion. MR has a high negative predictive value for bladder and rectal invasion (Rockall et al. 2006).

Cervical carcinoma spreads to the parametrium and tends to involve the parametrial lymph nodes and then extends to the obturator, internal, and external iliac chains. MRI like CT uses the size criteria for detection of nodal disease. A cut-off of short axis diameter of 10 mm is generally used for para-aortic and pelvic nodes. Eight millimeter is used as a cut-off value for the obturator nodes. The accuracy of MRI in nodal detection ranges between 76% and 88%. MRI and CT have low specificity for detection of metastatic lymph nodes. Recently ultra-small super paramagnetic iron oxide particles have been used to detect nodal metastases in normal size lymph nodes in patients with cervical and uterine cancers. This has been

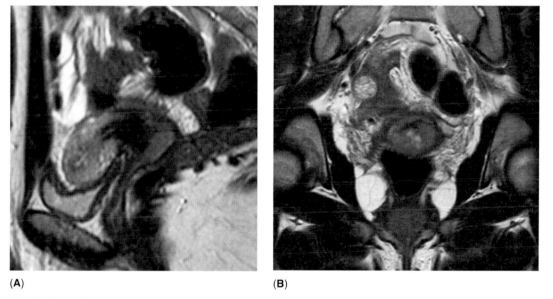

(A) **(B)**

Figure 18 (**A, B**) Sagittal and axial oblique T2-weighted MR scan shows an intermediate signal intensity cervical cancer involving the ecto-cervical lip on the left side with no extension into the surrounding parametrium.

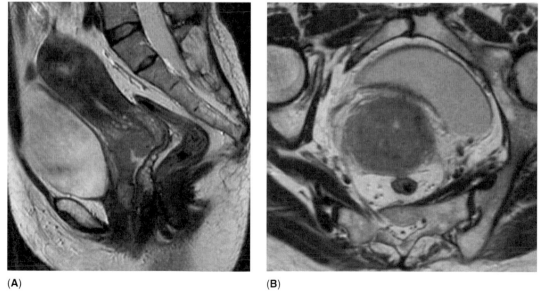

(A) **(B)**

Figure 19 (**A, B**) Sagittal and axial oblique T2-weighted MR scans show an intermediate signal intensity tumor involving the anterior cervical lip with involvement of the upper third of the vagina and extending into the right parametrium.

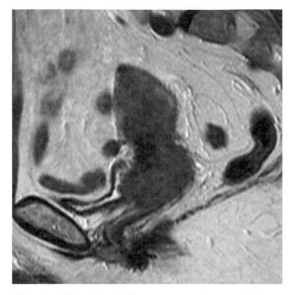

Figure 20 Sagittal T2-weighted MR scan shows a large cervical cancer with stage IV disease involving the posterior bladder wall.

shown to improve the sensitivity of detecting nodal metastases from 77% to almost 97% (Rockall et al. 2005). MRI has also been considered to be very useful for assessment of vaginal fistulas, which may be related to the primary tumor or a result of treatment.

DWI has a role at all levels of staging of cervical cancer by assessing the cellularity and ADC value of the tumor as well as for local nodal involvement and detection of recurrence. Poorly differentiated tumors have a higher cellularity and a low ADC value (Fig. 21). DWI has also been used quantitatively by measuring the ADC value and qualitatively by assessing the signal intensity on high *B*-value images to assess response to treatment (Charlotte et al. 2009).

FDG PET-CT
FDG PET-CT has also been extensively evaluated in assessment of nodal disease in patients with cervical cancer. This technique does not rely on the size criteria but is based on the utilization of glucose by malignant cells as well as involved lymph nodes (Fig. 22). In a recent study, the overall region-specific

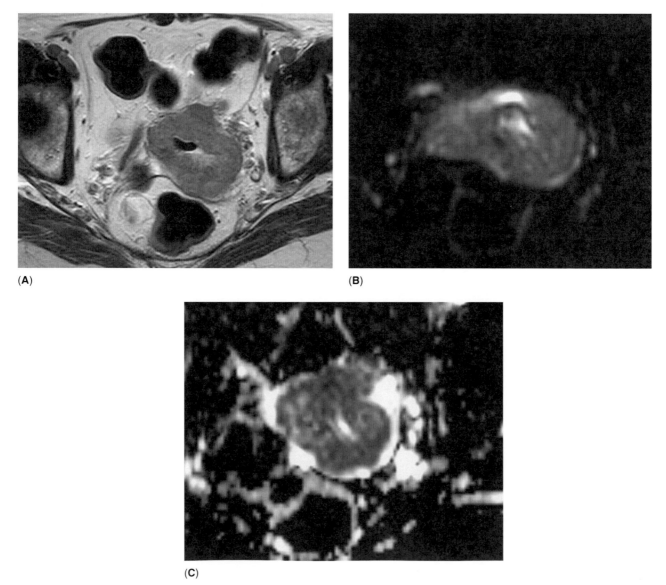

(A)

(B)

(C)

Figure 21 (A–C) Axial oblique T2-weighted scan of a cervical cancer showing restricted diffusion seen as high signal on the DWI scan and low signal on the corresponding ADC map.

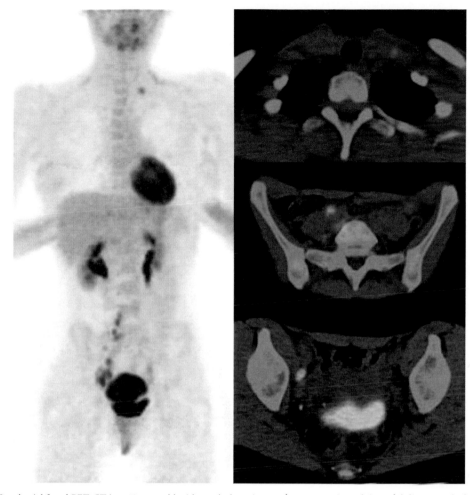

Figure 22 Coronal PET and axial fused PET-CT in a 40-year-old with cervical carcinoma shows extensive pelvic nodal disease and a left supra-clavicular node.

Table 3 RCOG RMI

Risk RMI	% Women	% Risk of cancer
Low 25	40	<3
Moderate 25–250	30	20
High >250	30	75

sensitivity, specificity, positive predictive value, negative predictive value, and accuracy of PET-CT have been quoted as 36.4%, 98.8%, 85.7%, 88.9%, and 88.7%, respectively (Chung et al. 2009). PET-CT has also been shown to have a very useful role in picking up distant nodal metastases and for detection of recurrent disease.

OVARIAN MALIGNANCY

The number of new cases of ovarian cancer in the USA in 2009 was over 21,000, with over 14,500 deaths (National Cancer Institute). Presenting symptoms are rather vague meaning that diagnosis is often at an advanced stage of disease. Imaging is used in the detection of ovarian cancer and surgical planning.

Ultrasound

Ultrasound is the main imaging modality used in the detection of ovarian cancer. Imaging features suggesting a malignant

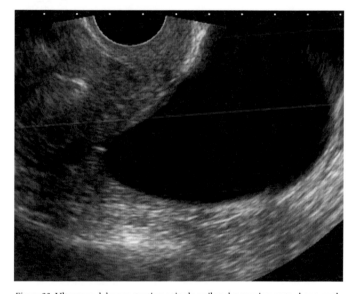

Figure 23 Ultrasound demonstrating a single unilocular ovarian cyst subsequently diagnosed as a cystadenoma.

diagnosis include solid or mixed cystic and solid lesions, bilateral disease, the presence of ascites and peritoneal deposits. Although a sensitive tool in the detection of an adnexal mass, ultrasound has rather low specificity. The risk of malignancy

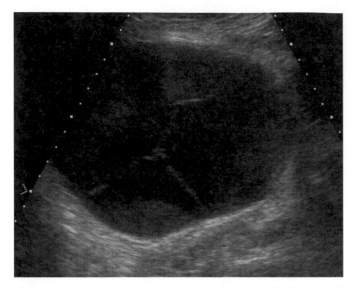

Figure 24 Ultrasound showing a simple ovarian cyst with fine internal septations.

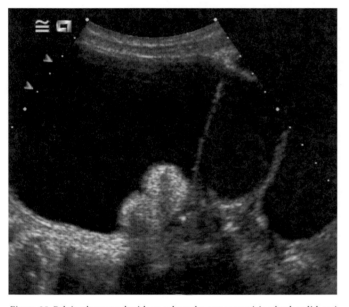

Figure 25 Pelvic ultrasound with an adnexal mass comprising both solid and septated cystic elements.

index (RMI) combines ultrasound with menopause status and the Ca125 level. RMI, ascribes a numerical value, which can be used to assess cancer risk (Table 3). Premenopausal women are ascribed a value of 1 compared with 3 for postmenopausal patients (Jacobs et al. 1990). Ultrasound is scored 0, 1, or 3 depending on the number of malignant indicators with 0 if no factors are present, 1 for one factor and 3 for two or more of the following: multilocular cyst; evidence of solid areas; evidence of metastases; presence of ascites; and/or bilateral lesions (Figs. 23–26). Ca125 is as per its value and interpretation is as in Table 3.

Trials of ultrasound as a screening test for ovarian cancer have to date demonstrated high levels of sensitivity but relatively low specificity with the result that ultrasound alone is not yet recommended for screening. Trials in high-risk populations are ongoing as are studies comparing serial Ca125 estimations with ultrasound (Menon et al. 2009).

Computed Tomography
This is usually performed with intravenous contrast agents. CT is the mainstay of ovarian cancer staging providing a rapid evaluation of chest, abdomen, and pelvis. The FIGO staging is outlined in Table 4.

Although FIGO staging of ovarian cancer is based on surgical findings and histopathology, imaging may be used for estimations of disease bulk and staging in more advanced disease. It should be noted that although liver metastases constitute stage IV disease this is only the case when they are parenchymal. Subcapsular or surface liver metastases, although dramatic in appearance only constitute stage III disease (Figs. 27–31).

The main limitation of CT in staging is that of spatial resolution in the detection of small peritoneal deposits. However, it is useful in predicting those patients less likely to benefit from a primary surgical approach to treatment i.e., those in whom optical debulking is likely to be unsuccessful. Indicators include significant disease in the upper abdomen, subcapsular liver deposits, and para-aortic lymph nodes above the renal vessels. For patients treated with primary chemotherapy, cytoreductive surgery is often

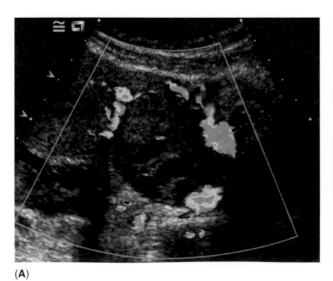

(A)

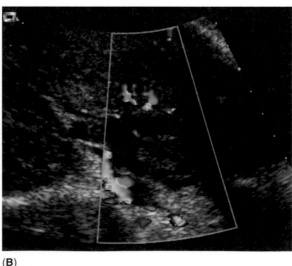

(B)

Figure 26 (**A, B**) Bilateral complex ovarian masses with cystic and solid elements with abnormal vascularity.

Table 4 Ovarian Cancer Staging

Stage I	Disease confined to one or both ovaries
Stage IA	Involves one ovary; capsule intact; no tumor on ovarian surface; no malignant cells in peritoneal washings or ascites
Stage IB	Involves both ovaries; capsule intact; no tumor on ovarian surface; negative washings
Stage IC	Tumor limited to ovaries with any of the following: capsule ruptured, tumor on ovarian surface, positive washings
Stage II	Pelvic extensions or implants
Stage IIA	Extension or implants onto uterus or fallopian tube; negative washings
Stage IIB	Extension or implants onto other pelvic structures; negative washings
Stage IIC	Pelvic extension or implants with positive peritoneal washings
Stage III	Microscopic peritoneal implants outside of the pelvis; or limited to the pelvis with extension to the small bowel or omentum
Stage IIIA	Microscopic peritoneal metastases beyond pelvis
Stage IIIB	Macroscopic peritoneal metastases beyond pelvis < 2 cm in size
Stage IIIC	Peritoneal metastases beyond pelvis >2 cm or lymph node metastases, including para-aortic nodes
Stage IV	Distant metastases to the liver or outside the peritoneal cavity

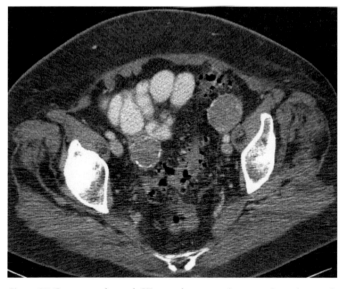

Figure 27 Contrast-enhanced CT scan demonstrating stage I ovarian carcinoma with small bilateral pelvic masses. There is no ascites and the remainder of the scan demonstrated no intra-abdominal disease.

considered if a partial response to treatment is seen after three cycles. In this respect, CT is used to accurately define the extent of post-treatment disease. Although a freehand technique is usually used to define response, many studies require formal RECIST evaluation (response evaluation criteria in solid tumors).

MRI

MRI serves two main roles in the work up of patients with ovarian cancer. Firstly, there is a diagnostic role as a good quality MRI can exclude some causes of complex ovarian cyst, e.g., dermoid and endometrioma (Figs. 32 and 33).

MRI can also be invaluable in surgical planning allowing multiplanar delineation of relationships of adjacent structures, e.g., bowel, ureters, and blood vessels. It can also give some indication of the type of malignancy. Anti-spasmolytics are routinely used to control bowel motion. Alternatively some scanners have motion correction sequences, e.g., BLADE (Fig. 34).

The place of DWI in ovarian cancer is still under consideration. Tumors of high cellularity are likely to show high signal intensity on high-*B* value images, however many ovarian tumors have significant cystic components in which there is free diffusion of water and hence low signal on high-*B* value sequences (Whittaker et al. 2009).

PET-CT

This is increasingly being used to accurately stage disease, which is apparently stage I or II to look for occult peritoneal deposits or lymph node disease. It is also used in the detection of recurrence as the similarity in attenuation of peritoneal deposits to bowel loops can make their detection difficult (Fig. 35).

PET-CT increases the conspicuity of abnormal lymph nodes in recurrent ovarian cancer.

Ovarian cancer staging is by the FIGO staging system and uses information obtained from surgery usually comprising of total abdominal hysterectomy, bilateral salpingo-ophorectomy, omentectomy, and peritoneal washings for cytology. The AJCC staging corresponds with that of FIGO.

VAGINAL CANCER

Vaginal cancer is a rare disease predominantly seen in elderly females with 70% to 80% occurring in women above the age of 60. The incidence of vaginal cancer in the USA is about 0.6 per 100,000. Invasive vaginal cancer is usually associated with vaginal intra-epithelial neoplasia (VAIN).

The majority of the vaginal cancers are squamous cell carcinoma; 5% to 10% of the vaginal cancers are adenocarcinomas.

Imaging

Superficial tumors do not require imaging for local staging (Table 5). However, MRI is the imaging modality, which is useful in staging the vaginal tumors and determining the extent of disease for surgical planning. The tumor is difficult to identify on CT. The tumor is intermediate signal on the T1W sequence and slightly high signal on the T2W sequence (Fig. 36). MRI can demonstrate the tumor spread in to the paracolpos fat, which implies stage II disease. Pelvic floor involvement, which implies stage III disease, is best seen on the coronal sequence. Stage IV disease is seen as involvement of the bladder and rectum. MRI can also demonstrate local pelvic nodal enlargement. MRI is also good for assessment of recurrent disease as well as colo-vaginal and vesico-vaginal fistulas.

CT is useful for assessing distant metastases in vaginal cancers.

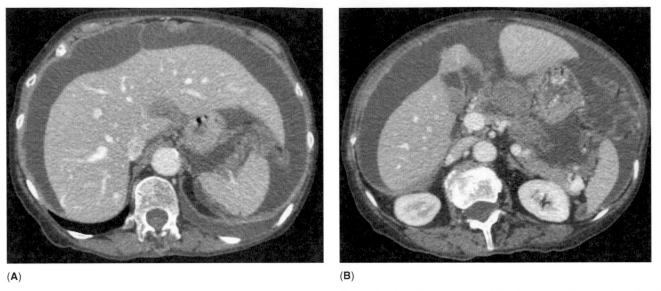

(A)   **(B)**

Figure 28 (**A, B**) Stage III ovarian carcinoma with ascites and peritoneal deposits affecting the visceral peritoneum and free floating within the peritoneal cavity.

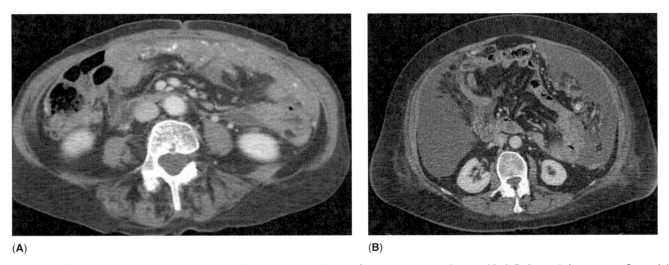

(A)   **(B)**

Figure 29 (**A, B**) Two examples of omental disease in stage III ovarian cancer. Figure **A** demonstrates a typical omental "cake" whereas **B** demonstrates fine nodular studding of the omentum.

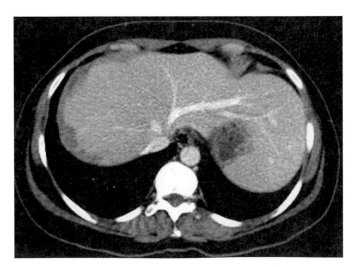

Figure 30 CT scan demonstrating subcapsular surface deposits on the liver. They are low attenuation peripheral masses which distort the serosal contour of the liver. This is considered as stage III disease within the FIGO categorization.

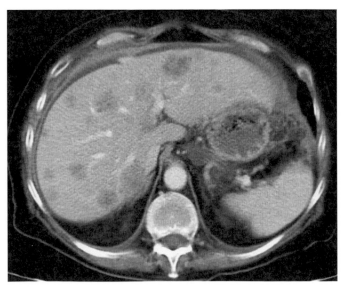

Figure 31 Parenchymal liver metastases in this example of stage IV disease are identified as multiple low attenuation deposits within the liver.

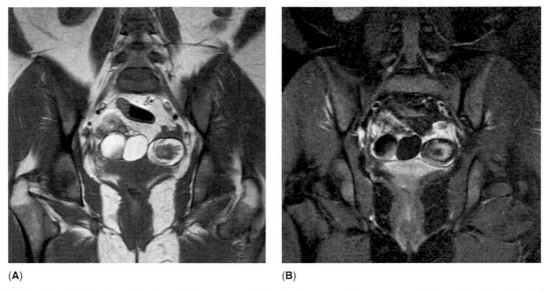

Figure 32 (**A, B**) MR imaging of bilateral ovarian dermoids demonstrates high signal return on T1 sequence with loss of signal on T1-weighted fat saturated imaging.

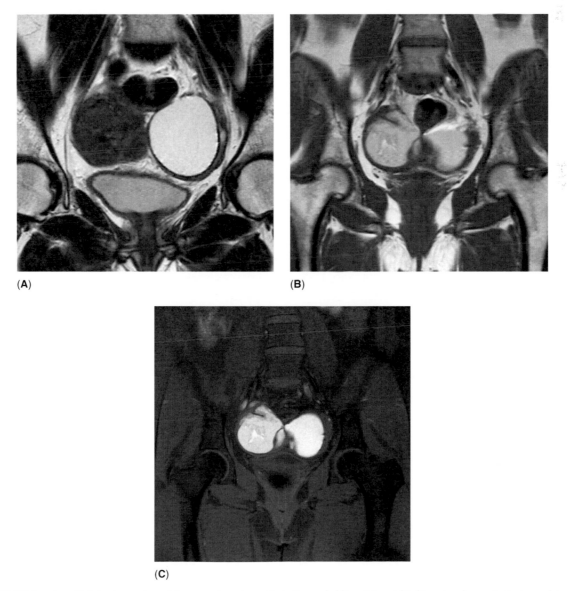

Figure 33 (**A–C**) MR imaging of bilateral complex pelvic masses in endometriosis. Coronal oblique T2-weighted imaging demonstrates two pelvic masses one of high signal and one of low signal (**A**). They are both high signal on T1-weighted and T1-weighted fat saturated images (**B, C**) indicating the presence of blood products. The T2 appearances indicate that these are of differing ages, a characteristic feature of endometriosis.

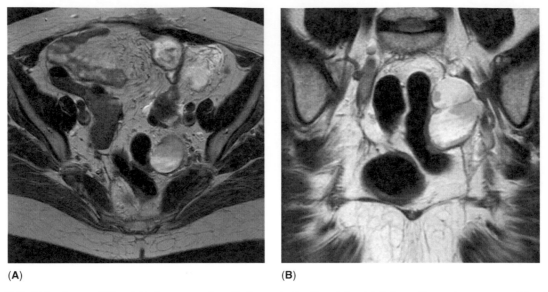

(A)   (B)

Figure 34 (**A, B**) Sagittal and coronal T2-weighted sequences elegantly demonstrating the relationship between the ovarian masses and the adjacent bowel.

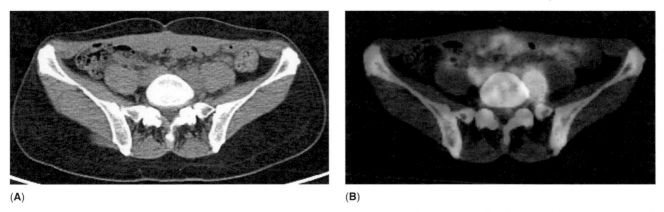

(A)   (B)

Figure 35 (**A, B**) Unenhanced CT and fused PET-CT in ovarian cancer. The common iliac lymphadenopathy is rendered considerably more conspicuous by the functional imaging.

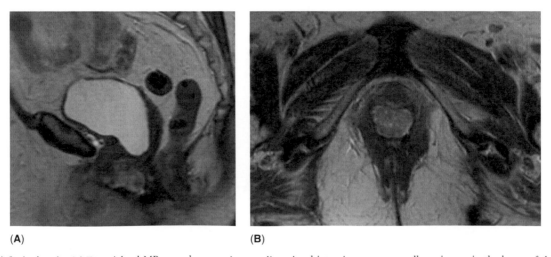

(A)   (B)

Figure 36 (**A, B**) Sagittal and axial T2-weighted MR scan shows an intermediate signal intensity squamous cell carcinoma in the lower of the vagina almost extending into the introitus.

VULVAL CANCER

Vulval carcinoma is a disease predominantly affecting older women. Early staging is related to the local extent of disease, which is readily evaluated by clinical examination (Table 6). Invasion of local structures is best assessed by MRI, as is inguinal and pelvic lymph node spread.

Ultrasound

There are some reports of the use of high-resolution ultrasound in the estimation of depth of invasion; however, this is operator dependent and not always clinically acceptable to patients. Ultrasound may be used for detection of inguinal and some iliac lymph nodes but views may be obscured by overlying bowel gas. Ultrasound-guided biopsy of lymph nodes, which are suspicious for invasion is possible with the drawback of false negative studies. This is because tumor does not uniformly infiltrate nodes with a resultant risk of sampling error.

Computer Tomography

The main role of CT is to identify distant metastases and record disease response to therapy. Standard contrast enhanced axial sequences are used. Combined CT and PET is still being evaluated but a role is anticipated in the more accurate staging of disease in patients for whom radical vulvectomy is planned.

Alternative functional imaging with sentinel lymphography is also under evaluation at present, potentially offering another means of staging.

MRI is increasingly being used to delineate the exact disease extent, depth of invasion, and involvement of adjacent structures, especially urethra and rectum (Fig. 37). The spatial resolution makes it impossible to accurately delineate stage IA disease but tumor can usually be identified when stromal invasion exceeds 2 to 3 mm. MRI has also been successfully used

Table 5 Vaginal Cancer-FIGO Staging

Stage 0	Carcinoma in situ
Stage I	Invasive carcinoma confined to the vagina
Stage IA	Tumor is <2 cm wide and <1 mm depth of invasion
Stage IB	Tumor is >2 cm wide and >1 mm depth of invasion
Stage II	Tumor invades para-vaginal tissues but not to the pelvic wall
Stage III	Extension to the pelvic wall
Stage IVA	Extension beyond the true pelvis or invasion of bladder or rectum
Stage IVB	Pelvic or inguinal lymphadenopathy or distant metastases

Table 6 Vulval Carcinoma Staging

Stage I	Tumor confined to the vulva
Stage IA	≤2 cm in size, confined to vulva or perineum, stromal invasion ≤1.0 mm negative nodes
Stage IB	>2 cm in size or stromal invasion >1.0 mm, confined to vulva or perineum, negative nodes
Stage II	Tumor of any size with extension to adjacent perineal structures (1/3 lower urethra, 1/3 lower vagina, anus) negative nodes
Stage III	Tumor of any size with or without extension to adjacent perineal structures (1/3 lower urethra, 1/3 lower vagina, anus) positive inguino-femoral lymph nodes
Stage IIIA	(i) With one lymph node metastasis (≥5 mm) (ii) One to two lymph node metastasis(es) (<5 mm)
Stage IIIB	(i) With two or more lymph node metastases (≥5 mm), or (ii) Three or more lymph node metastases (<5 mm)
Stage IIIC	With positive nodes with extracapsular spread
Stage IV	Tumor invades other regional (2/3 upper urethra, 2/3 upper vagina), or distant structures
Stage IVA	Tumor invades any of the following: (i) upper urethral and/or vaginal mucosa, bladder mucosa, rectal mucosa, or fixed to pelvic bone, or (ii) fixed or ulcerated inguino-femoral lymph nodes
Stage IVB	Any distant metastasis including pelvic lymph nodes

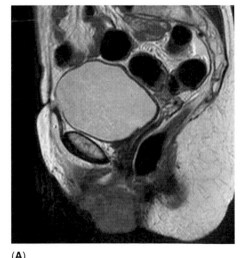 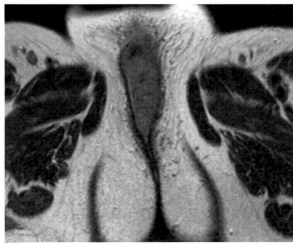

(A)   (B)

Figure 37 (**A, B**) Sagittal and T2-weighted MR scan shows a large vulval tumor expanding into the introitus and involving the clitoris. The tumor is seen clear of the lower part of the urethera.

for the identification of lymph node metastases, although the recognized size criteria are not always reliable in small volume disease. Work with USPIO MR contrast agents has demonstrated some improvements in sensitivity and specificity but they are not universally used.

ACKNOWLEDGMENT
We would like to acknowledge Dr. T. Barwick for providing the PET-CT images for the chapter.

REFERENCES
Ascher SM, Reinhold C (2002) Imaging of the endometrium. *Radiol Clin N Am* **40**:563–76.
Cabrita S, Rodrigues H, Abreu R, et al. (2008) Magnetic resonance imaging in pre-operative assessment of endometrial carcinoma. *Eur J Gynaecol Oncol* **29**(2):135–7.
Charlotte SW, Andy C, Linda C, et al. (2009) Diffusion weighted MR imaging of female pelvic tumours: a pictorial review. *Radiographics* **29**:759–74.
Chung HH, Park NH, Kim JW, et al. (2009) Role of integrated PET-CT in pelvic lymph node staging of cervical cancer before radical hysterectomy. *Gynecol Obstet Invest* **67**(1):61–6.
Fujii S, Matsusue E, Kigawa J, et al. (2008) Diagnostic accuracy of apparent coefficient diffusion in differentiating from benign from malignant uterine endometrial cavity lesions-initial results. *Eur Rad* **18**(2):384–9.
Hricak H, Rubenstein LV, Gherman GM, et al. (1991) MR imaging evaluation of endometrial carcinoma: results of NCI co-operative study. *Radiology* **179**:829–32.
Jacobs I, Oram D, Fairbanks J, et al. (1990) A risk of malignancy index incorporating Ca-125, ultrasound and menopause status for accurate pre-operative diagnosis of the ovarian cancer. *Br J Obstet Gynaecol* **97**:922–9.
Kanat-Pektas M, Gungor T, Mullamahmoutoglu L (2008) The evaluation of endometrial tumours by transvaginal and Doppler ultrasonography. *Arch Gynecol Obstet* **277**(6):695–9.
Kim SH, Kim HD, Song YS, et al. (1995) Detection of deep myometrial invasion in endometrial carcinoma: comparison of transvaginal ultrasound, CT and MR. *J Comput Assist Tomogr* **19**:766–72.
Kitajima K, Murakami K, Yamasaki E, et al. (2009) Accuracy of integrated FDG PET/contrast enhanced in detecting pelvic and para-aortic lymph node metastases in patients with uterine cancer. *Eur Radiol* **19**(6):1529–36.
Levine D, Gosink B, Johnson L (1995) Change in endometrial thickness in post-menopausal women undergoing hormone replacement therapy. *Radiology* **197**:603–8.
Menon U, Gentry-Maharaj A, Hallett R, et al. (2009) Sensitivity and specificity of multimodal and ultrasound screening for ovarian cancer, and stage distribution of detected cancers: results of the prevalence screen of the UK Collaborative Trial of Ovarian Cancer Screening (UKCTOCS). *Lancet Oncol* **10**:327–40L.
National Cancer Institute. www.cancer.gov.
Ortashi O, Jain S, Emmanuel O, et al. (2008) Evaluation of sensitivity, specificity, positive and negative predictive values of pre-operative magnetic resonance imaging for staging endometrial cancer. A prospective study of 100 cases at the Dorset cancer centre. *Euro J Obstet Gynecol Reprod Biol* **137**(2):232–5.
Pecorelli S (2009) Revised FIGO staging for carcinoma of the vulva, cervix, and endometrium. *Int J Gynecol Obstet* **105**(2):103–4.
Rockall AG, Gosh S, Babar S, et al. (2006) Can MRI rule out bladder and rectal invasion in cervical cancer to help select patients for limited EUA? *Gynaecol Oncol* **101**(2):244–9.
Rockall AG, Sohaib SA, Harisinghani MG, et al. (2005) Diagnostic performance of nano-particle enhanced magnetic resonance imaging in diagnosis of lymph nodes metastases in patients with endometrial and cervical cancer. *J Clin Oncol* **23**(12):2813–21.
Walsh JW, Jones CM III (1992) Diagnostic imaging techniques in gynaecologic oncology. In: Hoskins WJ, Perez CA, Young RC, eds. *Gynaecological Oncology: Principles and Practice*. Philadelphia: JB Lippincott, pp. 443–63.
Yang WT, Walkden SB, Ho S, et al. (1996) Transrectal ultrasound in evaluation of cervical carcinoma and comparison with computed tomography and magnetic resonance imaging. *Br J Radiol* **69**:610–16.

6 Sigmoidoscopy, cystoscopy and stenting
Louis J. Vitone, Peter A. Davis, and David J. Corless

PROCTOSCOPY, RIGID AND FLEXIBLE SIGMOIDOSCOPY
Indications

Proctoscopy and sigmoidoscopy form part of the routine examination of patients who present with lower gastrointestinal symptoms and should always be preceded by a digital rectal examination (DRE). DRE is an invaluable part of the clinical examination which may identify rectal tumors in the lower and middle rectum, and may identify pelvic masses in both males and females. It also provides independent clinical assessment relating to the presence of blood, melena, mucus, or pus in the rectum.

Patients presenting with rectal bleeding or a change in bowel habit should undergo either a DRE with rigid sigmoidoscopy followed by (i) barium enema and flexible sigmoidoscopy, or (ii) CT colonography and flexible sigmoidoscopy, or (iii) a colonoscopy. The choice of investigation(s) is not only dependent on a patient's clinical requirement but also often dictated by available resources and physician/radiologist expertise. In addition, patients presenting with vulvar carcinoma extending to the perineum should have an ano-rectal assessment. Rigid sigmoidoscopy can be used to assess the distal sigmoid colon and rectum and is useful in the conservative decompression of a sigmoid volvulus. Similarly, flexible sigmoidoscopy can confirm lesions from the proximal descending colon to the rectum, to obtain tissue biopsy, and in the follow-up of patients who have undergone colonic resections. Sigmoidoscopy remains an important adjunct in the assessment of complex gynecological or pelvic disease and in excluding rectal involvement. Proctoscopy is particularly useful in assessing the anal canal and lower rectum, and has a major diagnostic and therapeutic role in the outpatient assessment of hemorrhoids.

In the United Kingdom, physicians performing lower gastrointestinal endoscopy should be familiar with the British Society of Gastroenterology guidelines available for download (http://www.bsg.org.uk/clinical-guidelines/endoscopy/index.html) and must undergo the appropriate training in accordance with the Joint Advisory Group on Gastrointestinal Endoscopy (http://www.thejag.org.uk/) available through the National Endoscopy Training Program (http://www.jets.nhs.uk/). In the United States and Britain, gynecologic oncologists often perform these procedures in the OR as part of an examination under anesthesia to evaluate pelvic disorders.

Preoperative Preparation

Proctoscopy and rigid sigmoidoscopy can be performed in the outpatient department without any special preparation. Bowel preparation in most instances is unnecessary but, in some cases, feces in the rectum may limit views and the advancement of the proctoscope or rigid sigmoidoscope. In these cases, either a glycerin suppository or a phosphate enema can be used prior to the examination. Flexible sigmoidoscopy is usually carried out in the endoscopy suite with or without sedation. Adequate bowel preparation of the left colon and rectum is usually provided by a regimen of clear fluids for 24 hours and either a phosphate enema or, less commonly, one to two sachets of a purgative such as sodium picosulfate taken the previous day.

Instrumentation
Proctoscopy

The proctoscope (Fig. 1) has an internal obturator aiding insertion with an adjacent light source. There is no requirement to insufflate the rectum with air. After adequate lubrication, it is inserted into the rectum with the obturator in place, until the sphincter resistance is overcome, after which the obturator is removed. The lower rectal mucosa is visualized on slowly withdrawing the proctoscope with attention to the hemorrhoidal cushions, dentate line, and anal epithelium. It is helpful to the physician if the patient is asked to "bear down" as this may help demonstrate prolapsing mucosa and hemorrhoids, the latter can be banded or injected with a sclerosant.

Rigid Sigmoidoscope

The rigid sigmoidoscope (Fig. 1) is approximately 25-cm long with a 19-mm internal diameter and an internal obturator to aid insertion. It has a detachable eyepiece, which allows instruments to be passed along the shaft, and a circumferential light source. Bellows attached to the distal end are used to insufflate the rectum with air. Newer instruments are disposable, being made of self-lubricating plastic when run under water. Useful appendages are a punch biopsy, grasping forceps, and suction tubing.

Flexible Sigmoidoscope

The flexible sigmoidoscope (Fig. 2) is 70 to 110 cm long and consists of a control head with eyepiece and controls, a multi-channel flexible shaft, and a controllable tip. The flexible shaft contains fiberoptic channels carrying the optics and light source to the visual field, as well as channels for suction, irrigation, and insufflation of the colon, and the passage of instruments such as biopsy forceps. Movement of the tip in two planes is produced by pulling wires operated at the control head. The eyepiece can be attached to a video camera and the image viewed on a monitor. The "stack system" is shown in Figure 3. Immediately after use, instruments should be washed in fresh disinfectant in accordance with the manufacturers' instructions.

Operative Procedure
Rigid Sigmoidoscope

Rigid sigmoidoscopy can be performed with relative ease in the outpatient clinic. Patients are usually placed in the left

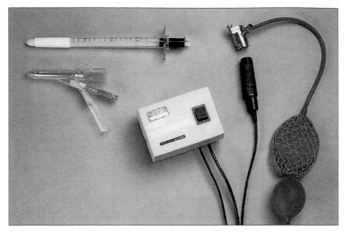

Figure 1 Proctoscope and rigid sigmoidoscope.

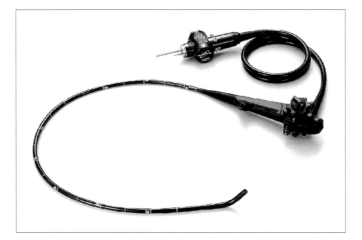

Figure 2 Flexible sigmoidoscope or colonoscope.

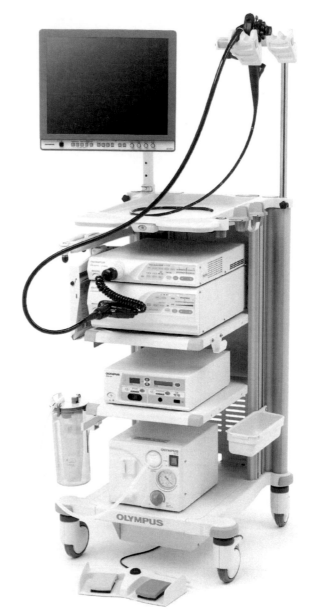

Figure 3 A stack system with high definition video monitor and recorder, light source, video processor, insufflators, and flexible sigmoidoscopy.

lateral (Sims) position with hips and knees flexed and parallel on a couch or bed. The buttocks should ideally overhang the edge of the couch marginally thus providing better maneuverability of the sigmoidoscope. The more transverse the patient is positioned, the easier the examination will be. The prone knee-elbow or jack-knife position where the patient lays prone in an inverted position is a less commonly used alternative position. A DRE of the rectum should be performed prior to the sigmoidoscopy.

The light source should always be checked prior to the patient assuming position by connecting to an appropriate power source. The obturator of the sigmoidoscope should be removed prior to connecting the bellows' tubing with intervening disposable air filter to the sigmoidoscope. The eyepiece window can then be opened and the obturator passed through until the obturator tip protrudes from the sigmoidoscope tip. The sigmoidoscope is held in the right hand with the left hand holding the buttocks for insertion. An assistant may be required to help with buttock retraction. The instrument is lubricated with a water based lubricant and inserted into the anal canal, pointing toward the umbilicus with the obturator in place. When the instrument is felt to enter the rectum it is directed posteriorly and the obturator removed and the eyepiece window closed. Using the bellows the rectum is gently insufflated with air which allows the sigmoidoscope to be

advanced while visualizing the whole circumference of the lumen. As the sigmoidoscope is passed through the rectum at 4 cm from the anus, the rectum angulates posteriorly over the sling formed by puborectalis and into the hollow of the sacrum (Fig. 4). At this point the sigmoidoscope should be gently directed from the anterior to posterior position. Inspection of the whole mucosa can be achieved by rotating the instrument. Slight angulation of the sigmoidoscope laterally is required to negotiate the rectal valves. At approximately 12 cm from the anal verge, the sacral promontory produces a sharp anterior angulation of the rectum. At this point the sigmoidoscope should be directed antero-superiorly.

Negotiation of the instrument at the rectosigmoid junction should be carried out with care; it can be achieved using gentle insufflation and manipulation in order to find the lumen of the sigmoid colon. The best views are often obtained while withdrawing the sigmoidoscope and inspection of the mucosa with particular care around the horizontal rectal folds.

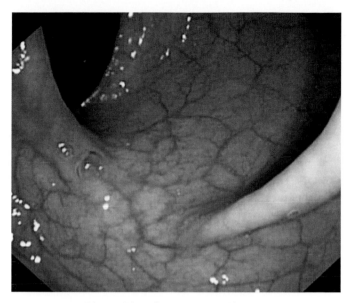

Figure 4 View of rectum at sigmoidoscopy.

Withdrawal assumes reversal of the aforementioned maneuvers. If the patient experiences pain at any point during the procedure, then the scope should be withdrawn and consideration given to termination of the examination. Documentation of the position reached should be made in centimetres from the anal verge. The patient's peri-anal region should be cleansed and the patient returned to a more comfortable position.

Rectal Biopsy

The sigmoidoscope is manipulated so that the lesion is at the tip of the instrument. The glass eyepiece is removed; although this causes deflation of the rectum, the lesion should still be in view. Punch biopsy forceps are passed along the sigmoidoscope and the biopsy is taken under direct vision. The jaws of the biopsy forceps are closed around the lesion and removal is aided by rotation of the closed forceps. Excessive bleeding at the site of the biopsy can easily be controlled with pressure from a cotton–wool swab or occasionally injection of 1 in 1000 adrenaline (epinephrine). Great caution should be taken if considering biopsy 8 cm or more proximal to the anal verge (level of peritoneal reflection) as the risk of perforation of flat lesions is significant with long, cumbersome biopsy forceps.

Polypectomy

Polyps with a long stalk can be removed using a diathermy snare technique through the rigid sigmoidoscope. The polyp is grasped with polyp-holding forceps which have been passed through the loop of a diathermy snare. The snare is then passed over the polyp and closure of the snare during application of diathermy coagulates the stalk. The polyp is then removed by the forceps and the excision site inspected for bleeding. It is important to avoid excessive traction on the forceps since this may result in removal of excess normal mucosa and hence perforation.

Flexible Sigmoidoscope

Patients are placed in the left lateral position on a couch or bed and a DRE is performed. Intravenous sedation and oxygen may be administered via a face mask or nasal prongs and a pulse oximeter attached to the patient. The tip of the sigmoidoscope is lubricated and inserted into the anal canal for a distance of 4 to 5 cm. Initially inspection usually reveals a red blur as the tip of the sigmoidoscope rests against the rectal mucosa. The rectum is gently inflated and the tip position adjusted and withdrawn until the lumen comes into view. It may be necessary to adjust the focus, wash the lens and suck out any residual fluid or feces to optimize the image. With gentle insufflation and guidance of the tip, the sigmoidoscope is advanced through the lumen and the rectosigmoid junction negotiated under direct vision. If the lumen or movement across the mucosa is not seen, then the sigmoidoscope should be withdrawn until the lumen once again comes into view. Looping of the sigmoidoscope prevents advancement and in such cases the instrument should also be withdrawn. In most patients, a combination of manipulation of the tip and twisting of the shaft (torque steering) should make it possible to examine the whole left colon. The best views are once again seen on slow withdrawal of the sigmoidoscope, keeping the lumen in view all the way and aspirating as much air as possible. Biopsy can also be performed on withdrawal. The lesion is cleaned by injecting water down the irrigation channel and biopsy forceps are passed through the instrument port. The biopsy is taken under direct vision, the closure usually performed by an assistant who then removes the forceps while the operator directs the sigmoidoscope and the position of the biopsy. Lesions that macroscopically represent a cancer can be biopsied and marked adjacently with indigo blue dye. This is a helpful adjunct in identifying the tumor and determining resection margins during surgery. However, the latter can be left to a later date as colonoscopic examination is recommended pre-operatively to exclude synchronous colonic lesions. The incidence of perforation with a flexible sigmoidoscope is extremely low, but if the patient complains of excessive pain or discomfort then the examination should cease.

Postoperative Care

No special postoperative care is necessary after routine sigmoidoscopy. After a polypectomy or biopsy the patient should be observed for signs of excessive bleeding or perforation. Barium enema or CT colonography should not be performed for 10 days after biopsy because of the risk of extravasation of contrast. Patients who have been sedated require postoperative monitoring in a designated recovery area.

CYSTOSCOPY AND STENTING
Indications

Cystoscopy is the single most common urological procedure and is used in the investigation of urinary symptoms. Patients who present with urological symptoms such as frequency, dysuria, and hematuria undergo cystoscopy for the diagnosis of lesions of the urethra and bladder. In addition, cystoscopy may be performed by gynecologic oncologists as part of the International Federation of Gynecology and Obstetrics preoperative staging for cervical carcinoma or where it is suspected that tumors may involve the bladder and urethra. It can also be used to perform retrograde ureterography to provide X-ray visualization of the ureter and collecting system and the placement of retrograde ureteric stents. Stents provide ureteric drainage and can also be used to identify the position of the ureter. Where retrograde stenting proves impossible the interventional radiologist may well be able to pass antegrade stents or, failing this, to insert bilateral nephrostomy tubes.

Preoperative Preparation

Rigid cystoscopy is carried out under general anesthesia or i.v. sedation in the operating theater or properly equipped outpatient facility with the patient in the lithotomy position. It is important to rule out severe osteoarthritis of the hips which may make examination impossible. Antibiotic prophylaxis is given if there is any evidence or suspicion of a urinary tract infection. Flexible cystoscopy is usually carried out in the endoscopy suite under local anesthesia. Lignocaine (lidocaine) gel inserted into the urethra acts as both lubricant and local anesthetic agent. If possible, the patient should void prior to examination to ensure the bladder is empty.

Instrumentation

Rigid Cystoscope

The rigid cystoscope (Fig. 5) is composed of a sheath, a bridge, and a telescope: It is 30-cm long. The sheath has both an inlet and an outlet port for irrigation and is attached to the bridge with a watertight lock. The endoscope is introduced into the sheath through the bridge, and is also fitted with a watertight lock. The telescope comprises a hollow metal cylinder containing a series of solid rod lenses and a magnifying eyepiece. In front of the eyepiece is a pillar connected to a fiberoptic light source which transmits light to the visual field. The bridge has one or two other ports for the introduction of biopsy forceps and electrodes, and a director which allows the passage of a ureteric catheter and its advancement into the ureteric orifice. Endoscopes with viewing angles of 0°, 30°, 70°, and 90° are available.

Flexible Cystoscope

The flexible cystoscope (Fig. 6) is 35 to 40 cm long and consists of a control head with eyepiece and controls, a multichannel flexible shaft, and a controllable tip. The flexible shaft contains fiberoptic channels carrying the optics and light source to the visual field, an irrigation channel, and a biopsy channel. Movement of the tip occurs in one plane and ranges from 145° to 180°, controlled by a deflecting level adjacent to the eyepiece.

Operative Procedure

Rigid Cystoscope

The patient is placed on the operating table in the lithotomy position. The cystoscope sheath is lubricated and introduced into the urethra. The female urethra is about 4 cm long and has a relatively uniform caliber from the meatus to the bladder outlet. Upon entering the bladder the telescope is removed to allow the residual urine and irrigant to drain from the bladder: this may be sent for cytological and bacteriological analysis. Approximately 50 ml of saline is inserted and the fundus of the bladder is identified by finding the air bubble. With incomplete distension the bladder mucosa appears rugated, but as the irrigant fluid distends the bladder the mucosa becomes smooth. The ureteric orifices are visualized on the inter-ureteric ridge at the superolateral corners of the trigone (Fig. 7). By regular sweeping of the cystoscope backward and forward and

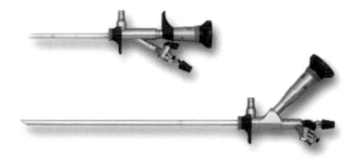

Figure 5 Rigid cystoscope.

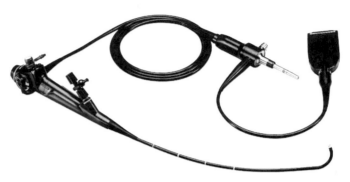

Figure 6 Flexible cystoscope.

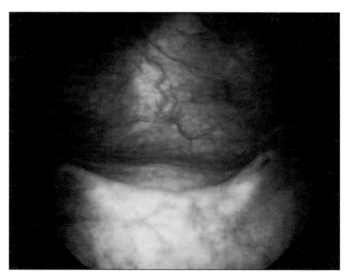

Figure 7 Ureteric orifices.

rotation of the endoscope the entire bladder mucosa can be visualized. Views of the anteroinferior bladder are obtained by suprapubic compression with the hand. At the completion of the examination, the irrigating fluid is evacuated from the bladder by removing the telescope and the instrument is slowly withdrawn. A bimanual examination of the pelvis is performed after the procedure.

Bladder Biopsy

Bladder biopsy (Fig. 8) is the procedure most commonly performed during cystoscopy. Biopsy forceps are introduced down the cystoscope sheath via a port in the bridge, sometimes together with a diathermy wire. This allows cup biopsies of the mucosa to be taken. If required, the biopsy sites are then cauterized with diathermy to prevent excessive bleeding.

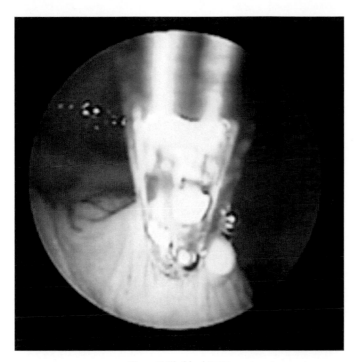

Figure 8 Bladder biopsy.

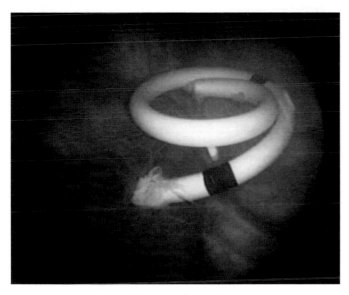

Figure 9 Distal end of a double J stent.

Ureteric Catheterization and Stenting

The instrumentation and stenting of ureters should only be performed by clinicians such as urologists or gynecologic oncologists since it is easy to damage the ureteric orifices and ureters. Ureteric catheterization and the placement of double J stents are achieved with the 30° telescope. There is a special port for the introduction of the stents which can be directed toward the ureteric orifices. A floppy-tipped, Teflon-coated guide wire is first placed into the ureteric orifice and advanced under fluoroscopic control into the renal pelvis. The double J stent is slid over the guide wire through the channel of the cystoscope and into the ureter (Fig. 9). The stent is radio-opaque and its position is monitored by fluoroscopic control. Excessive force used in insertion of the guide wire or stent should be avoided. The proximal and distal ends curl to form a J shape when they are correctly placed in the renal pelvis and bladder, respectively.

Flexible Cystoscope

The patient is placed on the operating table or bed in the "frog-leg" position. The cystoscope is lubricated and introduced into the urethra. The end of the cystoscope is passed into the bladder and deflected upward. The midline of the anterior bladder is examined by withdrawing the instrument until the bladder outlet is encountered. The cystoscope is then pushed back into the bladder, rotated 30° and withdrawn again. This process is continued until the entire bladder has been inspected. Biopsy of the bladder mucosa can also be achieved by the passage of biopsy forceps down the instrumental channel of the cystoscope.

Postoperative Care

No special postoperative measures are needed. Patients should be given general precautions including the recognition of early signs and symptoms of an infection.

ACKNOWLEDGMENTS

Daniel Wallaker and Hayley Kellett of Olympus Medical, UK, for their assistance in providing some of the images included in this chapter and Dr Laura Wilson, F2 General Surgery, Leighton Hospital, UK, for proofreading the manuscript.

BIBLIOGRAPHY

Calne RY, Pollard SG (1992) *Operative Surgery*. London: Gower.

Carter DC, Russell RCG, Pitt HA (1996) *Atlas of General Surgery*, 3rd edn. London: Chapman & Hall.

Corman ML (2005) *Colon and Rectal Surgery*, Philadelphia, Pennsylvania: Lippincott, Williams & Wilkins.

Cotton PB, Williams CB (2003) *Practical Gastrointestinal Endoscopy*, 5th edn. Oxford: Blackwell.

Jackson E, Fowler JR (1992) *Urologic Surgery*. Mastery of Surgery Series. New York: Little, Brown.

Reuter HJ (1987) *Atlas of Urological Endoscopy: Diagnosis and Treatment*. New York: Thieme.

7 Tumor markers
Ranjit Manchanda, Ian Jacobs, and Usha Menon

INTRODUCTION

A tumor marker is defined as a molecule or substance produced by or in response to neoplastic proliferation, which enters the circulation in detectable amounts. It indicates the likely presence of cancer or provides information about its behavior. Since the description of Bence-Jones proteins well over a century ago, a variety of substances have been investigated as potential tumor markers and advances in molecular biology and technology continually add to this list.

Tumor markers can be broadly classified into tumor-specific antigens and tumor-associated antigens. Two examples of strictly tumor specific antigens are the idiotypes of immunoglobulins of B cell tumors and certain neo-antigens of virus induced tumors. The vast majority of tumor markers are in reality tumor-associated antigens. In many cases, they are initially described as highly tumor specific with subsequent studies uncovering their presence in multiple cancers and in normal adult or fetal tissues. On the basis of size, tumor-associated antigens can be divided into low-molecular weight tumor markers (~<1000 Da) and macromolecular tumor antigens (Suresh 1996). It is the macromolecular tumor markers that form the largest sub group and have been most useful in the clinical management of cancer.

A marker's performance depends on its sensitivity (proportion of cancers detected by a positive test) and specificity (proportion of those without cancer identified by a negative test). An ideal tumor marker should have a 100% sensitivity, specificity, and positive predictive value (PPV). However, in practice such a marker does not exist. As the majority of markers are tumor associated rather than tumor specific, and are elevated in multiple cancers, benign and physiological conditions, they lack specificity. Additionally, varying sensitivity means that a normal result may not exclude malignancy. Hence, in most diseases, tumor markers contribute to differential diagnosis but are not themselves diagnostic. They may also have an important role to play in screening, surveillance, predicting prognosis, and determining therapeutic efficacy.

A wide variety of macromolecular tumor antigens, including enzymes, hormones, receptors, growth factors, biological response modifiers, and glycoconjugates, have been investigated as potential tumor markers. Despite significant research the number of clinically useful markers is limited. Two important reasons include poor study design and a lack of standardized methodologies. To overcome significant past reporting deficiencies in published literature, reporting recommendations for tumor marker prognostic studies (REMARK) have recently been proposed (McShane et al. 2005), and five phases for biomarker development have been suggested (Pepe et al. 2001). General guidelines on the application and use of tumor markers have been developed by a number of multidisciplinary groups following critical appraisal of available evidence (Duffy et al. 2005, Screening for ovarian cancer: recommendations and rationale 1994, Vasey et al. 2005, NIH consensus conference 1995) and are summarized elsewhere (Sturgeon et al. 2008). However, meta-analyses of tumor markers (such as Cochrane reviews) are lacking. The focus of this chapter is largely limited to tumor markers that are detectable in the blood and are clinically relevant to female genital tract malignancies.

OVARIAN AND FALLOPIAN TUBE CANCER

Women have approximately a 1% to 2% life time risk for developing ovarian cancer (OC) and it represents 4% of total incident cancers in women. Epithelial ovarian cancer (EOC) accounts for around 80% to 85% of all OC. These may be serous, mucinous, endometrioid, clear cell, transitional, and undifferentiated. Traditionally serous tumors are the commonest, present at advanced stages and have the poorest outcomes (Seidman et al. 2004). However, in the reproductive age group germ cell tumors, granulosa cell/sex-cord tumors, mucinous and endometrioid tumors are more common. Only a few tumor markers have been validated for clinical use with the best known among them being cancer antigen 125 (CA125).

Biochemical Markers in Ovarian Cancer
CA125

CA125 was first described by Bast in 1981. It is a 200 kD glycoprotein recognized by the OC125 murine monoclonal antibody (Bast et al. 1981). The CA125 structure includes two major antigenic domains: domain A (binds monoclonal antibody OC125) and domain B (binds monoclonal antibody M11) (Nustad et al. 1996). The present second-generation heterologous CA125-II assay incorporates M11 and OC125 antibodies, while the original homologous assay was with OC125 alone. A number of CA125 assays which correlate well with each other are currently in clinical use (Davelaar et al. 1998).

CA125 is widely distributed in adult tissues and lacks specificity for OC. A routinely used cut-off value of 35 kU/L is based upon the distribution of values in 99% of 888 healthy men and women (Bast et al. 1983). However, CA125 values can show wide variation, with lower levels (20 U/ml) found in postmenopausal women (Bon et al. 1996, Zurawski et al. 1988, Alagoz et al. 1994, Bonfrer et al. 1997b). Levels are raised in pregnancy with peak values occurring in the first trimester (112 kU/L, 65 kU/L correspond to 99th and the 96th centile, respectively) (El-Shawarby et al. 2005, Sarandakou et al. 2007) and postpartum (Gocze et al. 1988, Jacobs and Bast 1989, Fiegler et al. 2005, Spitzer et al. 1998, Takahashi et al. 1985, Urbancsek et al. 2005) and returning to normal by 10 weeks after delivery (Spitzer et al. 1998). Menstruation (Jacobs and Bast 1989, Grove et al. 1992) as well as benign gynecological conditions (pelvic inflammatory disease, fibroids, and endometriosis) increase CA125. Higher values are reported for Caucasian compared to African or Asian women (Pauler et al. 2001). Caffeine intake, hysterectomy, and smoking in some (Pauler et al. 2001) but not all reports (Green et al. 1986, Tuxen et al. 1999) were associated with lower CA125 levels (Pauler et al. 2001). Non-gynecological conditions (tuberculosis, cirrhosis, ascites, hepatitis, pancreatitis, peritonitis, pleuritis) and other cancers (breast, pancreas, lung, and colon cancer) can also cause an elevated CA125.

Raised levels were found in 25% of 59 stored serum samples collected five years before OC diagnosis (Zurawski et al. 1988), suggesting that CA125 is elevated in preclinical disease. An elevated CA125 (>35 U/ml) has been found in 85% of EOC (Bast et al. 1983, Canney et al. 1984): 50% stage I and >90% stage II to IV cancer (Jacobs and Bast 1989). CA125 levels are more frequently elevated in serous cancers as compared to mucinous/borderline tumors (Jacobs and Bast 1989, Tamakoshi et al. 1996, Vergote et al. 1987).

Role of CA125 in Screening

CA125 is currently being investigated as a screening tool in a number of clinical trials. Though on its own serum CA125 has low specificity, elevated CA125 on primary screening assessed with repeat CA125 and transvaginal ultrasound (TVS) (multimodal screening) can increase specificity to 99.9% and is associated with four operations for each OC detected (Jacobs et al. 1993, 1999). Ovarian morphology has been used to refine algorithms for interpreting TVS in postmenopausal women with elevated CA125 (Menon et al. 1999, 2000). Over the last decade, CA125 interpretation in the context of screening has been further improved by a more sophisticated approach incorporating age, menopausal status, and the rate of change of CA125 values over time (Menon et al. 2005, Skates et al. 1995, 2003). This computerized algorithm called the Risk of Ovarian Cancer Algorithm (ROCA) increases CA125 sensitivity by correctly identifying women with normal but rising levels as increased risk, and improves specificity by classifying women with static but elevated levels as low risk. For a target specificity of 98%, the ROCA achieved 86% sensitivity for detecting preclinical EOC (Skates et al. 2003). This approach is part of the UK Collaborative Trial of Ovarian Cancer Screening (UKCTOCS) in the general population (Menon et al. 2009) and the U.S. Cancer Genetics Network (CGN) pilot trial and the UK Familial Ovarian Cancer Screening Study (UKFOCSS) of high-risk women.

A randomized controlled trial (RCT) in 21,935 women provided preliminary evidence of improved survival with screening, with a median survival of 72.9 months found in screened and 41.8 months in control arms (Jacobs et al. 1999). Subsequently, a number of prospective trials have used CA125 alone or in combination with ultrasound to screen for OC. A detailed review of these studies has been published elsewhere (Rosenthal and Jacobs 2006, Rosenthal et al. 2006). In the Japanese Shizuoka Cohort Study of Ovarian Cancer Screening (SCSOCS) (82,487 low-risk postmenopausal women), the proportion of stage I OC was higher in the screened group (63%) than in the control group (38%) but did not reach statistical significance (Kobayashi et al. 2007). Two large RCTs in low-risk postmenopausal women are currently evaluating the mortality impact of OC screening. These are expected to report in 2015. (A) UKCTOCS: 202,638 postmenopausal women randomized in a 1:1:2 ratio to annual screening with CA125 using ROCA (multimodal screening), screening with TVS and control groups. Screening is expected to continue till 2011 and follow-up till 2014. Recently reported prevalence screen results found sensitivity and PPV for primary ovarian and tubal cancers to be 89.4% and 43.3% for multimodal screening and 84.9% and 5.3% for ultrasound screening. When the analysis was restricted to primary invasive epithelial ovarian and tubal cancers, the sensitivity and PPV were 89.5% and 35.1% for multimodal and 75.0% and 2.8% for ultrasound arms, respectively. Of the overall screen detected invasive EOC, 48% were stage I/II (Menon et al. 2009). (B) Prostate Lung Colorectal and Ovarian Cancer Screening Trial (PLCO): 78,000 women randomized to annual screening with TVS and CA125 (interpreted using a cut-off of ≥35 U/ml) or control groups. Recently reported results from the first four rounds of screening 34,261 postmenopausal women reported 89 invasive ovarian/peritoneal cancers, of which 60 were screen detected. Only 28% of screen-detected cases were stage I/II. The overall ratio of surgeries per screen-detected cancers was 19.5:1, having decreased over the years from 34% in the first year of screening to 15% to 20% in subsequent years (Partridge et al. 2009).

The sensitivity and effectiveness of screening in women at high risk for familial OC is still not established (Jacobs 2005). In addition, primary peritoneal cancer is a phenotypic variant of familial OC and both CA125 and ultrasound are not reliable in detecting early-stage disease (Karlan et al. 1999). Annual screening with CA125 and TVS has not been found to be effective for early stage disease (Hermsen et al. 2007). However, a recent re-analysis of earlier published data showed preliminary evidence of a change in stage distribution between prevalence and incident screen detected cancers in high-risk women undergoing annual screening (Manchanda et al. 2009). More frequent three-to-four monthly screening using the ROCA for CA125 interpretation is being evaluated in Phase 2 of the UKFOCSS as well as the CGN and Gynecological Oncology Group (GOG) (Greene et al. 2008) trials in the United States. In the CGN trial five OCs (following 38 surgeries) were detected in 2343 high-risk women undergoing three monthly screening. Two of these were prevalent screen (one early, one late stage) and three (all early stage) were incident screen detected cancers (Skates et al. 2007).

Though screening can detect asymptomatic early-stage disease (Kobayashi et al. 2007), and there is preliminary evidence of a survival benefit (Jacobs et al. 1999), the mortality impact of OC screening or the proportion of early cancers that will be detected is not yet known.

It is yet to be established whether screening will detect a significant number of early-stage high-grade serous carcinomas or be limited to better prognostic low-grade type-1 cancers. As screening is not yet proven to have clinical benefit, the current recommendation is that it should only be carried out within the context of a clinical trial.

Role of CA125 in Differential Diagnosis

Accurate discrimination between benign and malignant adnexal masses permits women with benign lesions to be managed conservatively or operated by general gynecologists while ensuring women with cancer are triaged to cancer centers for management by multidisciplinary teams and surgery by gynecological oncologists. CA125 alone has a pooled sensitivity and specificity of 78% for differentiating benign from malignant adnexal masses (Myers et al. 2006), with higher values achieved in postmenopausal women.

A variety of modalities have been used to improve CA125 performance. The "Risk of Malignancy Index" (RMI), a product of serum CA125 with an ultrasound-based ovarian morphology score (U) and menopausal status (M) (Jacobs et al. 1990), achieved a sensitivity of 85%, specificity of 97% (Jacobs et al. 1990). It has been validated in numerous prospective and retrospective studies (Andersen et al. 2003, Aslam et al. 2000, Bailey et al. 2006, Davies et al. 1993, Ma et al. 2003, Manjunath et al. 2001, Morgante et al. 1999, Tingulstad et al. 1996, Ulusoy et al. 2007). RMI sensitivity can be improved by increasing the RMI cut-off (Bailey et al. 2006, Davies et al. 1993, Ma et al. 2003), using artificial neural networks (ANN) (Timmerman et al. 1999), or modifying the RMI calculation (Manjunath et al. 2001, Morgante et al. 1999). Performance has also been improved by addition of specialist US and MRI for RMI cut-off between 25 and 1000 (van Trappen et al. 2007) or using an "ovarian crescent sign" (Yazbek et al. 2006). Ultrasound-based pattern recognition models have been found to be superior to CA125 alone (Timmerman et al. 2005, 2007). However, recent analyses suggest RMI performance is comparable to most logistic regression/ANN models (Timmerman et al. 2007, Van Holsbeke et al. 2007). The use of a panel of markers to improve CA125 performance is discussed later in the chapter.

Assessment of Prognosis. Serum CA125 level is a strong prognostic factor for OC and inversely related to overall survival and progression free survival (Gupta and Lis 2009). Preoperative serum CA125 levels correlate with tumor stage, volume and grade, and cut-offs of both 30 and 65 kU/L have been reported to be independent predictors of survival in early stage (Obermair et al. 2007, Paramasivam et al. 2005, Petri et al. 2006) but not advanced disease (Petri et al. 2006, Hogdall et al. 2002). Postoperative serum CA125 level is an independent prognostic factor for survival (Gupta and Lis 2009). In addition, the rate of fall of CA125 following treatment (Canney et al. 1984, van der Burg et al. 1988, Buller et al. 1992, Peters-Engl et al. 1999, Riedinger et al. 2006), absolute values following the first, second, or third courses of chemotherapy (Lavin et al. 1987, Mogensen 1992, Redman et al. 1990, Rustin et al. 1989, Fayers et al. 1993), CA125 half-life (20 days being most commonly used), and time to normalization or slope of exponential regression curve have also been found to correlate well with survival (Gupta and Lis 2009, Verheijen et al. 1999). A minority of studies have found no (Clark et al. 2001) or limited time dependent (Peters-Engl et al. 1999) prognostic correlation with survival. The European Group on Tumor Markers recommends that CA125 levels after the third course of initial chemotherapy be used for prediction (Duffy et al. 2005).

A recent report reconfirmed CA125 as a strong independent prognostic factor for high-risk, early-stage EOC following complete response to chemotherapy (Kang et al. 2009). The CA125 half-life and nadir during induction chemotherapy are independent predictors of outcome (Riedinger et al. 2006). Pre-maintenance chemotherapy patients with baseline CA125

values ≤10 U/ml have greater progression free survival compared to those with higher levels in the normal range (Markman et al. 2006). Post-chemotherapy CA125 level is a good predictor of overall and progression free survival (Gupta and Lis 2009). Patients with normal serum CA125 levels (≤35 U/ml) at relapse (recurrence) have a better prognosis than patients with elevated levels (Makar et al. 1993).

Monitoring Response to Treatment and Detection of Recurrence. Serial serum CA125 forms part of most standard protocols for monitoring therapy (Duffy et al. 2005, Sturgeon et al. 2008). Levels correlate with clinical course of EOC (Bast et al. 1983, Hawkins et al. 1989, Tuxen et al. 2001, 2002) and may also be of benefit for some AFP and human chorionic gonadotropin (hCG) negative germ cell tumors (Patterson and Rustin 2006). However, there is lack of consensus on how to define response to treatment resulting in different definitions being proposed (Tuxen et al. 2001, Rustin et al. 1996a, 2004, Gronlund et al. 2004). It is also important to adjust statistical estimates for assay and biological variation (Tuxen et al. 2000, 2001). This also applies to other markers like tissue polypeptide antigen (TPA), carcinoembryonic antigen (CEA), CA15-3, and CA54 (Soletormos et al. 1996).

Serial CA125 measurements are being used to detect recurrent disease with recommendations to follow patients every two to four months for two years and then less frequently (Sturgeon et al. 2008). Radiological imaging was not found to provide additional benefit over CA125 and clinical examination in detecting recurrence (Fehm et al. 2005). Various CA125-based definitions for recurrence have been suggested, such as 50% or 100% increase, increase from below to above reference range and doubling of upper limit of normal level (Tuxen et al. 2001, Rustin et al. 1996b, 2001). The latter definition has been adopted by the GCIG (Gynaecological Cancer Inter Group). A time of three to four months (range 1–15 months) has been reported between CA125 increase and clinical detection of progressive disease (Tuxen et al. 2001, Rustin et al. 1996b, Cruickshank et al. 1991). However, the U.K. Medical Research Council (MRC) sponsored OV05 trial (EORTC 55955/MRC OVO5) reported no survival benefit on commencing treatment on the basis of rising CA125 levels in the absence of other indicators of disease recurrence (Rustin and van der Burg 2009).

HE4

Human epididymis protein 4 (HE4) is a glycoprotein found in epididymis epithelium. Increased serum HE4 levels and expression of HE4 (WFCD2) gene occur in OC (Drapkin et al. 2005, Grisaru et al. 2007), as well as lung, pancreas, breast, bladder, ureter transitional cell (Galgano et al. 2006), and endometrial cancers (Huhtinen et al. 2009). HE4 is not increased in endometriosis (Huhtinen et al. 2009, Montagnana et al. 2009) and has fewer false positive results with benign disease compared to CA125 (Hellstrom et al. 2003). A retrospective report (67 invasive and 166 benign masses) found HE4 to have a higher sensitivity (73%) compared to CA125 (43.3%) for 95% specificity in distinguishing between benign and malignant ovarian masses and addition of HE4 to CA125 further improved sensitivity to 76.4% (Moore et al. 2008). HE4 performed better than CA125 alone in premenopausal women as well as for stage I OC (Moore et al. 2008).

Recently a prospective study in 531 patients evaluated separate premenopausal and postmenopausal logistic regression algorithms incorporating CA125 and HE4 for the differential diagnosis of adnexal masses (Moore et al. 2009). The sensitivity and specificity in the postmenopausal group were 92.3% (95% CI, 85.9–96.4) and 75.0% (95% CI, 66.9–81.4), respectively. In premenopausal women the sensitivity and specificity were 76.5% (95% CI, 58.8–89.3) and 74.8% (95% CI, 68.2–80.6), respectively. Although HE4 has been evaluated for differential diagnosis of OC (Moore et al. 2008), its efficacy in screening is still unknown.

Carcinoembryonic Antigen (CEA)

CEA is a 180 kDa glycoprotein, initially described as a tumor marker for gastrointestinal, prostate, and lung cancers (Icard et al. 1994). As a tumor marker for OC its utility is limited by its low sensitivity (16–25%) and PPV (14–37%) (Onsrud 1991, Roman et al. 1998, Tuxen et al. 1995). However, raised levels have been reported in endometrioid, mucinous, and Brenner tumors (Soletormos et al. 1996). An added benefit is that it is not elevated in benign and inflammatory adnexal masses or pregnancy.

Osteopontin

Higher plasma osteopontin levels are reported in OC cases compared to healthy controls, benign ovarian disease, and non-gynecological cancers (Kim et al. 2002, Nakae et al. 2006). Osteopontin levels correlate with advanced stage disease, presence of ascites, bulky disease, poor prognosis metastatic disease, and recurrence (Nakae et al. 2006, Brakora et al. 2004, Bao et al. 2007), but not histologic type (Nakae et al. 2006). It may serve as an adjunct to CA125 in differential diagnosis and monitoring recurrence.

CA-19-9

CA-19-9, an antigen, is more frequently elevated in mucinous (76%) than serous (27%) OCs (Gocze et al. 1988, Terracciano et al. 2005). It is a useful tool to monitor women with cancer in pregnancy as its levels in pregnancy do not exceed the normal cut-off of 37 kU/L (Hohlfeld et al. 1994, Kobayashi et al. 1989).

It has higher sensitivity than CA125 in diagnosing borderline mucinous (Ayhan et al. 2007) and CA125 negative invasive mucinous cancers (Gadducci et al. 2004). In combination with CA125 it has been found to distinguish between good (stage IA) and poor (stage IC) prognosis early-stage disease (Muramatsu et al. 2005).

Alpha-fetoprotein (AFP)

AFP (70 kDa glycoprotein) is synthesized initially in the yolk sac and subsequently in the fetal liver and intestine (Gitlin et al. 1972). AFP is increased in pregnancy, benign liver disease, liver, gastric, pancreatic, colon, and bronchogenic malignancies. AFP accurately predicts the presence of yolk sac elements in mixed germ-cell tumors (Olt et al. 1990), and levels are increased in most endodermal sinus/yolk sac tumors, 33% to 62% immature teratomas, and 12% dysgerminoma and embryonal tumors (Lu and Gershenson 2005, Kawai et al. 1992). Data regarding benefit in prognostication are conflicting, but it is of value in monitoring treatment and detecting early relapse (Chow et al. 1996, Ayas et al. 2007).

Inhibin, Activin and Related Peptides

Inhibin is a heterodimeric glycoprotein with two isoforms: inhibin-A (αβA) and inhibin-B (αβB). The initial Monash assay detected immunoreactive inhibin, which consisted of a number of inhibin-related peptides in addition to biologically active inhibin dimers. Specific immunoassays for inhibin isoforms are now available. The pro-αC assay measures precursor forms of inhibin. Activin is a dimer of the two-beta subunits of inhibin. It has three isoforms: activin-A (βAβA), activin-B (βB βB), and activin-AB (βA βB). Serum inhibin is elevated in ovarian granulosa cell (GCT)/sex cord/stromal tumors and has a useful role in differential diagnosis and surveillance of these malignancies (Lappohn et al. 1989, Boggess et al. 1997, Cooke et al. 1995, Jobling et al. 1994, Geerts et al. 2009). GCT secret both inhibin-A and inhibin-B though the latter is more common (Petraglia et al. 1998, Yamashita et al. 1997). Inhibin is considered more reliable and superior to estradiol in monitoring and predicting recurrence in GCTs (Boggess et al. 1997, Pectasides et al. 2007, Healy et al. 1993). Müllerian inhibitory substance is an emerging new marker for GCTs, which may be more specific than inhibin-B and of value in monitoring treatment and detecting recurrence (Geerts et al. 2009). Epithelial mucinous OCs may also have increased inhibin levels (Burger et al. 1996). Inhibin in combination with CA125 was found to detect most tumor types with a sensitivity and specificity of 95% (Robertson et al. 2004). High levels of activin-A have also been reported, particularly in undifferentiated tumors (Welt et al. 1997).

Kallikreins

Kallikreins are serine proteases (Diamandis and Yousef 2002), some of which are part of an enzymatic cascade activated in ovarian and other cancers. A number of recent publications suggest kallikriens (4, 5, 6, 7, 8, 9, 10, 11, 13, 14, and 15) may have a role in detection, diagnosis, monitoring, and prognostication of OC. Biomarker panels including Kallikriens 5, 7, and 10, along with CA125 have been found to be useful predictors of response to therapy, short term (one year) survival, progression free survival and overall survival (Oikonomopoulou et al. 2008). The role of kallikreins is still evolving and requires further research.

Cytokines

A number of cytokines like M-CSF, interleukins (IL6, IL7, IL10, sIL-2R), tumor necrosis factor, and immunosuppressive acidic protein have been evaluated as potential biomarkers. M-CSF was found to have high specificity for malignant ovarian germ-cell tumors, particularly dysgerminomas (Suzuki et al. 1998). Levels correlated with stage and prognosis (Chambers et al. 1997, Price et al. 1993, Scholl et al. 1994), and used in a combination of markers, it has been found to be of benefit in early detection (Suzuki et al. 1993, 1995, Skates et al. 2004), but not in monitoring recurrence (Gadducci et al. 1998). IL-7 in combination with CA125 accurately predicts 69% of the OCs, without falsely classifying patients with benign pelvic mass (Lambeck et al. 2007). IL-6 correlates with clinical disease and survival and though of prognostic significance is not better than CA125 (Foti et al. 1999, Scambia et al. 1995). IL-10 may be a good surrogate marker for tumor grade (Mustea et al. 2009).

Cancer Associated Serum Antigen

Cancer-associated serum antigen (CASA) is elevated levels in 38% to 73% of OCs, and has slightly higher specificity but much lower sensitivity than CA125 for OC. CASA has not been found to significantly add to the discriminative value of CA125 in the differential diagnosis of adnexal masses (Hogdall et al. 2000). A few studies suggest that CASA may be useful in monitoring and prognostication of disease. It may be superior to CA125 for detection of small-volume recurrent OC (McGuckin et al. 1990, Ward et al. 1993). Multivariate analysis found CASA was better than other prognostic factors except age for predicting survival (Ward et al. 1993, Hogdall et al. 1996), and useful in predicting second line chemoresistance and survival (Gronlund et al. 2005, 2006) and survival following recurrence (Gronlund et al. 2005).

Human Chorionic Gonadotropin (hCG)

Elevated hCG levels are found in a number of ovarian germ cell tumors and gestational trobhoblastic neoplasia (GTN). hCG has a lower sensitivity than other markers in current use for diagnosing OC, with the exception of germ-cell tumors with a chorionic component (Mann et al. 1993). Elevated hCG was found to be a significant predictor of overall survival along with stage and AFP in patients with malignant GCTs (Murugaesu et al. 2006). Serum and urinary (urinary βcore fragment, hCGβcf) hCG have also been shown to be strong independent prognostic indicators for EOC (Vartiainen et al. 2001).

Proteomics

The proteomic approach is based on the hypothesis that malignant transformation of tissue will be reflected in a detectable diagnostic protein biosignature. High-throughput mass spectrometry (MS) techniques such as surface-enhanced laser desorption ionization time-of-flight and matrix-associated laser desorption ionization time-of-flight have the potential to identify patterns or changes in thousand of proteins under 20 kDa, using algorithms based on sophisticated bioinformatics approaches. Following an initial report by Petricoin (Petricoin et al. 2002), a number of studies have reported high diagnostic sensitivities and specificities using MS generated profiles, compared to established biomarkers (Petricoin et al. 2002, Zhang et al. 2004, Rai et al. 2002, Lopez et al. 2007). Most have used blood samples to detect markers for differential diagnosis of OC, while few have also used ascitic fluid (Gortzak-Uzan et al. 2008, Kuk et al. 2009), urine (Petri et al. 2009) and tissue (Bengtsson et al. 2007, Li et al. 2009). A detailed review of these has recently been published elsewhere (Cadron et al. 2009). Although these approaches appear promising, a number of reports indicate potential problems and limitations related to cross-platform reliability, reproducibility, and standardization of sample handling and pre-analytical processing. Proteomic-based approaches require further refinement including cross validation utilizing strict protocols to minimize variation and optimize reproducibility (Timms et al. 2007, Bast et al. 2005, Fushiki et al. 2006, Oh et al. 2005) as well as prospective, large well-designed, multicenter clinical trials for validation (van der Merwe et al. 2007, Chan et al. 2006).

Other Marker Panels

Over the years a number of studies have evaluated the potential of a panel of markers to improve the diagnostic accuracy of CA125. However, increased sensitivity is often associated with decreased specificity. In mucinous OC markers like TATI, CA19-9, CA72-4 supplement serum CA125 (Stenman et al. 1995). More recent authors using sophisticated statistical methodologies like multivariable regression analysis, artificial neural networks, classification regression tree analysis, and mixture discriminate analysis have developed models incorporating serum biomarker panels which outperform CA125 alone. Some of the more recent panels investigated are listed in Table 1.

HE4 has emerged as an important marker in some panels (Moore et al. 2008, 2009, Havrilesk et al. 2008). A number of other panels which do not include HE4 have also found similarly high sensitivities and specificities for diagnosing OC including early-stage disease: TTR, TF, ApoA1 (Kozak et al. 2005, Nosov et al. 2009, Su et al. 2007); CA72-4, CA15-3, MCSF in combination with CA125 (Skates et al. 2004, Chan et al. 2006); IGF-II, OPN (osteopontin), leptin, and prolactin without CA125 (Mor et al. 2005); and the same four markers with CA125 and MIF (Kim et al. 2009, Visintin et al. 2008). However, a variety of methodological deficiencies in the latter study has been described (McIntosh et al. 2008). Although over 20 different marker panels have been reported in the literature, they have been developed and evaluated in the context of differential diagnosis and their performance as a screening test in asymptomatic women is as yet unknown and needs to be assessed. Further research is also needed to cross validate these results and ensure reproducibility as performance may vary with sample sets. It is also important to compare their performance to other methodologies used for differential diagnosis such as RMI, ultrasound-based algorithms, ANN, and regression models.

CERVICAL CANCER

In the United Kingdom, approximately 2700 cases and 1000 deaths from cervical cancer occur annually (CRUK 2007a). Over 90% of the cases of high grade cervical intraepithelial neoplasia occur in women under 45, with peak incidence occurring in the 25 to 29 year's age group. On the other hand, the incidence of invasive cervical cancer after the age of 25 is evenly spread across age groups, with 42% to 46% found in reproductive ages (CRUK 2007b,c, Reis et al. 2007).

Cervical cancer screening is one of the most successful public health interventions in the developed world and serological tumor markers do not currently play a role in this. However, a variety of serum markers have been investigated in assessing prognosis, monitoring response to treatment and detecting recurrence.

Squamous Cell Carcinoma Antigen

Squamous cell carcinoma (SCC) (Kato and Torigoe 1977) has two isoforms: SCC1 (neutral isoform) and SCC2 (acidic isoform). Elevated serum levels are more common in women with well-differentiated (78%) and moderately differentiated carcinoma (67%) than in those with poorly differentiated tumors (38%) (Crombach et al. 1989a), confirming that it is a marker for squamous cell differentiation. It has low diagnostic sensitivity for early-stage disease (Chmura et al. 2009). Around 24% to 53% of stage IB/IIA and 75% to 90% ≥stage-IIB squamous cell cervical cancers have raised

Table 1 Other Markers for Ovarian Cancer

Tumor marker	Description
Lactate dehydrogenase (LDH)	LDH has five isoforms, but mainly LDH-1, and LDH-2 contribute to elevated levels. It is less specific than AFP and hCG but has up to 60% sensitivity for non-seminomatous germ cell tumors and may be of use in monitoring as well as prognostication of disease
Tumor associated trypsin inhibitor (TATI)	TATI has more sensitivity for mucinous cancers, correlates well with tumor grade, and has been found to increase sensitivity in combination with CA125 (Medl et al. 1995, Peters-Engl et al. 1995). Elevated pre-operative levels have also been linked to a twofold increase in risk of death and lower 5 yr survival
Lysophosphatidic acid (LPA)	Bast demonstrated elevated levels of LPA in >90% of Stage-I/II ovarian cancers, <50% of whom had elevated CA125 levels (Bast et al. 1998). Recent reports reconfirm the correlation of raised plasma LPA with stage of ovarian cancer and indicate its potential as a useful marker particularly for early-stage disease (Sedlakova et al. 2008). However, further studies validating this are needed
Tetranectin	Tetranectin levels are reduced in patients with ovarian cancer inversely related to stage of disease. It is not useful as a stand-alone marker, but in combination with CA125 increases sensitivity without decreasing specificity. Levels correlate well with persistent disease, survival, chemoresistance to second line therapy and recurrence
Mesothelin	Mesothelin serum levels are elevated in ovarian cancers compared to benign ovarian tumors or normal controls (Hellstrom et al. 2008). Levels are found to correlate with stage of disease and elevated pre-treatment levels are associated with poor overall survival (Huang et al. 2006), and progression free survival (Cheng et al. 2009)
Cytokeratins: tissue polypeptide antigen (TPA), tissue polypeptide-specific antigen (TPS), and CYFRA 21-1)	TPA is a broad spectrum test that measures cytokeratins 8, 18, and 19, while TPS and CYFRA 21-1 are specific for cytokeratins 18 and 19, respectively. TPS is elevated in 50–77% of ovarian cancers studied (85% specificity) and levels correlate well with stage (Salman et al. 1995, Shabana and Onsrud 1994, Sliutz et al. 1995, Tempfer et al. 1998). It was found to be useful in monitoring (Salman et al. 1995, Shabana and Onsrud 1994) and predicting recurrence (Sliutz et al. 1995, Tempfer et al. 1998), though reports on role in prognosis are conflicting (Shabana and Onsrud 1994, van Dalen et al. 1999). CYFRA 21-1 has poor sensitivity for the differential diagnosis of adnexal masses and addition of CA125 did not improve diagnostic ability of the test
Cancer-associated antigen72-4 (CA72-4) or tumor-associated glycoprotein-72 (TAG-72)	Levels elevated in 50–67% of ovarian cancers (Scambia et al. 1990, Guadagni et al. 1995) with a better sensitivity than CA125 for mucinous tumors (Negishi et al. 1993, Hasholzner et al. 1996). CA72-4 has high specificity and has been found of value in combination with CA125
Prostasin	Prostasin levels are elevated in ovarian cancer and some data suggest it may be of benefit in detecting early-stage disease. In combination with CA125 achieved a sensitivity of 92% and specificity of 94% for non-mucinous ovarian cancer (Mok et al. 2001). Further studies are needed to explore and validate its potential either alone or in combination with CA125

SCC levels (Duk et al. 1990b, Gaarenstroom et al. 2000, Lozza et al. 1997, Gadducci al. 2007, Massuger et al. 1997). Levels also correlate significantly with stage and tumor volume (Brioschi et al. 1991, Crombach et al. 1989b, Yoon et al. 2007).

SCC levels positively correlate with lymph node metastasis. Sensitivities of 60% to 87% with specificities of 41% to 94% using different cut-offs ranging from 2 to 10 ng/ml have been described (Gaarenstroom et al. 2000, Yoon et al. 2007, Molina et al. 2005, Ogino et al. 2006, Avall-Lundqvist et al. 1992, Kim et al. 2005). Although elevated SCC levels may indicate lymph node involvement, a normal level cannot exclude it. A combination of CA125 and SCC was reported to have a PPV of 76% for lymph node involvement in stage IB/IIA disease (Massuger et al. 1997).

There are conflicting reports on the role of raised pre-treatment SCC as an independent prognostic factor for poor survival (Molina et al. 2005, Ogino et al. 2005, 2006, Bolger et al. 1997, Ngan et al. 1996). Elevated post-treatment SCC levels have also been reported to predict poor prognosis (Yoon et al. 2007, Bonfrer et al. 1997a). A role for SCC in identifying a subgroup who may need additional treatment has been advocated. However, trials evaluating the survival benefit of aggressive

treatment initiated by high pre-treatment SCC values have not yet been performed.

Serum SCC levels are useful in monitoring treatment of cervical cancer (Crombach et al. 1989b, Ogino et al. 2006, Schmidt-Rhode et al. 1988), predicting clinical response to therapy, identifying persistent or progressive disease (Hong et al. 1998, Scambia et al. 1994a) and detecting recurrence. Persistently elevated or rising post-treatment SCC levels are indicative of disease persistence or progression. Sensitivities between 56% and 86%, specificities between 83% and 100%, and lead times of up to 14 months (median 2–8 months) have been reported for detecting recurrent disease (Duk et al. 1990b, Brioschi et al. 1991, Schmidt-Rhode et al. 1988, Forni et al. 2007, Gitsch et al. 1992, Yazigi et al. 1991). The potential impact of earlier detection of recurrence on survival or treatment outcomes is unknown. However, recently in the presence of elevated markers, PET has been used to restage cervical cancer. This in turn could lead to treatment modifications resulting in improved two-year survival (Chang et al. 2004, Lai et al. 2004, 2007). SCC levels can predict disease recurrence (Molina et al. 2005, Ogino et al. 2006, Reesink-Peters et al. 2005), but reports regarding prediction of para-aortic node recurrence are conflicting (Ogino et al. 2005, Niibe et al. 2006).

CEA

CEA has a low sensitivity (up to 33%) for cervical cancer. However, a higher sensitivity (38%) and specificity (98%) for cervical adenocarcinoma has been reported (Ngan et al. 1996, Borras et al. 1995). Levels are reported to correlate with tumor stage, size, and lymph node involvement (Yoon et al. 2007, Molina et al. 2005). Although earlier reports suggested that it was not a prognostic marker and was of limited benefit in monitoring treatment (Ngan et al. 1996, Leminen et al. 1992), a recent publication indicates it may be of prognostic value in women with advanced cervical cancer (Chmura et al. 2009).

CA125

Serum CA125 levels are raised in 20% to 75% of women with cervical adenocarcinoma and found to correlate with stage, tumor size, stromal invasion, and lymph node involvement (Gadducci et al. 2007, Borras et al. 1995, Gocze et al. 1994), and to be of prognostic significance. However, lack of correlation with tumor stage has also been reported (Avall-Lundqvist et al. 1992). It may be of use in monitoring response, detecting recurrence (Borras et al. 1995, Leminen et al. 1992, Gocze et al. 1994), an indicator of poor survival (Gadducci et al. 2007, Avall-Lundqvist et al. 1992, Borras et al. 1995, Duk et al. 1990a), and predictor for lymph node metastases (Duk et al. 1990a).

CYFRA 21-1

Sensitivity for cervical cancer using CYFRA 21-1 has been found to range between 34% and 63%, with higher values reported for cervical adenocarcinoma and late stage disease (Tsai et al. 1996, Callet et al. 1998, Pras et al. 2002). Levels correlate with tumor size, stage, and nodal involvement (Gaarenstroom et al. 1995, 2000, Molina et al. 2005, Callet et al. 1998, Bonfrer et al. 1994), although no association with nodal status (Gaarenstroom et al. 2000) and histological type has also been reported (Ferdeghini et al. 1993). Reports include value in monitoring disease activity, response to treatment and recurrence (Callet et al. 1998), with rising values preceding disease progression in 61% to 90% of cases (Callet et al. 1998, Kainz et al. 1995). No significant association was detected on multivariate or Cox-regression analysis (Gaarenstroom et al. 2000, Molina et al. 2005).

Studies Comparing Markers

SCC was reported to be the tumor marker of choice for cervical cancer (Molina et al. 2005, Xiong et al. 2009), especially squamous cell carcinoma (Tsai et al. 1996, Xiong et al. 2009). CYFRA 21-1 may be better for adenocarcinoma (Ferdeghini et al. 1993). Both were reported to have a role in monitoring response and recurrence with SCC better than CYFRA 21-1 at detecting persistent disease and predicting lymph node metastasis, disease-free survival, or recurrence (Molina et al. 2005, Pras et al. 2002, Xiong et al. 2009). Reports indicate that combination assays of pre- and post-treatment CEA and SCC may be useful in prognostication and assessment of treatment response (Yoon et al. 2007). However, some studies have found CA125 and SCC but not CEA to be useful in monitoring treatment (CT) (Leminen et al. 1992). A combination of CA125, CA19-9, and CEA enabled detection of all cases with progressive disease, recurrence, or metastasis and also increased the

diagnostic sensitivity for cervical adenocarcinoma in one study (Borras et al. 1995). TPA has been found to be similar to SCC but better than TPS, CYFRA 21-1, or CTKRS 8-18 for cervical cancer (Ferdeghini et al. 1994).

GESTATIONAL TROPHOBLASTIC TUMORS/NEOPLASIA (GTT/GTN)

Gestational trophoblastic disease (GTD) comprises a wide spectrum of disorders with GTT or GTN representing the malignant end of the spectrum (Ngan and Seckl 2007). The U.K. incidence is 1 in 387 live births in Asian and 1 in 752 live births in non-Asian women (Tham et al. 2003). Although GTN may occur after any pregnancy, it is 2000 times more common following a molar pregnancy. Malignant transformation occurs in 16% complete and 0.5% partial molar pregnancies (Ngan and Seckl 2007, Seckl et al. 2000). Accurate diagnosis is paramount as it is almost always possible to cure GTN and preserve fertility. Survival rates of 98% have been reported over the last 10 years (Ngan and Seckl 2007).

Human Chorionic Gonadotropin

βhCG is an oncofetal antigen (glycoprotein), which consists of two subunits (α and β) and is normally secreted by the syncytiotrophoblast. While the β-subunit is distinct and responsible for its biologic and immunologic specificity, the α-subunit is common to other anterior pituitary hormones. It has a half-life of 24 to 48 hours, though this is much shorter for the individual subunits. In normal pregnancy, βhCG is largely intact and only hyperglycosylated in the first trimester. However, GTN is associated with the production of a number of different forms of βhCG such as free βhCG, core βhCG, nicked free βhCG, nicked hCG missing the βsubunit C-terminal peptide, hyperglycosylated βhCG, regular βhCG, and carboxyl terminal fragment forms (Mitchell and Seckl 2007). Hence, it is important to use hCG assays that detect all forms of βhCG. An inability to detect some hCG variants may lead to false negative test results, and miss detection of active disease or recurrence. This in turn could result in premature termination of treatment, increased recurrences, or even at times missed diagnoses. Heterophilic antibodies which have been found to occur in up to 3.4% of samples (Ward et al. 1997) may lead to false positive hCG (Phantom hCG) results (Rotmensch and Cole 2000).

The original radioimmunoassay (RIA) detected all forms βhCG (Birken et al. 1988, Vaitukaitis et al. 1972) but many of the new commercial assays are designed primarily for pregnancy application and do not necessarily detect the degraded molecules found in trophoblastic disease samples (Cole et al. 1994), which may lead to erroneous results. The Charing Cross hospital in the United Kingdom uses a non-commercial in house rabbit polyclonal antibody that detects all forms of hCG and routinely assays both serum and urine samples (Ngan and Seckl 2007).

βhCG is an "ideal tumor marker" for GTN as its levels are raised in almost all patients with trophoblastic disease and correlate with tumor burden and therapeutic response. It is very sensitive for small volume disease, and plays a primary role in the management of GTN. The FIGO diagnosis of GTN is dependent on serum hCG measurements: failure of hCG levels to regress in the absence of a normal pregnancy and with a history of either normal or abnormal pregnancy. Three of the four FIGO criteria for diagnosing GTN following molar pregnancy are dependent on hCG. In addition to diagnosis, hCG is also an integral part of GTN staging and risk scoring systems and is used for monitoring treatment and detecting recurrence (Ngan and Seckl 2007, Ngan et al. 2003a,b).

"Quiescent GTD" is defined as persistently low level of serum hCG, in the absence of clinical evidence of pregnancy or GTD. These cases do not respond to chemotherapy, and may not benefit from treatment, but do require long-term surveillance as they may subsequently develop malignant GTN (Kohorn 2002, Khanlian et al. 2003, Cole et al. 2006c). Two consecutive rising hCG titres with clinically or radiographically detectable disease would indicate need for treatment.

βhCG Variants
Hyperglycosylated hCG (hCG-H) or invasive trophoblast antigen (ITA) produced by invasive cytotrophoblasts is a potential new marker which can differentiate between invasive and non-invasive disease (Pandian et al. 2003, Seki et al. 2004). It has been found to have 100% sensitivity for discriminating quiescent GTD from active GTN/choriocarcinoma and accurately diagnose new or recurrent GTN/choriocarcinoma (Cole et al. 2006a,b). It could have a potential role in managing women with persistent low hCG levels (Khanlian and Cole 2006). Though preliminary reports are promising, further research is necessary.

Free βhCG to hCG ratio may be useful in distinguishing hydatidiform mole from choriocarcinoma (Fan et al. 1987, Ozturk et al. 1988) and a cut-off of >35% has been found to be of value in diagnosing placental site trophoblastic tumors (PSTTs) (Cole et al. 2006d), but these findings need further validation. PSTTs produce low levels of βhCG, and undetectable serum levels do not equate to lack of tumor (Rinne et al. 1999). Presence of β-core fragment in the urine may aid in the diagnosis of PSTT. Although serum βhCG levels in PSTT are low and do not correlate well with tumor volume, stage, or prognosis, it is still the best available marker for monitoring disease and treatment (Chang et al. 1999, Feltmate et al. 2001, Su et al. 1999).

Other Tumor Markers in GTN
Serum levels of Human placental lactogen (hPL) or human chorionic somatomammotropin (hCS) in GTN are lower than in normal pregnancy, and correlate with tumor burden by disappearing after treatment. If serum levels are elevated, hPL may serve as a tumor marker for monitoring PSTT.

ENDOMETRIAL CANCER
Around 93% of endometrial cancers occur in postmenopausal women. In the reproductive age group it is mainly linked to familial predisposition, obesity, or PCOS.

None of the serum markers have a well-established role in the clinical management of endometrial cancer.

Serum CA125 is elevated in 10% to 34% of patients with elevated levels detected in 61% to 100% of patients with advanced stage and 2% to 33% of those with early-stage disease (Gadducci et al. 1990, Powell et al. 2005). Preoperative CA125 levels have been found to correlate with stage, grade, depth of myometrial invasion, peritoneal cytology, and nodal involvement. Elevated CA125 levels have been reported to be

predictive of poor survival (Lundstrom et al. 2000, Sood et al. 1997, Denschlag et al. 2007, Scambia et al. 1994b). CA125 has been used for post-treatment surveillance and detecting recurrence (Scambia et al. 1994b, Cherchi et al. 1999, Hakala et al. 1995, Kurihara et al. 1998, Lo et al. 1997) but its value in monitoring uterine papillary serous carcinoma is uncertain (Abramovich et al. 1999, Price et al. 1998). Elevated levels have been found to occur in 50% relapsed and 5% disease free cases at follow-up. A combination of CA125 and CA19.9 can increase the sensitivity for detecting recurrence to 83% (12.8% false positive rate) (Cherchi et al. 1999). Although it has been suggested that serum CA125 may be useful in follow-up of patients with early-stage endometrial cancer, it has not been shown to add to clinical examination and imaging (Price et al. 1998).

VULVAR AND VAGINAL CANCER
Tumors of the vulva and the vagina are uncommon and only a few studies have described circulating markers in these cancers which include TPS, SCC, and UGF. There is currently no role for serological markers in the clinical management of these cancers.

SUMMARY
CA125 remains the most widely investigated and clinically used tumor marker for OC. Addition of TVS, use of the ROCA, and a multimodal screening approach has been found to improve its performance in screening. Though there is preliminary evidence of survival benefit, the mortality impact of screening is not yet known. It is currently being investigated as a screening tool in a number of clinical trials: UKCTOCS and PLCO in the low risk population, and UKFOCSS, CGN, and GOG trials in the high-risk populations. The current recommendation is for screening to be carried out only within the context of a clinical trial. As part of the RMI, CA125 is clinically used for the differential diagnosis of adnexal masses. RMI performance can be improved by addition of specialist US and MRI, and is comparable to most mathematical logistic regression or ANN models. The discriminatory ability of CA125 can also be enhanced by using it in a panel of markers (Table 2). Further cross validation of these marker panels to ensure reproducibility of results is needed. In addition, the efficacy of biomarker panels in screening has not yet been established. CA125 levels after the third course of initial chemotherapy can be used for prognostication. Serial CA125 measurements are used to monitor treatment and detect recurrence. However, no survival benefit was recently reported on commencing treatment on the basis of rising CA125 levels in the absence of other indicators of disease recurrence. HE4 is a promising new marker which has been found to improve the discriminatory ability of CA125 alone, particularly for early-stage disease. AFP may be of value in germ cell tumors; and inhibin in ovarian granulosa cell (GCT)/sex cord/stromal tumors. A number of other tumor markers such as cytokines, kallikreins, osteopontin, CEA, CA19.9, VEGF, TATI, TPA, Tetranectin, LASA, LPA, Prostasin, CA-72-4, Cytokeratins, leptin, prolactin, Glycodelin, activin, Apo A-1 have been investigated but are not yet routinely used in clinical practice. Proteomic-based approaches require further refinement, including cross

Table 2 Panels of Markers

Author	Model	No.	Markers	Findings
Zhang et al. 1999	ANN	4	CA125 II, CA72-4, CA15-3, and LASA	Increased sens (88%) vs. CA125 alone (68%) and spec (79%) comparable to CA125 (82%). Improved specificity to 82% in premenopausal women compared to 62% with CA125
van Haaften-Day et al. 2001	None	4	OVX1, CA125, M-CSF, CA125	Combination of all four increased sens (over CA125 alone) for all stages of disease
Skates et al. 2004	LR, MDA, classification tree	4	CA125II, CA72-4, CA15-3 and M-CSF	Sens early-stage dis were 45% for CA125II; 67% for CA125II and CA72-4; 70% for CA125II, CA72-4, and M-CSF; and 68% for all four markers. The panel of four markers increased sens of CA125 alone (45%) to 70%, while maintaining 98% specificity
Mor et al. 2005	LR analysis	4	IGF-II, OPN (osteopontin), leptin, prolactin	Combination of all four showed good performance: sens 95%, PPV 95%, spec 95%, and NPV 94%
Tsigkou et al. 2007		2	Total inhibin, CA125	Total inhibin—incr sens for mucinous tumors (94% vs. 82% for CA125). Combination of CA125 + total inhibin—inc sens for mucinous tumors to 100% and all ov ca to 99% at 95% spec
Su et al. 2007	Multivariable LR	4	CA125, apoA-I, TTR and TF	91% sensitivity for LMP, 89% sensitivity for ESOC for specificities of 92%. 95% sensitivity for mucinous ESOC
Visintin et al. 2008	LR analysis	6	Leptin, prolactin, osteopontin, IGF-II, MIF, and CA125	Four models (using 6 markers/4 markers) evaluated. Test set validated. 6 marker panel sens 95% with spec 99%, NPV 99.2, PPV 99.3 (vs. CA125 72% sens and 95% spec). 90% sens and 95% spec for early-stage disease
Moore et al. 2008	LR analysis	9	CA125, SMRP, HE4, CA72-4, activin, inhibin, osteopontin, EGFR, ERBB2 (Her2)	HE4 best single marker-highest sensitivity 72.9% (specificity 95%). Combined CA125 and HE4 yielded highest sensitivity 76.4% (specificity 95%). HE4 best for Stage I, HE4 + CA125 best overall. Addition of other markers did not greatly improve performance. Sens 76–79%, Spec 95%
Havrilesky et al. 2008	LR analysis	9	HE4, Glycodelin, MMP7, SLPI, Plau-R, MUC1, inhibin A, PAI-1, and CA125	HE4-best single marker for early- and late-stage dis. One-step marker panel: (a) 2 SD cutoff—(CA125, HE4, Glycodelin, Plau-R and MMP7→ sens 79% spec 93% early-stage dis and sens 86%, spec 94% late stage dis); (b) best cutoff (CA125, HE4, Glycodelin, Plau-R, MUC-1 and PAI-1 → sens 80.5%, spec 96.5% early-stage dis and sens 89 with spec 97% for late stage dis). Two-step marker analysis: (a) 2SD cut off (HE4 followed by panel-CA125, Glycodelin, Plau-R—any one positive → sens 74% spec 94% early-stage dis and sens 84%, spec 94% late stage dis); (b) best cutoff (HE4 followed by panel-CA125 positive or if any two of Glycodelin, MUC-1 or Plau-R tested positive → sens 77% with spec 97% early-stage dis and inc sens to 85% for late stage dis)
Zhang et al. 2007	ANN	4	CA125-II, CA72-4, CA15-3, MCSF (macrophage colony stimulating factor)	For specificity of 98%, the sensitivities for ANN and CA125II alone were 71% (37/52) and 46% (24/52) (*p* = 0.047), respectively, for detecting early-stage EOC, and 71% (30/42) and 43% (18/42) (*p* = 0.040), respectively, for detecting invasive early-stage EOC
Nosov et al. 2009	LR analysis	4	Apolipoprotein A-1, transthyretin, TF, CA125	Early-stage EOC sens 96%, spec 96% and AUC 0.99. Sens and spec of 98% for endometrioid early-stage EOC and 94% for serous early-stage EOC. Addition of CA125 improved performance of other three markers alone
Kim et al. 2009	LR analysis	6	Leptin, prolactin, osteopontin, IGF-II, MIF, CA125	Marker panel—sens 95.3% and spec 99.4%
Dieplinger et al. 2009		3	Afamin, ApolipoproteinA-IV (compared with CA125)	AUC: for a specificity of 90% sensitivity values of 92.4%, 42.4%, and 40.8% for CA125, afamin, and apoA-IV, respectively. Afamin, but not apoA-IV, added independent diagnostic information to CA125 and age. Afamin may be used as an adjunct to CA125
Moore et al. 2009	LR analysis	2	CA125 + HE4	Prospective validation of Moore 2008 model. Separate dual marker algorithms for pre- and postmenopausal groups. Postmenopausal cases-spec 75.0% (66.9–81.4) and sens 92.3% (85.9–96.4). Premenopausal cases-spec 74.8% (68.2–80.6), and sens 76.5% (58.8–89.3). Overall combined sens 88.7% (82.6–93.3%), spec 74.7% (69.8–79.2%) and NPV of 93.9% (90.5–96.4%)
Begum et al. 2009	LR analysis	2	Tetranectin (TN), CA125	TN, CA125, and menopausal status: AUC for invasive cancers 0.92 compared to 0.66 for borderline disease

Abbreviations: ANN, artificial neural network; dis,disease; LR, logistic regression; MDA, mixture discriminate analysis; NPV, negative predictive value; PPV, positive predictive value; sens, sensitivity; spec, specificity; TF, transferring.

validation utilizing strict protocols to minimize variation and optimize reproducibility, as well cross validation in large multicenter trials.

SCC is the commonest tumor marker used for cervical carcinoma. It is the best marker for squamous cell carcinoma. It has been found to have prognostic significance but whether it is of value in selecting a group of patients who will benefit from more aggressive treatment has not yet been established. Although of benefit in monitoring treatment and detecting recurrence, it is not clear whether early detection of recurrence will improve outcomes or survival. However, recent reports indicate a possible survival benefit from modified treatment of PET detected early recurrences in patients with elevated SCC. CA125 may be of added benefit in detecting and monitoring cases of adenocarcinoma and is of prognostic significance.

βhCG is the 'ideal tumor marker' for GTN, with elevated levels occurring in almost all patients with this condition. Levels correlate with tumor burden and therapeutic response and it plays a primary role in various aspects of disease management. Using hCG assays that detect all forms of βhCG minimizes false negative results. Hyperglycosylated hCG (hCG-H)/ invasive trophoblast antigen (ITA), is a new marker with a potential role in the diagnosis and management of choriocarcinoma. βhCG is still the best available marker for monitoring PSTT, though in the presence of elevated levels hPL may be of value in monitoring disease.

REFERENCES

Abramovich D, Markman M, Kennedy A, et al. (1999) Serum CA-125 as a marker of disease activity in uterine papillary serous carcinoma. *J Cancer Res Clin Oncol* **125**(12):697–8.

Alagoz T, Buller RE, Berman M, et al. (1994) What is a normal CA125 level? *Gynecol Oncol* **53**(1):93–7.

Andersen ES, Knudsen A, Rix P, et al. (2003) Risk of malignancy index in the preoperative evaluation of patients with adnexal masses. *Gynecol Oncol* **90**(1):109–12.

Aslam N, Tailor A, Lawton F, et al. (2000) Prospective evaluation of three different models for the pre-operative diagnosis of ovarian cancer. *BJOG* **107**(11):1347–53.

Avall-Lundqvist EH, Sjovall K, Nilsson BR, et al. (1992) Prognostic significance of pretreatment serum levels of squamous cell carcinoma antigen and CA 125 in cervical carcinoma. *Eur J Cancer* **28A**(10):1695–702.

Ayas S, Akoz I, Eskicirak E, et al. (2007) A case of endodermal sinus tumor associated with the first pregnancy and successful management of the second pregnancy: a case report and review of the literature. *Eur J Gynaecol Oncol* **28**(2):155–9.

Ayhan A, Guven S, Guven ES, et al. (2007) Is there a correlation between tumor marker panel and tumor size and histopathology in well staged patients with borderline ovarian tumors? *Acta Obstet Gynecol Scand* **86**(4):484–90.

Bailey J, Tailor A, Naik R, et al. (2006) Risk of malignancy index for referral of ovarian cancer cases to a tertiary center: does it identify the correct cases? *Int J Gynecol Cancer* **16**(Suppl 1):30–4.

Bao LH, Sakaguchi H, Fujimoto J, et al. (2007) Osteopontin in metastatic lesions as a prognostic marker in ovarian cancers. *J Biomed Sci* **14**(3):373–81.

Bast RC Jr, Badgwell D, Lu Z, et al. (2005) New tumor markers: CA125 and beyond. *Int J Gynecol Cancer* **15**(Suppl 3):274–81.

Bast RC Jr, Feeney M, Lazarus H, et al. (1981) Reactivity of a monoclonal antibody with human ovarian carcinoma. *J Clin Invest* **68**(5):1331–7.

Bast RC Jr, Klug TL, St John E, et al. (1983) A radioimmunoassay using a monoclonal antibody to monitor the course of epithelial ovarian cancer. *N Engl J Med* **309**(15):883–7.

Bast RC Jr, Xu FJ, Yu YH, et al. (1998) CA 125: the past and the future. *Int J Biol Markers* **13**(4):179–87.

Begum FD, Hogdall E, Kjaer SK, et al. (2009) Preoperative serum tetranectin, CA125 and menopausal status used as single markers in screening and in a risk assessment index (RAI) in discriminating between benign and malignant ovarian tumors. *Gynecol Oncol* **113**(2):221–7.

Bengtsson S, Krogh M, Szigyarto CA, et al. (2007) Large-scale proteomics analysis of human ovarian Cancer for Biomarkers. *J Proteome Res*.

Birken S, Armstrong EG, Kolks MA, et al. (1988) Structure of the human chorionic gonadotropin beta-subunit fragment from pregnancy urine. *Endocrinology* **123**(1):572–83.

Boggess JF, Soules MR, Goff BA, et al. (1997) Serum inhibin and disease status in women with ovarian granulosa cell tumors. *Gynecol Oncol* **64**(1):64–9.

Bolger BS, Dabbas M, Lopes A, et al. (1997) Prognostic value of preoperative squamous cell carcinoma antigen level in patients surgically treated for cervical carcinoma. *Gynecol Oncol* **65**(2):309–13.

Bon GG, Kenemans P, Verstraeten R, et al. (1996) Serum tumor marker immunoassays in gynecologic oncology: establishment of reference values. *Am J Obstet Gynecol* **174**(1 Pt 1):107–14.

Bonfrer JM, Gaarenstroom KN, Kenter GG, et al. (1994) Prognostic significance of serum fragments of cytokeratin 19 measured by Cyfra 21-1 in cervical cancer. *Gynecol Oncol* **55**(3 Pt 1):371–5.

Bonfrer JM, Gaarenstroom KN, Korse CM, et al. (1997a) Cyfra 21-1 in monitoring cervical cancer: a comparison with tissue polypeptide antigen and squamous cell carcinoma antigen. *Anticancer Res* **17**(3C):2329–34.

Bonfrer JM, Korse CM, Verstraeten RA, et al. (1997b) Clinical evaluation of the Byk LIA-mat CA125 II assay: discussion of a reference value. *Clin Chem* **43**(3):491–7.

Borras G, Molina R, Xercavins J, et al. (1995) Tumor antigens CA 19.9, CA 125, and CEA in carcinoma of the uterine cervix. *Gynecol Oncol* **57**(2):205–11.

Brakora KA, Lee H, Yusuf R, et al. (2004) Utility of osteopontin as a biomarker in recurrent epithelial ovarian cancer. *Gynecol Oncol* **93**(2):361–5.

Brioschi PA, Bischof P, Delafosse C, et al. (1991) Squamous-cell carcinoma antigen (SCC-A) values related to clinical outcome of pre-invasive and invasive cervical carcinoma. *Int J Cancer* **47**(3):376–9.

Buller RE, Berman ML, Bloss JD, et al. (1992) Serum CA125 regression in epithelial ovarian cancer: correlation with reassessment findings and survival. *Gynecol Oncol* **47**(1):87–92.

Burger HG, Robertson DM, Cahir N, et al. (1996) Characterization of inhibin immunoreactivity in post-menopausal women with ovarian tumours. *Clin Endocrinol (Oxf)* **44**(4):413–8.

Cadron I, Van Gorp T, Timmerman D, et al. (2009) Application of proteomics in ovarian cancer: Which sample should be used? *Gynecol Oncol*.

Callet N, Cohen-Solal Le Nir CC, Berthelot E, et al. (1998) Cancer of the uterine cervix: sensitivity and specificity of serum Cyfra 21.1 determinations. *Eur J Gynaecol Oncol* **19**(1):50–6.

Canney PA, Moore M, Wilkinson PM, et al. (1984) Ovarian cancer antigen CA125: a prospective clinical assessment of its role as a tumour marker. *Br J Cancer* **50**(6):765–9.

Chambers SK, Kacinski BM, Ivins CM, et al. (1997) Overexpression of epithelial macrophage colony-stimulating factor (CSF-1) and CSF-1 receptor: a poor prognostic factor in epithelial ovarian cancer, contrasted with a protective effect of stromal CSF-1. *Clin Cancer Res* **3**(6):999–1007.

Chan DW, Semmes OJ, Petricoin EF, et al. (2006) National Academy of Clinical Biochemistry Guidelines: The Use of MALDI-TOF Mass Spectrometry Profiling to Diagnose Cancer. Available from: http://www.aacc.org/NR/rdonlyres/45357D4E-FA88-4997-B8A6-74BFE31A3D49/0/chp4b_mass_spec.pdf accessed Jan 2008. [Cited January 2008].

Chang TC, Law KS, Hong JH, et al. (2004) Positron emission tomography for unexplained elevation of serum squamous cell carcinoma antigen levels during follow-up for patients with cervical malignancies: a phase II study. *Cancer* **101**(1):164–71.

Chang YL, Chang TC, Hsueh S, et al. (1999) Prognostic factors and treatment for placental site trophoblastic tumor-report of 3 cases and analysis of 88 cases. *Gynecol Oncol* **73**(2):216–22.

Cheng WF, Huang CY, Chang MC, et al. (2009) High mesothelin correlates with chemoresistance and poor survival in epithelial ovarian carcinoma. *Br J Cancer* **100**(7):1144–53.

Cherchi PL, Dessole S, Ruiu GA, et al. (1999) The value of serum CA 125 and association CA 125/CA 19-9 in endometrial carcinoma. *Eur J Gynaecol Oncol* **20**(4):315–7.

Chmura A, Wojcieszek A, Mrochem J, et al. (2009) Usefulness of the SCC, CEA, CYFRA 21.1, and CRP markers for the diagnosis and monitoring of cervical squamous cell carcinoma. *Ginekol Pol* **80**(5):361–6.

Chow SN, Yang JH, Lin YH, et al. (1996) Malignant ovarian germ cell tumors. *Int J Gynaecol Obstet* **53**(2):151–8.

Clark TG, Stewart ME, Altman DG, et al. (2001) A prognostic model for ovarian cancer. *Br J Cancer* **85**(7):944–52.

Cole LA, Butler SA, Khanlian SA, et al. (2006a) Gestational trophoblastic diseases: 2. Hyperglycosylated hCG as a reliable marker of active neoplasia. *Gynecol Oncol* **102**(2):151–9.

Cole LA, Dai D, Butler SA, et al. (2006b) Gestational trophoblastic diseases: 1. Pathophysiology of hyperglycosylated hCG. *Gynecol Oncol* **102**(2):145–50.

Cole LA, Khanlian SA, Giddings A, et al. (2006c) Gestational trophoblastic diseases: 4. Presentation with persistent low positive human chorionic gonadotropin test results. *Gynecol Oncol* **102**(2):165–72.

Cole LA, Khanlian SA, Muller CY, et al. (2006d) Gestational trophoblastic diseases: 3. Human chorionic gonadotropin-free beta-subunit, a reliable marker of placental site trophoblastic tumors. *Gynecol Oncol* **102**(2): 160–4.

Cole LA, Kohorn EI, Kim GS (1994) Detecting and monitoring trophoblastic disease. New perspectives on measuring human chorionic gonadotropin levels. *J Reprod Med* **39**(3):193–200.

Cooke I, O'Brien M, Charnock FM, et al. (1995) Inhibin as a marker for ovarian cancer. *Br J Cancer* **71**(5):1046–50.

Crombach G, Scharl A, Vierbuchen M, et al. (1989a) Detection of squamous cell carcinoma antigen in normal squamous epithelia and in squamous cell carcinomas of the uterine cervix. *Cancer* **63**(7):1337–42.

Crombach G, Wurz H, Herrmann F, et al. (1989b) The importance of the SCC antigen in the diagnosis and follow-up of cervix carcinoma. A cooperative study of the Gynecologic Tumor Marker Group (GTMG)]. *Dtsch Med Wochenschr* **114**(18):700–5.

Cruickshank DJ, Terry PB, Fullerton WT (1991) The potential value of CA125 as a tumour marker in small volume, non-evaluable epithelial ovarian cancer. *Int J Biol Markers* **6**(4):247–52.

CRUK (2007a) Latest UK Summary – Cancer Incidence 2004 and Mortality 2005. Available from: http://info.cancerresearchuk.org/images/pdfs/2004inc5 mortpdf. [Cited February 2008].

CRUK (2007b) UK Cancer Incidence statistics 2004. Available from: http://info.cancerresearchuk.org/cancerstats/incidence/ last updated August 2007. [Cited January 1, 2008].

CRUK (2007c) UK Cancer mortality statistics for common cancers. Available from: http://info.cancerresearchuk.org/cancerstats/mortality/cancerdeaths/ last update May 2007, accessed Jan 8. [Cited 2008].

Davelaar EM, van Kamp GJ, Verstraeten RA, et al. (1998) Comparison of seven immunoassays for the quantification of CA 125 antigen in serum. *Clin Chem* **44**(7):1417–22.

Davies AP, Jacobs I, Woolas R, et al. (1993) The adnexal mass: benign or malignant? Evaluation of a risk of malignancy index. *Br J Obstet Gynaecol* **100**(10):927–31.

Denschlag D, Tan L, Patel S, et al. (2007) Stage III endometrial cancer: preoperative predictability, prognostic factors, and treatment outcome. *Am J Obstet Gynecol* **196**(6):546 e1–7.

Diamandis EP, Yousef GM (2002) Human tissue kallikreins: a family of new cancer biomarkers. *Clin Chem* **48**(8):1198–205.

Dieplinger H, Ankerst DP, Burges A, et al. (2009) Afamin and apolipoprotein A-IV: novel protein markers for ovarian cancer. *Cancer Epidemiol Biomarkers Prev* **18**(4):1127–33.

Drapkin R, von Horsten HH, Lin Y, et al. (2005) Human epididymis protein 4 (HE4) is a secreted glycoprotein that is overexpressed by serous and endometrioid ovarian carcinomas. *Cancer Res* **65**(6):2162–9.

Duffy MJ, Bonfrer JM, Kulpa J, et al. (2005) CA125 in ovarian cancer: European Group on Tumor Markers guidelines for clinical use. *Int J Gynecol Cancer* **15**(5):679–91.

Duk JM, De Bruijn HW, Groenier KH, et al. (1990a) Adenocarcinoma of the uterine cervix. Prognostic significance of pretreatment serum CA 125, squamous cell carcinoma antigen, and carcinoembryonic antigen levels in relation to clinical and histopathologic tumor characteristics. *Cancer* **65**(8):1830–7.

Duk JM, de Bruijn HW, Groenier KH, et al. (1990b) Cancer of the uterine cervix: sensitivity and specificity of serum squamous cell carcinoma antigen determinations. *Gynecol Oncol* **39**(2):186–94.

El-Shawarby SA, Henderson AF, Mossa MA (2005) Ovarian cysts during pregnancy: dilemmas in diagnosis and management. *J Obstet Gynaecol* **25**(7):669–75.

Fan C, Goto S, Furuhashi Y, et al. (1987) Radioimmunoassay of the serum free beta-subunit of human chorionic gonadotropin in trophoblastic disease. *J Clin Endocrinol Metab* **64**(2):313–18.

Fayers PM, Rustin G, Wood R, et al. (1993) The prognostic value of serum CA 125 in patients with advanced ovarian carcinoma: an analysis of 573 patients by the Medical Research Council Working Party on Gynaecological Cancer. *Int J Gynecol Cancer* **3**(5):285–92.

Fehm T, Heller F, Kramer S, et al. (2005) Evaluation of CA125, physical and radiological findings in follow-up of ovarian cancer patients. *Anticancer Res* **25**(3A):1551–4.

Feltmate CM, Genest DR, Wise L, et al. (2001) Placental site trophoblastic tumor: a 17-year experience at the New England Trophoblastic Disease Center. *Gynecol Oncol* **82**(3):415–9.

Ferdeghini M, Gadducci A, Annicchiarico C, et al. (1993) Serum CYFRA 21-1 assay in squamous cell carcinoma of the cervix. *Anticancer Res* **13**(5C): 1841–4.

Ferdeghini M, Gadducci A, Prontera C, et al. (1994) Determination of serum levels of different cytokeratins in patients with uterine malignancies. *Anticancer Res* **14**(3B):1393–7.

Fiegler P, Kazmierczak W, Fiegler-Mecik H, et al. (2005) Why do we observe a high concentration of CA125 in mother's serum during pregnancy?. *Ginekol Pol* **76**(3):209–13.

Forni F, Ferrandina G, Deodato F, et al. (2007) Squamous cell carcinoma antigen in follow-up of cervical cancer treated with radiotherapy: evaluation of cost-effectiveness. *Int J Radiat Oncol Biol Phys* **69**(4):1145–9.

Foti E, Ferrandina G, Martucci R, et al. (1999) IL-6, M-CSF and IAP cytokines in ovarian cancer: simultaneous assessment of serum levels. *Oncology* **57**(3):211–5.

Fushiki T, Fujisawa H, Eguchi S (2006) Identification of biomarkers from mass spectrometry data using a "common" peak approach. *BMC Bioinformatics* **7**:358.

Gaarenstroom KN, Bonfrer JM, Kenter GG, et al. (1995) Clinical value of pretreatment serum Cyfra 21-1, tissue polypeptide antigen, and squamous cell carcinoma antigen levels in patients with cervical cancer. *Cancer* **76**(5):807–13.

Gaarenstroom KN, Kenter GG, Bonfrer JM, et al. (2000) Can initial serum cyfra 21-1, SCC antigen, and TPA levels in squamous cell cervical cancer predict lymph node metastases or prognosis? *Gynecol Oncol* **77**(1):164–70.

Gadducci A, Cosio S, Carpi A, et al. (2004) Serum tumor markers in the management of ovarian, endometrial and cervical cancer. *Biomed Pharmacother* **58**(1):24–38.

Gadducci A, Ferdeghini M, Castellani C, et al. (1998) Serum macrophage colony-stimulating factor (M-CSF) levels in patients with epithelial ovarian cancer. *Gynecol Oncol* **70**(1):111–4.

Gadducci A, Ferdeghini M, Prontera C, et al. (1990) A comparison of pretreatment serum levels of four tumor markers in patients with endometrial and cervical carcinoma. *Eur J Gynaecol Oncol* **11**(4):283–8.

Gadducci A, Tana R, Fanucchi A, et al. (2007) Biochemical prognostic factors and risk of relapses in patients with cervical cancer. *Gynecol Oncol* **107**(1 Suppl 1):S23–6.

Galgano MT, Hampton GM, Frierson HF Jr (2006) Comprehensive analysis of HE4 expression in normal and malignant human tissues. *Mod Pathol* **19**(6):847–53.

Geerts I, Vergote I, Neven P, et al. (2009) The role of inhibins B and antimullerian hormone for diagnosis and follow-up of granulosa cell tumors. *Int J Gynecol Cancer* **19**(5):847–55.

Gitlin D, Perricelli A, Gitlin GM (1972) Synthesis of -fetoprotein by liver, yolk sac, and gastrointestinal tract of the human conceptus. *Cancer Res* **32**(5):979–82.

Gitsch G, Kainz C, Joura E, et al. (1992) Squamous cell carcinoma antigen, tumor associated trypsin inhibitor and tissue polypeptide specific antigen in follow up of stage III cervical cancer. *Anticancer Res* **12**(4):1247–9.

Gocze PM, Szabo DG, Than GN, et al. (1988) Occurrence of CA 125 and CA 19-9 tumor-associated antigens in sera of patients with gynecologic, trophoblastic, and colorectal tumors. *Gynecol Obstet Invest* **25**(4):268–72.

Gocze PM, Vahrson HW, Freeman DA (1994) Serum levels of squamous cell carcinoma antigen and ovarian carcinoma antigen (CA 125) in patients with benign and malignant diseases of the uterine cervix. *Oncology* **51**(5):430–4.

Gortzak-Uzan L, Ignatchenko A, Evangelou AI, et al. (2008) A proteome resource of ovarian cancer ascites: integrated proteomic and bioinformatic analyses to identify putative biomarkers. *J Proteome Res* **7**(1):339–51.

Green PJ, Ballas SK, Westkaemper P, et al. (1986) CA 19-9 and CA 125 levels in the sera of normal blood donors in relation to smoking history. *J Natl Cancer Inst* **77**(2):337–41.

Greene MH, Piedmonte M, Alberts D, et al. (2008) A prospective study of risk-reducing salpingo-oophorectomy and longitudinal CA-125 screening among women at increased genetic risk of ovarian cancer: design and baseline characteristics: a gynecologic oncology group study. *Cancer Epidemiol Biomarkers Prev* **17**(3):594–604.

Grisaru D, Hauspy J, Prasad M, et al. (2007) Microarray expression identification of differentially expressed genes in serous epithelial ovarian cancer compared with bulk normal ovarian tissue and ovarian surface scrapings. *Oncol Rep* **18**(6):1347–56.

Gronlund B, Dehn H, Hogdall CK, et al. (2005) Cancer-associated serum antigen level: a novel prognostic indicator for survival in patients with recurrent ovarian carcinoma. *Int J Gynecol Cancer* **15**(5):836–43.

Gronlund B, Hogdall C, Hilden J, et al. (2004) Should CA-125 response criteria be preferred to response evaluation criteria in solid tumors (RECIST) for prognostication during second-line chemotherapy of ovarian carcinoma? *J Clin Oncol* **22**(20):4051–8.

Gronlund B, Hogdall EV, Christensen IJ, et al. (2006) Pre-treatment prediction of chemoresistance in second-line chemotherapy of ovarian carcinoma: value of serological tumor marker determination (tetranectin, YKL-40, CASA, CA 125). *Int J Biol Markers* **21**(3):141–8.

Grover S, Koh H, Weideman P, et al. (1992) The effect of the menstrual cycle on serum CA 125 levels: a population study. *Am J Obstet Gynecol* **167**(5):1379–81.

Guadagni F, Roselli M, Cosimelli M, et al. (1995) CA 72-4 serum marker – a new tool in the management of carcinoma patients. *Cancer Invest* **13**(2):227–38.

Gupta D, Lis CG (2009) Role of CA125 in predicting ovarian cancer survival—a review of the epidemiological literature. *J Ovarian Res* **2**:13.

Hakala A, Kacinski BM, Stanley ER, et al. (1995) Macrophage colony-stimulating factor 1, a clinically useful tumor marker in endometrial adenocarcinoma: comparison with CA 125 and the aminoterminal propeptide of type III procollagen. *Am J Obstet Gynecol* **173**(1):112–9.

Hasholzner U, Baumgartner L, Stieber P, et al. (1996) Clinical significance of the tumour markers CA 125 II and CA 72-4 in ovarian carcinoma. *Int J Cancer* **69**(4):329–34.

Havrilesky LJ, Whitehead CM, Rubatt JM, et al. (2008) Evaluation of biomarker panels for early stage ovarian cancer detection and monitoring for disease recurrence. *Gynecol Oncol* **110**(3):374–82.

Hawkins RE, Roberts K, Wiltshaw E, et al. (1989) The clinical correlates of serum CA125 in 169 patients with epithelial ovarian carcinoma. *Br J Cancer* **60**(4):634–7.

Healy DL, Burger HG, Mamers P, et al. (1993) Elevated serum inhibin concentrations in postmenopausal women with ovarian tumors. *N Engl J Med* **329**(21):1539–42.

Hellstrom I, Friedman E, Verch T, et al. (2008) Anti-mesothelin antibodies and circulating mesothelin relate to the clinical state in ovarian cancer patients. *Cancer Epidemiol Biomarkers Prev* **17**(6):1520–6.

Hellstrom I, Raycraft J, Hayden-Ledbetter M, et al. (2003) The HE4 (WFDC2) protein is a biomarker for ovarian carcinoma. *Cancer Res* **63**(13):3695–700.

Hermsen BB, Olivier RI, Verheijen RH, et al. (2007) No efficacy of annual gynaecological screening in BRCA1/2 mutation carriers; an observational follow-up study. *Br J Cancer* **96**(9):1335–42.

Hogdall CK, Hogdall EV, Hording U, et al. (1996) Use of tetranectin, CA-125 and CASA to predict residual tumor and survival at second- and third-look operations for ovarian cancer. *Acta Oncol* **35**(1):63–9.

Hogdall CK, Norgaard-Pedersen B, Mogensen O (2002) The prognostic value of pre-operative serum tetranectin, CA-125 and a combined index in women with primary ovarian cancer. *Anticancer Res* **22**(3):1765–8.

Hogdall EV, Hogdall CK, Tingulstad S, et al. (2000) Predictive values of serum tumour markers tetranectin, OVX1, CASA and CA125 in patients with a pelvic mass. *Int J Cancer* **89**(6):519–23.

Hohlfeld P, Dang TT, Nahoul K, et al. (1994) Tumour-associated antigens in maternal and fetal blood. *Prenat Diagn* **14**(10):907–12.

Hong JH, Tsai CS, Chang JT, et al. (1998) The prognostic significance of pre- and posttreatment SCC levels in patients with squamous cell carcinoma of the cervix treated by radiotherapy. *Int J Radiat Oncol Biol Phys* **41**(4):823–30.

Huang CY, Cheng WF, Lee CN, et al. (2006) Serum mesothelin in epithelial ovarian carcinoma: a new screening marker and prognostic factor. *Anticancer Res* **26**(6C):4721–8.

Huhtinen K, Suvitie P, Hiissa J, et al. (2009) Serum HE4 concentration differentiates malignant ovarian tumours from ovarian endometriotic cysts. *Br J Cancer* **100**(8):1315–9.

Icard P, Regnard JF, Essomba A, et al. (1994) Preoperative carcinoembryonic antigen level as a prognostic indicator in resected primary lung cancer. *Ann Thorac Surg* **58**(3):811–4.

Jacobs I (2005) Screening for familial ovarian cancer: the need for well-designed prospective studies. *J Clin Oncol* **23**(24):5443–5.

Jacobs I, Bast RC Jr (1989) The CA 125 tumour-associated antigen: a review of the literature. *Hum Reprod* **4**(1):1–12.

Jacobs I, Davies AP, Bridges J, et al. (1993) Prevalence screening for ovarian cancer in postmenopausal women by CA 125 measurement and ultrasonography. *BMJ* **306**(6884):1030–4.

Jacobs I, Oram D, Fairbanks J, et al. (1990) A risk of malignancy index incorporating CA 125, ultrasound and menopausal status for the accurate preoperative diagnosis of ovarian cancer. *Br J Obstet Gynaecol* **97**(10):922–9.

Jacobs IJ, Skates SJ, MacDonald N, et al. (1999) Screening for ovarian cancer: a pilot randomised controlled trial. *Lancet* **353**(9160):1207–10.

Jobling T, Mamers P, Healy DL, et al. (1994) A prospective study of inhibin in granulosa cell tumors of the ovary. *Gynecol Oncol* **55**(2):285–9.

Kainz C, Sliutz G, Mustafa G, et al. (1995) Cytokeratin subunit 19 measured by CYFRA 21-1 assay in follow-up of cervical cancer. *Gynecol Oncol* **56**(3):402–5.

Kang WD, Choi HS, Kim SM (2009) Value of serum CA125 levels in patients with high-risk, early stage epithelial ovarian cancer. *Gynecol Oncol*.

Karlan BY, Baldwin RL, Lopez-Luevanos E, et al. (1999) Peritoneal serous papillary carcinoma, a phenotypic variant of familial ovarian cancer: implications for ovarian cancer screening. *Am J Obstet Gynecol* **180**(4):917–28.

Kato H, Torigoe T (1977) Radioimmunoassay for tumor antigen of human cervical squamous cell carcinoma. *Cancer* **40**(4):1621–8.

Kawai M, Kano T, Kikkawa F, et al. (1992) Seven tumor markers in benign and malignant germ cell tumors of the ovary. *Gynecol Oncol* **45**(3):248–53.

Khanlian SA, Cole LA (2006) Management of gestational trophoblastic disease and other cases with low serum levels of human chorionic gonadotropin. *J Reprod Med* **51**(10):812–8.

Khanlian SA, Smith HO, Cole LA (2003) Persistent low levels of human chorionic gonadotropin: a premalignant gestational trophoblastic disease. *Am J Obstet Gynecol* **188**(5):1254–9.

Kim JH, Skates SJ, Uede T, et al. (2002) Osteopontin as a potential diagnostic biomarker for ovarian cancer. *Jama* **287**(13):1671–9.

Kim K, Visintin I, Alvero AB, et al. (2009) Development and validation of a protein-based signature for the detection of ovarian cancer. *Clin Lab Med* **29**(1):47–55.

Kim YT, Yoon BS, Kim JW, et al. (2005) Pretreatment levels of serum squamous cell carcinoma antigen and urine polyamines in women with squamous cell carcinoma of the cervix. *Int J Gynaecol Obstet* **91**(1):47–52.

Kobayashi F, Sagawa N, Nanbu Y, et al. (1989) Immunohistochemical localization and tissue levels of tumor-associated glycoproteins CA 125 and CA 19-9 in the decidua and fetal membranes at various gestational ages. *Am J Obstet Gynecol* **160**(5 Pt 1):1232–8.

Kobayashi H, Yamada Y, Sado T, et al. (2007) A randomized study of screening for ovarian cancer: a multicenter study in Japan. *Int J Gynecol Cancer*.

Kohorn EI (2002) Persistent low-level "real" human chorionic gonadotropin: a clinical challenge and a therapeutic dilemma. *Gynecol Oncol* **85**(2):315–20.

Kozak KR, Su F, Whitelegge JP, et al. (2005) Characterization of serum biomarkers for detection of early stage ovarian cancer. *Proteomics* **5**(17):4589–96.

Kuk C, Kulasingam V, Gunawardana CG, et al. (2009) Mining the ovarian cancer ascites proteome for potential ovarian cancer biomarkers. *Mol Cell Proteomics* **8**(4):661–9.

Kurihara T, Mizunuma H, Obara M, et al. (1998) Determination of a normal level of serum CA125 in postmenopausal women as a tool for preoperative evaluation and postoperative surveillance of endometrial carcinoma. *Gynecol Oncol* **69**(3):192–6.

Lai CH, Huang KG, See LC, et al. (2004) Restaging of recurrent cervical carcinoma with dual-phase [18F]fluoro-2-deoxy-D-glucose positron emission tomography. *Cancer* **100**(3):544–52.

Lai CH, Yen TC, Chang TC (2007) Positron emission tomography imaging for gynecologic malignancy. *Curr Opin Obstet Gynecol* **19**(1):37–41.

Lambeck AJ, Crijns AP, Leffers N, et al. (2007) Serum cytokine profiling as a diagnostic and prognostic tool in ovarian cancer: a potential role for interleukin 7. *Clin Cancer Res* **13**(8):2385–91.

Lappohn RE, Burger HG, Bouma J, et al. (1989) Inhibin as a marker for granulosa-cell tumors. *N Engl J Med* **321**(12):790–3.

Lavin PT, Knapp RC, Malkasian G, et al. (1987) CA 125 for the monitoring of ovarian carcinoma during primary therapy. *Obstet Gynecol* **69**(2):223–7.

Leminen A, Alftan H, Stenman UH, et al. (1992) Chemotherapy as initial treatment for cervical carcinoma: clinical and tumor marker response. *Acta Obstet Gynecol Scand* **71**(4):293–7.

Li XQ, Zhang SL, Cai Z, et al. (2009) Proteomic identification of tumor-associated protein in ovarian serous cystadenocarinoma. *Cancer Lett* **275**(1):109–16.

Lo SS, Cheng DK, Ng TY, et al. (1997) Prognostic significance of tumour markers in endometrial cancer. *Tumour Biol* **18**(4):241–9.

Lopez MF, Mikulskis A, Kuzdzal S, et al. (2007) A novel, high-throughput workflow for discovery and identification of serum carrier protein-bound peptide biomarker candidates in ovarian cancer samples. *Clin Chem* **53**(6):1067–74.

Lozza L, Merola M, Fontanelli R, et al. (1997) Cancer of the uterine cervix: clinical value of squamous cell carcinoma antigen (SCC) measurements. *Anticancer Res* **17**(1B):525–9.

Lu KH, Gershenson DM (2005) Update on the management of ovarian germ cell tumors. *J Reprod Med* **50**(6):417–25.

Lundstrom MS, Hogdall CK, Nielsen AL, et al. (2000) Serum tetranectin and CA125 in endometrial adenocarcinoma. *Anticancer Res* **20**(5C):3903–6.

Ma S, Shen K, Lang J (2003) A risk of malignancy index in preoperative diagnosis of ovarian cancer. *Chin Med J (Engl)* **116**(3):396–9.

Makar AP, Kristensen GB, Bormer OP, et al. (1993) Is serum CA 125 at the time of relapse a prognostic indicator for further survival prognosis in patients with ovarian cancer? *Gynecol Oncol* **49**(1):3–7.

Manchanda R, Rosenthal A, Burnell M, et al. (2009) Change in stage distribution observed with annual screening for ovarian cancer in BRCA carriers. *J Med Genet* **46**(6):423–4.

Manjunath AP, Pratapkumar Sujatha K, Vani R, et al. (2001) Comparison of three risk of malignancy indices in evaluation of pelvic masses. *Gynecol Oncol* **81**(2):225–9.

Mann K, Saller B, Hoermann R (1993) Clinical use of HCG and hCG beta determinations. *Scand J Clin Lab Invest Suppl* **216**:97–104.

Markman M, Liu PY, Rothenberg ML, et al. (2006) Pretreatment CA-125 and risk of relapse in advanced ovarian cancer. *J Clin Oncol* **24**(9):1454–8.

Massuger LF, Koper NP, Thomas CM, et al. (1997) Improvement of clinical staging in cervical cancer with serum squamous cell carcinoma antigen and CA 125 determinations. *Gynecol Oncol* **64**(3):473–6.

McGuckin MA, Layton GT, Bailey MJ, et al. (1990) Evaluation of two new assays for tumor-associated antigens, CASA and OSA, found in the serum of patients with epithelial ovarian carcinoma – comparison with CA125. *Gynecol Oncol* **37**(2):165–71.

McIntosh M, Anderson G, Drescher C, et al. (2008) Ovarian cancer early detection claims are biased. *Clin Cancer Res* **14**(22):7574; author reply 7–9.

McShane LM, Altman DG, Sauerbrei W, et al. (2005) REporting recommendations for tumor MARKer prognostic studies (REMARK). *Nat Clin Pract Oncol* **2**(8):416–22.

Medl M, Ogris E, Peters-Engl C, et al. (1995) TATI (tumour-associated trypsin inhibitor) as a marker of ovarian cancer. *Br J Cancer* **71**(5):1051–4.

Menon U, Gentry-Maharaj A, Hallett R, et al. (2009) Sensitivity and specificity of multimodal and ultrasound screening for ovarian cancer, and stage distribution of detected cancers: results of the prevalence screen of the UK Collaborative Trial of Ovarian Cancer Screening (UKCTOCS). *Lancet Oncol* **10**(4):327–40.

Menon U, Skates SJ, Lewis S, et al. (2005) Prospective study using the risk of ovarian cancer algorithm to screen for ovarian cancer. *J Clin Oncol* **23**(31):7919–26.

Menon U, Talaat A, Jeyarajah AR, et al. (1999) Ultrasound assessment of ovarian cancer risk in postmenopausal women with CA125 elevation. *Br J Cancer* **80**(10):1644–7.

Menon U, Talaat A, Rosenthal AN, et al. (2000) Performance of ultrasound as a second line test to serum CA125 in ovarian cancer screening. *BJOG* **107**(2):165–9.

Mitchell H, Seckl MJ (2007) Discrepancies between commercially available immunoassays in the detection of tumour-derived hCG. *Mol Cell Endocrinol* **260–262**:310–3.

Mogensen O (1992) Prognostic value of CA 125 in advanced ovarian cancer. *Gynecol Oncol* **44**(3):207–12.

Mok SC, Chao J, Skates S, et al. (2001) Prostasin, a potential serum marker for ovarian cancer: identification through microarray technology. *J Natl Cancer Inst* **93**(19):1458–64.

Molina R, Filella X, Auge JM, et al. (2005) CYFRA 21.1 in patients with cervical cancer: comparison with SCC and CEA. *Anticancer Res* **25**(3A):1765–71.

Montagnana M, Lippi G, Danese E, et al. (2009) Usefulness of serum HE4 in endometriotic cysts. *Br J Cancer* **101**(3):548.

Moore RG, Brown AK, Miller MC, et al. (2008) The use of multiple novel tumor biomarkers for the detection of ovarian carcinoma in patients with a pelvic mass. *Gynecol Oncol* **108**(2):402–8.

Moore RG, McMeekin DS, Brown AK, et al. (2009) A novel multiple marker bioassay utilizing HE4 and CA125 for the prediction of ovarian cancer in patients with a pelvic mass. *Gynecol Oncol* **112**(1):40–6.

Mor G, Visintin I, Lai Y, et al. (2005) Serum protein markers for early detection of ovarian cancer. *Proc Natl Acad Sci USA* **102**(21):7677–82.

Morgante G, la Marca A, Ditto A, et al. (1999) Comparison of two malignancy risk indices based on serum CA125, ultrasound score and menopausal status in the diagnosis of ovarian masses. *Br J Obstet Gynaecol* **106**(6):524–7.

Muramatsu T, Mukai M, Sato S, et al. (2005) Clinical usefulness of serum and immunohistochemical markers in patients with stage Ia and Ic ovarian cancer. *Oncol Rep* **14**(4):861–5.

Murugaesu N, Schmid P, Dancey G, et al. (2006) Malignant ovarian germ cell tumors: identification of novel prognostic markers and long-term outcome after multimodality treatment. *J Clin Oncol* **24**(30):4862–6.

Mustea A, Braicu EI, Koensgen D, et al. (2009) Monitoring of IL-10 in the serum of patients with advanced ovarian cancer: results from a prospective pilot-study. *Cytokine* **45**(1):8–11.

Myers ER, Bastian LA, Havrilesky LJ, et al. (2006) Management of adnexal mass. *Evid Rep Technol Assess (Full Rep)* **130**:1–145.

Nakae M, Iwamoto I, Fujino T, et al. (2006) Preoperative plasma osteopontin level as a biomarker complementary to carbohydrate antigen 125 in predicting ovarian cancer. *J Obstet Gynaecol Res* **32**(3):309–14.

Negishi Y, Iwabuchi H, Sakunaga H, et al. (1993) Serum and tissue measurements of CA72-4 in ovarian cancer patients. *Gynecol Oncol* **48**(2):148–54.

Ngan HY, Bender H, Benedet JL, et al. (2003a) Gestational trophoblastic neoplasia, FIGO 2000 staging and classification. *Int J Gynaecol Obstet* **83**(Suppl 1):175–7.

Ngan HY, Cheung AN, Lauder IJ, et al. (1996) Prognostic significance of serum tumour markers in carcinoma of the cervix. *Eur J Gynaecol Oncol* **17**(6):512–7.

Ngan HY, Odicino F, Maisonneuve P, et al. (2003b) Gestational trophoblastic diseases. *Int J Gynaecol Obstet* **83**(Suppl 1):167–74.

Ngan S, Seckl MJ (2007) Gestational trophoblastic neoplasia management: an update. *Curr Opin Oncol* **19**(5):486–91.

NIH consensus conference (1995) Ovarian cancer. Screening, treatment, and follow-up. NIH Consensus Development Panel on Ovarian Cancer. *JAMA* **273**(6):491–7.

Niibe Y, Kazumoto T, Toita T, et al. (2006) Frequency and characteristics of isolated para-aortic lymph node recurrence in patients with uterine cervical carcinoma in Japan: a multi-institutional study. *Gynecol Oncol* **103**(2):435–8.

Nosov V, Su F, Amneus M, et al. (2009) Validation of serum biomarkers for detection of early-stage ovarian cancer. *Am J Obstet Gynecol* **200**(6):639 e1–5.

Nustad K, Bast RC Jr, Brien TJ, et al. (1996) Specificity and affinity of 26 monoclonal antibodies against the CA 125 antigen: first report from the ISOBM TD-1 workshop. International Society for Oncodevelopmental Biology and Medicine. *Tumour Biol* **17**(4):196–219.

Obermair A, Fuller A, Lopez-Varela E, et al. (2007) A new prognostic model for FIGO stage 1 epithelial ovarian cancer. *Gynecol Oncol* **104**(3):607–11.

Ogino I, Nakayama H, Kitamura T, et al. (2005) The curative role of radiotherapy in patients with isolated para-aortic node recurrence from cervical cancer and value of squamous cell carcinoma antigen for early detection. *Int J Gynecol Cancer* **15**(4):630–8.

Ogino I, Nakayama H, Okamoto N, et al. (2006) The role of pretreatment squamous cell carcinoma antigen level in locally advanced squamous cell carcinoma of the uterine cervix treated by radiotherapy. *Int J Gynecol Cancer* **16**(3):1094–100.

Oh JH, Gao J, Nandi A, et al. (2005) Diagnosis of early relapse in ovarian cancer using serum proteomic profiling. *Genome Inform* **16**(2):195–204.

Oikonomopoulou K, Li L, Zheng Y, et al. (2008) Prediction of ovarian cancer prognosis and response to chemotherapy by a serum-based multiparametric biomarker panel. *Br J Cancer* **99**(7):1103–13.

Olt G, Berchuck A, Bast RC Jr (1990) The role of tumor markers in gynecologic oncology. *Obstet Gynecol Surv* **45**(9):570–7.

Onsrud M (1991) Tumour markers in gynaecologic oncology. *Scand J Clin Lab Invest Suppl* **206**:60–70.

Ozturk M, Berkowitz R, Goldstein D, et al. (1988) Differential production of human chorionic gonadotropin and free subunits in gestational trophoblastic disease. *Am J Obstet Gynecol* **158**(1):193–8.

Pandian R, Lu J, Ossolinska-Plewnia J (2003) Fully automated chemiluminometric assay for hyperglycosylated human chorionic gonadotropin (invasive trophoblast antigen). *Clin Chem* **49**(5):808–10.

Paramasivam S, Tripcony L, Crandon A, et al. (2005) Prognostic importance of preoperative CA-125 in International Federation of Gynecology and Obstetrics stage I epithelial ovarian cancer: an Australian multicenter study. *J Clin Oncol* **23**(25):5938–42.

Partridge E, Kreimer AR, Greenlee RT, et al. (2009) Results from four rounds of ovarian cancer screening in a randomized trial. *Obstet Gynecol* **113**(4):775–82.

Patterson DM, Rustin GJ (2006) Controversies in the management of germ cell tumours of the ovary. *Curr Opin Oncol* **18**(5):500–6.

Pauler DK, Menon U, McIntosh M, et al. (2001) Factors influencing serum CA125II levels in healthy postmenopausal women. *Cancer Epidemiol Biomarkers Prev* **10**(5):489–93.

Pectasides D, Pectasides E, Psyrri A (2007) Granulosa cell tumor of the ovary. *Cancer Treat Rev*

Pepe MS, Etzioni R, Feng Z, et al. (2001) Phases of biomarker development for early detection of cancer. *J Natl Cancer Inst* **93**(14):1054–61.

Peters-Engl C, Medl M, Ogris E, et al. (1995) Tumor-associated trypsin inhibitor (TATI) and cancer antigen 125 (CA125) in patients with epithelial ovarian cancer. *Anticancer Res* **15**(6B):2727–30.

Peters-Engl C, Obermair A, Heinzl H, et al. (1999) CA 125 regression after two completed cycles of chemotherapy: lack of prediction for long-term survival in patients with advanced ovarian cancer. *Br J Cancer* **81**(4):662–6.

Petraglia F, Luisi S, Pautier P, et al. (1998) Inhibin B is the major form of inhibin/activin family secreted by granulosa cell tumors. *J Clin Endocrinol Metab* **83**(3):1029–32.

Petri AL, Hogdall E, Christensen IJ, et al. (2006) Preoperative CA125 as a prognostic factor in stage I epithelial ovarian cancer. *Apmis* **114**(5):359–63.

Petri AL, Simonsen AH, Yip TT, et al. (2009) Three new potential ovarian cancer biomarkers detected in human urine with equalizer bead technology. *Acta Obstet Gynecol Scand* **88**(1):18–26.

Petricoin EF, Ardekani AM, Hitt BA, et al. (2002) Use of proteomic patterns in serum to identify ovarian cancer. *Lancet* **359**(9306):572–7.

Powell JL, Hill KA, Shiro BC, et al. (2005) Preoperative serum CA-125 levels in treating endometrial cancer. *J Reprod Med* **50**(8):585–90.

Pras E, Willemse PH, Canrinus AA, et al. (2002) Serum squamous cell carcinoma antigen and CYFRA 21-1 in cervical cancer treatment. *Int J Radiat Oncol Biol Phys* **52**(1):23–32.

Price FV, Chambers SK, Carcangiu ML, et al. (1998) CA 125 may not reflect disease status in patients with uterine serous carcinoma. *Cancer* **82**(9):1720–5.

Price FV, Chambers SK, Chambers JT, et al. (1993) Colony-stimulating factor-1 in primary ascites of ovarian cancer is a significant predictor of survival. *Am J Obstet Gynecol* **168**(2):520–7.

Rai AJ, Zhang Z, Rosenzweig J, et al. (2002) Proteomic approaches to tumor marker discovery. *Arch Pathol Lab Med* **126**(12):1518–26.

Redman CW, Blackledge GR, Kelly K, et al. (1990) Early serum CA125 response and outcome in epithelial ovarian cancer. *Eur J Cancer* **26**(5):593–6.

Reesink-Peters N, van der Velden J, Ten Hoor KA, et al. (2005) Preoperative serum squamous cell carcinoma antigen levels in clinical decision making for patients with early-stage cervical cancer. *J Clin Oncol* **23**(7):1455–62.

Reis LAG, Melbert D, Krapcho M, et al. (2007) SEER Cancer Statistics Review, 1975–2004. Available from: http://seer.cancer.gov/csr/1975_2004/, based on November 6 SEER data submission, posted to the SEER web site, 7. [Cited January 1, 2008].

Riedinger JM, Wafflart J, Ricolleau G, et al. (2006) CA 125 half-life and CA 125 nadir during induction chemotherapy are independent predictors of epithelial ovarian cancer outcome: results of a French multicentric study. *Ann Oncol* **17**(8):1234–8.

Rinne K, Shahabi S, Cole L (1999) Following metastatic placental site trophoblastic tumor with urine beta-core fragment. *Gynecol Oncol* **74**(2):302–3.

Robertson DM, Pruysers E, Burger HG, et al. (2004) Inhibins and ovarian cancer. *Mol Cell Endocrinol* **225**(1–2):65–71.

Roman LD, Muderspach LI, Burnett AF, et al. (1998) Carcinoembryonic antigen in women with isolated pelvic masses. Clinical utility? *J Reprod Med* **43**(5):403–7.

Rosenthal A, Jacobs I (2006) Familial ovarian cancer screening. *Best Pract Res Clin Obstet Gynaecol* **20**(2):321–38.

Rosenthal AN, Menon U, Jacobs IJ (2006) Screening for ovarian cancer. *Clin Obstet Gynecol* **49**(3):433–47.

Rotmensch S, Cole LA (2000) False diagnosis and needless therapy of presumed malignant disease in women with false-positive human chorionic gonadotropin concentrations. *Lancet* **355**(9205):712–5.

Rustin G, van der Burg ME (2009) A randomized trial in ovarian cancer (OC) of early treatment of relapse based on CA 125 level alone versus delayed treatment based on conventional clinical indicators (MRC OVO5/EORTC 55955 trials). *J Clin Oncol* **27**(15 Suppl)(5s):Abstract 1.

Rustin GJ, Gennings JN, Nelstrop AE, et al. (1989) Use of CA-125 to predict survival of patients with ovarian carcinoma. North Thames Cooperative Group. *J Clin Oncol* **7**(11):1667–71.

Rustin GJ, Marples M, Nelstrop AE, et al. (2001) Use of CA-125 to define progression of ovarian cancer in patients with persistently elevated levels. *J Clin Oncol* **19**(20):4054–7.

Rustin GJ, Nelstrop AE, McClean P, et al. (1996a) Defining response of ovarian carcinoma to initial chemotherapy according to serum CA 125. *J Clin Oncol* **14**(5):1545–51.

Rustin GJ, Nelstrop AE, Tuxen MK, et al. (1996b) Defining progression of ovarian carcinoma during follow-up according to CA 125: a North Thames Ovary Group Study. *Ann Oncol* **7**(4):361–4.

Rustin GJ, Quinn M, Thigpen T, et al. (2004) Re: New guidelines to evaluate the response to treatment in solid tumors (ovarian cancer). *J Natl Cancer Inst* **96**(6):487–8.

Salman T, el-Ahmady O, Sawsan MR, et al. (1995) The clinical value of serum TPS in gynecological malignancies. *Int J Biol Markers* **10**(2):81–6.

Sarandakou A, Protonotariou E, Rizos D (2007) Tumor markers in biological fluids associated with pregnancy. *Crit Rev Clin Lab Sci* **44**(2):151–78.

Scambia G, Benedetti Panici P, Foti E, et al. (1994a) Squamous cell carcinoma antigen: prognostic significance and role in the monitoring of neoadjuvant chemotherapy response in cervical cancer. *J Clin Oncol* **12**(11):2309–16.

Scambia G, Benedetti Panici P, Perrone L, et al. (1990) Serum levels of tumour associated glycoprotein (TAG 72) in patients with gynaecological malignancies. *Br J Cancer* **62**(1):147–51.

Scambia G, Gadducci A, Panici PB, et al. (1994b) Combined use of CA 125 and CA 15-3 in patients with endometrial carcinoma. *Gynecol Oncol* **54**(3):292–7.

Scambia G, Testa U, Benedetti Panici P, et al. (1995) Prognostic significance of interleukin 6 serum levels in patients with ovarian cancer. *Br J Cancer* **71**(2):354–6.

Schmidt-Rhode P, Schulz KD, Sturm G, et al. (1988) Squamous cell carcinoma antigen for monitoring cervical cancer. *Int J Biol Markers* **3**(2):87–94.

Scholl SM, Bascou CH, Mosseri V, et al. (1994) Circulating levels of colony-stimulating factor 1 as a prognostic indicator in 82 patients with epithelial ovarian cancer. *Br J Cancer* **69**(2):342–6.

Screening for ovarian cancer: recommendations and rationale (1994). American College of Physicians. *Ann Intern Med* **121**(2):141–2.

Seckl MJ, Fisher RA, Salerno G, et al. (2000) Choriocarcinoma and partial hydatidiform moles. *Lancet* **356**(9223):36–9.

Sedlakova I, Vavrova J, Tosner J, et al. (2008) Lysophosphatidic acid: an ovarian cancer marker. *Eur J Gynaecol Oncol* **29**(5):511–4.

Seidman JD, Horkayne-Szakaly I, Haiba M, et al. (2004) The histologic type and stage distribution of ovarian carcinomas of surface epithelial origin. *Int J Gynecol Pathol* **23**(1):41–4.

Seki K, Matsui H, Sekiya S (2004) Advances in the clinical laboratory detection of gestational trophoblastic disease. *Clin Chim Acta* **349**(1–2):1–13.

Shabana A, Onsrud M (1994) Tissue polypeptide-specific antigen and CA 125 as serum tumor markers in ovarian carcinoma. *Tumour Biol* **15**(6):361–7.

Skates SJ, Drescher CW, Isaacs C, et al. (2007) A prospective multi-center ovarian cancer screening study in women at increased risk. American Society of Clinical Oncology; 2007. *J Clin Oncol* **25**(18S):276s.

Skates SJ, Horick N, Yu Y, et al. (2004) Preoperative sensitivity and specificity for early-stage ovarian cancer when combining cancer antigen CA-125II, CA 15-3, CA 72-4, and macrophage colony-stimulating factor using mixtures of multivariate normal distributions. *J Clin Oncol* **22**(20):4059–66.

Skates SJ, Menon U, MacDonald N, et al. (2003) Calculation of the risk of ovarian cancer from serial CA-125 values for preclinical detection in post-menopausal women. *J Clin Oncol* **21**(Suppl 10):206–10.

Skates SJ, Xu FJ, Yu YH, et al. (1995) Toward an optimal algorithm for ovarian cancer screening with longitudinal tumor markers. *Cancer* **76**(Suppl 10):2004–10.

Sliutz G, Tempfer C, Kainz C, et al. (1995) Tissue polypeptide specific antigen and cancer associated serum antigen in the follow-up of ovarian cancer. *Anticancer Res* **15**(3):1127–9.

Soletormos G, Nielsen D, Schioler V, et al. (1996) Tumor markers cancer antigen 15.3, carcinoembryonic antigen, and tissue polypeptide antigen for monitoring metastatic breast cancer during first-line chemotherapy and follow-up. *Clin Chem* **42**(4):564–75.

Sood AK, Buller RE, Burger RA, et al. (1997) Value of preoperative CA 125 level in the management of uterine cancer and prediction of clinical outcome. *Obstet Gynecol* **90**(3):441–7.

Spitzer M, Kaushal V, Benjamin F (1998) Maternal CA-125 levels in pregnancy and the puerperium. *J Reprod Med* **43**(4):387–92.

Stenman UH, Alfthan H, Vartiainen J, et al. (1995) Markers supplementing CA 125 in ovarian cancer. *Ann Med* **27**(1):115–20.

Sturgeon CM, Duffy MJ, Stenman UH, et al. (2008) National Academy of Clinical Biochemistry laboratory medicine practice guidelines for use of tumor markers in testicular, prostate, colorectal, breast, and ovarian cancers. *Clin Chem* **54**(12):e11–79.

Su F, Lang J, Kumar A, et al. (2007) Validation of candidate serum ovarian cancer biomarkers for early detection. *Biomark Insights* **2**:369–75.

Su YN, Cheng WF, Chen CA, et al. (1999) Pregnancy with primary tubal placental site trophoblastic tumor—a case report and literature review. *Gynecol Oncol* **73**(2):322–5.

Suresh MR (1996) Classification of tumor markers. *Anticancer Res* **16**(4B):2273–7.

Suzuki M, Kobayashi H, Ohwada M, et al. (1998) Macrophage colony-stimulating factor as a marker for malignant germ cell tumors of the ovary. *Gynecol Oncol* **68**(1):35–7.

Suzuki M, Ohwada M, Aida I, et al. (1993) Macrophage colony-stimulating factor as a tumor marker for epithelial ovarian cancer. *Obstet Gynecol* **82**(6):946–50.

Suzuki M, Ohwada M, Sato I, et al. (1995) Serum level of macrophage colony-stimulating factor as a marker for gynecologic malignancies. *Oncology* **52**(2):128–33.

Takahashi K, Yamane Y, Yoshino K, et al. (1985) Studies on serum CA125 levels in pregnant women. *Nippon Sanka Fujinka Gakkai Zasshi* **37**(9):1931–4.

Tamakoshi K, Kikkawa F, Shibata K, et al. (1996) Clinical value of CA125, CA19-9, CEA, CA72-4, and TPA in borderline ovarian tumor. *Gynecol Oncol* **62**(1):67–72.

Tempfer C, Hefler L, Haeusler G, et al. (1998) Tissue polypeptide specific antigen in the follow-up of ovarian and cervical cancer patients. *Int J Cancer* **79**(3):241–4.

Terracciano D, Mariano A, Macchia V, et al. (2005) Analysis of glycoproteins in human colon cancers, normal tissues and in human colon carcinoma cells reactive with monoclonal antibody NCL-19-9. *Oncol Rep* **14**(3):719–22.

Tham BW, Everard JE, Tidy JA, et al. (2003) Gestational trophoblastic disease in the Asian population of Northern England and North Wales. *BJOG* **110**(6):555–9.

Timmerman D, Testa AC, Bourne T, et al. (2005) Logistic regression model to distinguish between the benign and malignant adnexal mass before surgery: a multicenter study by the International Ovarian Tumor Analysis Group. *J Clin Oncol* **23**(34):8794–801.

Timmerman D, Van Calster B, Jurkovic D, et al. (2007) Inclusion of CA-125 does not improve mathematical models developed to distinguish between benign and malignant adnexal tumors. *J Clin Oncol* **25**(27):4194–200.

Timmerman D, Verrelst H, Bourne TH, et al. (1999) Artificial neural network models for the preoperative discrimination between malignant and benign adnexal masses. *Ultrasound Obstet Gynecol* **13**(1):17–25.

Timms JF, Arslan-Low E, Gentry-Maharaj A, et al. (2007) Preanalytic influence of sample handling on SELDI-TOF serum protein profiles. *Clin Chem*.

Tingulstad S, Hagen B, Skjeldestad FE, et al. (1996) Evaluation of a risk of malignancy index based on serum CA125, ultrasound findings and menopausal status in the pre-operative diagnosis of pelvic masses. *Br J Obstet Gynaecol* **103**(8):826–31.

Tsai SC, Kao CH, Wang SJ (1996) Study of a new tumor marker, CYFRA 21-1, in squamous cell carcinoma of the cervix, and comparison with squamous cell carcinoma antigen. *Neoplasma* **43**(1):27–9.

Tsigkou A, Marrelli D, Reis FM, et al. (2007) Total inhibin is a potential serum marker for epithelial ovarian cancer. *J Clin Endocrinol Metab*.

Tuxen MK, Soletormos G, Dombernowsky P (1995) Tumor markers in the management of patients with ovarian cancer. *Cancer Treat Rev* **21**(3): 215–45.

Tuxen MK, Soletormos G, Dombernowsky P (2001) Serum tumour marker CA 125 in monitoring of ovarian cancer during first-line chemotherapy. *Br J Cancer* **84**(10):1301–7.

Tuxen MK, Soletormos G, Dombernowsky P (2002) Serum tumor marker CA 125 for monitoring ovarian cancer during follow-up. *Scand J Clin Lab Invest* **62**(3):177–88.

Tuxen MK, Soletormos G, Petersen PH, et al. (1999) Assessment of biological variation and analytical imprecision of CA 125, CEA, and TPA in relation to monitoring of ovarian cancer. *Gynecol Oncol* **74**(1):12–22.

Tuxen MK, Soletormos G, Rustin GJ, et al. (2000) Biological variation and analytical imprecision of CA 125 in patients with ovarian cancer. *Scand J Clin Lab Invest* **60**(8):713–21.

UKFOCSS. United Kingdom Familial Ovarian Cancer Screening Study (protocol). London: Gynaecological Cancer Research Centre, EGA Institute for Women's Health, University College London, United Kingdom http://www.instituteforwomenshealth.ucl.ac.uk/academic_research/gynaecological cancer/gcrc/ukfocss/.

Ulusoy S, Akbayir O, Numanoglu C, et al. (2007) The risk of malignancy index in discrimination of adnexal masses. *Int J Gynaecol Obstet* **96**(3):186–91.

Urbancsek J, Hauzman EE, Lagarde AR, et al. (2005) Serum CA-125 levels in the second week after embryo transfer predict clinical pregnancy. *Fertil Steril* **83**(5):1414–21.

Vaitukaitis JL, Braunstein GD, Ross GT (1972) A radioimmunoassay which specifically measures human chorionic gonadotropin in the presence of human luteinizing hormone. *Am J Obstet Gynecol* **113**(6):751–8.

van Dalen A, Favier J, Baumgartner L, et al. (1999) Prognostic significance of CA 125 and TPS levels after chemotherapy in ovarian cancer patients. *Anticancer Res* **19**(4A):2523–6.

van der Burg ME, Lammes FB, van Putten WL, et al. (1988) Ovarian cancer: the prognostic value of the serum half-life of CA125 during induction chemotherapy. *Gynecol Oncol* **30**(3):307–12.

van der Merwe DE, Oikonomopoulou K, Marshall J, et al. (2007) Mass spectrometry: uncovering the cancer proteome for diagnostics. *Adv Cancer Res* **96**:23–50.

van Haaften-Day C, Shen Y, Xu F, et al. (2001) OVX1, macrophage-colony stimulating factor, and CA-125-II as tumor markers for epithelial ovarian carcinoma: a critical appraisal. *Cancer* **92**(11):2837–44.

Van Holsbeke C, Van Calster B, Valentin L, et al. (2007) External validation of mathematical models to distinguish between benign and malignant adnexal tumors: a multicenter study by the International Ovarian Tumor Analysis Group. *Clin Cancer Res* **13**(15 Pt 1):4440–7.

van Trappen PO, Rufford BD, Mills TD, et al. (2007) Differential diagnosis of adnexal masses: risk of malignancy index, ultrasonography, magnetic resonance imaging, and radioimmunoscintigraphy. *Int J Gynecol Cancer* **17**(1):61–7.

Vartiainen J, Lehtovirta P, Finne P, et al. (2001) Preoperative serum concentration of hCGbeta as a prognostic factor in ovarian cancer. *Int J Cancer* **95**(5):313–6.

Vasey PA, Herrstedt J, Jelic S (2005) ESMO Minimum Clinical Recommendations for diagnosis, treatment and follow-up of epithelial ovarian carcinoma. *Ann Oncol* **16**(Suppl 1):i13–15.

Vergote IB, Bormer OP, Abeler VM (1987) Evaluation of serum CA 125 levels in the monitoring of ovarian cancer. *Am J Obstet Gynecol* **157**(1):88–92.

Verheijen RH, von Mensdorff-Pouilly S, van Kamp GJ, et al. (1999) CA 125: fundamental and clinical aspects. *Semin Cancer Biol* **9**(2):117–24.

Visintin I, Feng Z, Longton G, et al. (2008) Diagnostic markers for early detection of ovarian cancer. *Clin Cancer Res*.

Ward BG, McGuckin MA, Ramm LE, et al. (1993) The management of ovarian carcinoma is improved by the use of cancer-associated serum antigen and CA 125 assays. *Cancer* **71**(2):430–8.

Ward G, McKinnon L, Badrick T, et al. (1997) Heterophilic antibodies remain a problem for the immunoassay laboratory. *Am J Clin Pathol* **108**(4):417–21.

Welt CK, Lambert-Messerlian G, Zheng W, et al. (1997) Presence of activin, inhibin, and follistatin in epithelial ovarian carcinoma. *J Clin Endocrinol Metab* **82**(11):3720–7.

Xiong Y, Peng XP, Liang LZ, et al. (2009) Clinical significance of combined examination of pretreatment serum CYFRA21-1 and SCCAg in cervical cancer patients. *Chin J Cancer* **28**(1):64–7.

Yamashita K, Yamoto M, Shikone T, et al. (1997) Production of inhibin A and inhibin B in human ovarian sex cord stromal tumors. *Am J Obstet Gynecol* **177**(6):1450–7.

Yazbek J, Aslam N, Tailor A, et al. (2006) A comparative study of the risk of malignancy index and the ovarian crescent sign for the diagnosis of invasive ovarian cancer. *Ultrasound Obstet Gynecol* **28**(3):320–4.

Yazigi R, Munoz AK, Richardson B, et al. (1991) Correlation of squamous cell carcinoma antigen levels and treatment response in cervical cancer. *Gynecol Oncol* **41**(2):135–8.

Yoon SM, Shin KH, Kim JY, et al. (2007) The clinical values of squamous cell carcinoma antigen and carcinoembryonic antigen in patients with cervical cancer treated with concurrent chemoradiotherapy. *Int J Gynecol Cancer* **17**(4):872–8.

Zhang Z, Barnhill SD, Zhang H, et al. (1999) Combination of multiple serum markers using an artificial neural network to improve specificity in discriminating malignant from benign pelvic masses. *Gynecol Oncol* **73**(1):56–61.

Zhang Z, Bast RC Jr, Yu Y, et al. (2004) Three biomarkers identified from serum proteomic analysis for the detection of early stage ovarian cancer. *Cancer Res* **64**(16):5882–90.

Zhang Z, Yu Y, Xu F, et al. (2007) Combining multiple serum tumor markers improves detection of stage I epithelial ovarian cancer. *Gynecol Oncol* **107**(3):526–31.

Zurawski VR Jr, Orjaseter H, Andersen A, et al. (1988) Elevated serum CA 125 levels prior to diagnosis of ovarian neoplasia: relevance for early detection of ovarian cancer. *Int J Cancer* **42**(5):677–80.

8 Cone biopsy
Giuseppe Del Priore

INTRODUCTION

The cone biopsy—removal of a cone-shaped portion of the cervix—has been performed by gynecologists for decades. Several methods exist for obtaining this specimen. These include an electrosurgical technique, laser or scalpel method of excision. The electrosurgical technique referred to as the *loop electrosurgical excision procedure* (LEEP) or *loop excision of the transformation zone* (LETZ) has gained popularity. It has several advantages over the other methods. These include less immediate bleeding and discomfort. It is therefore possible to perform LEEP in the office without general anesthesia. Although the surgical margins are cauterized, it still provides a reasonable specimen for pathologic interpretation with no clinically significant limitations. The scalpel and LEEP techniques are also generally equivalent in their clinically significant outcomes (i.e., cure rates). However, the scalpel cone tends to be larger, which is of no particular advantage except perhaps when used in patients with adenocarcinoma of the endocervix. Since this histology may be multifocal, a larger specimen may be more likely to remove all of the lesions. As there may still be, on occasion, the need to perform a scalpel cone biopsy, all gynecologists should be familiar with both techniques.

INDICATIONS

Cone biopsy is indicated for the diagnosis or exclusion of microinvasive cervical cancer as suggested on a presurgical Papanicolaou (Pap) smear or colposcopic punch biopsy. It could also be used to exclude and possibly treat endocervical adenocarcinoma. As mentioned above, a large scalpel cone biopsy may be a better option for these women. Cone biopsy, preferably by LEEP, is also indicated for patients with high-grade squamous epithelial lesions on Pap smear but no identifiable colposcopic lesion. Some advocate cone biopsy for larger cancers (e.g., IA2) with separate lymphadenectomy. In these cases, the cone seeks to avoid the morbidity of the parametrectomy of radical surgery.

ANATOMIC CONSIDERATIONS
Vascular Supply

A small descending branch of uterine artery supplies the cervix. It can usually be found laterally in the vaginal portion of the cervix at 3 and 9 o'clock positions. Despite its apparent accessible location, lateral stay sutures to occlude these vessels do so in less than half of all cases.

Innervation

The nerves of the cervix arise from the hypogastric plexus. Specific branches from this plexus to the cervix are sometimes known as the utero-vaginal plexus that are found in the broad ligament. Even more distal, the uterine cervical ganglion may be identified in the paracervical tissue closest to the cervix. The autonomic sympathetic nerves arise from the sympathetic trunk originating in the nerve roots from T10 to L1. The parasympathetics arise from the roots of S2 to S4.

Muscles Involved

The cervix sits above the urogenital diaphragm and, as such, does not have any direct muscle connection. Retaining the cervix during a supracervical hysterectomy or removing part of it during a cone biopsy does not have a significant effect on pelvic physiology or prolapse.

Bony Landmarks

The cervix lies roughly in the plane of the ischial spine, being slightly anterior and inferior to it. It is important to consider the bony pelvic outlet when contemplating operating transvaginally on the cervix. For cone biopsies, only the most contracted pelvis would present a significant limitation. Often, cases that seem impossible in the office are found to be feasible during general anesthesia with proper assistance and retraction.

SURGICAL PROCEDURE
Loop Electrosurgical Incision

The LEEP procedure begins with the proper positioning of the patient's legs. The standard office examination table with stirrups is usually sufficient. A speculum that is large enough to hold the vaginal wall away from the cervix should be inserted. An insulated speculum is not necessary. In fact, if the insulated speculum has an undetected break in its insulation, it may allow for a high-energy discharge and patient injury. A suction apparatus for evacuating the copious amount of smoke produced is absolutely essential. This may either be built into the speculum or clipped on to a standard one. Hand-held wall suction (e.g., Yankauer) is generally not adequate as it is usually too large to fit into the vagina simultaneously with the LEEP device. Immediately before the actual procedure, colposcopy is used to identify the lesion. In obese patients, the finger of a latex glove with the tip cut off may be used to assist in retraction of the vaginal walls. It is pulled over the speculum in a "condom like" application.

Local anesthesia should be administered circumferentially with a narrow gauge (e.g., 27-gauge reinforced Potocky needle). Larger needles will lead to significantly more bleeding. Any local anesthetic with epinephrine 1:100,000 will do. Since water dissipates the electrosurgical current, excess stromal injections may make the procedure difficult. Discomfort from the local injection can be minimized by having the patient cough simultaneously with placing the needle on the surface of the cervix. The movement inferiorly of the cervix during this Valsalva maneuver is usually all that is needed for the needle to painlessly enter the cervix. The anesthetic should be administered early to allow sufficient time for it to take effect (Fig. 1).

Different electrosurgical units have various settings and power sources. The only important parameter is current density at the electrosurgical wire surface. This is the actual energy that the cervix receives and is dependent on the length of the wire loop in contact with the tissue, the diameter or gauge of the wire itself, and the current setting. The highest current density possible should be used to minimize drag through the tissue and, consequently, cautery artifact. However, too high a current density will result in the loop wire breaking much like an incandescent light bulb filament. If this should happen, completing the procedure will be more difficult as the operator will have to begin with a new wire loop in the middle of the specimen. Trial and error using inanimate specimens may be needed to find the maximal power settings depending on the combination of generator and loop wires used.

After infiltration of the cervix, the operator should choose a loop size and shape that can remove the colposcopically identified acetowhite lesion with clear margins but no larger than necessary to avoid excessive cervical damage. However, if the cone is diagnostic, then the entire transformation zone should be removed. The operator should practice the hand motion to be used before actually turning on the current. Once a comfortable hand motion has been determined, the colposcope, used to identify the lesion and transformation zone, may be removed unless it has a very low magnification setting, since using the loop wire under colposcopic vision is unnecessarily difficult. Once everything has been rechecked, the operator applies the pure cutting current and smoothly passes the loop wire through the cervix being careful not to touch the vaginal wall. The specimen may be grasped with a forceps and sent to pathology. A sample of the endocervical canal may be obtained at this point using an endocervical curette followed by a cytobrush and sent together to pathology. Alternatively, another smaller cone "top hat" may be obtained with a smaller wire loop LEEP device (Fig. 2). Although there is usually no immediate bleeding, late rebleeding can be reduced by prophylactically cauterizing the cone base. This should be done using a ball, needle tip or spatula tip cautery attachment. The current should be set on coagulation at a sufficiently high current setting or "spray" to exceed the capacitance of air. The ball or other suitable tip should then be held a few millimeters from the surface of the cone base to allow the current to arc across to the tissue for hemostasis. A small rim of endocervical canal should be left un-coagulated to allow the transformation zone to evert during healing. After the entire base is cauterized in this manner, ferric subsulfate (Monsel's) solution may also be applied. The patient should be instructed not to place anything in the vagina for at least two weeks and call for any signs

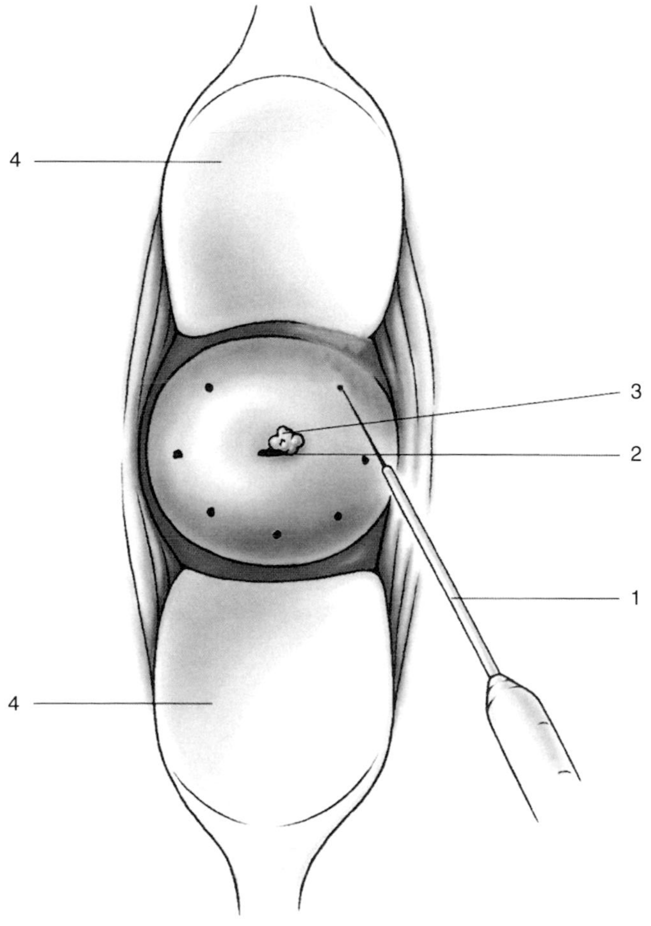

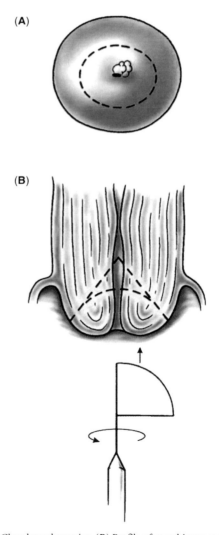

Figure 1 1 Reinforced shaft with thin needle; 2 Squamocolumnar junction; 3 Acetowhite epithelium; 4 Speculum blades.

Figure 2 (**A**) Clear lateral margins. (**B**) Profile of cone biopsy margins.

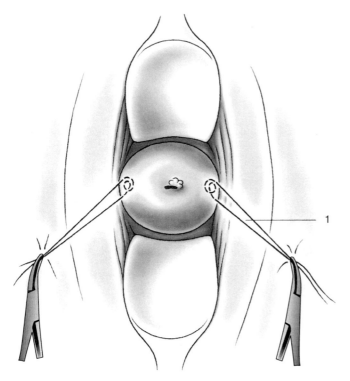

Figure 3A 1 Hemostat on drape.

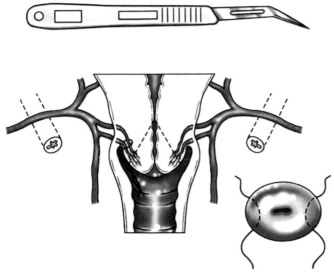

Figure 3B Cone to be excised.

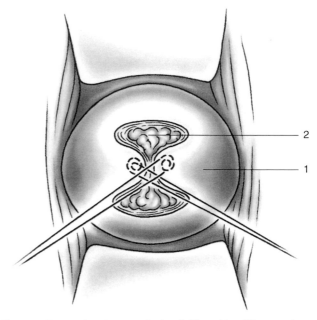

Figure 4 1 Ectocervix, 2 Hemostatic absorbable packing filling cone base.

or symptoms of infection. A routine postoperative visit is not necessary.

Scalpel "Cold Knife" Cone

Colposcopy should be used to identify the lesion. The scalpel cone biopsy does not require a special speculum with smoke evacuator. However, wall suction must be available since considerably more bleeding will be encountered. Because the procedure lasts longer than the LEEP and patient cooperation is

necessary to deal with the intraoperative bleeding, either general or regional anesthesia is usually required. No thromboembolic prophylaxis is needed. After positioning of the speculum, two lateral stay sutures are placed at approximately 3 and 9 o'clock positions. The sutures are placed in a figure-of-eight manner to help hold the cervix and reduce the blood supply by ligation of the cervical branch of the uterine artery. An absorbable suture of 0 or 00 is sufficient. These are held with hemostats attached to the drapes to help draw the cervix down into the lower vagina (Fig. 3A and 3B). As with the LEEP local anesthetic, circumferential injection of dilute vasopression, (e.g., 10 units/100cc NS) can be injected for added hemostasis. Starting posteriorly, using a large curved knife handle, the colposcopically identified acetowhite lesion is excised. Again, for diagnostic cones, the entire transformation zone should be removed. The base of the cone may be difficult to separate completely with the scalpel. Instead, curved scissors may be used for the last cut separating the specimen entirely. A sample of the endocervical canal may be obtained at this point using an endocervical curette and cyto-brush. Active bleeding may be controlled with cautery or fine 000 absorbable sutures on a small highly curved vascular needle. Prophylactic cautery of the base reduces delayed bleeding better than the occluding "Sturmdorf" sutures which turn the edge of the cervix over the excision base. Care must be taken not to occlude the os during any of these maneuvers. A cotton-tipped swab, placed in the os before any sutures, will help in avoiding this complication. Monsel's solution should be applied after hemostasis for prophylaxis against delayed bleeding. If hemostasis is still a problem, a commercial hemostatic agent, such as sheets of oxidized cellulose, may be used to tamponade the bleeding base and held in place by the lateral stay sutures. These sutures can be brought together over the midline and tied together (Fig. 4).

9 Radical abdominal hysterectomy

J. Richard Smith, Deborah C. M. Boyle, and Giuseppe Del Priore

INTRODUCTION

Radical abdominal hysterectomy is designed to remove the uterus, cervix, upper third of the vagina, either part or the whole of the parametrium, and the uterosacral and vesicouterine ligaments. In addition, the common iliac, internal iliac, external iliac, obturator, hypogastric, and presacral lymph nodes are also removed, as may be the paraaortic nodes.

This surgery is used for the management of stage IA2 and IB1 and IB2 tumors of the uterine cervix. It may be used by some surgeons for the management of stage IIA cervical tumors and occasionally in the management of vaginal cancer. It has been classified by Rutledge as radical abdominal hysterectomy types II and III (Piver et al. 1974). Staging of cervical cancer, carried out preoperatively, is not further discussed in this chapter. The choice of whether to perform this procedure or one of those described in chapters 8, 9, 10, and 27 depends on the surgeon's preference, with each operation tailored to the needs of the specific patient. The radicality of the planned procedure depends on the characteristics of the tumor.

Prior to surgery, the patient's bowel should be prepared using standard protocol. Consent for the specific procedure, including oophorectomy if planned, should have been obtained.

The procedure described here is an open approach. Many centers will adopt a laparoscopic or robotic approach but the dissection and order of the surgery are the same. Readers are referred to chapter 27 ("Robotic surgery") and chapter 26 ("Laparoscopy").

SURGICAL PROCEDURE

A general anesthetic is administered with or without an epidural anesthetic. The addition of a regional anesthetic allows better pain control postoperatively and facilitates surgery by reducing intraoperative blood loss.

The patient is then placed supine on the operating table. The bladder is catheterized with an indwelling Foley catheter and the vagina packed with a roll of gauze. Some surgeons insert the Foley catheter postoperatively, whilst others prefer to insert a suprapubic catheter at the end of the procedure. The authors' practice depends on the radicality of the procedure. In cases of stage IIA cervical cancer the vagina may be marked with cutting diathermy 2 to 3 cm away from the vaginal lesion to assist in later ensuring good resection margins.

The abdomen is opened using either a subumbilical, vertical midline incision or a large lower transverse, rectus muscle-cutting incision, dependent on the patient's desire for cosmesis (Fig. 1). It may be helpful to insert stay sutures to hold the peritoneum to the edges of the transverse skin incision.

After adequate exposure of the pelvis, the lymph nodes of the pelvis, the common iliac nodes and those above the bifurcation of the aorta are palpated, as is the liver.

The round ligament is then grasped, divided, and ligated close to the pelvic side-wall and the broad ligament opened to expose the retroperitoneal structures including the ureter attached to the medial aspect (Fig. 2).

The paravesical space is the first of the potential spaces to be developed during surgery (Fig. 3). This is achieved using blunt dissection with a combination of dissecting scissors and fingers or mounted pledgets. The dissection is commenced medial and slightly inferior to the external iliac vein. The paravesical space is bounded medially by the bladder and obliterated hypogastric artery and caudally by the ventral aspect of the cardinal ligament. The obturator muscle and fossa form the lateral border; this is dissected out later.

The pararectal space is then opened using a similar technique (Fig. 4). This space is bounded by the rectum medially, the sacrum ventrally, the pelvic side-wall, and internal iliac vessels laterally, and the cardinal ligament anteriorly. This allows the cardinal ligament and parametrium to be directly assessed by placing one's fingers in the newly opened paravesical and para-rectal spaces (Fig. 5).

Some clinicians perform the removal of the uterus first and others the lymphadenectomy. The choice is purely personal.

The lymphadenectomy is commenced at the bifurcation of the common iliac vessels, excising the loose lymphatic tissue overlying the internal and external iliac arteries and veins (Figs. 6 and 7). This is performed in a caudal direction, having first identified psoas muscle and the genitofemoral and lateral cutaneous nerve of the thigh. The dissection of the external iliac vessels continues caudally until the circumflex iliac vessels are encountered. Dissection in a cephalad direction allows clearance of common iliac and paraaortic nodes. Presacral nodes are also removed (Fig. 8).

Once the external iliac artery and vein are exposed they can be separated from the underlying tissue laterally. With gentle lateral (Fig. 9) and/or medial (Fig. 10) traction on the external iliac vessels the obturator fossa is now exposed. It is often helpful to sweep the external iliac vessels off the pelvic side-wall and approach the obturator fossa from the lateral side (Fig. 11). Great care must be taken to preserve the obturator nerve, and the dissection always becomes much easier once this structure has been identified (Figs. 12 and 13). Occasionally, the obturator artery and vein may require to be sacrificed to allow adequate dissection of the tissues posterior and lateral to the nerve. The ureter is further dissected from the peritoneum. Sharp dissection is employed to create the vesicouterine and vesicocervical spaces (Fig. 14). It is important to find the correct tissue plane since this facilitates easier and bloodless dissection. The uterine arteries are clamped, divided, and ligated close to their origins at the internal iliac arteries using either ligatures or hemoclips (Fig. 15). The ureteric tunnels are then deroofed, allowing exposure of the ureters and their

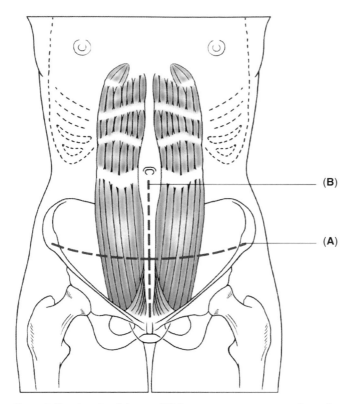

Figure 1 Opening the abdomen. (**A**) Low transverse rectus muscle cutting incision. (**B**) Vertical subumbilical incision.

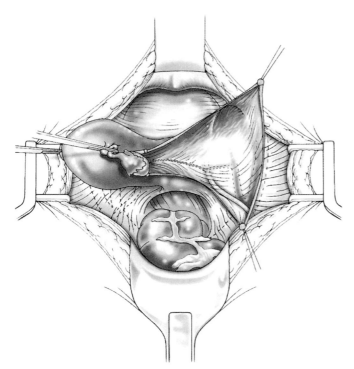

Figure 2 The round ligament is divided and the broad ligament opened.

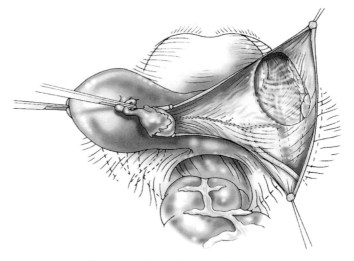

Figure 3 Developing the paravesical space.

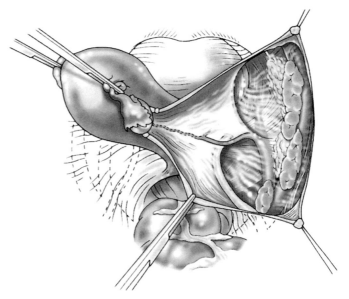

Figure 4 Developing the para-vesical and para-rectal spaces.

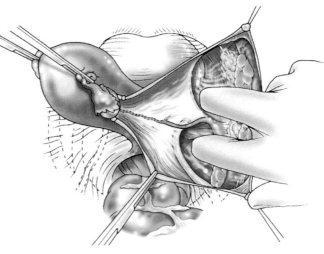

Figure 5 Palpating the parametrium directly.

separation from parametrial tissue (Fig. 16).This can be performed cephalad to caudal or vice versa. Roberts clamps or large hemoclips are helpful in minimizing hemorrhage. Whatever technique is used, bleeding tends to be brisk at this stage.

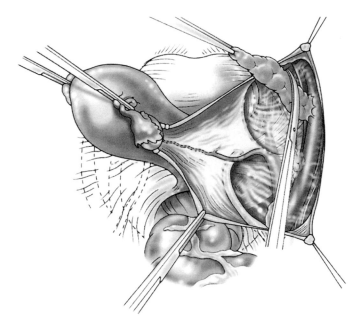

Figure 6 Pelvic lymphadenectomy.

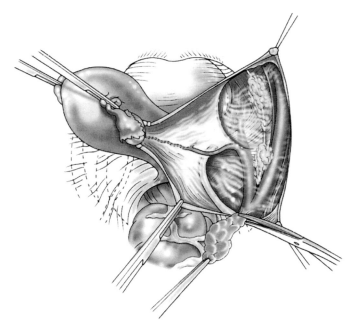

Figure 7 Pelvic lymphadenectomy: side-wall dissection.

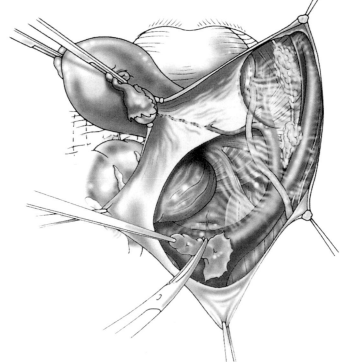

Figure 8 Presacral node removal.

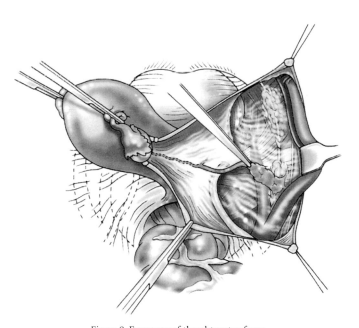

Figure 9 Exposure of the obturator fossa.

Harmonic scissors can be very useful at reducing hemorrhage at this stage.

The pararectal space is further developed from above from between the ureter medially and the internal iliac vessels later-ally (Fig. 17). The boundaries have been described above but the dissection now takes place to the level of the pelvic floor. The rectum is dissected away from the uterus, thus freeing it of its posterior visceral attachments (Fig. 18). This is best achieved by grasping the rectum between the fingers and lifting it in a cephalad direction and then entering the rectovaginal space by sharp dissection. The rectum is often much higher on the

uterus than is at first suspected and this technique minimizes the possibility of inadvertent rectal injury.

Clamping, division, and ligation of the utero-sacral ligaments then takes place (Figs. 19 and 20). Alternatively, Harmonic scis-sors can be used. These can either be performed midway along the ligaments or at the sacrum, depending on the size and nature of the tumor. The cardinal ligaments are then clamped, divided, and ligated, again either halfway between the cervix

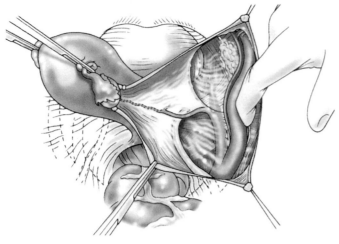

Figure 10 Exposure of the obturator fossa: lateral approach.

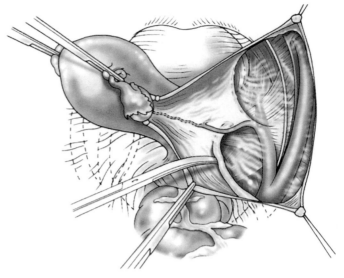

Figure 13 Exposure of the obturator fossa.

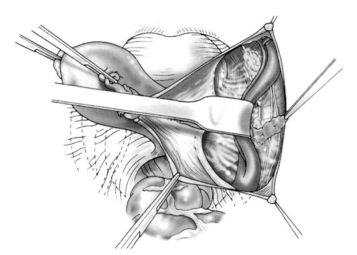

Figure 11 Exposure of the obturator fossa.

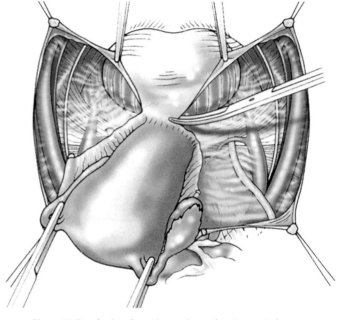

Figure 14 Developing the vesicouterine and vesicocervical spaces.

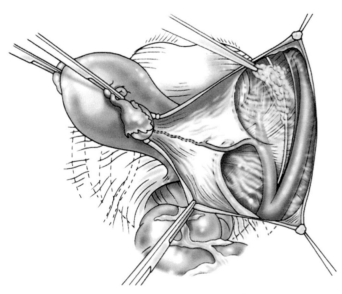

Figure 12 Exposure of the obturator fossa.

and the pelvic side-wall or at the pelvic side-wall, using the same criteria as with the uterosacral ligaments (Fig. 21). Again, Harmonic scissors can be used to effect this maneuver. These differing levels of radicality have been classified by Rutledge and the procedures just described are Rutledge II and III procedures (Piver et al. 1974) (Fig. 22).

The division of these ligaments causes the paravesical and pararectal spaces to be united (Figs. 23 and 24).

Right-angle clamps or cutting diathermy are applied to the vagina far enough caudally to allow removal of the upper third of the vagina (Fig. 25). As described above in cases of stage IIA tumor, the vagina may have been marked with diathermy at the start of the procedure to ensure adequate resection margins are obtained. The vagina is then incised and the uterus with

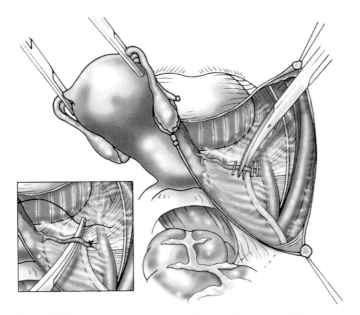

Figure 15 The uterine arteries are clamped and divided close to their origins.

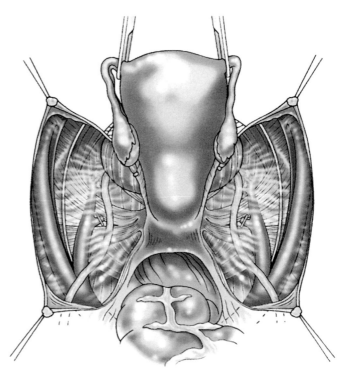

Figure 17 Further dissection of the pararectal space.

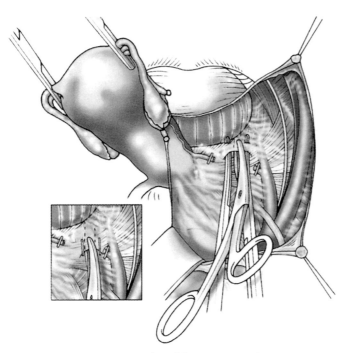

Figure 16 Deroofing of the ureteric tunnels.

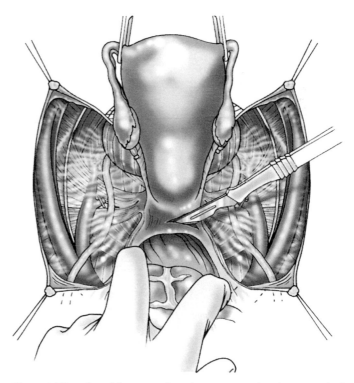

Figure 18 Dissection of the rectum from the uterus, opening the rectovaginal space.

parametrium and upper vagina is then removed. The upper edges of the vagina may be oversewn circumferentially with a locked-on suture to achieve hemostasis, while leaving the vagina open to act as a natural drain. It is also thought that this suturing allows the edges of the vagina to come together by direct apposition, thus minimizing the chances of vaginal mucosa being obscured from view during long-term follow-up. Direct closure of the vagina will inevitably leave some

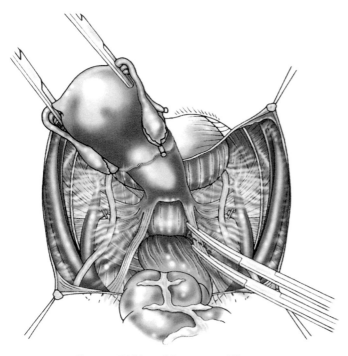

Figure 19 Division of the uterosacral ligaments.

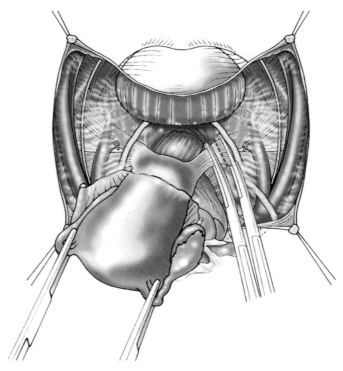

Figure 21 Division of the cardinal ligaments.

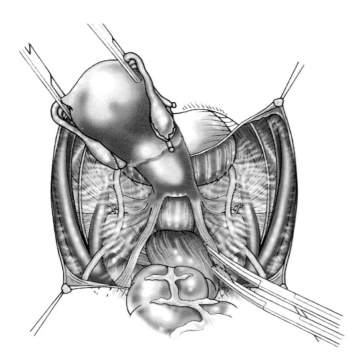

Figure 20 Division of the uterosacral ligaments.

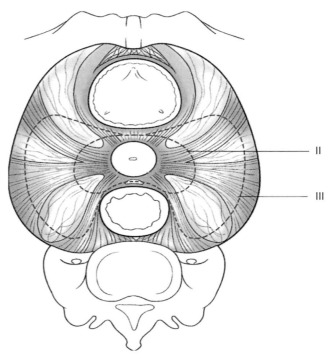

Figure 22 Rutledge II and III procedures, operative procedure.

vagina above the suture line and thus out of sight when inspected at follow-up.

At the end of the procedure, the skeletonized vessels, nerves, and ureters can be clearly seen. The paravesical and pararectal spaces are joined and the rectum is exposed to the level of the pelvic floor. Many surgeons leave a silastic drain with gravity drainage in situ at the end of the procedure, although the need for this is questionable. This will probably not be required for more than 24 hours (Fig. 26). Suction drainage has been shown not to reduce lympho cyst formation. A suprapubic

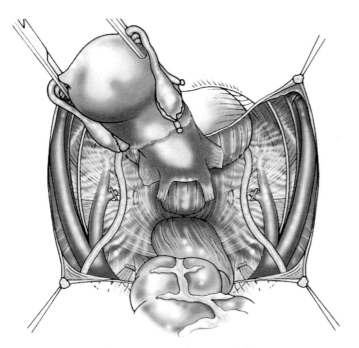

Figure 23 Pararectal spaces united.

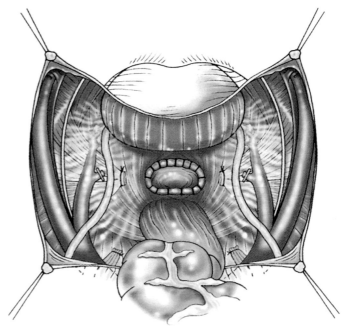

Figure 25 Division of the vagina.

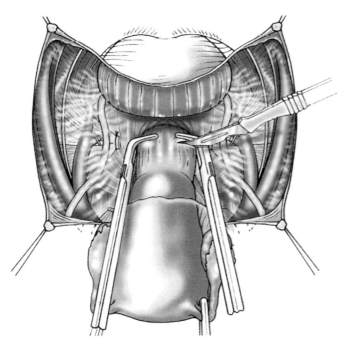

Figure 24 Paravesical spaces united.

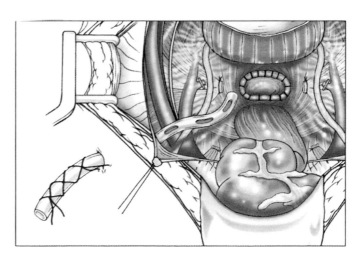

Figure 26 The completed procedure. A drain may be left in situ.

catheter may be inserted at this point. It is the authors' practice to use one when a Rutledge III procedure has been performed, since these patients are more likely to encounter urinary difficulties in the postoperative period. The abdomen is then closed with mass closure for vertical incision using a looped PDS suture; a fat suture can be used and the authors use clips to skin. Transverse muscle cutting incisions are closed in a mass closure involving anterior, posterior rectus sheath and parietal peritoneum, usually without attempting to repair the transected rectus muscles; again, clips to skin are used.

REFERENCE

Piver MS, Rutledge FN, Smith JP (1974) Five classes of extended hysterectomy for women with cervical cancer. *Obstet Gynecol* **44**:265–72.

10 Laparoscopically assisted vaginal radical hysterectomy

Daniel Dargent[†] and Michel Roy

INTRODUCTION

When surgeons considered treating cancers of the cervix in ways other than by cauterization or similar palliative tools, the vaginal hysterectomy was the first technique used (Recamier 1829). However, at the turn of the 19th century the abdominal approach became common, as a consequence of two simultaneous changes. First, even if it was more risky than vaginal surgery, abdominal surgery was no longer a death sentence. Second, the concept of radical surgery, introduced by Halsted in the field of breast cancer, was also spreading to the management of all other malignancies. The first "radical hysterectomy" performed by Clark in 1895 included, as a true Halstedian operation, an extirpation of the parauterine tissues and pelvic lymph nodes. Just before Clark devised the radical abdominal hysterectomy, Pavlik in Czechoslovakia (1889) and Schuchardt in Germany (1893) had described a method enabling the removal of the parauterine tissues at the same time as the uterus, while maintaining a vaginal approach. However, the removal of the pelvic lymph nodes could obviously not be included in this operation.

The abdominal and vaginal techniques were used concurrently in middle Europe at the end of the 19th century. Wertheim became the champion of the first technique and Schauta the defender of the second. The long and hard fight between the two surgeons ceased when Wertheim's book (1911) was published. Despite higher rates of pre- and post-operative complications, the survival rates obtained by Wertheim were far higher than those noted by Schauta in his book of 1908. With Marie Curie's subsequent discovery of radium in 1910, surgery was no longuer a treatment option until the 1930s and 1940s.

Surgery found a new place in the management of cervical cancer as a tool to solve the problem of positive lymph nodes that were not managed by radiotherapy. Leveuf in France (1931) and Taussig in the United States (1935) proposed a combination of radiation therapy and pelvic lymphadenectomy in order to improve outcomes. This idea was the first step toward the reintroduction of radical surgery, whose official beginning was 1945, the year in which JV Meigs delivered his first paper about the new Wertheim operation. Since the highlight of the new radical surgery was systematic pelvic lymphadenectomy, the vaginal approach clearly could not benefit from the revival of such surgery.

The Revival of Radical Vaginal Hysterectomy—Role of Laparoscopy

Following an idea first expressed by Navratil, the Indian surgeon Suboth Mitra (1959) proposed a new combined approach and can be considered as the spiritual father of the new era of vaginal surgery in the management of cervical cancer. In the Suboth Mitra operation, a systematic pelvic lymphadenectomy was first carried out through a bilateral abdominal extraperitoneal incision, then a vaginal radical hysterectomy (VRH) after Schauta. In spite of the two successive surgical interventions, the operation remained less dangerous than the abdominal radical hysterectomy (ARH) because it did not include a large and lengthy opening of the peritoneal cavity. During the 1970s, postoperative morbidity was three times less after the Suboth Mitra operation than after the Meigs operation. Therefore we used it (Dargent 1991) for the high surgical risk patients as today does Massi (Savino et al. 2001). But we did not extend the indications to the standard surgical risk patients.

In order to increase the area of application of the VRH it was proposed (Dargent 1987) to replace the bilateral abdominal incision by the laparoscopic tool for performing the systematic pelvic dissection which is part of the radical hysterectomy since the Meigs publication. So was born the concept of "Celio-Schauta" or laparoscopically assisted vaginal radical hysterectomy (LAVRH), a concept derived from laparoscopically assisted vaginal hysterectomy (LAVH). LAVH includes four variants. In variant 0, the laparoscope is only used for assessing the peritoneal cavity before performing the vaginal hysterectomy. In variant 1, the round ligaments and the infundibulo-pelvic ligaments (and the peritoneal adhesions if needed) are divided with the laparoscope. In variant 2, one pushes up to the level of the uterine arteries. In variant 3, the paracervical ligaments as well are divided with the laparoscope. In variant 4, the entire operation is carried out with the laparoscope including incision and closure of the vagina. A similar classification can be used for the LAVRH.

From 1986 to 1992 the LAVRH type 0 Celio-Schauta was our daily practice. The laparoscope was used for assessing the pelvic cavity, the organs it contains and the lymph nodes along the pelvic side walls in the retro-peritoneal spaces. After having performed the systematic pelvic lymphadenectomy, the vaginal approach was used and the VRH was performed following the technique of Schauta using either the German variant (Stoeckel 1928) whose radicality is like the Piver 2 ARH or the Austrian variant (Amreich 1924) whose radicality is like the Piver 3 ARH. The first operation was selected for the smallest tumors (<2 cm in size), and the second one was reserved for the biggest ones (2 cm in size or more).

From 1992 a handful (Dargent and Mathevet 1992, Kadar and Reich 1993, Roy et al. 1996, Schneider et al. 1996, Pomel et al. 2003) of papers were published concerning variants of LAVRH one could designate as the variant 3 in that meaning that the laparoscope was not only used for performing the indispensable systematic pelvic lymphadenectomy but for

---

[†]Deceased.

dividing the uterine arteries and the paracervical ligaments as well. The common feature of these techniques was the quest for radicality which could be greatly increased thanks to the laparoscope. Indeed, one of the technical difficulties the vaginal approach is clamping the parametrium close to the pelvic side wall because of the oblique angle. Conversely, the laparoscope, with its magnification, helps the surgeon removing parametrial tissue potentially containing nodes and leaving only vessels, nerves, and connective tissue. This makes possible clamping of the parametrium away from the pelvic side wall and therefore limiting the damage to bladder and rectal innervation. The operation we describe in the following pages is a variant of these LAVRH type 3.

SURGICAL PROCEDURE

The aim of the radical hysterectomy operation, whichever approach is chosen, is to retrieve part of the vagina and the parauterine tissues, together with the uterus itself. The ventral and dorsal surfaces of the vagina and the tissues closed to the uterus are also in close proximity with the bladder floor and the ureters from the ventral surface of the specimen when opening the vesico-vaginal space on the midline and the paravesical spaces on either side in order to locate the bladder pillars and divide them after identification of the ureters. The dorsal aspect of the specimen is freed when the rectal pillars are divided (a much simpler step of the operation).

Laparoscopic Operation

The laparoscopic part of the LARVH is usually done using the classical transumbilical transperitoneal route.

Four tracars are used: two 10 mm for the umbilical and suprapubic opening and two 5 mm placed laterally in the pelvis. In the transperitoneal approach, inspection of the peritoneal surfaces, liver, pelvic organs is carried out. When obvious peritoneal invasion is seen around the cervix, or gross pelvic node metastasis are encountered, the radical hysterectomy is aborted and para-aortic dissection is carried out to rule out metastasis in the para-aortic area.

The search and removal of the sentinel lymph nodes (SLN) is performed and sent for frozen section (see chapter 18) and the pelvic lymphadenectomy is done. If one of the SLN is positive, the radical hysterectomy is aborted.

The medial aspect of the iliac vessels is easily cleaned (Fig. 1). The lateral aspect is a little more difficult; however, it can be achieved laparoscopically as effectively as it is at laparotomy, if not better. The iliac vessels are detached from the psoas muscle and pushed medially. The opened space is cleaned out until the obturator nerve is identified (Fig. 2).

The last step of the laparoscopic procedure is dividing the uterine arteries and preparing the cardinal ligament (Fig. 3). Rather than cutting the ligament laparoscopically, its lateral part is emptied of the lymph node-bearing tissues which are in the vascular network of the ligament. This emptying is done by gentle teasing of the adipose tissue between the vessels. Among the vessels handled are the uterine arteries which are accompanied by lymphatic channels. A superficial uterine vein can accompany the artery as well (Fig. 3).

Vaginal Surgery

The original Schauta operation started with a Schuchardt incision (deep left lateral episiotomy) in order to enlarge the field of dissection and to more easily open the left pararectal space. Nowadays, the Schuchardt is rarely used for three main reasons. First, the vaginal radical approach should not be chosen when the volume of the cervical tumor exceeds 2.5 to 3 cm, and in those cases, there is no need for removal of the entire parametrial tissue. Furthermore, distal parametrectomy is performed laparoscopically, so only proximal parametrium needs to be removed vaginally. The second reason is the risk of metastasis in the incision (Beranger et al. 2004, Bader et al. 2006). The third reason is the discomfort of the patient and the risk of vaginal hematoma. In the post-operative period, the most important site of pain used to be the vaginal incision.

So after the cervix is grasped with clamps, determination of the vaginal margin (Fig. 4) is made roughly 1 to 2 cm from the cervix, depending on the size and location of the tumor. The inferior brim of the head of the prolapse is infiltrated using diluted synthetic vasopressin, primarily for prophylactic hemostasis but also to separate the two parts of the fold.

Dividing the vagina is done in four stages. The anterior aspect is treated first (Fig. 5). It is the most difficult step, because the bladder floor is drawn inside the vaginal fold one pulls on. All the layers of the vaginal wall must be cut, without injury to the bladder wall. Treating the posterior aspect is

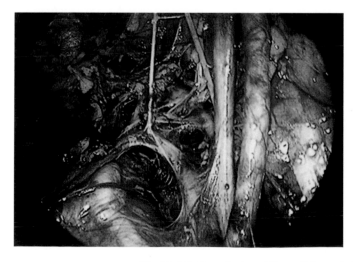

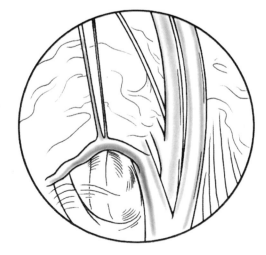

Figure 1 Laparoscopic view of the medial aspect of the common iliac bifurcation.

easier because of the tissue present between the rectum and vagina. On the lateral aspects only the mucosa is cut (Fig. 6) in order to keep the relationship between the vaginal cuff and the underlying structures, that is, the paracervical ligaments. Compare this with the anterior and posterior surfaces, where the goal was separating the cuff from the underlying organs, that is, the bladder and rectum.

Once the vaginal cuff is separated it is grasped using Chrobak forceps (Fig. 7) and pulled downward. Traction reveals the supravaginal septum, a pseudomembrane made by

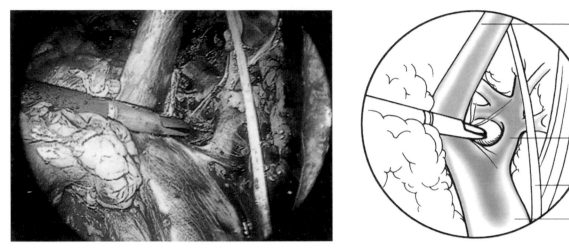

Figure 2 Laparoscopic view of the lateral aspect of the common iliac venous convergence: the obturator nerve crosses the gluteal vessels. 1 Common iliac vein; 2 Obturator nerve; 3 Internal iliac vein; 4 External iliac vein.

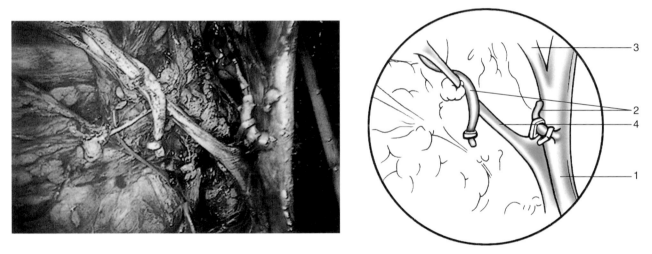

Figure 3 Laparoscopic view after transection of uterine artery: A superficial uterine vein will be cut next. 1 Internal iliac artery; 2 Uterine artery; 3 Superior vesical artery; 4 Uterine vein.

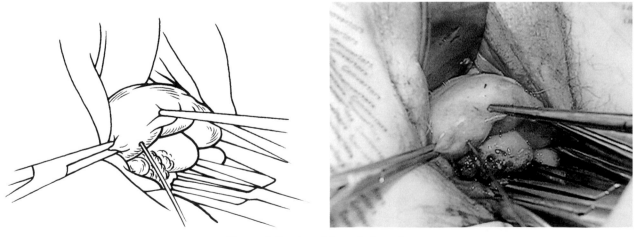

Figure 4 Infiltration of the vaginal margin.

condensation of the connective fibers joining the bladder floor to the vagina. This pseudo-aponeurosis has to be opened on the midline close to the base of the trigone (Fig. 8). Once the aponeurosis has been opened (use the scissors perpendicularly to the vagina), the areolar tissue of the vesicovaginal space is visible and a tunnel can be made and enlarged to the level of

the vesicovaginal peritoneal fold (this is possible using the scissors parallel to the vagina).

Next the vesicovaginal space is opened, together with the paravesical space.

To open the paravesical spaces, two forceps are applied to the brim of the vagina (at positions 1 o'clock and 3 o'clock for the

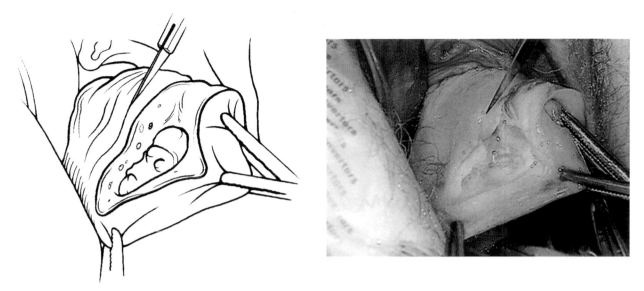

Figure 5 The Schauta operation: separation of the vaginal cuff on the ventral (anterior) aspect; the incision is full thickness.

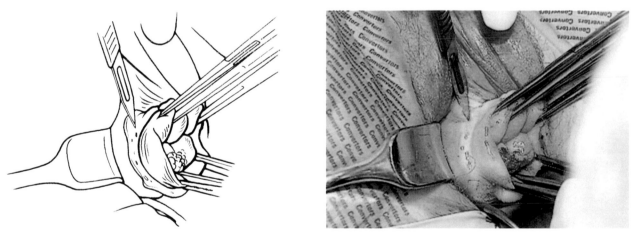

Figure 6 Separation of the vaginal cuff on the lateral aspect; the incision is more superficial.

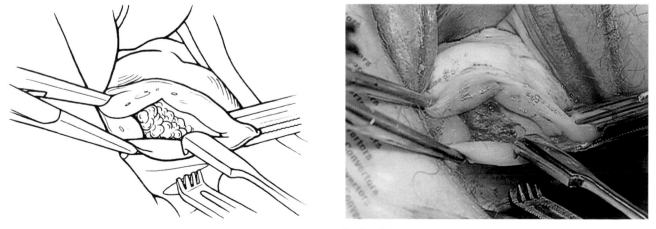

Figure 7 Grasping the vaginal cuff with the forceps.

left side, 11 o'clock and 9 o'clock for the right side). Pulling on the forceps reveals a depression located close to the most lateral instrument (Fig. 9). Deepening this depression by blunt use of Metzenbaum's scissors oriented laterally and ventrally (Fig. 10) opens the paravesical space, into which is introduced a micro-Breiski retractor. The structure interposed between this retractor and the previously opened vesicovaginal space is the bladder pillar, inside which the contour of the ureter can be identified while palpating the pillar against the retractor. The characteristic "snap" of the ureter is evinced (Fig. 11).

While appropriate exposure is maintained with the retractors, the inferior brim of the pillar, which appears vertical, is opened with the tip of the scissors and its lateral fibers are separated using the same scissors (Fig. 12). After a new palpatory assessment (make sure the ureter is located, laterally to the isolated part of the pillar) the fibers of the pillar are cut (Fig. 13). The paravesical space becomes wider, and a broader retractor is introduced. The lateral aspect of the "knee" of the ureter becomes visible (Fig. 14). The medial fibers of the pillar can then be cut to release the ventral aspect of the paracervical

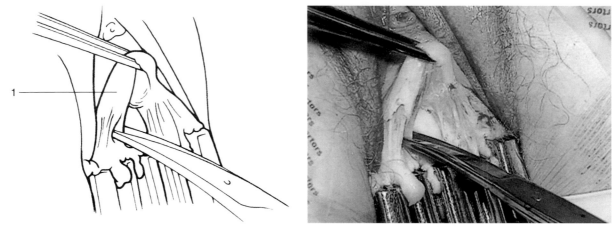

Figure 8 Opening the vesicovaginal space on the midline. 1 Bladder.

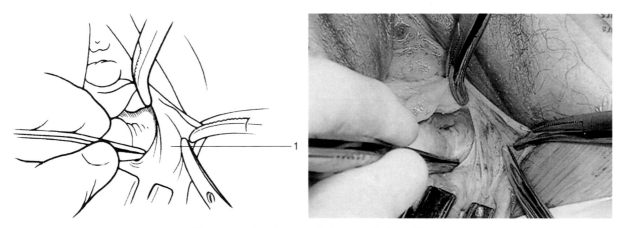

Figure 9 Opening the paravesical space. 1 Bladder pillar.

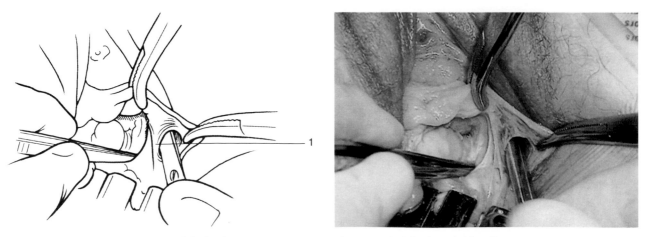

Figure 10 Evincing the entry into the paravesical space on the left side. 1 Bladder pillar.

ligament (Fig. 15): this enables location of the arch of the uterine artery in the para-isthmic window (a space whose inferior brim is the superior edge of the paracervical ligament). The descending branch of the arch is tugged and the already divided artery arrives in the operative field with a staple at the cut end (Fig. 16).

After freeing the ventral aspect of the specimen, the surgeon moves to the dorsal aspect. The first step is opening the pouch of Douglas (Fig. 17). The recto-uterine ligaments are then divided, at a point equidistant between the uterus and the recto-sigmoid. Cutting at this level is easy (no preventive clamping is needed) and leads directly to the dorsal aspect of the para-isthmic window, the ventral aspect of which has been identified previously. The tip of a right angle forceps is pushed into the window from back to front.

Two clamps can be put onto the cardinal ligament. The first one is placed medially, and traction is exerted. The second clamp (which has a slightly greater curvature) is placed

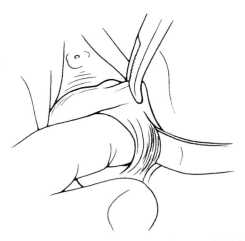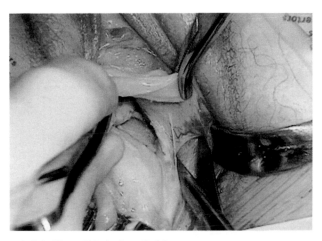

Figure 11 Palpation of the bladder pillar on the left side to elicit the "snap" of the ureter.

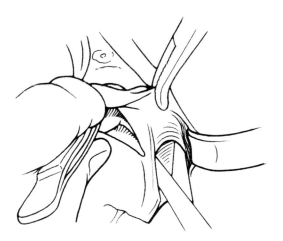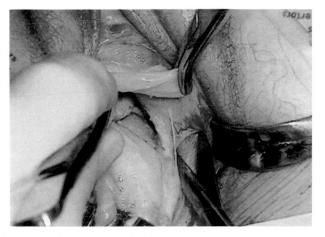

Figure 12 Separation of the lateral part of the bladder pillar on the left side.

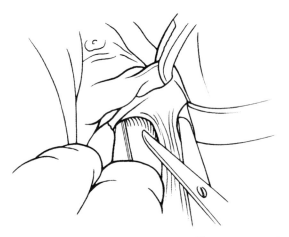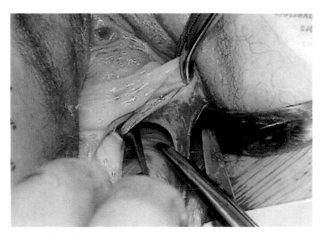

Figure 13 Cutting the lateral part of the bladder pillar.

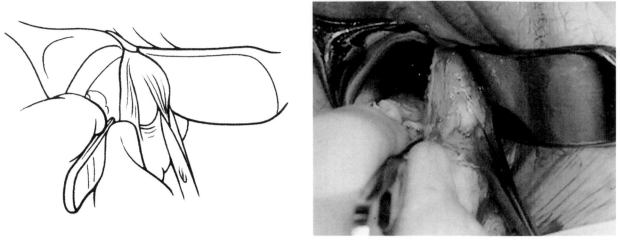

Figure 14 Further division of the lateral fibers of bladder pillar on left side: the knee of the ureter is visible.

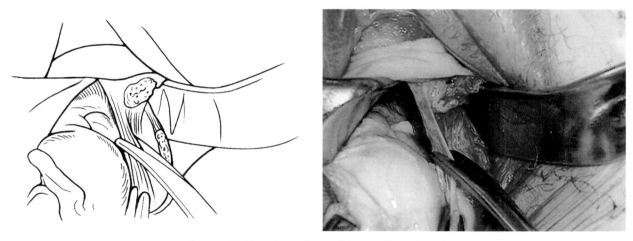

Figure 15 Division of medial part of bladder pillar on left side.

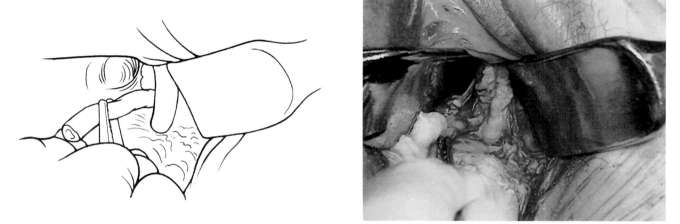

Figure 16 Pulling on the descending branch of arch of uterine artery on left side.

laterally; the convexity of its curvature lies in contact with the "knee" of the ureter (Fig. 18).

Following transection of the ligaments the uterine body can be turned in a dorsal direction, and the adnexa can be left in place or removed, depending on the age of the patient (Fig. 19). The vagina is closed with interrupted sutures after careful evaluation of intra-peritoneal hemostasis. A Foley catheter is left in place for 3 to 5 days. Since hemostasis can be difficult to assess vaginally, we go back laparoscopically for inspection of the dissected areas, to complete hemostasis and to make sure of the integrity of the bladder and the ureters.

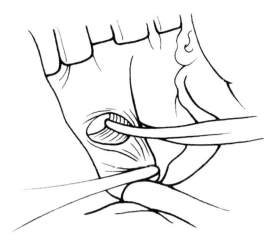
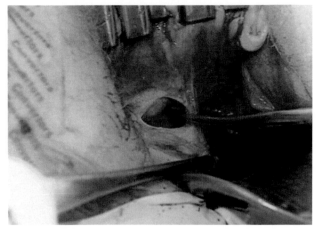

Figure 17 Opening the pouch of Douglas and the rectal pillar.

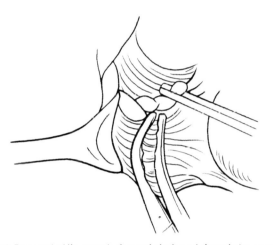
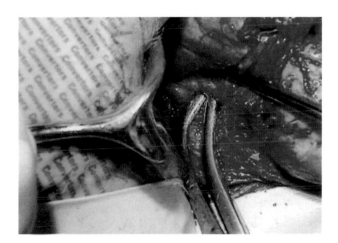

Figure 18 Paracervical ligament is clamped, the lateral clamp being put underneath the tip of the "knee" of the ureter. The vagina is closed without a drain or gauze. A Foley catheter is left in place for three to five days. Since hemostasis can be difficult to assess vaginally, we go back laparoscopically for inspection of the dissected areas, to complete hemostasis and to make sure of the integrity of the bladder and the ureters.

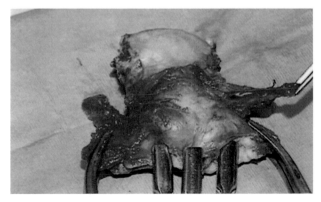

Figure 19 The removed specimen with proximal parametrium and uterine arteries is lacking here, having been removed during the laparoscopic procedure.

Post-operative Course—Complications

The LAVRH is performed in three hours including two hours for the laparoscopic part and localization and retrieval of the sentinel nodes, and one hour roughly for the vaginal part. Preservation of the bladder floor and ureters is the main concern. Injuries can occur which are easily detected because of urine leakage. They can usually be fixed without having recourse to laparotomy. If the injury concerns the ureter(s) or the bladder floor close to the ureteric orifices, stents should be used. Other per-operative problems are not specific. The post-operative course is usually simple. The patient can get up the night of surgery or on post-op day one. The return to normal diet is rapid. Resuming normal urinary bladder function can take time. We recommend leaving the bladder catheter in place for three to five days. Post-micturition residuals must be done and self-catheterization is taught to the patient when indicated and she can be discharged home when there is no significant residual ($2 \times <100\,cm^3$) or self-catheterization is understood. Post-operative complications are similar to those that can occur after all extended pelvic surgery. Bleeding is the first complication, but usually less than with the abdominal approach (Roy and Plante, 2011). It occurs most of the time in the first 48 hours post-op. The incidence of bleeding is lowered by laparoscopic re-evaluation of the abdomen after the vagina is closed. Post-operative pelvic collections of various nature can be observed as a consequence of occult bleeding during the first post-operative days or as consequence of accumulation of lymphatic fluid in the successive weeks. Fistulas are generally the consequence of undiagnosed injuries and symptoms appear in the first hours following the surgery. Fistulas linked to tissues necrosis and occurring later in the post-operative course are practically unknown after VRH unlike ARH. Nevertheless it is mandatory to investigate by an intravenous pyelogram if injury is suspected.

Urinary, bowel, and sexual sequelaes can occur. The first ones are the most concerning. The urinary bladder voiding difficulties observed in the immediate post-operative period can persist at least in form of loss of the feeling of the need to urinate and a prolonged time to void. In the extreme forms self-catheterization is the treatment. A micturition calendar and bio-feedback usually are enough. The same is for constipation which can be the consequence of neurogenic rectal atony and preexisting anal problems. Non-irritant laxatives and bio-feedback are the two pillars of the management.

The complication rates of LAVRH depend essentially on the "learning curve effect". In the literature of the early 1990s, the rate of urinary injuries and/or fistulas was around 10%. In the literature of the early 2000s, the rates are much lower. In the Quebec City experience (Renaud et al. 2000), 7 complications were observed among 91 patients of which 3 were among the first 25 cases and 4 among the following 77 cases. In the Jena experience (Hertel et al. 2003), 65% of the complications occurred for the first 100 cases versus 35% for the 100 following cases. Other publications (Querleu et al. 2002) do not mention any severe complications with the exception of one post-radiotherapy ureteral stenosis in a series of 95 patients who had LAVRH.

Endpoints—Indications

The data of the recent literature enable us to define the indications for the LAVRH. In our own series (unpublished data), the actuarial disease free five year survival was 94.2% in a series of 216 patients affected by cervical cancer stage N0, pIA2, and pIB1 submitted to Celio-Schauta or LAVRH between December 1986 and May 2002. For stages IB2 and higher the results are not as good. In the Jena series (Hertel et al. 2003), the actuarial disease free five year survival was under 70% for stage IB2 and under 60% for stages IIA and IIB. In stage IB1, a clear cut-off exists between the tumors less than 2 cm in size and the others. In our own experience (unpublished data), the disease-free five year survival was 100% for the 144 patients with tumors less than 2 cm in size versus 87.5% for the 72 patients with tumors 2 cm or more in size. Among the patients with the biggest tumors followed three years or more, the number of recurrences was 4 out of 23 after the VRH type Schauta-Amreich versus 3 out of 11 after VRH type Schauta-Stoeckel and 3 out of 19 after VRH type Schauta-Stoeckel preceded by a paracervical lymphadenectomy carried out as a complement of the laparoscopic pelvic lymphadenectomy which was performed in all cases.

The radical vaginal hysterectomy should not be performed for stage IB2 and more. Clinical examination and magnetic resonance imaging (MRI) are the keys of this first selection. The team from Jena (Hertel et al. 2003) proposes going further and rejecting the cases with lympho vascular space involvement and also pN1. The first risk factor is assessed on the initial large biopsy specimen. The second one can be evidenced at the initial imaging. If not, the frozen sections done on the sentinel nodes retrieved laparoscopically give the answer. Such a selection could provide a 98% rate of five year disease-free survival. Furthermore this result can be obtained at the price of

the least aggressive of the VRH techniques, that of Stoeckel. Our data seem to demonstrate that the parametrial lymphadenectomy performed during the laparoscopic part of the surgery significantly lower the risk of recurrences.

CONCLUSIONS

LAVRH at the light of the published data is equivalent to ARH in the management of early cervical cancer for the chances of cure. The evidence is level B (consistent retrospective and prospective surveys). Perioperatively, blood loss is significantly less (Roy and Plante, 2011). Concerning the post-operative comfort LAVRH offers better than ARH (level A). The minimally invasive surgery, at first sight, seems to be more "patient friendly" but classical surgery has changed a lot since the new tool appeared and has been developed further: new incisions, new instruments (Ligasure®, Biclamp®, Ultracision®), new wound closure techniques, new analgesic strategies, make post-operative course much less painful than it was.

REFERENCES

Amreich AI (1924) Zur Anatomie und Technik der erweiterten vaginalem Carzinom Operation. *Arch Gynäkol* **122**:497.

Bader AA, Bjelic-Radisic V, Tamussimo KF, et al. (2006) Recurrence in a Schuchardt incision after Schauta-Amreich operation for cervical cancer. *Int J Gynecol Cancer* **16**:1479.

Barranger E, Hugol D, Darai E (2004) Metastasis on a Schuchardt incision after Schauta-Amreich operation for cervical carcinoma. *Gynecol Oncol* **92**:1006.

Clark JG (1895) A more radical method for performing hysterectomy for cancer of the uterus. *Bull Johns Hopkins Hosp* **6**:120.

Dargent D (1987) A new future for Schauta's operation trough presurgical retroperitoneal pelviscopy. *Eur J Gynaecol Oncol* **8**:292.

Dargent D (1991) Treatment of the cancers of the ecto-cervix and vagina with preservation of the uterus and adnexae. *Cah Oncol* **1**:21.

Dargent D, Kouakou N, Adeleine P (1991) L'operation de Schauta 90 ans apres. *Lyon Chir* **87**:324.

Dargent D, Mathevet P (1992) Radical laparoscopic vaginal hysterectomy. *J Gynecol Obstet Biol Reprod (Paris)* **21**:709.

Hertel H, Kohler C, Michels W, et al. (2003) Laparoscopic-assisted radical vaginal hysterectomy (LARVH): prospective evaluation of 200 patients with cervical cancer. *Gynecol Oncol* **90**:505.

Kadar N, Reich H (1993) Laparoscopically assisted radical Schauta hysterectomy and bilateral laparoscopic pelvic lymphadenectomy for the treatment of bulky stage IB carcinoma of the cervix. *Gynaecol Endosc* **2**:135.

Leveuf J (1931) L'envahissement des ganglions lymphatiques dans le cancer du col de l'uterus. *Bull & Mem Soc Nat De Chir* **57**:662.

Meigs JV (1945) Wertheim operation for carcinoma of the cervix. *Am J Obstet Gynecol* **49**:542.

Mitra S (1959) Extraperitoneal lymphadenectomy and radical vaginal hysterectomy for cancer of the cervix (Mitra technique). *Am J Obstet Gynecol* **78**:191.

Pavlik K (1889) O extirpaci cele dălohy a casti vaziva panvicniho. *Casopis Lekaru Ceskych* **XVIII**:28.

Pomel C, Atallah D, Le Bouedec G, et al. (2003) Laparoscopic radical hysterectomy for invasive cervical cancer: 8-year experience of a pilot study. *Gynecol Oncol* **91**:534.

Querleu D, Narducci F, Poulard V, et al. (2002) Modified radical vaginal hysterectomy with or without laparoscopic nerve-sparing dissection: a comparative study. *Gynecol Oncol* **85**:154.

Recamier JCA (1829) Ablation de l'uterus cancereux. In: *Recherche sur le traitement du cancer*. Paris: Gabon, pp. 519–29.

Renaud MC, Plante M, Roy M (2000) Combined laparoscopic and vaginal radical surgery in cervical cancer. *Gynecol Oncol* **79**:59.

Roy M, Plante M, Renaud MC, et al. (1996) Vaginal radical hysterectomy versus abdominal radical hysterectomy in the treatment of early-stage cervical cancer. *Gynecol Oncol* **62**:336.

Roy M, Plante M. Place of Schauta's radical vaginal hysterectomy. *Best Practice & Research Clinical Obstetrics and Gynaecology* **25**:227-37

Savino L, Borruto F, Comparetto C, et al. (2001) Radical vaginal hysterectomy with extraperitoneal pelvic lymphadenectomy in cervical cancer. *Eur J Gynaecol Oncol* **22**:31–5.

Schauta F (1908) *Die erweiterte vaginale Totalextirpation des Uterus beim Kollumkarzinome.* Vienna: J. Safar.

Schneider A, Possover M, Kamprath S, et al. (1996) Laparoscopy-assisted radical vaginal hysterectomy modified according to Schauta-Stoeckel. *Obstet Gynecol* **88**:1057.

Schuchardt K (1893) Eine neue methode der gebärmutterexstirpation. *Zbl Chir* 1131.

Stoeckel W (1928) *Die vaginale Radikaloperation des Collumkarzinomes.* *Zbl Gynäkol* **52**:39.

Taussig FJ (1935) The removal of lymph nodes in cancer of the cervix. *Am J Roentgenol* **34**:354.

Wertheim (1911) Die erweiterte abdominale Operation bei Carcinoma Colli Uteri. Berlin: Urban & Schwarzenberg.

11 Radical vaginal trachelectomy
Marie Plante and Michel Roy

INTRODUCTION

Cervical cancer frequently affects young women in their reproductive years, often before they have had the chance to begin or complete their family plans. So, in terms of quality of life, fertility preservation has become a major issue in the management of young women with early-stage cervical cancer (Plante 2000).

Vaginal radical trachelectomy (VRT) is a new conservative fertility-preserving surgical procedure for the treatment of selected cases of early-stage cervical cancer. This procedure has the advantage of preserving the uterine body which in turns allows preservation of childbearing potential. This surgery has been described and first published by Professor Daniel Dargent from Lyon, France (Dargent et al. 1994). The procedure has been performed for over 20 years and over 600 women have undergone this procedure worldwide. More than 250 pregnancies have been reported and more than 150 healthy babies have been born so far. The majority of patients have delivered by elective Cesarean Section and approximately two-thirds were at term. The main obstetrical problem is the risk of premature second trimester birth or miscarriage. Oncologic results are also reassuring as the risk of recurrences remains <5% (Plante 2008). This procedure is now accepted as a valid alternative to the radical hysterectomy procedure in young women with early-stage disease who wish to preserve their fertility.

INDICATIONS

The eligibility criteria have not changed significantly since first proposed (Roy and Plante 1998). As data accumulate, these criteria are subject to change in the future.

1. Desire to preserve fertility
2. No clinical evidence of impaired fertility
3. Lesion size <2.0 to 2.5 cm
4. FIGO stage IA1 with vascular space invasion (VSI), IA2 to IB1
5. Squamous cell or adenocarcinoma
6. No involvement of the upper endocervical canal as determined by colposcopy and/or magnetic resonance imaging (MRI)
7. No metastasis to regional lymph nodes

ANATOMICAL CONSIDERATION
Vascular Supply

The blood supply to the cervix is assured by the *cervical* (or descending) branch of the uterine artery, and by the *vaginal* artery which originates from either the hypogastric, the uterine or the superior vesical artery. At the level of the upper endocervix, these two arteries form a network of anastomosis and a rich vascular plexus. At the isthmus, the uterine artery also forms a loop often referred to as the *cross* of the uterine artery. This is an important landmark because all efforts should be made to preserve the uterine artery in order to assure a good vascular supply to the uterine body, particularly in the event of a pregnancy. The venous supply follows the arterial one (Fig. 1).

Uterovaginal Endopelvic Fascia

The endopelvic fascia refers to the reflections of the superior fascia of the pelvic diaphragm upon the pelvic viscera. This thin layer thus encase respectively the urethra and bladder (urethrovesical fascia), the vagina and lower uterus (uterovaginal fascia), and the rectum (rectal fascia). The uterovaginal endopelvic fascia is of particular importance as it lies in close proximity to the pelvic peritoneum. The former is an avascular space that should be defined when mobilizing the bladder base at the time of VRT, but the anterior pelvic peritoneum itself should not be entered (Fig. 2).

Cardinal (Mackenrodt) Ligament

The cardinal ligament is composed of condensed fibrous tissue and some smooth muscle fibers. It extends from the lateral aspect of the uterine isthmus toward the pelvic wall. This fibrous sheath contains the ureter, the uterine vessels and associated nerves, the lymphatic channels and lymph nodes draining the cervix, and some fatty tissue. It is commonly referred to as the *parametrium*. The cardinal ligament is in continuity anteriorly to the uterovaginal endopelvic fascia and posteriorly, fibers are integrated with the uterosacral ligament. Since VRT is performed in patients with small lesions, only the medial part (i.e., ~2 cm) of the cardinal ligaments is usually taken at the time of a VRT (Fig. 3).

Uterosacral Ligaments

These ligaments are true ligaments of musculofascial consistency that run from the upper part of the cervix to the sides of the sacrum. They contribute to the uterine support together with the cardinal ligaments. Only the proximal part of the uterosacral ligaments is taken at the time of VRT so as to leave adequate uterine support (Fig. 3).

PROCEDURE
Anatomical Relationship

It is of paramount importance to understand the relationship between the ureter, the uterine artery, and the cardinal ligament (parametrium), and picture the relationship between the bladder base and the lower uterine segment when performing radical vaginal surgery. When a radical hysterectomy is done *abdominally*, the uterus is pulled upward bringing with it the parametrium and the uterine vessels, while the bladder base is mobilized downward. Therefore,

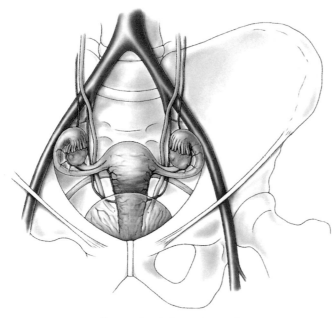

Figure 1 Cervical vascular supply.

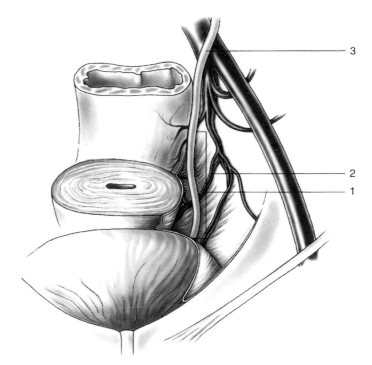

Figure 3 1 Cardinal ligament; 2 Uterine artery; 3 Ureter.

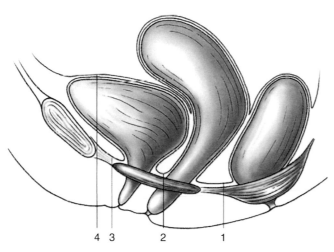

Figure 2 1 Rectal fascia; 2 Uterovaginal fascia; 3 Pelvic peritoneum; 4 Urethrovesical fascia.

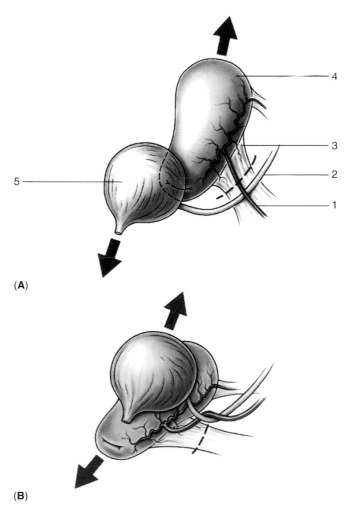

Figure 4 Comparison of (**A**) abdominal and (**B**) vaginal approaches to radical hysterectomy (after Dr Hélène Roy). The *arrows* indicate the direction of traction; the *dotted line* indicates the level of excision of the parametrium. 1 Uterine artery; 2 Ureter; 3 Parametrium; 4 Uterus; 5 Bladder.

the uterine vessels lie *above* the concavity of the ureters as the ureters run into the parametrial tunnel to enter the bladder base. Thus, after mobilization, the ureters end up lateral and below the parametrium (Fig. 4A). When the radical hysterectomy is done *vaginally*, the relationship between the structures is completely the opposite. The uterus is pulled downward and the bladder base along with the ureter is mobilized upward. As such, the uterine vessels end up *below* the concavity or the "knee" of the ureter and after mobilization, the ureter courses above the parametrium (Fig. 4B).

Vaginal Cuff Preparation
A rim of vaginal mucosa is delineated circumferentially clockwise using 8 to 10 straight Kocher clamps placed at regular interval. For small lesions, 1 to 2 cm of vaginal mucosa is sufficient. To reduce bleeding from the edges of the vaginal mucosa, 20 to 30 cm³ of a xylocaine 1% solution mixed with epinephrine 1:100,000 is used to inject the vaginal mucosa between each Kocher clamp. A circumferential incision is then made

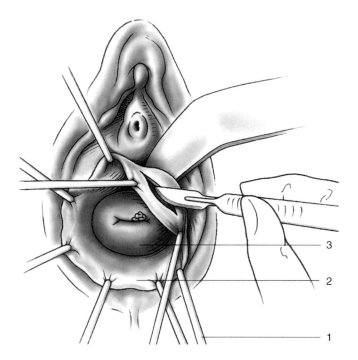

Figure 5 Vaginal cuff preparation: incision (after Dr Hélène Roy). 1 Straight Kocher clamps; 2 Vaginal mucosa; 3 Cervix.

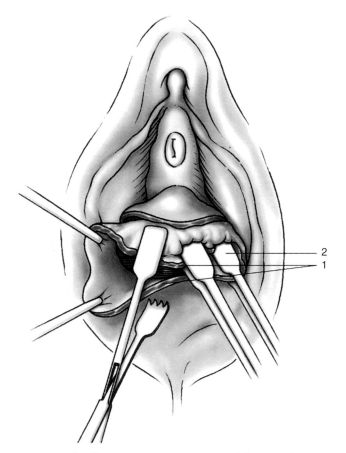

Figure 6 Vaginal cuff preparation: placing the clamps (after Dr Hélène Roy). 1 Anterior and posterior vaginal mucosa covering cervix; 2 Chrobak clamps.

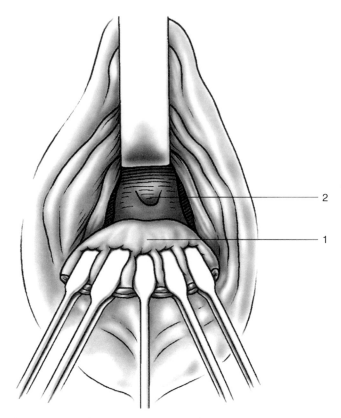

Figure 7 Opening the vesico-uterine space (after Dr Hélène Roy). 1 Exocervix; 2 Uterine isthmus.

Identification of the Vesico-uterine Space

This space is opened by directing Metzenbaum scissors perpendicular to the cervix. Care is taken not to enter the peritoneum as in a simple vaginal hysterectomy. The space should be avascular and allows one to easily palpate the anterior surface of the endocervix and isthmus and see the whitish body of the uterus and the bladder base. When the space is stretched with a narrow Deaver, the anterior bladder pillars lie on each side of the space as vertical strands of tissue (Fig. 7).

Opening of the Paravesical Space (Description for the Patient's Left Side)

The Chrobak clamps are pulled toward the patient's right side. Straight Kocher clamps are placed onto the vaginal mucosa at 1 and 3 o'clock and stretched out. An areolar opening is seen just medial and slightly anterior to the 3 o'clock clamp. The space is *blindly* entered using Metzenbaum scissors, with the tips pointing upward and outward. The space is widened by rotating the scissors under the pubic bone in a semicircular rotating motion to the patient's right side (Fig. 8).

Identification and Mobilization of the Ureter

A small retractor is placed in the left pvesical space and rotated under the symphysis pubis pulling the bladder pillars and the bladder medially. The knee of the ureter is located on the lateral aspect of the bladder pillars which act as pseudo-ligaments (Fig. 9). Holding the Chrobak clamps between the palms of both hands, the surgeon's right index finger (or the back of a surgical instrument) is placed in the left paravesical space and the left index finger in the vesico-uterine space. The surgeon's

with a scalpel just above the Kocher clamps (Fig. 5). Finally, the edges of the vaginal mucosa are grasped with five or six Chrobak clamps in order to completely cover the exocervix and allow a good traction onto the specimen (Fig. 6).

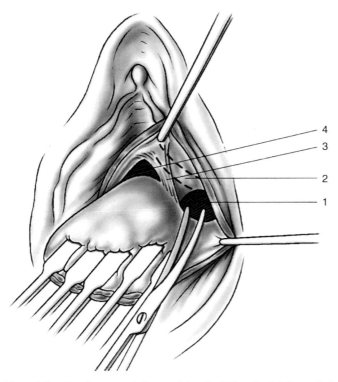

Figure 8 Opening the paravesical space (after Dr Hélène Roy). 1 Paravesical space; 2 Ureter; 3 Bladder pillars; 4 Vesico-uterine space.

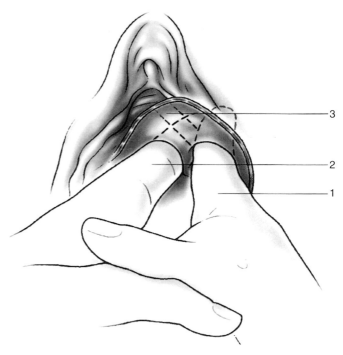

Figure 10 To avoid damage to the ureter, it must be clearly seen and palpated (after Dr Hélène Roy). 1 Right index in paravesical space; 2 Ureter; 3 Left index in vesico-uterine space.

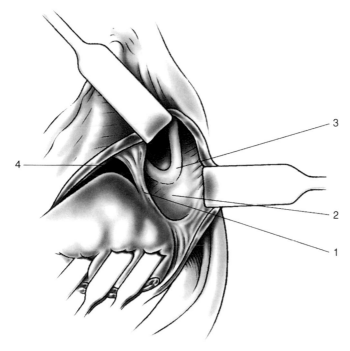

Figure 9 The "knee" of the ureter is exposed on the lateral aspect of the bladder pillars (after Dr Hélène Roy). 1 Bladder pillars; 2 Paravesical space; 3 Knee of ureter; 4 Vesico-uterine space.

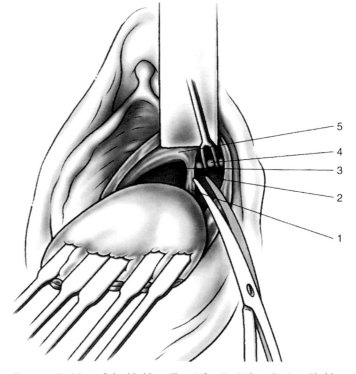

Figure 11 Excision of the bladder pillars (after Dr Hélène Roy). 1 Bladder pillars; 2 Paravesical space; 3 Vesico-uterine space; 4 Ureter; 5 Bladder base.

fingers are then pulled down gently until the "click" is *heard* and the ureter is *felt* rolling under the fingers (Fig. 10).

Section of the Bladder Pillars

To avoid damage, the ureter has to be seen and palpated unequivocally. With Metzenbaum scissors, the bladder pillars are stretched open and dissected carefully until the ureter is seen (Fig. 11). Once the ureter has been safely mobilized

upward, the bladder pillars can be excised midway between the bladder base and the anterior aspect of the specimen (Fig. 11). The ureter is then freed laterally from its posterior attachment to allow its mobilization upward (Fig. 11). Medial dissection of the ureter should be avoided because of the risk of injury to the bladder base. This maneuver allows the ureter and the bladder base to be mobilized upward as well.

Section of the Cardinal Ligament (Proximal Parametrium)

After opening the posterior cul-de-sac, the proximal aspect of the uterosacral ligament is excised. After careful re-identification of the ureter and the cross of the uterine artery, two curved Heaney clamps are used to secure the cardinal ligament or proximal parametrium. The first Heaney clamp is placed medially and with gentle traction the second Heaney is placed more distally to get wider parametrium, having the ureter safely mobilized upward (Fig. 12). The cervico-vaginal branch of the uterine artery is then identified at the level of the isthmus, clamped, excised, and ligated. Care should be taken to carefully identify and preserve the cross of the uterine artery (Fig. 13).

Excision of the Specimen

Steps 5 to 8 are performed on the patient's right side. The cervix is then amputated with a scalpel held perpendicular to the specimen at about 1 cm from the isthmus (Fig. 14). The new exocervix appears gradually (Fig. 14). An endocervical curettage (ECC) of the residual endocervical canal is done afterward. The trachelectomy specimen is sent for immediate frozen section to assess the level of the tumor in relation to the endocervical resection margin. At least 8 to 10 mm of free endocervical canal should be obtained, otherwise additional endocervix should be removed, or the trachelectomy should be aborted and a radical vaginal hysterectomy (Schauta) completed instead. Indications and methods of frozen section of vaginal trachelectomy specimen have recently been reviewed (Chênevert et al. 2009).

Prophylactic Cervical Cerclage and Closure of the Vaginal Mucosa

The posterior cul-de-sac is first closed with a purse-string suture of Chromic 2-0 suture. A permanent cerclage is then placed using a non-resorbable Prolene-0 suture starting at 6 o'clock to have the knot lying posteriorly. Sutures are placed at the level of the internal os and not too deeply within the cervical stroma. When tying the knot, a uterine probe can be left in the cervical os to avoid tightening the knot too much as this may cause cervical stenosis (Fig. 15). The edges of the vaginal mucosa are sutured to the residual exocervical stroma (and not to the endocervical tissue) with interrupted figure-of-eight. Sometimes, excess vaginal mucosa has to be excised to facilitate the closure. Sutures should not be placed too close to the new cervical os to avoid burying the cervix making follow-up examinations more difficult (Fig. 16).

Trachelectomy Specimen

Ideally, the cervical specimen should be at least 1 cm long, with 1 cm of vaginal mucosa and 1 to 2 cm of parametrium. Figure 17 shows a cervix with a small exophytic lesion (A); figure B shows a lateral view of the trachelectomy specimen demonstrating the endocervical cut margin, proximal parametria (stretched by the Debakey instruments), and vaginal cuff (suture) covering the cervical lesion; figure C shows the appearance of the cervix after suturing of the vaginal mucosa to the residual exocervix.

Cervical Appearance After a Trachelectomy Procedure

With time, the new cervix gradually resumes an almost normal appearance except for its shorter length. It therefore remains

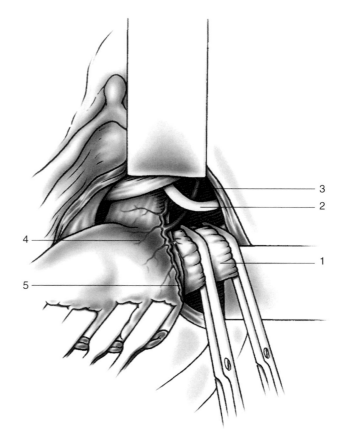

Figure 12 Excision of the parametrium (after Dr Hélène Roy). 1 Parametrium; 2 Ureter; 3 Uterine artery; 4 Isthmus with cross of uterine artery; 5 Descending branch of uterine artery.

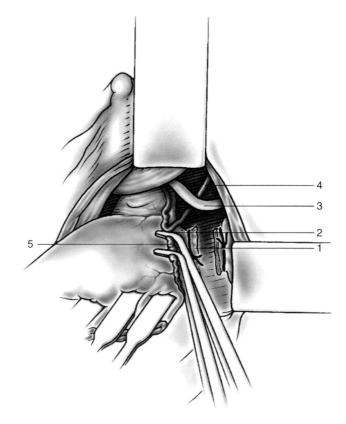

Figure 13 Care is needed to preserve the cross of the uterine artery (after Dr Hélène Roy). 1 Excised parametrium; 2 Cross of the uterine artery; 3 Ureter; 4 Uterine artery; 5 Descending branch of uterine artery.

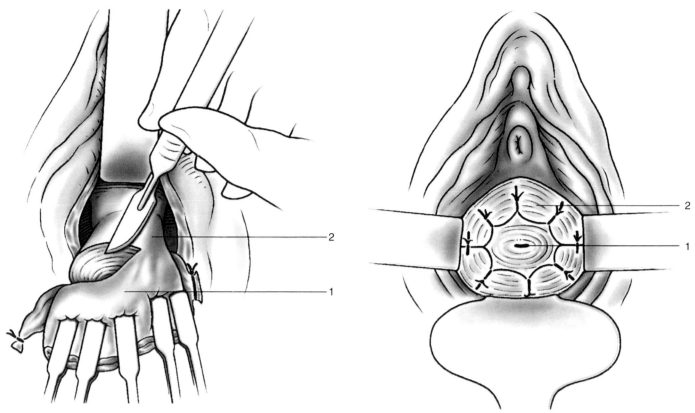

Figure 14 Excision of the cervix (after Dr Hélène Roy). 1 Trachelectomy specimen; 2 Residual endocervix.

Figure 16 Closure of vaginal mucosa (after Dr Hélène Roy). 1 New external os; 2 New ectocervix.

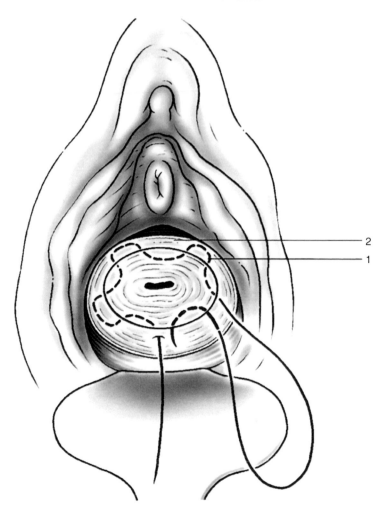

Figure 15 Placing the cervical cerclage (after Dr Hélène Roy). 1 Suture; 2 New ectocervix.

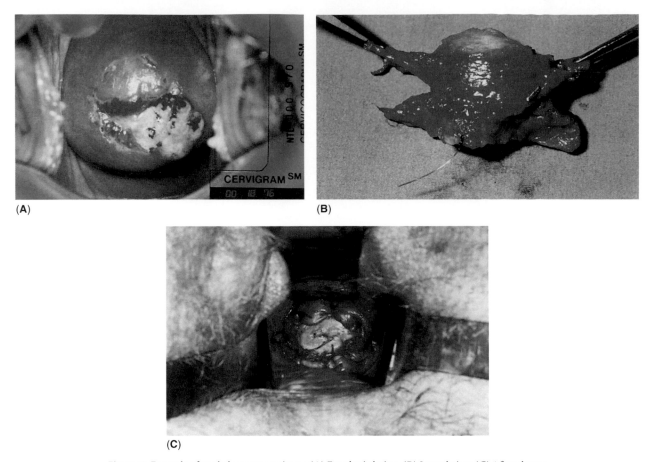

Figure 17 Example of trachelectomy specimen. (**A**) Exophytic lesion. (**B**) Lateral view. (**C**) After closure.

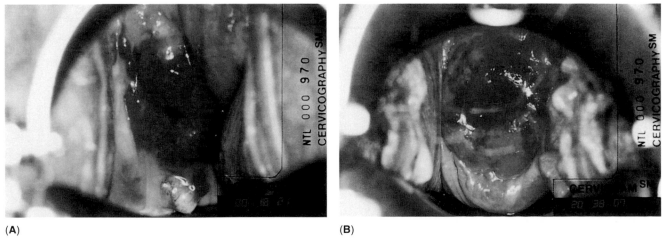

Figure 18 Postoperative appearance. (**A**) Six months after RVT. (**B**) First trimester of a subsequent pregnancy.

accessible for monitoring with colposcopic examination, cytology and ECC. Figure 18 shows pictures of the cervix six months after a trachelectomy (A) and in the first trimester in a patient who became pregnant after the procedure (B).

RESULTS
The radical trachelectomy procedure has gained wider acceptance and recognition over the years. Data totalizing over 600 cases have recently been summarized elsewhere and will be briefly reviewed here (Plante 2008, Gien 2010).

Oncologic Results

Over 600 cases of vaginal radical trachelectomies have been reported so far in the literature (Plante 2008, Gien 2010). The recurrence rate has remained below 5% and the death rate is in the range of 2% to 3%. This is comparable to the overall outcome following the standard radical hysterectomy for similar size lesions. Recent data confirms that lesions measuring >2 cm are statistically associated with a higher risk of recurrence (Plante 2011). Neoadjuvant chemotherapy followed by fertilty-preserving radical trachelectomy has been proposed as an alternative in those patients. Available data suggest excellent tumor response and preservation of fertility in most cases (Plante 2006)

Approximately 10% of patients are found to have lymph node metastasis (Plante 2011). The majority are detected intraoperatively and in such cases, the trachelectomy is usually abandoned in favor of definite chemo-radiation. When lymph node metastasis are identified on final pathology, adjuvant chemo-radiation is usually recommended postoperatively.

The use of preoperative pelvic MRI has become a mandatory part of the preoperative evaluation to carefully assess the extent of endocervical tumor extension, and reduce the chances of abandoning the trachelectomy because of inability to clear a safe endocervical margin at the time of surgery (Plante 2011).

Obstetrical Results

Over 256 pregnancies have been reported (Plante 2008). The rate of first trimester loss is in the range of 18% which is comparable to the rate in the general population. However the rate of second trimester loss is slightly <10% which is higher than in the general population. It is believed to be secondary to the short cervix and less effective mucus plug which normally acts as a natural barrier against ascending infection. Subacute chorioamnionitis probably eventually leads to premature contractions and premature labor and delivery. It is unknown at this point whether prophylactic cultures and antibiotic coverage is beneficial. Some authors suggest the routine injection of prophylactic steroids to hasten fetal lung maturation in case of premature delivery (Bernardini et al. 2003). Others have suggested the use of progesterone supplements, reduction of physical activities, monitoring of the cervical length with serial endovaginal ultrasounds, prophylactic antibiotics, etc. (Jolley 2007). None of the above recommendations have been shown to improve outcome. However, serial ultrasounds is probably the most sensible method to monitor cervical length and predict the risk of premature deliveries. Ideally, a multidisciplinary team including a gynecologic oncologist, a maternal–fetal medicine and a neonatologist should be involved in the care and evaluation of pregnant women post trachelectomy. It is reassuring that in a large series of 106 pregnancies, 75% of pregnant women post vaginal trachelectomy reaching the third trimester actually delivered at term (Plante 2011).

Fertility Results

Following a radical trachelectomy procedure, up to 80% of women attempting to conceive have been successful (Plante 2011). The estimated cumulative fertility rate is in the range of 55% (Bernardini et al. 2003). The majority of women experiencing fertility problems are due to causes unrelated to the trachelectomy issues (ovulatory dysfunction, endometriosis, male factor, etc.). However, cervical stenosis, which occurs in up to 10% to 15% of women post trachelectomy, may be a cause of infertility in up to 40% of infertility problems (Plante 2011). Managing the tight pinpoint stenosis causes special challenges for the infertility specialist and often limits the possibility of intrauterine insemination (IUI) and embryo transfer (ET) following in vitro fertilization (IVF). New options and tools have been developed to assist the infertility specialist in dealing with those obstacles (Noyes 2009). Women undergoing fertility-preserving surgery in the hope of conceiving often experience a high level of anxiety postoperatively and may require emotional support (Carter 2008).

SUMMARY

The radical trachelectomy has now been performed for approximately 20 years. Data are accumulating indicating that the procedure is oncologically safe in well selected cases: young women, small lesions, limited endocervical extension, and limited VSI. Obstetrically data are also accumulating indicating that the two-third of the patients can anticipate a normal pregnancy and delivery near term. However, the risk of premature second trimester loss or delivery is higher than in the general population and these pregnancies should probably be managed jointly with a fetal–maternal medicine consultant.

Thus, the radical trachelectomy procedure truly offers a valuable alternative to young women with small lesions who wish to preserve their fertility potential. In the future, even more conservative procedures such as conization alone or simple trachelectomy with lymph node assessment may be sufficient in women with very early lesions and in the absence of high-risk features (Rob et al. 2007).

REFERENCES

Bernardini M, Barrett J, Seaward G, Covens A (2003) Pregnancy outcome in patients post radical trachelectomy. *Am J Obstet Gynecol* **189**:1378–82.

Carter J, Sonoda Y, Chi DS, Raviv L, Abu-Rustum N (2008) Radical trachelectomy for cervical cancer: postoperative physical and emotional adjustment concerns. *Gynecol Oncol* **111**:151–7.

Chênevert J, Têtu B, Plante M, et al. (2009) Indication and method of frozen section in vaginal radical trachelectomy. *Int J Gynecol Pathol* **28**:480–8.

Dargent D, Brun J-L, Roy M, Mathevet P, Remy I (1994) La trachélectomie élargie (T.E.). Une alternative à l'hystérectomie radicale dans le traitement des cancers infiltrants développés sur la face externe du col utérin. *J Obstet Gynecol* **2**:285–92.

Dargent D, Franzosi F, Ansquer Y, et al. (2002) Extended trachelectomy relapse: plea for patient involvement in the medical decision. *Bull Cancer* **89**:1027–30.

Gien LT and Covens A (2010). Fertility-sparing options for early stage cervical cancer. *Gynecol Oncol* **117**: 350–7.

Jolley JA, Battista L, Wing DA (2007). Management of pregnancy after radical trachelectomy: case reports and systematic review of the literature. *Am J Perinatol* **24**:531–9.

Noyes N, Abu-Rustum N, Ramirez P, Plante M (2009) Options in the management of fertility-related issues after radical trachelectomy in patients with early-stage cervical cancer. *Gynecol Oncol* **114**:117–20.

Plante M (2000) Fertility preservation in the management of gynecologic cancers. *Curr Opin Oncol* **12**(5):497–507.

Plante M, Gregoire J, Renaud MC et al. (2011) The vaginal radical trachelec-tomy: an update of a series of 125 cases and 106 pregnancies. Gynecol Oncol in press.

Plante M (2008) Vaginal radical trachelectomy: an update. *Gynecol Oncol* **111**:S105–10.

Plante M, Lau S, Brydon L, et al. (2006) Neoadjuvant chemotherapy followed by vaginal radical trachelectomy in bulky stage IB1 cervical cancer: case report. *Gynecol Oncol* **101**:367–70.

Rob L, Charvat M, Robova H, et al. (2007) Less radical fertility-sparing surgery than radical trachelectomy in early-stage cervical cancer. *Int J Gynecol Cancer* **17**:304–10.

Roy M, Plante M (1998) Radical trachelectomy in the treatment of early stage cervical cancer. *Am J Obstet Gynecol* **179**:1491–6.

12 Radical abdominal trachelectomy

Laszlo Ungar, Laszlo Palfalvi, Deborah C. M. Boyle,
Giuseppe Del Priore, and J. Richard Smith

FIGO STAGING

The traditional management of invasive cervical carcinoma has naturally depended on the stage of the tumor (Table 1). As outlined above, conization is suitable management for cervical intraepithelial neoplasia (CIN) and stage IA1 tumors. It is also probably adequate management for the majority of stage IA2 tumors. Table 2 shows the papers published relating to extra-cervical spread of microinvasive tumors, suggesting that the majority will be adequately managed by conization. Most gynecologic oncologists would qualify this, depending on whether lymphovascular permeation was present. If it was, they might proceed to a radical hysterectomy and pelvic lymphadenectomy. As can be seen from the table, this practice is not based strictly on evidence. It should be noted that, according to current FIGO definitions, some of the tumors referred to in the table would now be staged beyond IA2 by virtue of their lateral dimensions; however, this serves further to confirm that radical hysterectomy is overtreatment in many cases. Practice will also vary depending on the woman's desire to retain fertility. Traditionally, stage IB1, IB2, and IIA tumors have been managed by radical hysterectomy and pelvic lymphadenectomy, although many centers now utilize primary chemo-radiotherapy for stage IB2 and IIA tumors. Stage IIB, III, and IV tumors are managed by radiotherapy, chemotherapy, and surgery, either singly or in combination, and dependent upon the individual center and the individual patient. Units vary on their policy for commencing radiotherapy depending on the number of lymph nodes involved.

An increasing number of younger women are being diagnosed with invasive cervical cancer. This is probably a result of the cervical smear program, which enables women to be detected both at an earlier stage in their malignancy and at an earlier age. The increasing number of young patients has made many wonder whether a less radical treatment than a radical hysterectomy and pelvic lymphadenectomy could be offered, while still maintaining a high cure rate and allowing preservation of fertility.

The late Daniel Dargent and Michel Roy describe in chapter 10 the radical vaginal hysterectomy. Expertise in this procedure is the prerequisite to having the skill required for a new technique he has described for removal of exophytic tumors—stages IA2 to IIA—which were unsuitable for treatment by conization; he called this procedure "radical vaginal trachelectomy". It involves removal of the cervix, parametrium, and upper vagina via the vaginal route. Patients also undergo a pelvic lymphadenectomy performed laparoscopically prior to the trachelectomy (this operation is fully described by Plante and Roy in chapter 11). This procedure requires considerable skill in both vaginal and laparoscopic techniques. Many gynecological oncologists have acquired laparoscopic skills to complement their open surgical skills, but few have been trained to perform Schauta's radical vaginal hysterectomy. For these reasons, we have been involved in developing an abdominal approach to radical trachelectomy which is technically similar to a traditional radical hysterectomy, but still offers prospects for future fertility.

When considering more conservative surgery than has previously been the norm for a given condition, one has to consider both the pathology of the disease and its mode of metastasis. The spread of squamous cervical carcinoma is predominantly lateral; it may be continuous, where the tumor spreads in a confluent manner toward the pelvic sidewall, or discontinuous, with vessel or parametrial node involvement.

Vertical spread of cervical cancer is much less common than lateral spread. In Burghardt's series of 395 women, there were no cases of vertical spread in any stage IB or IIA tumors (Burghardt 1991). In the case of stage IIB tumors, there were 11 out of 220 cases (20%) of spread to the uterine corpus, while other workers quote figures of 26% (Mitani et al. 1964) and 24% (Ferraris et al. 1988). Age may be an important factor in spread to the uterine body. Baltzer (1978) found that in women under the age of 50 the vertical spread of stage IIB tumors was 9.5%, whereas in women over 50 years old the figure rose to 32%.

ANATOMICAL CONSIDERATIONS
Fertility

To retain fertility without the need for assisted conception techniques, a woman must retain her ovaries, fallopian tubes, uterus, a residuum of cervix with a patent cervical os and a functioning vagina. With the use of assisted conception and ovum donation techniques, a woman requires as an absolute minimum to have retained her uterus and perhaps a tiny slither of cervix to retain a cervical cerclage suture.

VASCULAR CONSIDERATIONS

The uterus is supplied by three pairs of arteries: the uterine, ovarian, and vaginal arteries, the latter two via collaterals. Viability of the uterus can certainly be maintained in the absence of uterine arteries, and it used to be thought only if there is no interruption of the ovarian or vaginal arterial supply. At the Society of Gynaecologic Oncologists Meeting in New Orleans in February 1996, the membership in an interactive session were asked to vote on how many vessels they felt were required for uterine preservation: the majority felt that the uterus required three of its six supplying vessels to remain viable. Interestingly, we now know that uterine viability may be

Table 1 The International Federation of Obstetrics and Gynaecology (FIGO) Staging of Cervical Cancer

Stage	Extent
0	Intraepithelial neoplasia
I	The carcinoma is strictly confined to the cervix; extension to the uterine corpus should be disregarded
IA	Preclinical carcinomas of the cervix (i.e., those diagnosed by microscopy only). All gross lesions even with superficial invasion are stage IB. Invasion is limited to measured stromal invasion with a maximum depth of 5 mm and no wider than 7 mm. Measurement of the depth of invasion should be from the base of the epithelium, either surface or glandular, from which it originates. Vascular space involvement, either venous or lymphatic, should not alter the staging
IA1	Minimal microscopically evident stromal invasion. The stromal invasion is no more than 3 mm deep and no more than 7 mm in diameter
IA2	Lesions detected microscopically that can be measured. The measured invasion of the stroma is deeper than 3 mm but no >5 mm, and the diameter is no wider than 7 mm
IB	Clinical lesions confined to the cervix, or preclinical lesions greater than stage IA
IB1	Clinical lesions not >4 cm in size
IB2	Clinical lesions >4 cm in size
II	Involvement of the vagina except the lower third, or infiltration of the parametrium. No involvement of the pelvic side-wall
IIA	Involvement of the upper two-thirds of the vagina, but not out to the side-wall
IIB	Infiltration of the parametrium, but not out to the side-wall
III	Involvement of the lower third of the vagina. Extension to the pelvic side-wall. On rectal examination there is no cancer-free space between the tumor and the pelvic side-wall. All cases with a hydronephrosis or non-functioning kidney should be included, unless this is known to be attributable to another cause
IIIA	Involvement of the lower third of the vagina, but not out to the pelvic side-wall if the parametrium is involved
IIIB	Extension on to the pelvic side-wall and/or hydronephrosis or non-functional kidney
IV	Extension of the carcinoma beyond the reproductive tract
IVA	Involvement of the mucosa of the bladder or rectum
IVB	Distant metastasis or disease outside the true pelvis

Table 2 Results of Pelvic Lymphadenectomy in Microinvasive Carcinomas (65 mm Invasion, Early Stromal Invasion Excluded)

Author, Year	No. depth (%)	Maximal size (%)	CLS involvement (%)	Confluent pattern (%)	Lymph-node involvement	Died of disease
Roche and Norris 1975	30	5 mm	57	37	0	–
Sedlis et al. 1979	74	5 × 3 > 8 mm	NS	22.5 (of 133 cases)	0	–
Lohe et al. 1978	37	5 × 10 mm	NS	NS	0	–
Taki et al. 1979	55	3 mm	0	0	0	–
Hasumi et al. 1980	29	3.1–5 mm	11.1	100	4	–
van Nagell et al. 1983	52	3.1–5 mm			3	–
Creasman et al. 1985	32	5 mm	15.6 (of 95 cases)	20 (of 96 cases)	0	–
Simon et al. 1986	69	5 × 12 mm	6.6 (of 105 cases)	NS	1	–
Maiman et al. 1988	30	3.1–5 mm				
Kolstad 1989	63	5 mm	16.1 (of 411 cases)	NS	1	–
Burghardt et al. 1991	39	5 × 10 mm	NS	NS	0	–
Creasman et al. 1998	51	5 mm	25	NS	0	–

Abbreviations: CLS, capillary-like space; NS, not stated.
Source: Adapted from Burghardt 1993.

maintained by the ovarian arteries alone, as demonstrated in approximately 200 cases of radical abdominal trachelectomy already undertaken.

ONCOLOGICAL CONSIDERATIONS

Any form of radical surgery for treatment of cervical carcinoma requires the removal of at least the cervix, some of or all the parametrium and upper vagina coupled with pelvic lymphadenectomy. The extent of parametrial resection required is still a subject of controversy (Hagen et al. 2000). Pelvic lymphadenectomy should involve removal of the paracervical, presacral, obturator, internal, external, and common iliac nodes and possibly also the para-aortic nodes. A full

description of Dargent's vaginal radical hysterectomy technique is given in chapter 10. Plante and Roy describe the vaginal approach to radical trachelectomy in chapter 11. Laparoscopic lymphadenectomy techniques are described in chapters 10 and 26.

Figure 1 demonstrates the tumor requiring to be removed and the vascular supply to the uterus. In our technique for performing a radical abdominal trachelectomy, the abdomen is opened in standard fashion, through either a midline incision or a modified Cherney's incision, and the operation proceeds initially like a standard radical abdominal hysterectomy. The dissection commences by dividing the round ligaments, opening the broad ligament, paravesical, and pararectal spaces

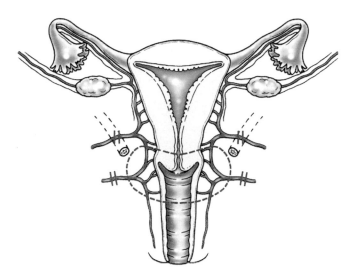

Figure 1 The area to be removed during the procedure.

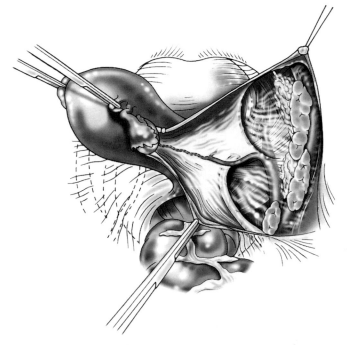

Figure 3 The internal iliac and uterine arteries are skeletonized.

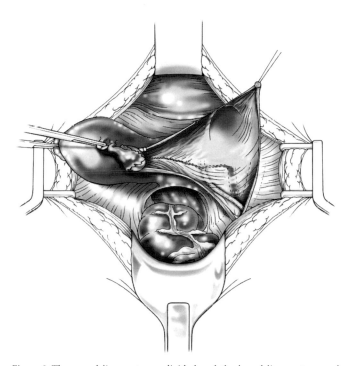

Figure 2 The round ligaments are divided and the broad ligament opened onto the pelvic side-wall.

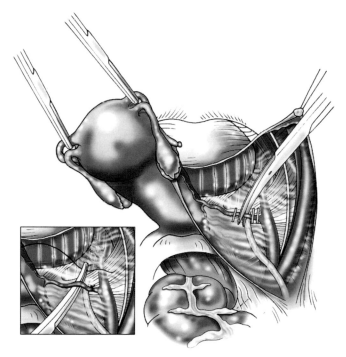

Figure 4 The uterine artery is divided close to its origin following application of hemoclips or ligation (see the inset).

(Fig. 2). The ovarian pedicles must be handled with great care and preserved at all costs. The external iliac, common iliac, internal iliac, and obturator nodes are removed (Fig. 3). The ureter is dissected from its entry into the pelvis until it runs under the uterine artery. The dissection of the anterior division of the internal iliac artery into the superior vesical and uterine vessels is continued with skeletonization of the proximal part of these vessels (Fig. 4). The uterine artery is ligated at its origin. The ureteric tunnels are then opened and dissected and the bladder deflected anteriorly (Fig. 5). In method 1, the rectovaginal septum is opened to the level of the pelvic floor. The uterosacral ligaments are divided close to the sacrum and the vagina and parametrium are then incised. The uterus, cervix, upper third of vagina, and parametrium are then swung superiorly, still attached to the ovarian pedicle

(Fig. 6). This allows excision of the cervix, parametrium, and upper vagina (Fig. 7). A small residuum of cervix may be left as the site for inserting a cervical cerclage suture. In method 2, it is also possible to cut across the cervix/cervicouterine junction (Fig. 8), and to place the uterus still attached to the ovarian vessels into the abdomen (Fig. 9). One can then undertake the opening of the rectovaginal septum and radical removal of cervix, parametrium, and vagina without the danger of damaging the uterus (Fig. 10); the authors have utilized both

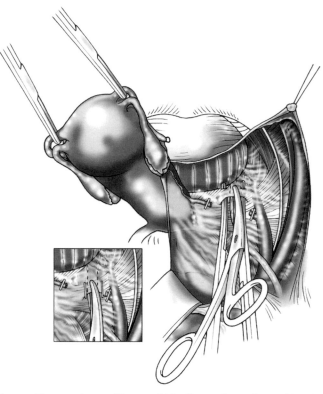

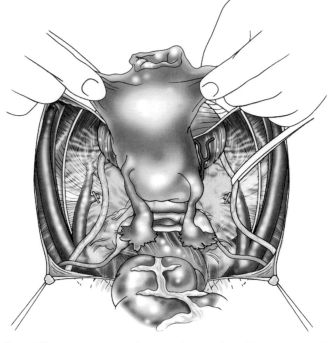

Figure 7 The uterus, cervix, and parametrium are shown here, swung superiorly with the ovaries and uterine tubes attached.

Figure 5 The ureteric tunnel is opened. Bleeding can be profuse at this point and the application of hemoclips or the use of Lotus harmonic scissors may be helpful. (Lotus company address is S.R.A. Developments Ltd., Bremridge House, Ashburton, South Devon TQ13 7JK, UK.)

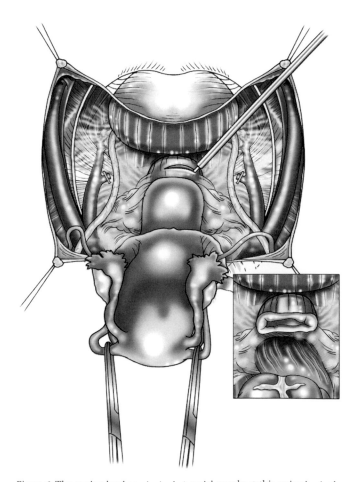

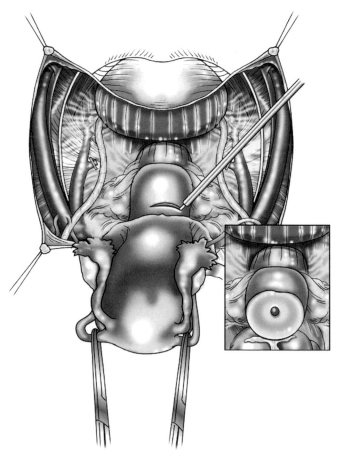

Figure 8 The uterocervico junction is transected.

Figure 6 The vagina has been incised. Arterial supply at this point is via the ovarian vessels alone.

methods. Whichever method is used, frozen section histological examination is performed on tissue from the upper surface of the cervix, to ensure adequate resection margins, and also from the lymph nodes. If the cervix demon-

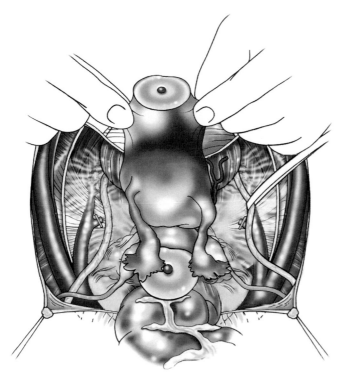

Figure 9 Insertion of the cervical suture with the knot placed posteriorly. This allows the uterus to be placed in the abdomen prior to completion of the trachelectomy.

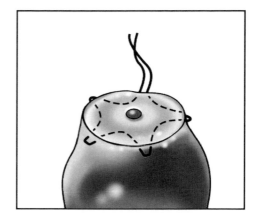

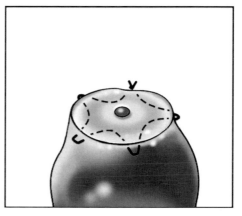

Figure 11 Insertion of cervical suture with care to apply the knot posteriorly.

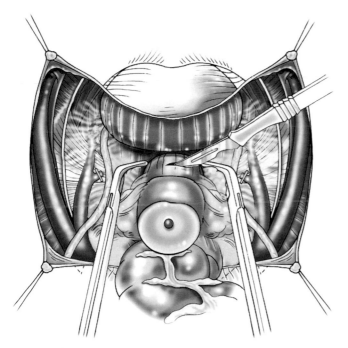

Figure 10 The parametrium is clamped, divided, and ligated. Alternatively Lotus harmonic scissors may be used.

strates inadequate resection margins or the pelvic lymph nodes contain tumor, the procedure is abandoned and a full radical hysterectomy performed.

Assuming the margins to be acceptable, if a thin plate of cervix has been retained a cervical cerclage suture may be inserted.

Prolene (Ethicon) can be used with the knot tied so as to lie posteriorly (Fig. 11). This allows for the possibility of easy removal by a vaginal route via the Pouch of Douglas, should this ever be required. In addition it prevents potential bladder irritation by the knot. The vast majority of cases have been performed without use of a cerclage suture, even though in many of the cases the cervix has been removed in its entirety. The next step is to reanastomose the cervical plate/lower part of the uterus to the vagina. The authors have utilized two methods, one being insertion of a circumferential single-layer running suture between uterus and vaginal cuff (Figs. 12 and 13), the other being insertion of six interrupted sutures running from the outside of the vagina to the inside, then through the cervical plate from inside to outside. If this method is used it is made easier by moistening the vicryl sutures with lubricating jelly. After the six sutures are inserted, the uterus is "parachuted" into position and the sutures ligated (Figs. 14 and 15). Figure 16 shows the end result. The abdomen is then closed in the standard fashion.

Criticism of our procedure is not oncological, since our operation, in terms of clearance, is virtually the same as a radical hysterectomy and, we believe, has equal capacity to deliver clearance of tumor. Either a proportion of or all the parametrium can be removed, depending upon the tumor being excised.

The authors have now performed the operation in approximately 150 women. The last time the data were fully analyzed for the presentation at the SGO, Palm Springs (2007).

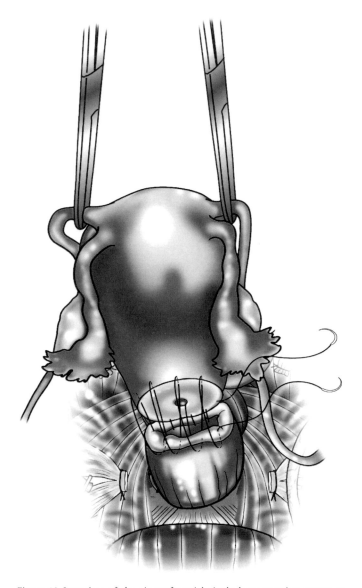

Figure 12 Insertion of the circumferential single layer running suture to achieve final end result.

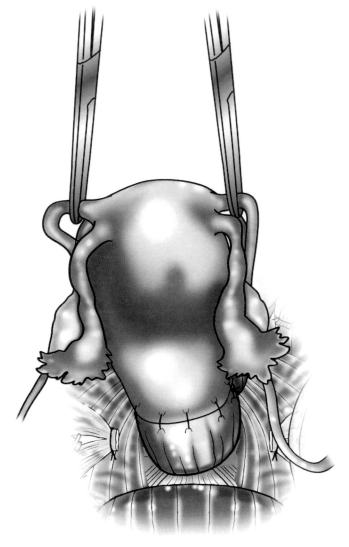

Figure 13 Insertion of the circumferential single layer running suture to achieve final end result.

Ninety-one patients were recruited; eighty-three completed the procedure. Seven were abandoned after positive pelvic nodes (six patients were stage IB2, and one was stage IB1) and one had involvement of the cervical uterine margin. Of the 83 who completed the procedure, 11 were stage IA2, 54 stage IB1, and 18 stage IB2.

During follow-up one patient subsequently underwent a hysterectomy owing to an abnormal Papanicolaou smear result (the histology in this case was negative). The median follow-up was 30 months (range 4–99 months). Normal menses resumed within 12 weeks in 95.2% of women. There were two recurrences (2.4%). One had a rapidly growing exophytic stage IB1 SCC, had negative lymph nodes with good margins but had a large vaginal recurrence at six months. The other had a 5-cm stage IB2 glassy cell adenocarcinoma with LVSI and perineural spread positive. She developed a recurrence 14 months later. In the original series, two women have been delivered of live, healthy babies by cesarean section with no complications (Palfalvi et al. 2003). The babies weighed 3200 and 3350 g despite the reliance on ovarian vessels alone. Doppler flow studies in pregnancy not

surprisingly showed massively increased flow via these vessels. In a further report of three cases of radical abdominal trachelectomy one other baby has been delivered and that baby's mother was reported as being pregnant again (Rodriguez et al. 2001). In the total series of 83, there have been five term deliveries, one pre-term at 36 weeks and in 2007 there were three ongoing gestations. There were four spontaneous first trimester miscarriages.

In addition, five women have undergone the procedure during pregnancy between 7 and 18 weeks. Two had spontaneous first trimester miscarriage two days post-procedure and one had a second trimester miscarriage three weeks post-procedure. Two were delivered by elective Caesarean Section at 39 weeks (Ungar et al. 2006).

In summary, radical abdominal hysterectomy offers an oncologically sound procedure with a good chance of cure, but fertility is not preserved. It is this operation which is most commonly performed and has the best follow-up data. Radical vaginal trachelectomy requires advanced vaginal and laparoscopic surgical skills. It has, however, been proved that fertility follows such surgery, and so far, at least for tumors of <2 cm diameter the long-term survival data look impressive.

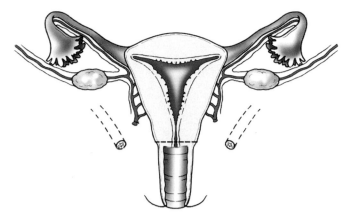

Figure 16 Shows an overview of the final result.

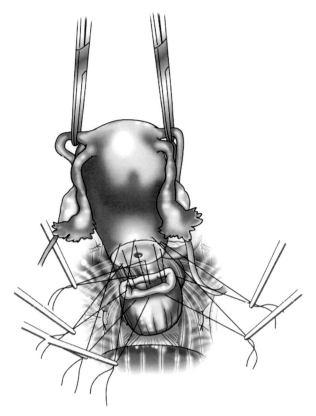

Figure 14 Insertion of six interrupted sutures to allow the uterus to be parachuted back into position to achieve the final end result.

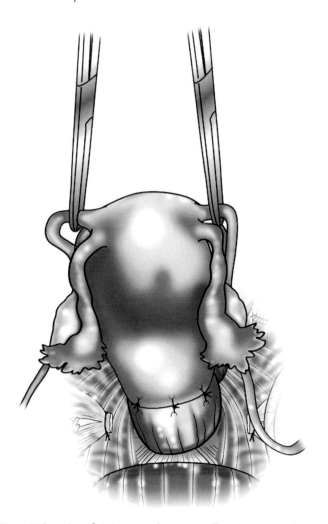

Figure 15 Insertion of six interrupted sutures to allow the uterus to be parachuted back into position to achieve the final end result.

In larger tumors recurrences have occurred (Dargent et al. 2000). Radical abdominal trachelectomy appears to be oncologically sound, and is perhaps more accessible in technical terms than radical vaginal trachelectomy. Fertility is preserved and despite limited follow-up data, we believe long-term survival rates should be similar to those in radical abdominal hysterectomy.

REFERENCES

Baltzer J (1978) Die operative Behandlung des Zervixcarcinoms. Klinische, histologische und tumormetrische Untersuchungsergebnisse einer kooperativen Studie an vier Universitätsfrauenkliniken bei 1092 Patientinnen mit Zervixcarcinom (dissertation). Munich: University of Munich.

Burghardt E (1993) Cervical cancer. In: Burghardt E, Webb MJ, Monaghan JM, Kindermann G, eds. *Surgical Gynecologic Oncology*. New York: Thieme, p. 306.

Burghardt E, Girardi F, Lahousen M, et al. (1991) Microinvasive carcinoma of the uterine cervix. *Cancer* **67**:1037–45.

Creasman WT, Fetter BF, Clarke-Paterson DL, et al. (1985) Management of stage 1A carcinoma of the cervix. *Am J Obstet Gynecol* **153**:164–72.

Creasman WT, Zaino RJ, Major FJ, et al. (1998) Early invasive carcinoma of the cervix (3–5 mm invasion): risk factors and prognosis. *Am J Obstet Gynecol* **178**:62–5.

Dargent D, Martin X, Sacchetoni A, et al. (2000) Laparoscopic radical vaginal trachelectomy: a treatment to preserve the fertility of cervical carcinoma patients. *Cancer* **88**:1877–82.

Ferraris G, Lanza A, Re A, et al. (1988) The significance of lymph node status at pelvic, common iliac and para-aortic levels. *Bailliere's Clin Obstet Gynaecol* **2**:913–20.

Hagen B, Shepherd JH, Jacobs IJ (2000) Parametrial resection for invasive cancer. *Int J Gynecol Cancer* **10**:1–6.

Hasumi K, Sakamoto A, Sugano H (1980) Microinvasive carcinoma of the uterine cervix. *Cancer* **45**:928–31.

Kolstad P (1989) Follow-up study of 232 patients with stage Ia1 and 411 patients with Ia2 squamous cell carcinoma of the cervix (microinvasive carcinoma). *Gynecol Oncol* **33**:265–72.

Lohe KJ, Burghardt E, Hillemans HG, et al. (1978) Early squamous cell carcinoma of the uterine cervix: clinical results of a cooperative study in the management of 419 patients with early stromal invasion and microcarcinoma. *Gynecol Oncol* **6**:31–5.

Maiman MA, Fruchter RG, DiMaio TM, et al. (1988) Superficially invasive squamous cell carcinoma of the cervix. *Obstet Gynecol* **72**:399–403.

Mitani Y, Jimi S, Iwasaki H (1964) Carcinomatous infiltration into the uterine body in carcinoma of the uterine cervix. *Am J Obstet Gynecol* **89**:984.

Palfalvi L, Ungar L, Boyle DCM, et al. (2003) Announcement of healthy baby boy born following abdominal radical trachelectomy. *Int J Gynecol Cancer* **13**:249.

Roche WD, Norris HJ (1975) Microinvasive carcinoma of the cervix: the significance of lymphatic invasion and confluent patterns of stromal growth. *Cancer* **36**:180–6.

Rodriguez M, Guimares O, Rose PG (2001) Radical abdominal trachelectomy and pelvic lymphadenectomy with uterine conservation and subsequent pregnancy in the treatment of early invasive cervical cancer. *Am J Obstet Gynecol* **185**:370–4.

Sedlis A, Sall S, Tsukada Y, et al. (1979) Microinvasive carcinoma of the uterine cervix: a clinical–pathologic study. *Am J Obstet Gynecol* **133**:64–74.

Simon NL, Gore H, Shingleton HM, et al. (1986) Study of superficially invasive carcinoma of the cervix. *Obstet Gynecol* **68**:19–24.

Taki I, Sugimori M, Matsuyami T, et al. (1979) Treatment of microinvasive carcinoma. *Obstet Gynecol Surv* **34**:839–43.

Ungar L, Smith JR, Palfalvi L, Del Priore G (2006) Abdominal radical trachelectomy during pregnancy to preserve pregnancy and fertility. *Obstet Gynecol* **108**:811–4.

van Nagell JR Jr, Greenwell N, Powell DF, et al. (1983) Microinvasive carcinoma of the cervix. *Am J Obstet Gynecol* **145**:981–91.

BIBLIOGRAPHY

Schauta R (1908) *Die erweiterte vaginale Totalextirpation des Uterus beim Kollumkarzinom.* Vienna: Safar.

Smith JR, Boyle D, Corless D, et al. (1997) Abdominal radical trachelectomy: a new approach to the management of early cervical cancer. *Br J Obstet Gynaecol* **104**:1196–200.

Ungar L, Palfalvi L, Hogg R, et al. (2005) Abdominal radical trachelectomy: a fertility preserving option for women with early cervical cancer. *Br J Obstet Gynaecol* **112**:366–9.

13 Central recurrent cervical cancer: the role of exenterative surgery
John M. Monaghan

INTRODUCTION

The procedure of pelvic exenteration was first described in its present form by Brunschwig in 1948. Over the years, it has been used mainly in the treatment of advanced and recurrent carcinoma of the cervix (Barber 1969). Its primary role at the present time is the management of the numerous patients who develop recurrent cancer of the cervix following primary radiotherapeutic treatment (Disaia and Creasman 1981). It has been estimated that between one-third and one-half of patients with invasive carcinoma of the cervix will have residual or recurrent disease after treatment. Approximately one quarter of these cases will develop a central recurrence which may be amenable to exenterative surgery. However, pelvic exenteration as a therapy for recurrent cancer of the cervix has not been widely accepted and many patients will succumb to their disease having been through the process of radiotherapy followed by chemotherapy and other experimental treatments without being given the formal opportunity of a curative procedure. The published results of exenterative procedures show an acceptable primary mortality of approximately 3% to 4% and an overall survival/cure rate of 30% to 60% (Hockel and Dornhofer 2006). The procedure is also applicable to a wide range of other pelvic cancers including cancer of the vagina, vulva and rectum, both for primary and secondary diseases. It is less often applicable to ovarian epithelial cancers and melanomas and sarcomas because of their tendency for widespread metastases.

The surgery involved is extensive, and postoperative care is complex; as a consequence, the operation has become part of the repertoire of the advanced gynecological oncologist working in a center with a wide experience of radical surgery. The procedure does demand of the surgeon considerable expertise and flexibility: virtually no two exenterations are identical, and considerable judgment and ingenuity are required during the procedure in order to achieve a comprehensive removal of all tumor. With small recurrences, more limited procedures may be carried out with a degree of conservation of structures in and around the pelvis. With extensive procedures and particularly following extensive radiotherapy, complete clearance of all organs from the pelvis (total exenteration) together with widespread lymphadenectomy may be essential in order to achieve a cure. There is now considerable evidence that even in patients with node metastases at the time of exenteration a significant survival rate can be achieved.

Selection of the Patient for Exenterative Surgery

Exenterative surgery should be considered for both advanced primary pelvic carcinoma and recurrent disease. Many patients will be eliminated from the possibility of surgery at an early stage because of complete fixity of the tumor mass to the bony structures of the pelvis. The only exception to this rule is the rare circumstance in which a vulval or vaginal cancer is attached to one of the pubic rami: the ramus can be resected and a clear margin around the cancer obtained. In general terms exenterative surgery should not be used as a palliative, except perhaps in the presence of malignant fistulas in the pelvis when it may significantly improve the quality of the patient's life without any significant extension to her life. It is important that the surgical team including nurses and ancillary workers are confident in their ability to manage not only the extensive surgery involved but also the difficult, testing and sometimes bizarre complications that can sometimes occur after exenteration. The average age of patients who are subject to exenteration is 50 to 60 years, but the age range is wide—from early childhood through to the eighth or ninth decade.

PATIENT ASSESSMENT

It is frequently difficult following radiotherapeutic treatment to be certain that the mass palpable in the pelvis is due to recurrent disease and not to radiation reaction or persistent scarring associated with infection or the effects of adhesion of bowel to the irradiated areas.

In recent years both computed tomography (CT) and magnetic resonance imaging (MRI) have been used extensively in the preoperative assessment of patients for many oncological procedures. The considerable difficulties of assessing CT scans in patients who have had preceding surgery or radiotherapy are a particular problem in patients being assessed for exenteration. Some clinicians feel that CT scanning is useful (Crawford et al. 1996), whereas the author has not found the level of reliability to be acceptable. There will be many individual variations from center to center depending upon the skills available to the clinician. A tissue diagnosis is essential prior to embarking on exenterative surgery, and needle biopsy, aspiration cytology, or even open biopsy at laparotomy will be required. As distant metastases tend to occur with recurrent and residual disease, it is sometimes helpful to perform scalene node biopsies and radiological assessments of the pelvic and para-aortic lymph nodes together with fine-needle aspiration, in order to assist with the assessment. PET scans are used in some centers. The mental state of the patient is also important, but should not in itself be a bar to the performance of such surgery.

Absolute Contraindications

If there are metastases in extra-pelvic lymph nodes, abdominal viscera, lungs, or bones there appears to be little value in performing such major surgery (Stanhope and Symmonds 1985). However, there is evidence that patients with pelvic lymph node metastases may well survive, and a good quality of life is reported in a small but significant percentage of such patients. Local resection of pelvic side-wall vasculature together with the lymphatic ray has been shown to achieve salvage in selected patients (Austin and Solomon 2009).

Relative Contraindications

- Pelvic side-wall spread: if the tumor has extended to the pelvic side-wall either in the form of direct extension or nodal metastases the prospects of a cure are extremely small and the surgeon must decide whether the procedure will materially improve the patient's quality of life. The triad of unilateral uropathy, renal non-function or ureteric obstruction together with unilateral leg edema and sciatic leg pain is an ominous sign. The prospects of a cure are poor; readers are, however, referred to chapter 14 for possible combination therapies. Perineural lymphatic spread is not visible on CT and can be a major source of pain and eventual death.
- Obesity has always been a problem with all surgical procedures, producing many technical difficulties as well as postoperative respiratory and mobilization problems. In the present day obesity is almost endemic in some societies markedly increasing the complexity of surgery and recovery. The more massive the surgery the greater are these problems.

Type of Exenteration

In North America, the majority of exenterations performed are total; in the author's series approximately half of his exenterations have been of the anterior type, removing the bladder, uterus, cervix and vagina, but preserving the rectum (Fig. 1). For very small, high lesions around the cervix and lower uterus and bladder, it may be possible to carry out a more limited procedure (a supralevator exenteration) retaining considerable parts of the pelvic floor. Posterior exenteration (abdominal perineal procedure) is rarely performed by gynecological oncologists as this procedure tends to be the province of the general surgeon.

Preoperative Preparation

Probably the most important part of the preoperative preparation is the extensive counseling needed to make certain that the patient and her relatives, particularly her partner, understand fully the extent of the surgery and the marked effect it will have upon normal lifestyle, in particular the loss of normal sexual function when the vagina has been taken out. The transference of urinary and bowel function to the chosen type of diversionary procedure should be discussed, as should the possibility of reconstructive surgery of the vagina and bladder, and the significant risks of such extensive surgery must be honestly explained. During the course of this counseling the patient should be seen by a stoma therapist. The author finds it ideal for the patient to meet others who have had the procedure, to discuss on a woman-to-woman basis the real problems and feelings about exenteration.

The patient is usually admitted to hospital two to three days prior to the planned procedure to undergo high-quality bowel preparation. With the modern alternative liquid diets and antibiotic therapy, complete cleaning of the small and large bowel can be achieved very rapidly. The anesthesiologist responsible for the patient's care will see the patient and explain the process of anesthesia. The author prefers to carry out all radical surgery under a combination of epidural or spinal analgesia together with general anesthesia. Cardiac and blood gas monitoring is essential. Although the majority of patients do not require intensive care therapy, its availability must be ensured prior to the surgical procedure. Prophylaxis against deep venous thrombosis is usually organized by the ward team utilizing a combination of modern elastic stockings and low-dose heparin which is initiated immediately following surgery.

The Final Intraoperative Assessment

The final decision to proceed with exenteration will not be made until the abdomen has been opened and assessment of the pelvic side-wall and posterior abdominal wall has been made,

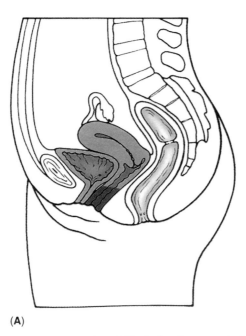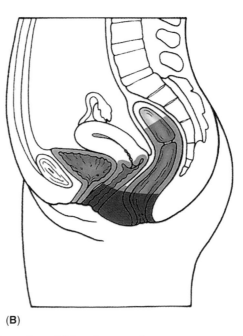

(A)   (B)

Figure 1 The limits of resection for (**A**) anterior and (**B**) total exenteration.

utilizing frozen sections where necessary. As laparoscopic surgery has extended its application, it has become inevitable that its use has extended to exenterative surgery. The value of laparoscopic techniques in the early assessment of the extent of disease is clear. However, its use for the totality of exenterative surgery is limited by the need to develop neovaginas and bladders (Schneider et al. 2009). Similarly, robotic surgery may have a place in some aspects of radical gynecological surgery (Magrina and Zanagnolo 2008). In the author's practice the procedure is performed by a single team. If plastic surgical procedures such as the formation of a neovagina are planned, then a second plastic surgical team will carry out the necessary operation at the same time as the diversionary procedures are being performed by the primary team.

OPERATIVE PROCEDURE

Once the patient has been anesthetized and placed in the supine position in the operating theater the abdomen is opened using either a longitudinal midline incision extending above the umbilicus, or a high transverse (Maylard) incision (Fig. 2) cutting through muscles at the interspinous level. Exploration of the abdomen will confirm the mobility of the central tumor mass; thereafter the para-aortic lymph nodes and pelvic side-wall nodes are dissected (Fig. 3) and sent for frozen section examination. Once the frozen sections show no extension of tumor the procedure of total exenteration can begin. At the same time as this initial intraoperative assessment the experienced exenterative surgeon will have opened

tissue planes, including the paravesical, pararectal, and presacral spaces to a deep level (Figs. 4 and 5) in the pelvis in order to become familiar with the full extent of the tumor. The dissection is achieved by opening the broad ligament: this can be done directly or the round ligament can be ligated and divided first. These dissections can be carried out without any significant blood loss and will yield considerable information. If it is not possible to proceed with the operation the abdomen may be closed at this stage as no significant trauma has been

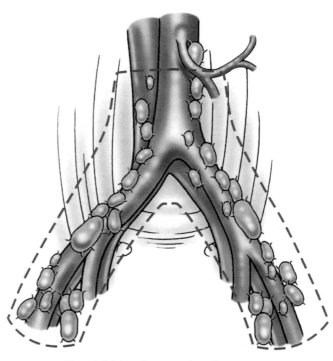

Figure 3 Pelvic and para-aortic node assessment.

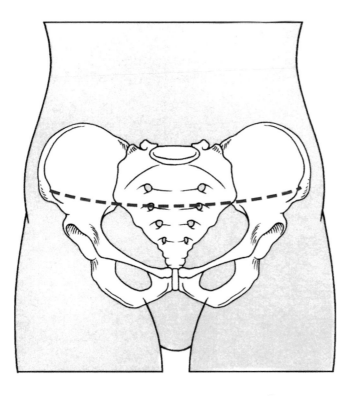

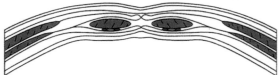

Figure 2 A Maylard or high transverse incision.

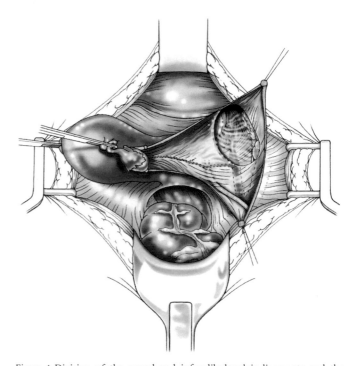

Figure 4 Division of the round and infundibulopelvic ligaments and the beginning of the lateral pelvic dissection.

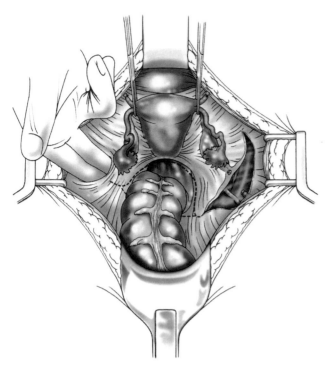

Figure 5 Deepening the lateral pelvic dissection to reveal the pelvic spaces.

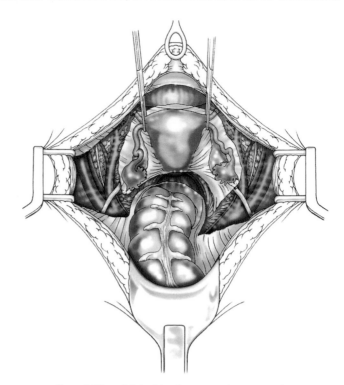

Figure 6 The pelvic incision for an anterior exenteration.

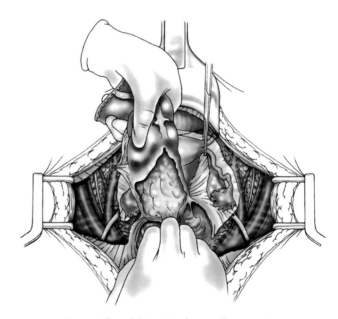

Figure 7 The pelvic incision for a total exenteration.

inflicted by the surgeon. Considerable experience and judgment are required in order to make this decision. Often the most difficult decision is to stop operating. Very occasionally, for example with some vulval cancers, resection of pubic bones may be attempted, but in general terms if there is bony involvement of tumor the procedure should be abandoned.

Total and Anterior Exenteration

After the comprehensive manual and visual assessment of the pelvis and the abdominal cavity, the surgeon proceeds by dividing the round ligament (if it is not already divided), drawing back the infundibulopelvic ligament and opening up the pelvic side-wall (Fig. 6). The line of incision for removal of the entire pelvic organs begins at the pelvic side-wall, over the internal iliac artery, and will pass forward through the peritoneum of the upper part of the bladder, meeting with the similar lateral pelvic side-wall incision at the opposite side. The sigmoid colon will be elevated and at a suitable point will be transected, the peritoneal incision will be continued around the brim of the pelvis—with identification of the ureter as it passes over the common iliac artery—and will meet up with the similar incision on the opposite side. After the round ligaments have been divided and tied and the pelvic side-wall space opened, the infundibulopelvic ligament can also be identified, divided, and tied. The incision is continued posteriorly and the ureters are separated and identified. If an anterior exenteration is to be performed the peritoneal dissection will be brought down into the pelvis to run across the anterior part of the rectum, just above the pouch of Douglas; this will allow a dissection from the anterior part of the rectum passing posteriorly around the uterosacral ligaments to the sacrum, releasing the entire anterior contents of the pelvis. For a total exenteration the dissection is even simpler: the mesentery of the sigmoid colon is opened and individual vessels clamped, divided, and tied. The colon is divided, usually with

a stapling device which allows the sealed ends of the colon to lie, without interfering with the operation in the upper abdomen (Fig. 7). A dissection posterior to the rectum is then carried out from the sacral promontory, deep behind the pelvis; this dissection is rapid and simple and permits complete separation of the rectum from the sacrum. This allows complete and usually bloodless removal of the rectal mesentery including lymph nodes. Anteriorly, the bladder is dissected with blunt dissection from the cave of Retzius resulting in the entire bladder with its peritoneal covering falling posteriorly. This dissection is carried down to the pelvic floor, isolating the urethra as it passes through the pelvic floor (perineal diaphragm). As dissection is carried posteriorly into the

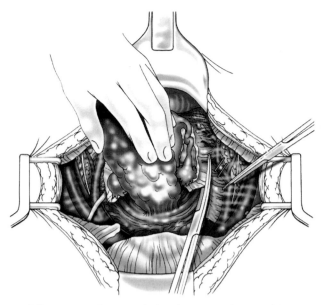

Figure 8 Exenteration clamps applied to the anterior division of the internal iliac arteries.

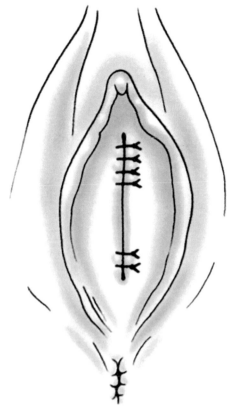

Figure 10 Closure of the pelvic floor musculature.

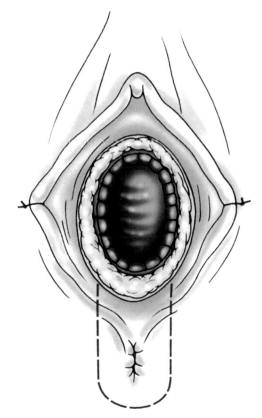

Figure 9 The perineal incisions for anterior and total exenterations.

paravesical spaces, the uterine artery and the terminal part of the internal iliac artery will become clearly visible. By steadily deepening this dissection, the anterior division of the internal iliac will be isolated and the tissues of the lower obturator fossa identified; at this point, large exenteration clamps may be placed over the anterior division of the internal iliac artery and its veins (Fig. 8). The ureter by this time will have been divided a short distance beyond the pelvic brim. The pelvic phase of the procedure is at this point completed and the perineal phase is now to be carried out.

The patient is placed in the extended lithotomy position and an incision made to remove the lower vagina (for an anterior exenteration) or the lower vagina and rectum (for a total exenteration) (Fig. 9). Anteriorly the incision is carried through above the urethra just below the pubic arch to enter the space of the cave of Retzius which has been dissected in the pelvic procedure. The dissection is carried laterally and posteriorly, dividing the pelvic floor musculature, and the entire block of tissue is then removed through the inferior pelvic opening. Small amounts of bleeding will occur at this point, usually arising from the edge of the pelvic floor musculature. These can be picked up by either isolated or running sutures which will act as a hemostat.

Once the perineal dissection has been completed and hemostasis achieved, the surgeon's choice will depend on the preoperative arrangements made with the patient. If in the preoperative assessment period it was decided by the clinician and the patient that a neovagina should be formed, then at this point either the primary surgeon or the plastic surgeon will initiate the development of a neovagina. This may be in the form of a myocutaneous graft using the gracilis muscle (see chapter 32) or a Singapore graft may be used from alongside the vulva; other possible techniques involve the development of a skin graft placed within an omental pad, or transposition of a segment of sigmoid colon in order to form a sigmoid neovagina. For many patients, however, the desire to have a new vagina is a very low priority and it is surprising how frequently patients will put off these decisions until well after the time of exenteration. Surviving the cancer appears to be their uppermost desire. To this end the careful closure of the posterior parts of the pelvic musculature, a drawing together of the fat (Fig. 10) anterior to that and a careful closure of the skin is all that is required. It is usually possible to preserve the clitoris, the clitoral fold and significant proportions of the anterior parts of the labia minora and labia majora so that when recovery is finally made the anterior part of the genitalia has a completely normal appearance. On some occasions patients will be able to have a neovagina formed some significant period of time following the exenteration. This is becoming the predominant pattern in the author's experience of some 89 cases.

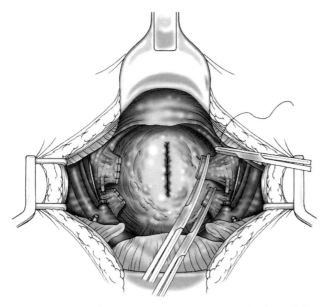

Figure 11 Suture of the internal iliac arteries and lateral pelvic pedicle.

Once the perineal phase is finished the legs can be lowered so that the patient is once more lying supine and attention can be addressed to dealing with the pedicles deep in the pelvis. All that remains following a total exenteration will be the two exenteration clamps on either side of the pelvis and a completely clean and clear pelvis. The pelvic side-wall dissection of lymph nodes can be completed before dealing with the clamps and any tiny blood vessels that require hemostasis are ligated. As the exenteration clamps are attached to the distal part of the internal iliac arteries it is important that comprehensive suture fixation is carried out (Fig. 11). This is usually readily and easily done, although occasionally the large veins of the pelvic wall can provide difficulties and the use of mattress sutures may be necessary in order to deal with these complex vascular patterns. Having completed the dissection of the pelvis, the clinician now moves to produce either a continent urinary conduit or a Wallace or Bricker ileal conduit, and if the procedure has been a total exenteration a left iliac fossa stoma will be formed (see chapters 28 and 29).

Dealing with the Empty Pelvis
A problem which must be avoided is that of small bowel adhesion to the tissues of a denuded pelvis. This is particularly important when patients have previously had radiotherapy, as the risk of fistula formation in these circumstances is extremely high. A variety of techniques have been utilized to deal with this potentially life-threatening complication, including the placing in the pelvis of artificial materials such as Merselene (Ethicon, Edinburgh, UK), Dacron (DuPont) and Gortex sacs (WL Gore & Associates, Flagstaff, Arizona, USA), or even using bull pericardium.

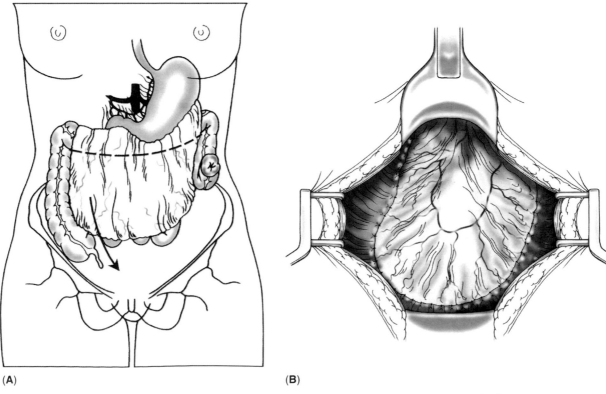

(A)   (B)

Figure 12 Development of the "omental pelvic floor": (**A**) omental incision, (**B**) soft "trampoline" area.

The author's predecessor Stanley Way used a "sac technique" bringing together precut flaps of peritoneum to cover the denuded pelvis (Way 1974). This sac technique in which he manufactured a bag of peritoneum allowed the entire abdominal contents to be kept above the pelvis. This resulted in an empty pelvis, which from time to time became infected and generated a new problem, that of the empty pelvis syndrome. Intermittently over the years patching with the peritoneum has been used. From time to time procedures such as bringing gracilis muscle flaps into the empty pelvis have been carried out to deal with the difficulty of a devitalized epithelium due to previous radiation.

The mobilization of the omentum from its attachment to the transverse colon leaving a significant blood supply from the left side of the transverse colon and allowing the formation of a complete covering of the pelvis by a soft "trampoline" of omentum which will then stretch, completely covering and bringing a new blood supply into the pelvis.

The technique involves separating the omentum from the transverse colon using a powered autosuture; this allows a broad pedicle to remain at the left-hand end of the transverse colon, maintaining an excellent blood supply to the omentum. This is brought down to the right side of the large bowel, dropping into the pelvis immediately to the left side of the ileal conduit which is anchored just above the sacral promontory. By careful individual suturing around the edge of the pelvis and sometimes by refolding the omentum upon itself, a complete covering of the true pelvis with a soft central "trampoline" area can be generated (Fig. 12). A suction drain is inserted below the omentum, which when activated will draw the omentum down into soft contact with the pelvic floor. The small bowel can thus come into contact with an area with a good blood supply, obviating the risk of adherence and subsequent fistula formation. At the end of the procedure the bowel is carefully oriented to make sure that no hernia can develop and the abdomen is closed with a mass closure. The stomas are dressed in theater and their appliances put in place. The patient leaves the operating theater into recovery or ITU and is then transferred back to the ward at the appropriate time.

POSTOPERATIVE CARE

The postoperative care of exenterations is straightforward, essentially being a matter of maintaining good fluid balance, good hemoglobin levels, and ideally a significant flow of urine of 2.5 to 3.5 L/day. Bowel function often returns at the usual time of two to four days following the procedure, and a nasogastric tube (the author's preference) can be removed after three to four days; the return to oral intake, beginning with simple fluid, is initiated on the third day. During and following the procedure prophylactic antibiotic cover is maintained, as is subcutaneous heparin cover as prophylaxis against deep venous thrombosis. Mobilization should be rapid. Patients are usually discharged 10 to 15 days postoperatively, once they are used to dealing with the stomas and the ileal conduit tubes have been removed.

RESULTS OF EXENTERATION

Most series show that the five-year survival rate following exenteration is of the order of 40% to 60%; these figures depend very largely upon the selection of patients (Robertson et al. 1994, Goldberg et al. 2006). A figure that is rather more difficult to obtain is the exact number of patients who are assessed for exenteration but fail at one of the many hurdles that the patient must face before finally undergoing the procedure. It is therefore likely that the final, truly salvageable figure is an extremely low percentage. The value of exenteration procedures in patients who have lymph node involvement has been shown to be low but significant, and it is now many clinicians' practice to carry on with an exenterative procedure even in circumstances where one or two pelvic lymph nodes are involved by tumor.

REFERENCES

Austin KK, Solomon MJ (2009) Pelvic exenteration with en bloc iliac vessel resection for lateral pelvic wall involvement. *Dis Colon Rectum* **52**(7):1223–33.

Barber HRK (1969) Relative prognostic significance of preoperative and operative findings in pelvic exenteration. *Surg Clin North Am* **49**(2):431–7

Brunschwig A (1948) Complete excision of the pelvic viscera for advanced carcinoma. *Cancer* **1**:177.

Crawford RAF, Richards PJ, Reznek RH, et al. (1996) The role of CT in predicting the surgical feasibility of exenteration in carcinoma of the cervix. *Int J Gynecol Cancer* **6**:231–4.

Disaia PJ, Creasman WT (1981) *Clinical Gynaecologic Oncology; Cancer of the Cervix, Pelvic Exenteration*, Chapters 2–8. New York: Mosby, pp. 82–8.

Goldberg GL, Sukumvanich P, Einstein MH, et al. (2006) Total pelvic exenteration: The Albert Einstein College of Medicine/Montefiore Medical Center Experience (1987 to 2003). *Gynecol Oncol* **101**(2):261–8.

Hockel M, Dornhofer N (2006) Pelvic exenteration for gynecologic tumours; achievements and unanswered questions. *Lancet Oncol* **7**(10):837–47.

Magrina JF, Zanagnolo VL (2008) Robotic surgery for cervical cancer. *Yonsei Med J* **49**(6):879–85.

Robertson G, Lopes A, Beynon G, et al. (1994) Pelvic exenteration: a review of the Gateshead experience 1974–1992. *Br J Obstet Gynaecol* **96**:1395–9.

Schneider A, Kohler C, Erdemoglu E (2009) Current developments for pelvic exenteration in gynecologic oncology. *Curr Opin Obstet Gynecol* **21**(1):4–9.

Stanhope CR, Symmonds RE (1985) Palliative exenteration—what, when and why? *Am J Obstet Gynecol* **152**:12–16.

Way S (1974) The use of the sac technique in pelvic exenteration. *Gynecol Oncol* **2**:476–81.

14 Total mesometrial resection
Michael Höckel

INTRODUCTION

About 40% of cervical cancer patients are diagnosed with early macroscopic disease, i.e., FIGO stages IB to IIA, being candidates for surgical treatment with radical hysterectomy, an operation which is conceptually over 100 years old (Wertheim 1912, Quinn et al. 2006). Although various modifications have been applied since the introduction of abdominal radical hysterectomy by Wertheim in the early 20th century, such as the vaginal approach, systematic pelvic and para-aortic lymph node dissection, extension of the paracervical dissection by including the "vesicouterine ligament", tailoring the radicality of the pericervical dissection, autonomic nerve sparing, fertility preserving, minimally invasive techniques, and recently robotic assistance, the principles on which these operations are based have remained essentially unchanged (Dornhöfer and Höckel 2008, Zakashansky et al. 2008). These are: (i) surgical anatomy deduced with regard to tissue function, and (ii) a model of local tumor spread assuming isotropic intra- and transcervical permeation with microscopic and occult disease preceding the macroscopic tumor front. Consequently, for radical treatment the tumor is resected with a ubiquitous metrically defined margin of intra- and paracervical tumor-free tissue (Piver et al. 1974, Querleu and Morrow 2008). Close margins are regarded an indication for adjuvant radiation (Viswanathan et al. 2006). Moreover, it is anticipated that surgical treatment is not sufficient to control discontinuous local and metastatic pelvic disease (Sedlis et al. 1999, Peters et al. 2000).

We have suggested revisiting the surgical anatomy for cancer treatment in general from embryonic development (ontogenetic anatomy) and established the *compartment theory of local tumor spread* (Höckel et al. 2005, 2009). The theory states that malignant solid tumors are confined for a relatively long phase during their natural course to a permissive compartment which can be deduced from embryonic development as mesenchymal differentiation product of the corresponding anlage[a]. Compartment borders are tumor suppressive. For transgression into adjacent compartments of different embryonic origin phenotypical changes are necessary, which evolve relatively late during malignant progression. Local relapses may arise from remnants of the compartment remaining in situ after treatment harboring or recruiting residual tumor (stem) cells.

The compartment theory sets up the new principles of radicality for surgical tumor treatment, namely the resection of the tumor bearing compartment with intact borders. Non-lymphatic adjacent tissues of embryologically different

---

[a]An anlage or primordium is defined in embryology as first discernable epithelium-mesenchyme complex with a fixed morphogenetic determination.

compartments can safely be retained despite their close proximity to the tumor front. Compartment resection should result on the one hand in maximum local tumor control without adjuvant radiation and on the other hand in minimal treatment-related morbidity. Only at the site of intra-compartmental resection, which may be indicated to preserve functional aspects of the morphogenetic unit, a metrically defined tumor-free resection margin has to be achieved. *Total mesometrial resection (TMMR)* is the translation of this principle for the surgical treatment of early cervical cancer.

ONTOGENETIC SURGICAL ANATOMY

We have identified the uterovaginal (Müllerian) compartment in the adult female by following the differentiation and maturation of the Müllerian anlage mesenchyme, that is, the paramesonephric–mesonephric complex connected to the deep urogenital sinus (Höckel et al. 2005). The complex topography of the Müllerian compartment is highlighted in Figure 1.

The cranial part of the compartment is located intraperitoneally, consisting of the Fallopian tubes, mesosalpinx, uterine corpus, and broad ligament. The retro- and subperitoneal caudal part is represented by the cervix, the vagina (except its distal part), and enveloping mesotissue, designated as mesometrium. The mesometrium tapers off with bilateral wings made up of dorsolaterally directed supply tissue with the uterine and vaginal arteries and veins, lymphatic drainage and a few lymph nodes (termed "vascular mesometrium"), and dorsally directed suspensory and fatty tissue fused to the anterior and lateral mesorectum (termed "ligamentous mesometrium"). The vascular mesometrium is adherent to the bladder and its mesentery anterolaterally and is traversed by the ureters. The ligamentous mesometrium is a semi-cylindrical tissue sheet attached to the mesorectum following the pelvic curvature sagittally. It is composed of parts of the posterior broad ligaments, uterosacral ligaments, the rectouterine and rectovaginal ligaments, and the rectovaginal septum. Laterally, the plexus hypogastricus inferior adheres to the ligamentous mesometrium. Dorsally and inferiorly it is continuous with the endopelvic fascia of the pelvic wall and floor. The subperitoneal part of the Müllerian compartment is a distinct arterial-capillary territory covered by continuous lamellae. Venous drainage of the uterovaginal compartment is connected to the lower urinary tract. The deep uterine and vaginal veins fuse with the bladder veins.

SURGICAL PROCEDURE
Indications

Carcinoma of the uterine cervix, FIGO stages IB and IIA; FIGO stage IIB if tumor size is not larger than 5 cm and bladder muscularis infiltration can be excluded.

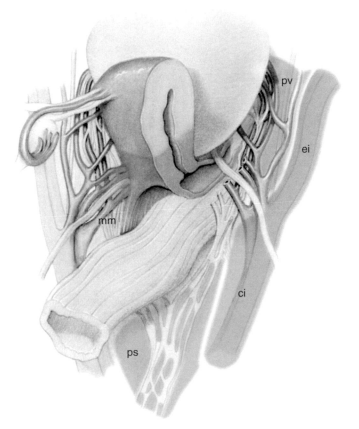

Figure 1 Schematic representation of the Müllerian compartment (*green*) and the draining pelvic lymph node basins (*red*) deduced from ontogenetic surgical anatomy. To display the topographic relations the right half of the compartment and the complete pelvic peritoneal covering are omitted and the visceral branches of the internal iliac vessel system have been spread. *Abbreviations*: pv, paravisceral; ei, external iliac; ci, common iliac; ps, presacral; mm, mesometrial. *Source*: Höckel et al. 2009, Figure 1.

Contraindications
Medical conditions compromising operability.

Treatment Goals
- Local tumor control through extirpation of the uterovaginal (Müllerian) compartment with a wide tumor-free vaginal margin
- Regional tumor control through clearance of lymph node basins specified by embryologically deduced pelvic visceroparietal compartments
- Eventually ascending para-aortic lymph node dissection for M(LYM) control

Technique
TMMR is performed in defined steps as previously published (Höckel et al. 2005, 2009), illustrated with Figures 2–21.

Step 1 (Fig. 2)
Hypogastric midline laparotomy is performed with left circumcision of the umbilicus. In obese patients and for para-aortic lymph node dissection epigastric advancement of the incision may be necessary.

Step 2 (Fig. 3)
Peritoneal incisions above the psoas muscles, in the para-aortic gutters, and along the radix mesenterii are done to gain access to the pelvic and mid-abdominal retroperitoneum.

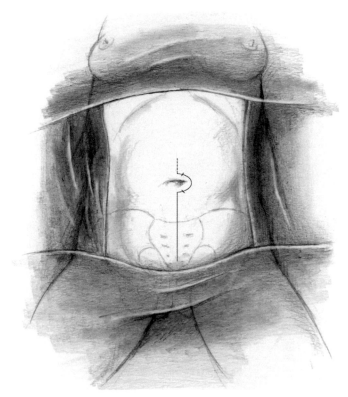

Figure 2 Laparotomy (after E.W. Hanns). *Source*: Höckel et al. 2009, Webappendix Figure 1.

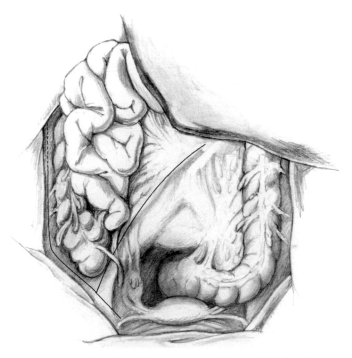

Figure 3 Peritoneal incisions (after E.W. Hanns). *Source*: Höckel et al. 2009, Webappendix Figure 2.

Step 3 (Fig. 4)
At the pelvic brim the infundibulopelvic ligaments and ureters are exposed. The superior hypogastric plexus is identified between the mesosigma and the bifurcation of the aorta.

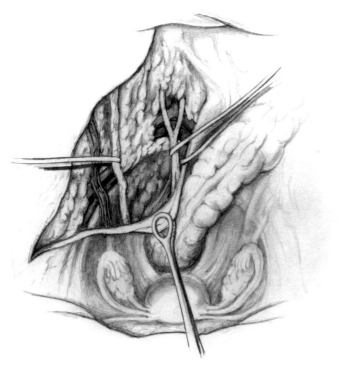

Figure 4 Exposition of the superior hypogastric plexus (after E.W. Hanns). *Source*: Höckel et al. 2009, Webappendix Figure 3.

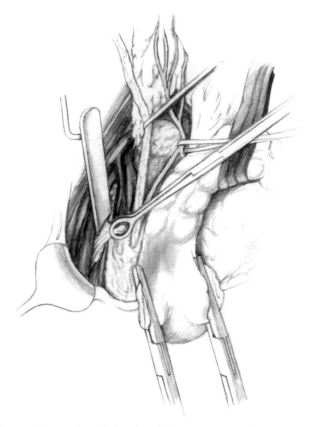

Figure 6 Therapeutic pelvic lymph node dissection, part I (after E.W. Hanns). *Source*: Höckel et al. 2009, Webappendix Figure 5.

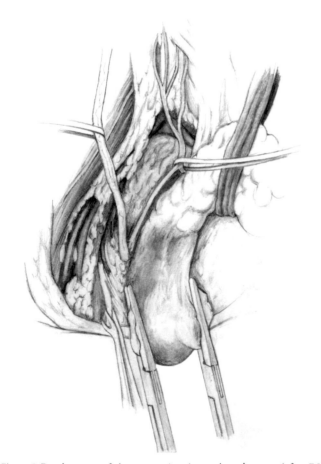

Figure 5 Development of the presacral and paravisceral spaces (after E.W. Hanns). *Source*: Höckel et al. 2009, Webappendix Figure 4.

muscles. The lateral pelvic parietal regions are separated by this maneuver from the combined urogenital mesentery. The hypogastric nerves and the upper parts of the inferior hypogastric plexus are exposed as well.

Step 5 (Fig. 6)
Complete lymph node dissection is performed along the external iliac vessels, internal iliac vessels, and within the obturator fossa above and below the obturator nerve, and presciatically down to the ischial spine.

Step 6 (Fig. 7)
Access to the anterior subperitoneal space is gained by sharp separation of the bladder from the cervix and the proximal vagina after incision of the vesicouterine peritoneal fold.

Step 7 (Fig. 8)
The bilateral vascular mesometrium containing the uterine arteries and superficial veins, lymphatics and a few small lymph nodes is completely separated from the "bladder mesentery". The prevesical ureters are exposed medially.

Step 8 (Fig. 9)
The vascular mesometrium is sealed and dissected at the level where the uterine vessels branch from the internal iliac vessel system.

Step 9 (Fig. 10)
The deep uterine veins are ligated and cut at their branching from the vesical veins.

Step 4 (Fig. 5)
The presacral space is developed to the level of S2, the paravisceral spaces are developed to the pubo- and iliococcygeus

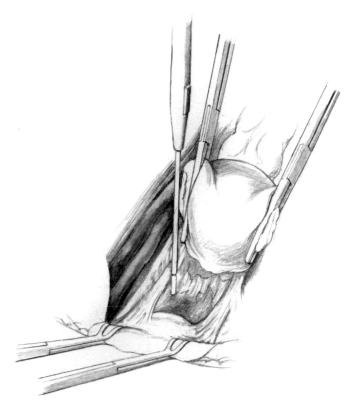

Figure 7 Separation of the uterovaginal compartment from the bladder compartment (after E.W. Hanns). *Source*: Höckel et al. 2009, Webappendix Figure 6.

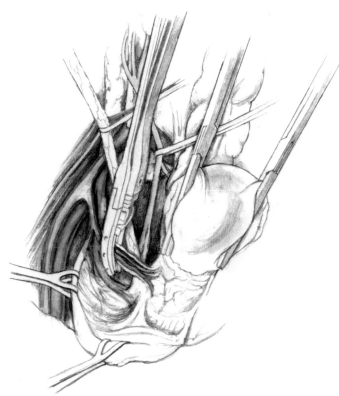

Figure 9 Sealing of the vascular mesometrium at the branching site of the uterine vessels from the internal iliac vessels (after E.W. Hanns). *Source*: Höckel et al. 2009, Webappendix Figure 8.

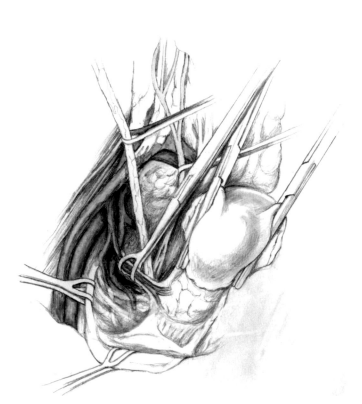

Figure 8 Separation of the vascular mesometrium from the "bladder mesentery" (after E.W. Hanns). *Source*: Höckel et al. 2009, Webappendix Figure 7.

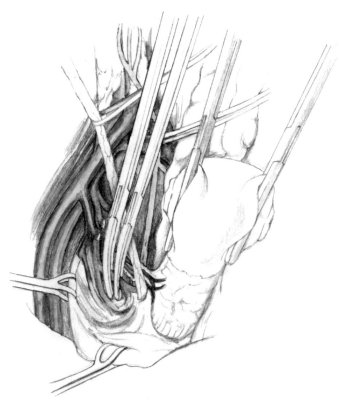

Figure 10 Transection of the deep uterine veins (after E.W. Hanns). *Source*: Höckel et al. 2009, Webappendix Figure 9.

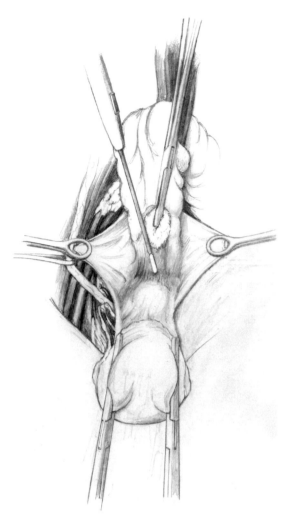

Figure 11 Incision of the rectouterine peritoneum (after E.W. Hanns). *Source*: Höckel et al. 2009, Webappendix Figure 10.

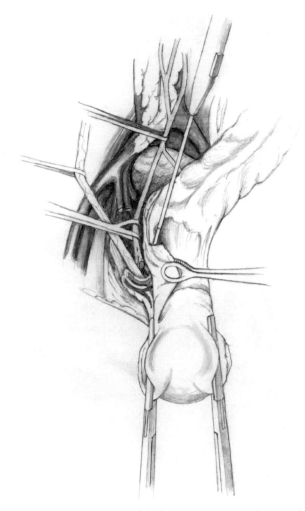

Figure 12 Lateral mobilization of the hypogastric nerves and proximal inferior hypogastric plexus from the ligamentous mesometrium and transection of the posterior leaf of the broad ligament (after E.W. Hanns). *Source*: Höckel et al. 2009, Webappendix Figure 11.

Step 10 (Fig. 11)

Access to the posterior subperitoneum is obtained by sharp separation of the anterior mesorectum from the upper central ligamentous mesometrium after incision of the rectouterine peritoneal fold.

Step 11 (Fig. 12)

After lateral mobilization of the inferior hypogastric plexus the cranial part of the ligamentous mesometrium corresponding to the posterior leaf of the broad ligament is transected.

Step 12 (Fig. 13)

Sealing and dissection of the ligamentous mesometrium is continued caudally at the lateral mesorectum (uterosacral ligaments).

Step 13 (Fig. 14)

The ligamentous mesometrium is sealed and dissected at the anterior mesorectum (rectovaginal ligaments and septum).

Step 14 (Fig. 15)

After flipping the vascular mesometrium above the ureter the vesicovaginal venous connections and condensed connective tissue crossing the prevesical ureters are clamped and transected over a protecting groove. Subsequently, the distal ureters can be completely mobilized laterally.

Step 15 (Fig. 16)

After clamping the vagina with a wide margin to the most caudal tumor extension the anterior vaginal wall is incised. The transverse colpotomy is advanced and completed after sealing the dissection site.

Step 16 (Fig. 17)

Comprehensive pelvic lymph node dissection is continued by removing the lymph nodes along the common iliac and gluteal vessels. The lumbar branch of the lumbosacral trunk, the proximal sciatic nerve, and the parietal branches of the internal iliac vessels are exposed.

Step 17 (Fig. 18)

Presacral lymph node dissection is performed, caudally to the level of S2. The superior hypogastric plexus and the hypogastric nerves are mobilized and preserved.

Step 18 (Fig. 19)

Ascending para-aortic lymph node dissection is added in the case of intraoperatively detected pelvic lymph node metastases. The cranial border of the paracaval, interaortocaval, and para-aortic lymph node dissection is set to the level of the inferior mesenteric artery if the lymph nodes do not contain

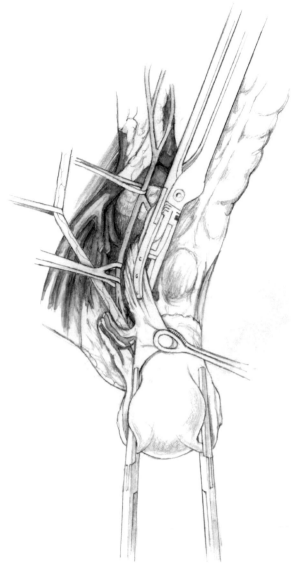

Figure 13 Continued dissection of the ligamentous mesometrium (uterosacral ligament) (after E.W. Hanns). *Source*: Höckel et al. 2009, Webappendix Figure 12.

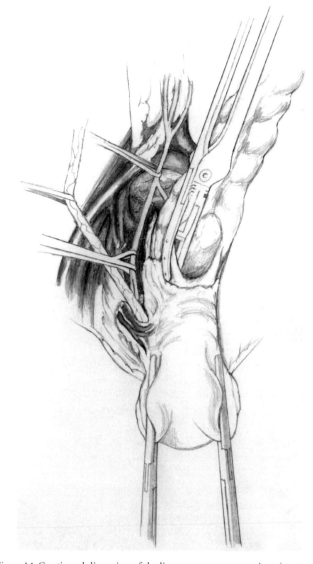

Figure 14 Continued dissection of the ligamentous mesometrium (rectovaginal ligaments and septum) (after E.W. Hanns). *Source*: Höckel et al. 2009, Webappendix Figure 13.

metastases. It will be elevated to the left renal vein if para-aortic lymph node metastases are detected with frozen section histological investigation.

Step 19 (Fig. 20)
The bladder and rectum peritoneum flaps are sutured together to support the mobilized pelvic ureters. The sigmoid colon is refixed to the parietal peritoneum at the site of the connatal adhesions.

Step 20 (Fig. 21)
After suprapubic cystostomy the laparotomy is closed with a running Smead-Jones suture. The skin is stapled.

Pathological Evaluation
- Histopathological diagnosis of pretreatment biopsies
- Intraoperative frozen section evaluation of
  - external iliac and paravisceral lymph node fractions
  - ascending periaortic lymph node fractions in the case of pelvic lymph node metastases

  - vaginal (intracompartmental) margin of the TMMR specimen
  - eventually compartmental border of the TMMR specimen at the site of fibrotic fixation to adjacent non-Müllerian tissues
- Preparation and investigation of the formalin-fixed TMMR specimens and topographically specified lymph node fractions according to the protocol of the Cancer Committee of the College of the American Pathologists (Kurman and Amin 1999).

OUTLOOK
TMMR holds a great potential to improve the therapeutic index of surgical cervical cancer therapy. Although standardized TMMR may be applied for the treatment of cervical cancer stages IB, IIA, and selected IIB, the new principles of surgical radicality are also compatible with fertility-preserving mesometrial resection for very early disease. Mesometrial resections should also be feasible for the minimally invasive and robotic performance.

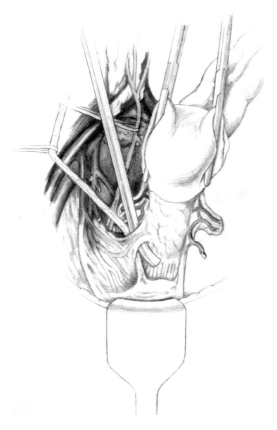

Figure 15 Transection of the paraureteral vesicovaginal venous connections and mobilization of the prevesical ureters (after E.W. Hanns). *Source*: Höckel et al. 2009, Webappendix Figure 14.

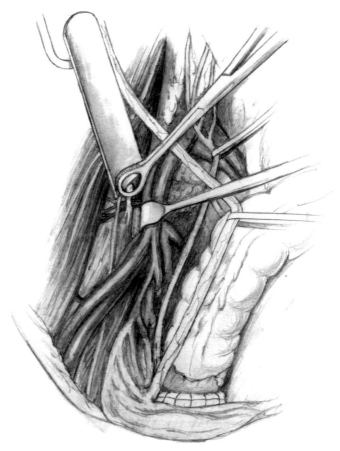

Figure 17 Therapeutic pelvic lymph node dissection, part II (after E.W. Hanns). *Source*: Höckel et al. 2009, Webappendix Figure 16.

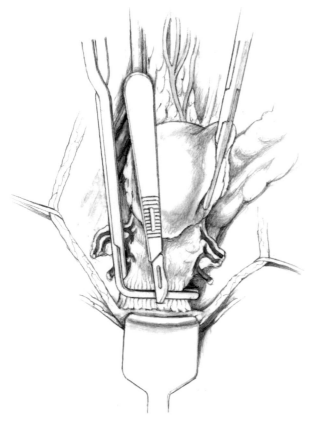

Figure 16 Colpotomy (after E.W. Hanns). *Source*: Höckel et al. 2009, Webappendix Figure 15.

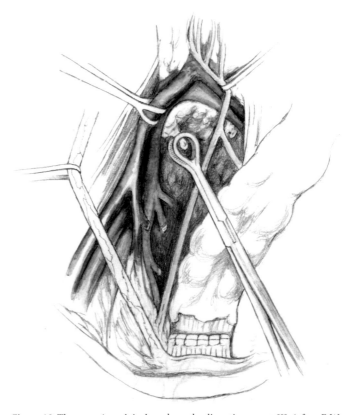

Figure 18 Therapeutic pelvic lymph node dissection, part III (after E.W. Hanns). *Source*: Höckel et al. 2009, Webappendix Figure 17.

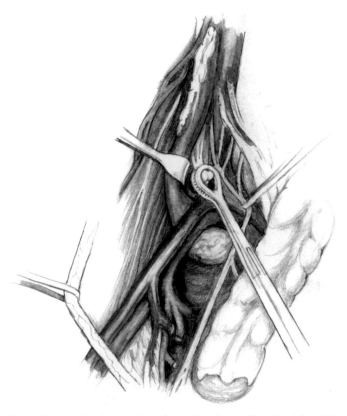

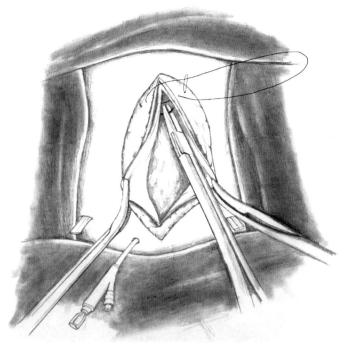

Figure 21 Laparotomy closure (after E.W. Hanns). *Source*: Höckel et al. 2009, Webappendix Figure 20.

Figure 19 Ascending therapeutic periaortic lymph node dissection (after E.W. Hanns). *Source*: Höckel et al. 2009, Webappendix Figure 18.

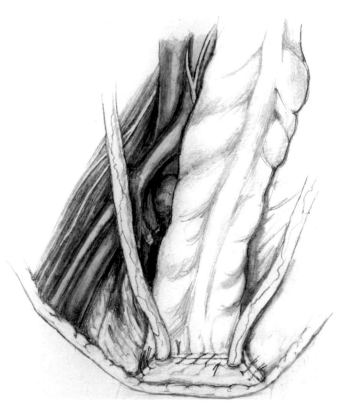

Figure 20 Vesicorectal peritoneal bridge (after E.W. Hanns). *Source*: Höckel et al. 2009, Webappendix Figure 19.

REFERENCES

Dornhöfer N, Höckel M (2008) New developments in the surgical therapy of cervical carcinoma. *Ann N Y Acad Sci* **1138**:233–52.

Höckel M, Horn LC, Fritsch H (2005) Association between the mesenchymal compartment of uterovaginal organogenesis and local tumor spread in stage IB-IIB cervical carcinoma: a prospective study. *Lancet Oncol* **6**:751–6.

Höckel M, Horn LC, Manthey N, et al. (2009) Resection of the embryologically defined uterovaginal (Müllerian) compartment and pelvic control in patients with cervical cancer: a prospective analysis. *Lancet Oncol* **10**:683–92.

Kurman RJ, Amin MB (1999) Cancer Committee College of American Pathologists. Protocol for the examination of the specimens from patients with carcinomas of the cervix. A basis for checklists. *Arch Pathol Lab Med* **123**:55–61.

Peters WA, Liu PY, Barrett RJ, et al. (2000) Concurrent chemotherapy and pelvic radiation therapy compared with pelvic radiation alone as adjuvant therapy after radical surgery in high-risk early-stage cancer of the cervix. *J Clin Oncol* **18**:1606–13.

Piver MS, Rutledge F, Smith JP (1974) Five classes of extended hysterectomy for women with cervical cancer. *Obstet Gynecol* **44**:265–72.

Querleu D, Morrow CP (2008) Classification of radical hysterectomy. *Lancet Oncol* **9**:297–303.

Quinn MA, Benedet JL, Odicino F, et al. (2006) 26th annual report on the results of treatment in gynecological cancer. *Int J Gynecol Obstet* **95**:S43–S103.

Sedlis A, Bundy BN, Rotman MZ, et al. (1999) A randomized trial of pelvic radiation therapy versus no further therapy in selected patients with stage IB carcinoma of the cervix after radical hysterectomy and pelvic lymphadenectomy: a Gynecologic Oncology Group study. *Gynecol Oncol* **73**:177–83.

Viswanathan AN, Lee H, Hanson E, et al. (2006) Influence of margin status and radiation on recurrence after radical hysterectomy in stage IB cervical cancer. *Int J Rad Oncol Biol Phys* **65**:1501–7.

Wertheim E (1912) The extended abdominal operation for carcinoma uteri (based on 500 operative cases). *Am J Obstet Dis Women Child* **66**:169–232.

Zakashansky K, Bradley WH, Nezhat FR (2008) New techniques in radical hysterectomy. *Curr Opin Obstet Gynecol* **20**:14–19.

15 Laterally extended endopelvic resection
Michael Höckel

INTRODUCTION

We have shown that for cancer of the lower female genital tract (cervix, vagina, vulva) tumors are confined to permissive compartments during extended phases of their natural course and proposed the *compartment theory of local tumor spread* (Höckel et al. 2005, 2009). The permissive compartments are established as morphogenetic units by differentiation from a common precursor tissue through embryonic development. The theory postulates that proliferation and migration of tumor cells are primarily suppressed at the compartment borders. However, during malignant progression tumors may evolve the ability to transgress into adjacent compartments of different embryonic origin. This initial focal process is accompanied by local inflammation and adherence of compartment borders to the adjacent tissue. Compartment transgression usually obeys a hierarchical order according to embryonic kinship. Local recurrences arise from tumor (stem) cells interacting with stromal remnants of the tumor-associated tissue compartments remaining in situ after primary therapy.

Locally advanced large primary tumors are more likely to transgress compartment borders and to spread within multiple pelvic visceral compartments. Locally recurrent tumors not only are advanced in malignant progression but also grow in a tissue landscape which may have been altered through the previous anti-cancer treatment. Particularly after surgical therapy, compartment borders may have been damaged and substituted by scar tissue, which appears to be associated with a loss of their barrier function facilitating neoplastic transgression (Höckel and Dornhöfer 2005). Therefore, local tumor relapses are often multi-compartmental even at small sizes. According to the theory of compartmental tumor spread, radical surgical treatment of a malignant neoplasm mandates its resection within the intact borders of the corresponding tissue or organ compartment. Most advanced primary and recurrent tumors necessitate multi-compartmental resection for local tumor control.

Exenteration has been used for six decades to treat selected mostly irradiated patients with locally advanced and recurrent cancer of the lower and middle female genital tract. The mainstay for treatment success in terms of locoregional control and survival is the resection of the pelvic tumor with microscopically clear margins (R0). New ablative techniques based on ontogenetic surgical anatomy termed *laterally extended endopelvic resection* (*LEER*) aim at increasing the curative resection rate even of tumors extending to and fixed to the pelvic side wall (Höckel and Dornhöfer 2006).

For pelvic multivisceral resection, the dissection planes of exenteration have been adjusted to the borders of the combined compartments of the pelvic organ system. Pelvic exenteration is thus performed as a combination of at least two of the following procedures: total mesorectal excision, total mesometrial resection, and total mesovesical resection. In the case of lateral tumor fixation the inclusion of pelvic side wall and floor muscles, such as obturator internus muscle, pubococcygeus, iliococcygeus and coccygeus muscles, and eventually of the internal iliac vessel system assures completeness of the resected compartments. Depending on the extent of caudal tumor propagation, LEER is carried out through an abdominal or abdominoperineal approach.

LEER is usually combined with a therapeutic pelvic and periaortic lymph node dissection unless this treatment for regional tumor control has been performed by previous surgery. For reconstruction or substitution of the pelvic functions lost due to LEER, a broad spectrum of procedures has to be available comprising ileum and transverse colon conduits, ileum neobladder, ileocecal and transverse colon pouches, rectal J-pouches, colorectal anastomosis or colostomy, rectus abdominis musculocutaneous flaps, and sigmoid colon neovagina. Therapeutic angiogenesis of the denuded and mostly irradiated pelvis preferably by an omentum majus flap is essential. In abdomino-perineal LEER procedures vulvovaginal and perineal reconstruction is accomplished with fasciocutaneous and musculocutaneous flaps, such as pudendal thigh flaps, gracilis flaps, and gluteal thigh flaps (Höckel and Dornhöfer 2008). General principles include using no irradiated tissue for reconstruction and to set safety over comfort in all situations of potential surgical compromise. Secondary healing is used as primary surgical strategy in situations where therapeutic angiogenesis is not applicable.

ONTOGENETIC SURGICAL ANATOMY

The uterovaginal compartment as the adult differentiation product of the Müllerian anlage has been described in chapter 14 on "Total mesometrial resection". The adult uterovaginal compartment is fused anterolaterally to the lower urinary tract compartment and posteriolaterally to the anorectal compartment. As the primordia of these adjacent compartments appear earlier in development than the Müllerian system, the ureters, bladder, and rectum are already established when the paramesonephric–mesonephric complex connects to the deep urogenital sinus (Fig. 1). Further differentiation leads to focally dense fibrous connections as well as venous connections between the three visceral compartments in the female pelvis. Whereas the lower urinary tract compartment has a bilateral neurovascular supply—the corresponding mesotissues are located laterally and deep to the vascular mesometrium—the rectum is mainly vascularized axially within the circular mesorectum. The bilateral urogenital mesentery is only loosely connected laterally to the paravisceral fat body of the ischiopubic pelvic side wall. Likewise, the mesorectum is attached to the presacral parietal surface

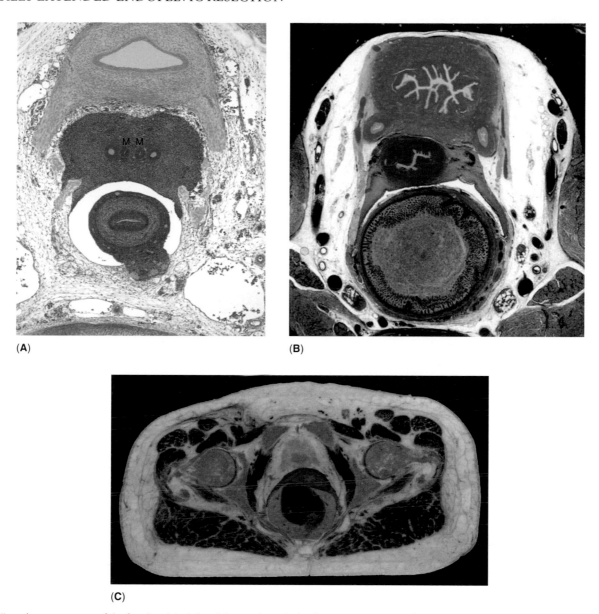

Figure 1 Visceral compartments of the female pelvis deduced from embryonic development. Transverse pelvic sections at the level of the ureterovesical junction of a nine weeks old embryo (**A**), 24 weeks old fetus (**B**), and an adult woman (**C**). The uterovaginal (Müllerian) compartment is highlighted in red, the pelvic urinary tract compartment in blue, and the rectal compartment in brown. Autonomic nerves are colored *yellow*. MM, Müllerian ducts. Laterally extended endopelvic resection (LEER) extirpates the Müllerian compartment en bloc with the pelvic urinary tract compartment and/or the rectal compartment. *Source:* Höckel et al. 2006, Figure 2.

tissues only by areolar tissue. Knowing the tissue architecture by following the endopelvic development allows the surgeon to expose and dissect along the intact borders of all three pelvic visceral compartments. The blood vessels of the urogenital mesentery are continuous with the internal iliac vessel system. The autonomic nerves branch from the inferior hypogastric plexus. The bilateral fixation structures are directed posteriorly encasing the mesorectum and fusing with the parietal endopelvic fascia. Developmentally, these tissues are mainly derived from the paramesonephric–mesonephric complex. Therefore, we suggest the term "ligamentous mesometrium/mesocolpos" for them. Deep and lateral to the fusion zones of the ligamentous mesometrium with the parietal endopelvic fascia the following structures forming the pelvic floor and side wall are located: pubococcygeus, iliococcygeus, and coccygeus muscles, obturator internus muscle, proximal sciatic nerve with its sacral trunk and piriformis muscle (Fig. 2).

SURGICAL PROCEDURE
Indications
- Post-irradiation local recurrences of uterovaginal cancer
- Locally advanced primary disease and post-surgical relapses without a radiotherapeutic treatment option

Contraindications
- Distant metastases except <3 para-aortic lymph node metastases
- Tumor size >5 cm in irradiated pelvis
- Parietal involvement at the site of the sciatic foramen
- Insufficient fitness to tolerate the operation and cope with its sequelae

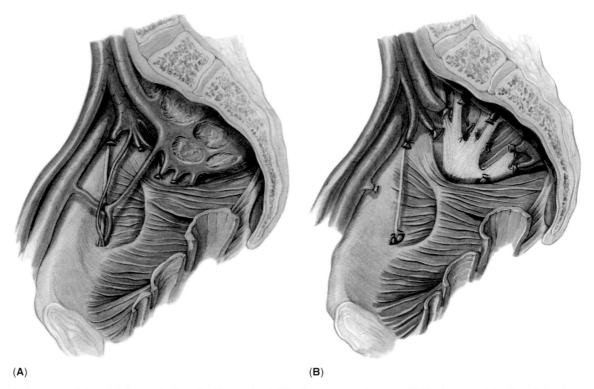

(A)　　　　　　　　　　　　　　　　**(B)**

Figure 2 Surgical anatomy of the pelvic floor and side wall with regard to LEER. If the tumor to be resected is fixed to the pelvic side wall the obturator internus, pubococcygeus, iliococcygeus, and coccygeus muscles (**A**) and eventually the internal iliac vessel system (**B**) are removed to assure completeness of the resected visceral compartments. Tumor fixation to the sites of the iliac vessels, lumbosacral trunk and sciatic nerve is regarded as contraindication for LEER (after N. Lechenbauer). *Source*: Höckel et al. 2006, Figure 3.

TECHNIQUE

The patient is informed about the potential minimal and maximal version of the operation with respect to resection and reconstruction. Forty-eight hours before surgery mechanical bowel cleaning is begun. Using a central venous access, total parenteral nutrition is established and a broad-spectrum antibiotic combination (e.g., ampicillin with clavulanic acid and metronidazole) is infused. Bilateral stoma sites in the epigastric and hypogastric regions are marked. If a gluteal thigh flap is considered for reconstruction the course of the inferior gluteal artery branch at the posterior thigh is drawn on the skin.

In addition to standard surgical instruments for radical hysterectomy, Cobb periosteal dissectors and vessel tourniquets are required. Surgical access is achieved through a hypogastric and epigastric midline laparotomy circumventing the umbilicus. In very obese patients, an abdominoinguinal incision can be helpful; this is made by advancing the laparotomy to the middle of the inguinal region at the side of the recurrence and separating the origin of the rectus abdominis muscle without severing the inferior epigastric vessels (Fig. 3). For low recurrences, additional perineal incisions at the vaginal introitus (possibly including the anus) are necessary.

The surgical techniques of the most extensive version of LEER, the laterally extended total pelvic evisceration are illustrated in Figures 4 to 13. Pelvic wall and floor resection is performed at the left side in this example.

All peritoneal adhesions are lysed and the abdominal and pelvic intraperitoneal regions are systematically explored by inspection and palpation. Biopsies are taken from suspicious sites.

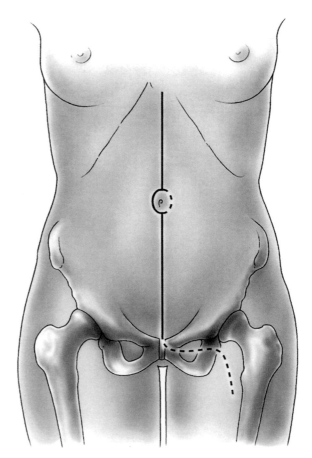

Figure 3 In most cases LEER is performed through a hypo- and epigastric midline laparotomy. In very obese patients a modified abdominoinguinal incision can be advantageous (after E. W. Hanns).

If intraperitoneal tumor dissemination can be excluded, the retroperitoneal pelvic and midabdominal regions are exposed. On both sides the paracolic and pelvic parietal peritoneum is incised along the psoas muscles and the round ligaments are separated. The peritoneum at the base of the small bowel mesentery is dissected and the duodenum is mobilized against the vena cava and aorta. The small bowel and the right and transverse colon are packed into a bowel bag. The anterior visceral peritoneum of the bladder is incised and the space of Retzius is entered. The paravisceral and presacral spaces are developed as far as the location of the recurrent tumor allows. Intralesional dissection should be strictly avoided. Both ureters are liberated. Selective periaortic and pelvic lymph node dissection is performed as dictated by the extent of earlier operations and the intraoperative findings.

If lymphatic tumor dissemination cannot be demonstrated in frozen sections, LEER is started. A tourniquét is placed around the vena cava inferior at the level of the origin of the inferior mesenteric artery. The aorta abdominalis is mobilized at that site so that it can be easily undermined by a large vessel clamp. Temporary (up to 30 minutes) occlusion of the large vessels facilitates the control of severe bleeding at later steps of the operation (Fig. 4).

The infundibulopelvic ligaments are divided and the ureters are cut as low as possible in the pelvis. Biopsies of the distal ureters are examined with frozen sections to exclude neoplastic infiltration. Stents are inserted into the ureters. The mesosigmoid is skeletized and the blood vessels are ligated at the rectosigmoidal transition. The bowel continuity is interrupted at this site using a gastrointestinal stapler (Fig. 5). The sigmoid colon is included into the bowel bag. At the right pelvic wall the urogenital mesentery containing the visceral branches of

the internal iliac vessels, the pelvic autonomic nerve plexus, and the subperitoneal dense connective tissue is completely divided.

The left internal iliac artery is ligated and divided where it branches off from the common iliac artery (Fig. 6). Thereafter, all parietal branches of the iliac vessel system are transected between hemoclips or clamps: the ascending lumbar vein, superior gluteal artery and vein, inferior gluteal artery and vein, and internal pudendal artery and vein (Fig. 7). The internal iliac vein can now be divided at its bifurcation as well. The lumbosacral plexus and the piriform muscle are exposed by this maneuver. In the case of severe hemorrhage the aorta should be clamped immediately below the origin of the inferior mesenteric artery and the prelaid tourniquét around the vena cava should be closed.

The internal obturator muscle is incised at the site of the obturator nerve (Fig. 8). This nerve can be preserved in most cases; rarely, it has to be divided if it is incorporated in the tumor. The muscle is separated from the acetabulum and the obturator membrane by use of a Cobb periosteal dissector (Fig. 9). Below the ischial spine the obturator muscle which leaves the endopelvis at this point is divided again, with ligation or sealing of the muscle stump (Fig. 10). The separated endopelvic part of the obturator muscle in continuity with the attached iliococcygeus and pubococcygeus muscles is retracted medially exposing the ischiorectal fossa.

A superficial incision is made below the lumbosacral plexus between the ischial spine and the fourth sacral body and the

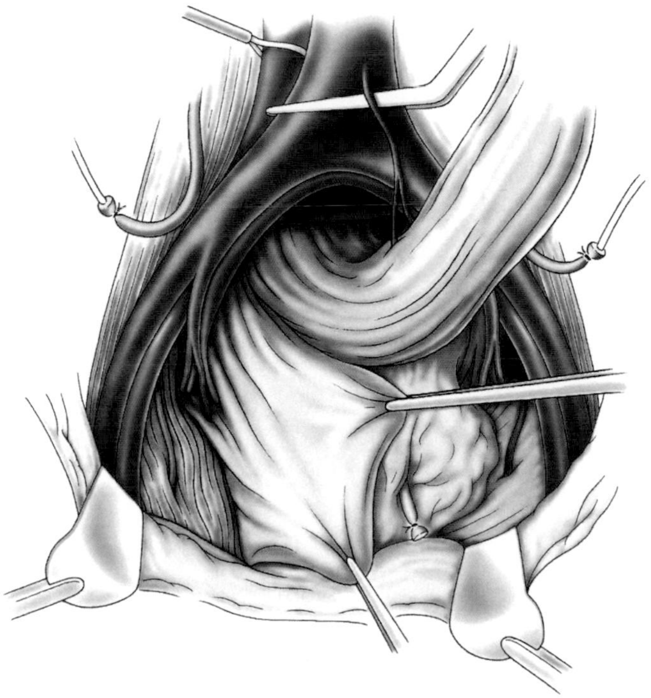

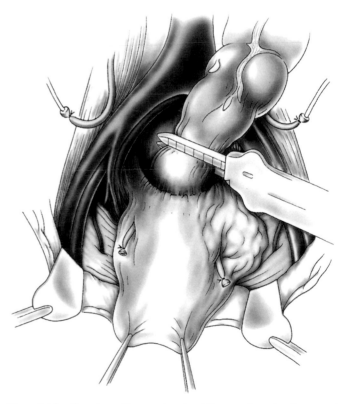

Figure 4 Placement of a tourniquet around the vena cava inferior and of a large vessel clamp on the aorta abdominalis at the level below the origin of the inferior mesenteric artery to prepare for temporary large vessel occlusion during later steps of the operation (after E. W. Hanns).

Figure 5 After the retroperitoneum is entered the paravisceral and presacral spaces are completely developed at the tumor-free pelvic side wall (*right*). These spaces can only be developed in part on the side of the recurrent disease (*left*). Following selective periaortic and pelvic lymph node dissection both ureters are transected as deep in the pelvis as possible and stented. The bowel continuity is interrupted at the rectosigmoid transition (after E. W. Hanns).

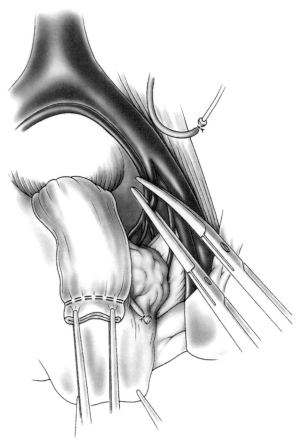

Figure 6 Ligation of the internal iliac artery (after E. W. Hanns).

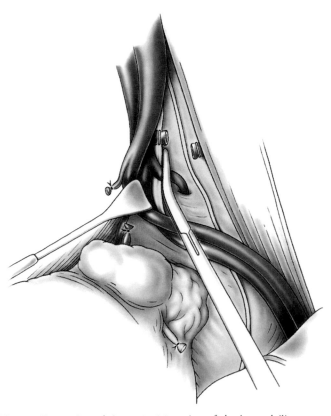

Figure 7 Transection of the parietal branches of the internal iliac artery and vein after retracting the common/external iliac vessels medially as a prerequisite for the ligation of the internal iliac vein (after E. W. Hanns).

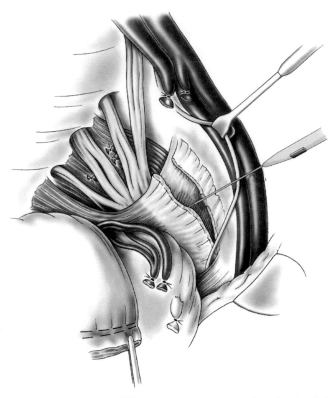

Figure 8 Ventral incision of the obturator internus muscle at the site of the obturator nerve which is retracted (after E. W. Hanns).

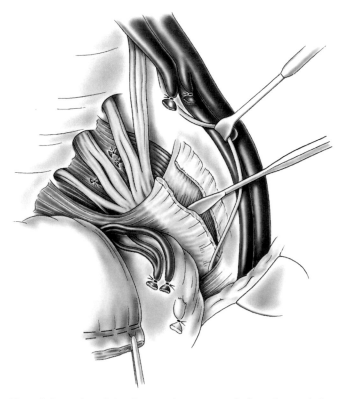

Figure 9 Separation of the obturator internus muscle from the acetabulum and obturator membrane with a Cobb periosteal dissector (after E. W. Hanns).

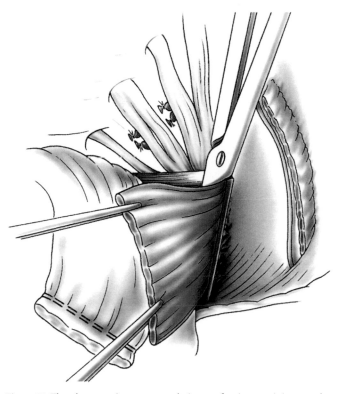

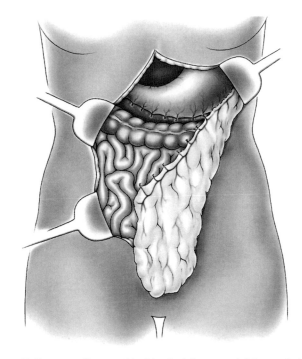

Figure 12 Omentum flap nourished by the left gastroepiploic vessels (after E. W. Hanns).

Figure 10 The obturator internus muscle is cut after its remaining part has been clamped at the lesser sciatic foramen (after E. W. Hanns).

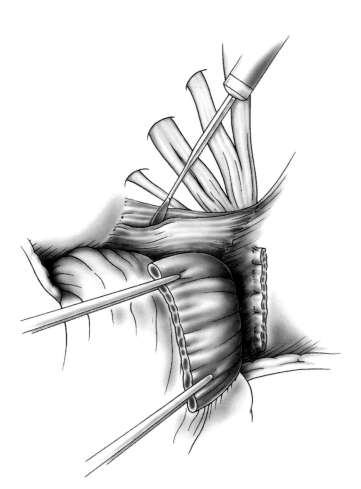

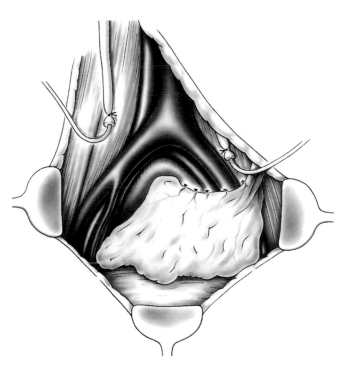

Figure 13 Omentum flap transposed to the pelvis for therapeutic angiogenesis (after E. W. Hanns).

Figure 11 Elevation of the coccygeus muscle from the sacrospinous ligament with a Cobb periosteal dissector (after E. W. Hanns).

coccygeus muscle is elevated from the sacrospinous ligament with a Cobb periosteal dissector (Fig. 11).

At the level of the ischiorectal fossa the lateral vaginal wall is identified and incised. The anterior vaginal wall and urethra are transected. The anal canal is mobilized from the posterior vaginal wall which is divided after clamping or sealing as well. The anorectal transition is separated with an articulated stapling instrument. Now the complete specimen of the laterally extended total pelvic evisceration consisting of the urethra, bladder, vagina, uterus and adnexa, rectum at the left side en bloc with the complete endopelvic urogenital mesentery, the coccygeus, iliococcygeus, pubococcygeus, and the internal obturator muscles can be removed and examined with frozen sections for tumor margins. If necessary the caudal dissection can be shifted further downward to include the vaginal introitus, urethral meatus vulva, and anus by secondary access from the perineum.

To improve wound healing in the irradiated pelvis an omentum flap nourished by the ipsilateral gastroepiploic artery is elevated (Liebermann-Meffert and White 1983), transposed to the pelvis along the paracolic gutter, and fixed to the pelvic surface (Figs. 12 and 13). The inclusion of the anus and anal canal into the laterally extended pelvic evisceration necessitates the reconstruction of the perineum and pelvic floor. This can be accomplished together with the formation of a neovagina if desired by the patient by the use of gluteal thigh (Hurwitz et al. 1981), gracilis (McGraw et al. 1976), and rectus abdominis musculocutaneous (Taylor et al. 1984) flaps or pudendal thigh flaps (Wee and Joseph 1989). For supravesical urinary diversion either a conduit or a continent pouch is constructed from non-irradiated colon segments (see chapter 29). Fecal diversion is accomplished by an end sigmoidostomy (see chapter 28).

The laparotomy is closed with a running Smead-Jones suture and skin stapling.

OUTLOOK
LEER holds significant potential to improve locoregional tumor control in advanced primary and recurrent uterovaginal cancer without a radiotherapeutic treatment option. Selected patients including those with tumors fixed to the pelvic side wall and hydronephrosis traditionally not considered for surgical therapy can be salvaged.

REFERENCES
Höckel M, Dornhöfer N (2005) The hydra phenomenon of cancer. Why tumors recur locally after microscopically complete resection. *Cancer Res* **65**:2997–3002.

Höckel M, Dornhöfer N (2006) Pelvic exenteration for gynaecological tumours: achievements and unanswered questions. *Lancet Oncol* **7**:837–47.

Höckel M, Dornhöfer N (2008) Vulvovaginal reconstruction for neoplastic disease. *Lancet Oncol* **9**:559–68.

Höckel M, Horn LC, Fritsch H (2005) Association between the mesenchymal compartment of uterovaginal organogenesis and local tumor spread in stage IB–IIB cervical carcinoma: a prospective study. *Lancet Oncol* **6**:751–6.

Höckel M, Horn LC, Manthey N, et al. (2009) Resection of the embryologically defined uterovaginal (Müllerian) compartment and pelvic control in patients with cervical cancer: a prospective analysis. *Lancet Oncol* **10**: 683–92.

Hurwitz DJ, Swartz WW, Mathes SJ (1981) The gluteal thigh flap: a reliable sensate flap for the closure of buttock and perineal wounds. *Plast Reconstr Surg* **68**:521–32.

Liebermann-Meffert D, White H (1983) Protective and reconstructive surgery with the omentum in man. In: Liebermann-Meffert D, White H, eds. *The Greater Omentum*. Berlin: Springer, pp. 211–329.

McGraw JB, Massey FM, Shanklin KD, et al. (1976) Vaginal reconstruction with gracilis myocutaneous flaps. *Plast Reconstr Surg* **58**:176–83.

Taylor GI, Corlett RJ, Boyd JB (1984) The versatile deep inferior epigastric (inferior rectus abdominis) flap. *Br J Plast Surg* **37**:330–50.

Wee JT, Joseph VT (1989) A new technique of vaginal reconstruction using neurovascular pudendal-thigh flaps: a preliminary report. *Plast Reconstr Surg* **83**:701–9.

16 Vaginectomy
John M. Monaghan

INTRODUCTION

The procedure of vaginectomy, or colpectomy, whether partial or complete is rarely performed but has very clear indications and very significant benefits. The procedure is most commonly indicated where there is residual vaginal intra-epithelial neoplasia (VAIN) in the upper vagina after hysterectomy. While it is relatively rare for hysterectomies to be performed in the treatment of cervical pre-malignancy [cervical intraepithelial neoplasia (CIN)], without the benefit of preoperative colposcopy to localize and delineate the disease, there remain a small but important group of patients where a "cut through" of cervical pre-malignancy is identified on post-hysterectomy pathology. As a consequence, this incomplete removal of the lesion will result in persistently abnormal smears in the post-operative period. If hysterectomy is indicated for CIN, then ideally this should be performed vaginally in conjunction with colposcopy to reduce the likelihood of the CIN and any associated VAIN being incompletely excised. In a small minority of patients (<2%), the transformation zone may naturally extend onto the vaginal vault. If such patients have had a hysterectomy for CIN without accurate colposcopy, then there is a risk of leaving part of the lesion behind. Due to the prevalent habit of closure of the vaginal vault the lesion may be included in the suture line resulting in the risk of an occult focus of CIN developing into a cancerous lesion with time.

PRE-OPERATIVE ASSESSMENT

As noted above, the majority of patients presenting with post-hysterectomy lesions will be identified by the use of vault smears in follow-up. Identification of the true site of the source of the abnormal smear may present colposcopic difficulties. Colposcopy with biopsy of any identified lesion is a usually performed as an outpatient.

Once biopsy confirmation of a pre-cancerous lesion is available, it is important to fully identify the whole extent of the lesion in the vagina so that a tailored procedure can be planned and the patient may understand the extent of the surgery and its impact upon her sexual function. Where a complete vaginectomy is contemplated, replacement of function should be planned with Plastic Surgical colleagues for the development of a neo-vagina (see chapter 9).

If the lesion or lesions can be seen and fully outlined, then a local excisional procedure performed vaginally is the best management method (see below). If the lesion cannot be fully visualized or it extends into the "dog-ears" at the angles of the vaginal vault, then a more extensive surgical procedure via an abdominal approach is the only realistic choice. Some authorities have recommended radiotherapy but the editor feels that this is not indicated as there is a very significant vaginal morbidity after treatment, often without clearance of the vault lesion, whereas with partial colpectomy there is a good prospect of a reasonable return to normal vaginal function without the attendant post-radiotherapy vaginal morbidity of atrophy and scarring, coupled with the reassurance of histopathological confirmation of clearance of the lesion.

Colpectomy is not an adequate procedure for invasive carcinoma of the vagina but is of great value in treating microinvasive lesions. In those patients with an upper vaginal lesion and who have a uterus, a hysterocolpectomy is performed—a much simpler procedure than colpectomy after hysterectomy.

ANATOMIC CONSIDERATIONS

The close relationship of the vagina to the bladder anteriorly and to the rectum posteriorly clearly require great care when dissecting the vaginal mucosa from its supporting tissues. The close relationship of the ureters to the dog-ears of the vaginal remnant requires careful consideration and attention during the procedure. For clinicians experienced in vaginal reconstructive surgery the identification of the clear tissue planes beneath the vaginal mucosa does not present problems. Special regard has to be taken below the urethra and also when dealing with the inevitably scarred areas at the vaginal vault.

THE VAGINAL PROCEDURE
Instruments

The instruments in the general gynecology set will be required together with colposcopy to identify smaller lesions in the upper vagina.

The Operation

1. Identification of the lesion. The patient is placed in a lithotomy position, cleansed, draped and the bladder emptied. A bimanual and rectal examination is performed to exclude the possibility of a discrete invasive lesion lying above the suture line at the vaginal vault. A colposcopic assessment of the upper vagina is performed followed by mapping of the lesion using Lugol's iodine. Infiltration of the sub-epithelial tissues with a solution of 1% local anesthetic with adrenaline 1:200,000 helps to define tissue planes and reduce minor bleeding. Access to the vault is best achieved by use of a large Sim's retractor placed in the posterior vagina, with a smaller vaginal retractor placed in the anterior vagina which may be moved laterally during the course of the procedure as required.

2. The incision. A 2-cm vaginal epithelial incision is made just inferior to the posterior margins of the lesion. This incision should give good clearance of the identified lesion and provide a rim of normal tissue which may be grasped by instruments to manipulate the tissue being dissected. It is vital not to generate "crush artifacts" in the lesion which may present diagnostic difficulties for the pathologist. It is important to "work upward" so that any bleeding does not interfere with the surgeon's view of the operative field. A toothed dissector is

AN ATLAS OF GYNECOLOGIC ONCOLOGY, INVESTIGATION AND SURGERY

used to apply traction to the skin flap anteriorly, while the blunted scissors are used to develop the sub-epithelial plane further toward the vaginal vault and laterally (Fig. 1). The skin edges are incised further around the circumference of the mapped lesion as the development of the tissue planes continues. Attention is required not to "button-hole" the specimen, as this will increase the possibility of leaving diseased tissue remnants behind. Eventually, the incision is completed around the entire lesion, with the only attachment remaining being a thin strip at the vaginal vault with underlying scar tissue. Applying firm traction to the vaginal skin, the attachments at the vaginal vault are now boldly cut from right to left including the "dog-ears" within the specimen, eventually releasing the entire specimen and without damage to the underlying structures (Fig. 2). In leaving the scarred tissue at the vaginal vault and "dog-ears" till last, the risk of injury to the underlying rectum, bladder, and ureters is kept to an absolute minimum, while increasing the likelihood of achieving complete excision of the entire lesion with a single specimen.

3. *Dealing with the denuded vault.* If the peritoneal cavity has been entered at the vaginal vault during the procedure, then this can be either left open or closed using a continuous stitch. Individual vessels can be dealt with using a combination of sutures or diathermy. Once hemostasis is achieved, the denuded tissue at the vaginal vault is left unsutured to re-granulate, and a bacteriostatic soaked vaginal pack and trans-urethral urinary catheter inserted for 24 hours.

Post-operative Care
No special attention is required, and the patient can be discharged home following removal of the pack and catheter. Satisfactory urinary function should be checked prior to discharge.

THE ABDOMINAL PROCEDURE
Instruments
The instruments for a radical hysterectomy will be required (see chapter 9).

Preoperative Preparation
Identification of the lesion and biopsy should be as described above.

The patient should be prepared as for a radical hysterectomy with normal cross matching of blood and simple bowel preparation. An additional procedure to mark the inferior aspect of the vaginal lesion with a marker stitch, which will be useful later during the operation to confirm adequate excision. A firm vaginal pack is inserted following anesthesia to facilitate dissection of the vagina from the bladder and the rectum, and a catheter on free drainage with a small (5 ml) balloon should be inserted into the bladder.

The Operation
Frequently, adhesions from previous surgery have to be cleared before it is possible to fully visualize the pelvic structures. As in the radical hysterectomy procedure, a self-retaining retractor should be used but without the lower blade, which should be replaced by a dynamic Morris retractor held by the second assistant. This allows the peritoneum and the bladder to be manipulated in order to give better vision and access. As a

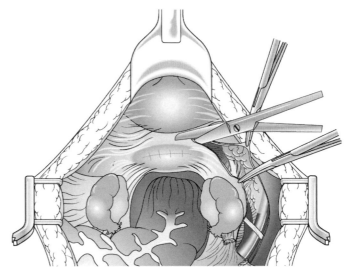

Figure 1 Releasing the vaginal edges.

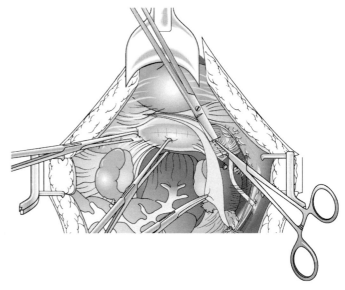

Figure 2 Excising the vaginal skin at the vault.

result of the previous surgical intervention, there can be considerable scarring particularly at the angles of the vaginal vault overlying the ureters.

1. *The incision.* The abdomen is opened via a longitudinal midline incision; low transverse incisions give more limited access and should not be used.

2. *Identifying the ureters.* After clearing obstructions and adhesions from previous surgery, the ureters should be identified as they pass along the pelvic side wall behind the peritoneum. The peritoneum at the brim of the pelvis is opened along a line between the remnant of the round ligament and the infundibulo-pelvic ligament. Using the fingers, the retroperitoneal space is opened and the ureter identified and separated from the overlying peritoneum.

3. *Dealing with the scar tissue at the angles of the vault.* The uterine artery should be identified as far laterally as possible and then divided and drawn medially. This will have the effect of identifying the entrance to the ureteric tunnel at its lateral end. This area is often surrounded by dense scarring from the previous surgery; however, if the ureteric tunnel can be

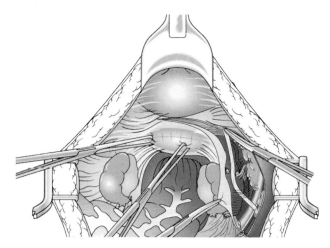

Figure 3 Dividing the roof of the ureteric tunnel.

accurately defined, the scar overlying it can be cut with confidence and without trauma to the ureter.

4. *Identifying the medial end of the ureteric tunnel.* Now, the uppermost point of the vagina must be palpated and a transverse incision made in the peritoneum so that the bladder can be separated from the anterior surface of the vagina. It may be necessary to use sharp dissection in order to identify the correct plane. Once this has been identified, the bladder should be pushed down in the midline; this will have the effect of making the scar tissue and the fascia overlying the ureteric tunnel laterally more prominent.

5. *Incising the roof of the ureteric tunnel.* The ureter can be identified as it passes into the bladder. If this is possible Bonney's scissors should be gently introduced over the upper surface of the ureter and, using a separating movement without cutting, the scissors are gently insinuated laterally to appear at the lateral end of the ureteric tunnel. This dissection may be performed from medial to lateral or in the reverse direction. It is important not to kink or to nip the ureter in the edges of the scissors; the simple maneuver of lifting the scissors while in the tunnel will allow a good view of the entire length of the ureter. A medium straight tissue forceps is then placed over the scissors and the ureteric tunnel and the scar tissue incised (Fig. 3). The pedicle is then tied, as it carries some veins and small arteries to and from the bladder. At this point, there may still be a few strands of fascia passing across the ureter; these should be divided and the tissue plane between the ureter and the vagina identified. The cardinal ligament is now visible below and medial to the ureter. Sharp dissection may still be required if there has been extensive scarring from the previous surgery. The upper vagina is revealed very quickly and the ureters dislocated laterally. The firm pack in the vagina greatly facilitates this dissection.

6. *Releasing the vagina posteriorly.* An incision is made in the peritoneum at the upper posterior part of the vagina. This incision is then extended laterally over the remnants of the uterosacral ligaments. The rectum is now easily pushed away from the posterior surface of the vagina by passing the fingers down into the recto-vaginal space.

7. *Removing the vagina.* At this point, having released the ureters laterally, the bladder anteriorly, and the rectum posteriorly, the surgeon can decide just how much vagina he wishes to remove. The uterosacral and then the paracolpos is grasped and clamped in Zeppelin clamps and the chosen length of vagina removed. If the requirement is to remove the upper part of the vagina to excise VAIN, no further dissection is necessary and the vagina can be opened at this point to confirm placement of the original marker stitch and adequate excision of tissue. If a total vaginectomy is necessary. The abdominal dissection should be extended down the vagina to the pelvic floor. Thereafter, the patient is put in lithotomy position and the lower vagina dissected free from the urethra and bladder anteriorly and the rectum posteriorly. Great care should be exercised when dissecting below the urethra as the fascia is very dense and the dissection must be very accurate. Having joined up with the abdominal dissection, the entire vagina can be removed. Bleeding around the pelvic floor is readily dealt with.

8. *Draining the vagina.* The space left behind after vaginectomy will vary in size depending on the extent of the procedure. Following partial vaginectomy there is no need for special drainage procedures except to leave the vaginal remnant open. However, after total vaginectomy either a vaginal passive drain or a suction drain should be put in place. This may be augmented by a pelvic suction drain brought out abdominally if it has been necessary to perform an extensive dissection in the pelvis. It is the author's experience that remarkably little drainage is necessary.

9. Where it has been decided that a neovagina should be developed this part of the procedure will immediately follow the vaginectomy (see chapter 32).

Complications

The main postoperative problems following this procedure will be similar to those following radical hysterectomy, particularly bladder dysfunction and difficulties in initiating micturition.

Post-operative Care

The patient should be managed in the same manner as the radical hysterectomy patient, particular emphasis being placed on bladder care, and in the long-term continued surveillance of any remnants of vaginal tissue remaining.

17 Radical vulvar surgery
John M. Monaghan

INTRODUCTION

When Basset published his monograph on the surgical treatment of cancer of the clitoris in 1912, he outlined the major criteria for the operative management of cancer of the vulva which was utilized worldwide for most of the 20th century. Basset outlined the importance of the metastases to the groin and the equal importance of removing the lymphatic ray connecting the primary tumor on the vulva with the primary lymph node drainage site in the groin. It is important to remember that although Basset outlined these surgical maneuvers, all his work was performed on cadavers and the procedure was rarely used in live subjects.

In the 1920s, Victor Bonney (1920) continued the tradition of radical vulvectomy and groin node dissection in British patients. However, it was Stoekel, working initially in Munich, and later in Berlin, who demonstrated the need for individualization of surgical treatment. Stoekel, in his seminal monograph of 1930, outlined every known variant of surgical treatment, many of which have later been "rediscovered" by other experts around the world. Closer to home, Stanley Way, working in Gateshead in the 1940s, re-confirmed the importance of the lymphatic ray and the drainage of the vulva, and suggested that a wide local excision of the lesion on the vulva should be combined with an extensive dissection of the skin of the suprapubic area and the groin (Way 1948). Unfortunately, although the cure rates for cancer of the vulva improved markedly when radical treatment was adopted, the adverse effects of such massive surgery were that patients spent a considerable time in hospital and were left with large wounds requiring intensive nursing care. Interestingly, the long-term result of these large wounds was frequently a remarkably satisfactory cosmetic effect.

As a consequence of the realization that not all patients required such radical surgery, in the latter part of the 20th century, moves toward individualization of care, first outlined by Stoekel in 1930, were resurrected. It is now common practice to accurately stage the cancer of the vulva with careful measurement, both clinical and pathological, and based on these measurements, to determine exactly the most appropriate surgical procedure to achieve high cure rates with minimal adverse cosmetic effect.

ANATOMIC CONSIDERATIONS
Blood Supply

The blood supply to the vulva is derived from the internal pudendal artery, a terminal branch of the anterior division of the hypogastric artery (internal iliac artery). A contribution from the superficial and deep external pudendal artery originating from the femoral artery is of variable amount. The internal pudendal artery continues as the posterior labial vessels that supply the posterior part of the labia majora, labia minora, and the vestibule. The anterior labial branches of the external pudendal vessels and the small arteries of the ligamentum teres, a branch of the inferior epigastric, may also contribute to the blood supply.

Nerve Supply

The nerve supply of the vulva is derived from a variety of sources. The mons pubis and upper labia majora are innervated by the ilioinguinal nerve and the genital branch of the genitofemoral nerve. The superficial perineal branches of the pudendal nerve supply the labia majora and the structures of the external genitalia. The deep branches supply the clitoris, vestibular bulb, and muscles of the region.

Lymphatic Drainage

Most carcinomas of the vulva affect the labia majora and minora. The second commonest site is the clitoris. All these skin areas have a lymphatic drainage which passes in a narrow ray through the groin into the superficial inguinal lymph nodes and then through the cribriform fascia into the femoral nodes, which are in close proximity to the femoral artery and vein immediately below the fossa ovale. While the superficial groin nodes are disparate and variable in their position, the femoral nodes are more constant, lying in close proximity to the vessels. The drainage from the femoral nodes then passes cranially through the inguinal ligament to enter the lymphatics of the external iliac system.

Alternative Routes of Lymph Drainage

In the past, there was concern that lymphatic drainage may occur directly through the perineal membrane into the external iliac lymphatic system, but this has been disproved in a variety of studies. However, it will be noted that retrograde spread may sometimes occur down into the nodes alongside the saphenous vein when the nodes of the femoral group are heavily involved with tumor.

INDICATIONS

Over many years it has been demonstrated that for virtually all patients with truly invasive cancer of the vulva it is mandatory not only to perform a wide local excision of the tumor on the vulva, but also to remove the groin nodes. This broad instruction initially generated by Basset in 1912 has been modified and made more sophisticated due to an understanding of the metastatic spread patterns depending on the depth of invasion of the tumor. Careful measurement of tumor invasive depths has demonstrated that where the tumor invades for <1 mm, that is, stage IA, then the risk of nodal metastases is zero. In these circumstances a wide local excision of the lesion on the vulva is all that is required. For any depth of invasion beyond 1 mm the risk of nodal metastases rises markedly and it is vital that all patients should be subjected to groin node dissection.

Initially, this instruction was interpreted as requiring a radical excision of the lesion on the vulva in continuity with the lymphatic ray and the groin node dissection itself. Stoekel (1930) and other authors since, have demonstrated that because of the initial pattern of metastatic spread, that is, embolization rather than permeation of lymphatic vessels, it is possible to leave behind the skin bridge between the groin and the vulva, and by carrying out separate groin dissections the patient can safely and confidently be cured of her condition (Grimshaw et al. 1993). For all small tumors, where there is no clinical involvement of the groin nodes, the use of separate groin incisions is now the preferred method of management.

It has also been shown where a tumor is placed laterally on the vulva, that is, that the tumor does not impinge on a line drawn below the clitoris, or behind a line drawn through the fourchette, then the patient need only be subjected to a unilateral (ipsilateral) groin node dissection. The risk of contralateral groin node spread is vanishingly small.

Role of the 'En bloc' Dissection

It is the author's belief that when groin nodes are obviously grossly involved that a full radical vulvectomy with an en bloc dissection of the groin nodes is the optimal management. The reason for this is that once nodes are filled with metastatic tumor there will be stasis in the lymphatic ray and a high risk of leaving active tumor behind if separate incisions are used.

Pelvic Node Dissection

In the past, the pelvic nodes were also routinely dissected, but these should only be dissected and/or included in a treatment field, when there is gross involvement of the groin nodes and where there is clear evidence of tumor continuity through the femoral canal into the external iliac system. Few modern series will be able to comment on survival data for patients with positive pelvic nodes. In the author's early series when this dissection was commonly performed 19% of patients with positive pelvic nodes survived five years.

Identification of Lymphatic Spread and Nodal Involvement

The techniques available for identification of involved groin nodes have been many and various. It has been known for many years that palpation is of very limited value and modern imaging techniques, including computed tomography (CT), nuclear magnetic resonance (NMR) imaging, ultrasound, and lymphangiography, have all demonstrated variable results. Philip Disaia et al. (1979) described the use of a "sentinel node" technique for determining metastatic spread to the groin nodes. The concept was perfect but the difficulties in identifying the true sentinel node made its use uncertain. More recently, Levenbach et al. (2001) have demonstrated that by injecting a vital blue dye into the leading edge of the tumor it is possible to pick up blue nodes in the groin, which can be regarded as the sentinel nodes for the remainder of the groin lymphatics. Although this blue dye technique confirmed the presence of a sentinel node or nodes, it was not of the quality required for its general use as guidance as to whether the groin nodes should be dissected or not. In a number of centers following its use in breast cancer, sentinel node identification using a radiolabeled material (technetium) has been elevated to the point at which one can confidently utilize the sentinel node technetium technique in order to determine the involvement or otherwise of the groin nodes (De Cicco et al. 2000). If the sentinel node is negative when removed, then the clinicians may be able to dispense with a formal groin node dissection, thus markedly reducing the morbidity for the patient. If the groin node shows involvement then a formal dissection of the groin is mandatory. The most difficult aspect of the use of sentinel node assessment is the possibility of micrometastases being missed by the examining pathologist. One technique, now commonly utilized, is to perform cytokeratin immunohistochemical staining in cytologically negative sentinel nodes. These techniques were utilized in two large observational trials of sentinel node mapping in early stage vulvar cancer – GROINSV-1 and GOG-173 (ate van der Zee, J Clin Oncol 2008:26; 884). Both clinical trials were performed to assess whether sentinel node assessment would be a reasonable surrogate of pathology in the groin. The determinant of failure was an unacceptable rate of false negatives – that is, the situation where the sentinel node was identified and histologically negative, yet tumor deposits were identified in the non-sentinel nodes. In both studies, the false negative predictive value was about 2–4%. Whether triage by sentinel node status can avert lymphadenectomy completely is the subject of the ongoing GROINSV-II trial. As sentinel node assessment has moved to be the norm in the work-up of the patient occasional reports of recurrence after negative sentinel nodes have been reported. In spite of these reports, the use of sentinel node assessment is now considered de rigeur for vulval cancer patients (Knopp et al. 2008).

SURGICAL PROCEDURE

Patient Preparation

All patients should be admitted one to two days prior to surgery. Blood is typed and cross-matched and consent obtained. It is important that the patient understands fully all real and potential complications of the surgery as wound breakdown continues to occur in spite of many modifications, and that some femoral nerve bundles may be resected during the groin dissection leaving anesthesia and paraesthesia over areas of the anterior thigh.

Thromboembolic Prophylaxis

The average age of patients developing vulval cancer is in the late seventh decade and the risk of developing thromboembolic disease is high. It is important to initiate thromboembolic prophylaxis shortly before surgery and to maintain it using a variety of methods until the patient is fully ambulant. The use of subcutaneous heparin, anti-thromboembolic stockings, and intraoperative muscle pumps are all of great value (see chapter 2). Early mobilization following surgery, however, remains the cornerstone of efforts to reduce thromboembolic risks.

The patient is placed in the supine position on the operating table with the ankles separated by approximately 20 cm. This allows the groin folds to be opened and gives easy access for the groin dissection.

Skin Incision

For the vast majority of patients separate groin node dissections will be performed. The incision should run from

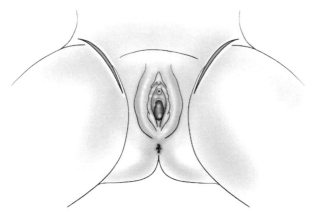

Figure 1 The incision used in the "triple incision" technique.

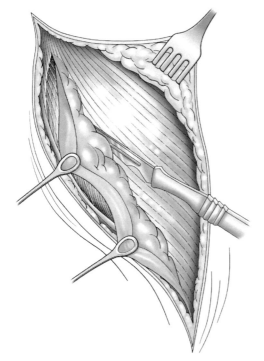

Figure 2 Incising the fat and fascia down to the external oblique aponeurosis and the sartorious muscle.

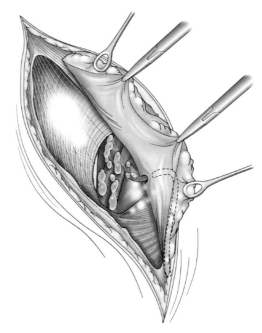

Figure 3 The medial edge of the sartorius fascia is elevated by forceps.

approximately 4 cm medial to the anterior superior iliac spine down to a point some 4 cm below the pubic tubercle. Although it is common for surgeons to use a single incision, the author has found that by performing a double incision, leaving a skin strip approximately 1 cm wide along the length of this incision, will allow easier manipulation of the block of lymph nodes which will be dissected below this incision. The incision is carried down in a manner which allows a triangular block of tissue to be removed down to the superficial fascia. When outlining the incision it is important to utilize bony landmarks and to ignore natural skin folds, which may be very variable, particularly in obese patients. Figure 1 shows the incisions to the groin and vulva.

Defining the Fascial Planes in the Groin Incisions
The thin strip of skin in the groin is picked up using tissue forceps so that the whole block of tissue in the groin can be maneuvered during the dissection. Gentle tension is put on the upper edge of the skin incision with the left hand and the

surgeon incises in a slightly angular fashion upward, down to the level of the aponeurosis of the external oblique muscle above the groin. In a similar fashion, the fascia over the sartorious muscle that forms the lateral boundary of the femoral triangle can now be identified in a similar manner. The fascia over the sartorious muscle is incised longitudinally from just below the anterior superior iliac spine to the lower apex of the femoral triangle (Fig. 2). Small vessels in the fat and on the muscle surface may be cut and should be meticulously identified and tied or diathermied.

Division of the Saphenous Vein
In the lower part of the femoral triangle the saphenous vein may be identified as it curves inferiorly. It can be easily isolated where it lies above the fascia lata and is then divided and ligated at the apex of the lower part of the dissection.

Some surgeons preserve the saphenous vein, dissecting it out and cleaning it in its superficial passage, and then identifying it as it drops through the fossa ovale. The author does not believe that cutting the saphenous vein significantly increases the risk of lymphedema.

Developing the Deep Dissection
The medial edge of the incised fascia over the sartorious muscle is now picked up using two small Spencer Wells clips (Fig. 3). Strands of the femoral nerve can now be seen in the soft tissue at the medial side of the sartorious muscle and should be preserved wherever possible. On the medial side of the sartorious muscle the femoral artery will be identified and should be cleaned from the lower part of the femoral triangle cranially to the inguinal ligament. This meticulous cleaning will then reveal the femoral vein lying on the medial side of the femoral artery. The saphenous vein will now be noted to be passing from the superficial lymph node area through the fossa ovale into the femoral vein, roughly at its midpoint in the exposed femoral triangle. The saphenous vein should be clamped close to its entry into the femoral vein as shown in Figure 4. With the surgeon's left hand raising the block of

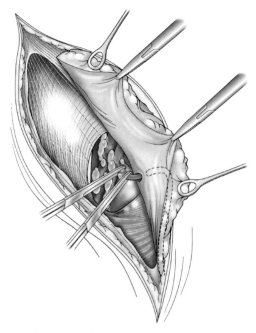

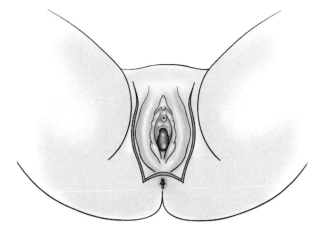

Figure 6 The vulvar incision to be used when there is a small tumor and the removal of associated skin changes is required, such as VIN.

Figure 4 The saphenous vein is identified as it passes through the fossa ovale from the superficial compartment.

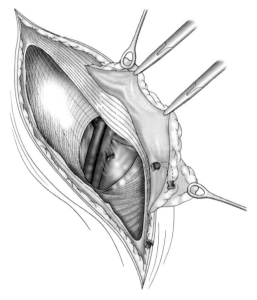

Figure 5 The superficial groin nodes are removed en bloc and the final cleansing of the femoral vessels can be achieved.

tissue containing the superficial lymph nodes, the femoral vein can be seen lying on the medial side of the femoral artery with the divided saphenous vein passing through the fossa ovale, which is now turned over to reveal its underside. Meticulous cleaning of all tissue around the femoral artery and vein will remove all the femoral lymph nodes. This cleansing should be carried out up to the inguinal ligament and occasionally the node of Cloquet or Rosenmuller will be identified as it fills the femoral canal. In normal circumstances this will be the upper limit of the nodal dissection.

Cleaning the Adductor Muscles
The block of tissue elevated by the surgeon containing all superficial and femoral nodes can now be put on tension by drawing it medially, and the surgeon continues a dissection

under the fascia covering the adductor muscles on the medial side of the femoral vein. This dissection will continue through to the outer part of the adductor muscles over a distance of approximately 5 to 6 cm. Small veins that enter the muscles may require ligating at this point but most of the tissue plane is avascular. The dissection is completed by cutting through small amounts of fat on the medial side of the elevated block of tissue, and the comprehensive dissection of the groin nodes has been achieved (Fig. 5). The completely cleansed femoral triangle will now be lying open. The two skin edges will lie together very closely without any tension. It is important first of all to put in place a small suction drain. The author finds it valuable to utilize a continuous fat stitch, drawing together the subcutaneous fat, and thereafter the skin incisions can be easily stapled in a linear fashion.

The fat stitch assists in making the sutured incision airtight. Once the suction drain is activated, the skin will depress into the defect generated by removal of the groin nodal mass. This suction should be maintained for some days until drainage reduces markedly or ceases altogether.

The Vulval Incision
The most important element in performing radical vulvectomy is to be certain of performing a wide excision of the tumor. The margin generally recommended is 2 cm, and it is important to remember that this 2 cm margin must not only occur laterally and medially, but also deeply, so that the dissection should be carried down to the superficial fascia below the fat layers.

Where the tumor lies close to the urethra or anus it may not always be possible to gain the full 2 cm margin, but it is important to remember that the terminal urethra can be sacrificed and extension of the incision closer to the anus will be achievable without compromising continence. Figure 6 shows the incisions which can be utilized in a small tumor with extensive skin change affecting most of the vulva. The use of posterior releasing incisions may only be necessary where the tumor is very large and apposition of the skin is not so easily achieved at the end of the dissection.

The author would recommend that the incision begins anteriorly some 2 cm above the clitoris, passing in an elliptical fashion, providing the 2 cm margin around the tumor, and also performed in a similar fashion on the opposite side in order to produce a symmetrical result. In those circumstances where the

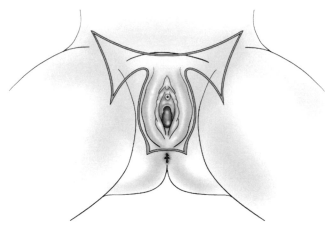

Figure 7 Skin incisions for the "butterfly incision".

tumor is small and laterally placed it may be possible to perform a hemivulvectomy and ipsilateral groin node dissection achieving a high chance of cure with an excellent cosmetic result.

However, the preservation of vulval skin on the opposite side may increase the risk of new tumor occurring in the future.

During radical vulvectomy surgery, significant vessels will be identified around the clitoral base, and posteriorly the deep labial branches of the internal pudendal artery. These three sites are the major sources of bleeding. It may be necessary to utilize square mattress sutures in dealing with the bleeding around the clitoral base, but the pudendal vessels can normally be dealt with by simple clipping and tying. Diathermy and tying of small vessels below the skin in other parts of the vulva should be meticulous achieving a high level of hemostasis.

Primary closure of the vulval wound is easily achieved utilizing a series of interrupted sutures. The vertical mattress suture is particularly helpful where the tissues are deep due to excessive fat.

It may be necessary in a small number of patients to perform an en bloc dissection and this will result in removal of the skin in the skin bridge between the groin and the vulva. This is best achieved using a variation of the skin incision shown above, sometimes described as the "butterfly incision" (Fig. 7).This incision will give a comprehensive dissection of the lymphatic ray and resulting in an en bloc dissection of the groin and vulval lesion.

Pelvic Node Dissection

As noted above, the indications for removing the pelvic nodes are rare. In order to achieve a margin when the groin nodes are involved it may be necessary to dissect the pelvic nodes, although in many practices radiotherapy is utilized as an adjuvant treatment to extend the field of management.

If the pelvic nodes are to be dissected, they are best approached following the completion of the groin phase. The incision to access the pelvic nodes is made some 2 cm above the inguinal ligament (Fig. 8) in a line along the external oblique aponeurosis. A second incision is now made deep to this along the line of the internal oblique muscle fibers, roughly at right angles to the first incision. The second incision is taken down through transversalis muscle to the peritoneum. The peritoneum is kept intact, and using the fingers, it is gently

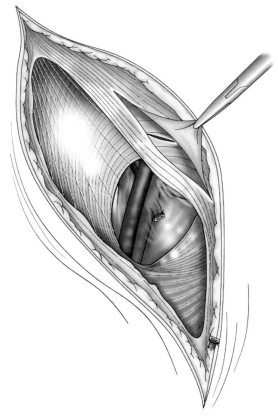

Figure 8 The external oblique aponeurosis is incised superolaterally.

swept medially revealing the brim of the pelvis and the external iliac vessels.

Using appropriate retraction the entire external iliac, obturator, and internal iliac nodes to the common iliac can be dissected.

It is sometimes prudent to split the inguinal ligament to improve access but care to identify and sometimes ligate the inferior epigastric artery is necessary at this time.

The wounds in the muscles are repaired in reverse order to achieve a strong closure with minimal risk of hernia development.

REFERENCES

Basset A (1912) Traitement chirurgical operatoire de l'epi-thelioma primitif du clitoris. *Rev Chir (Paris)* **46**:546.

Bonney V (1920) In: Berkeley C, Bonney V, eds. *A Textbook of Gynaecological Surgery.* London: Cassell, p. 122.

De Cicco, Sideri M, Bartolomei M, et al. (2000) Sentinel node biopsy in early vulvar cancer. *Br J Cancer* **82**(2):295–9.

Disaia PJ, Creasman WT, Rich WM (1979) An alternate approach to early cancer of the vulva. *Am J Obstet Gynecol* **133**:825–30.

Grimshaw RN, Murdoch JB, Monaghan JM (1993) Radical vulvectomy and bilateral inguinal-femoral lymphadenectomy through separate incisions— experience with 100 cases. *Int J Gynecol Cancer* **3**:18–23.

Knopp S, Nesland JM, Trope C (2008) SLNB and the importance of microme-tastases in vulvar Squamous cell carcinoma. *Surg Oncol* **17**:219–25.

Levenbach C, Coleman RL, Burke TW, et al. (2001) Intraoperative lymphatic mapping and sentinel node identification with blue dye in patients with vulvar cancer. *Gynecol Oncol* **83**(2):276–81.

Monaghan JM, Hammond IG (1984) Pelvic node dissection in the treatment of vulval carcinoma—is it necessary? *Br J Obstet Gynaecol* **91**:270–4.

Stoekel W (1930) Zur Therapie des Vulvakarzinoms. *Zentralbl Gynakol* 1:47–71.

Way S (1948) The anatomy of the lymphatic drainage of the vulva, and its influence on the radical operation for carcinoma. *Ann R Coll Surg Engl* **3**:187.

18 Sentinel lymph node biopsy

Michael Frumovitz, Robert L. Coleman, and Charles M. Levenback

INTRODUCTION

Advances in surgical management among the solid tumors have developed in response to a variety of catalysts over the years. One of these has been the pursuit of surgical precision—balancing maximal survival against morbidity of therapy. This relatively recent concept derives from a combination of an improved understanding of disease biology and the identification of effective adjuvant therapies, which have allowed modification of traditional surgical paradigms and procedures. Lymphatic mapping and sentinel node identification, new to gynecologic malignancies, represents one of these advances, which among diseases, such as malignant melanoma and breast cancer, have radically altered classic surgical practices once deemed "the final achievement of surgery" (Way 1951). Integration of lymphatic mapping into triage and management has dramatically improved treatment precision by offering better disease characterization with the potential for reduced toxicity through less radical intervention. "Proof-of-principle" studies are currently being undertaken. The purpose of this chapter is to introduce the concept of lymphatic mapping and sentinel node identification as it is being developed among the gynecologic cancers and to report on the early, albeit promising, experience, particularly in vulvar and cervical malignancy.

WHAT IS LYMPHATIC MAPPING?

Lymphatic mapping is simply documentation of the regional lymphatic spillways from an organ of interest. While obvious in our current understanding of the metastatic process, the role of the regional lymphatics and their direct relationship with the major anatomic structures was somewhat elusive in early studies and anatomical dissections. Limited by evaluation of putrefied and fixed tissue, reliable identification of the lymphatic channels to the regional lymph nodes was a major challenge for early anatomists. Painstaking dissections led to the production of remarkable drawings of lymphatic anatomy, which served as reference materials for future generations of surgeons who ultimately designed operative procedures to remove these "at risk" sites. Indeed, the "en bloc" resection of these "at risk" nodal basins championed by Halsted is heralded as one of the first great advances in the primary surgical treatment of solid tumors (Halsted 1997). To aid the visualization of individual lymphatic vessels, various dyes have been developed and used, including early adoption of a number of mercurial compounds. While an important adjuvant, this dye technique most likely contributed to some early erroneous depictions of lymphatic anatomy, such as Sappey's illustration of vulvar lymphatics crossing the labiocrural fold (Parry-Jones 1963) (Fig. 1). Subsequent development of more lymphotrophic dyes, techniques of administration, and study of live tissues provided a more "functional" understanding of the regional lymphatics. Focused on gynecology, these functional

pathways have been well characterized by Plentl and Friedman (1971) in their landmark monograph, *Lymphatic Anatomy of the Female Genital Tract.*

HISTORICAL PERSPECTIVE

The purpose of clinical lymphatic mapping is identification of the node or nodal group that receives the principal and primary flow from the target organ (Fig. 2). Theoretically, these tissues hold the highest promise for disease characterization, as they should represent the first localization and highest statistical risk for early metastatic spread. In the early 20th century, the French gynecologists Leveuf and Godard (1923) studied the lymphatic anatomy of the cervix by injecting Gerotti blue into the cervices of neonatal cadavers. They found that the injected dye reproducibly drained to a lymph node usually found in the obturator space or at the bifurcation of the iliac vessels. They named this the *principal* lymph node. The term *sentinel node* is most often credited to Ernest Gould, who proposed that the lymph node found at the junction of the anterior and posterior facial veins was the first and most important basin for patients with parotid cancer (Gould et al. 1960). Based on observations in 28 patients, he reasoned that if a negative node in this anatomic region was found it would be unlikely that other regional nodes would contain disease and thus, one could forego a full neck dissection. However, it was Ramon Cabanas (1997), who combined the concepts of regional lymphatic flow and selective regional node identification into the technique of modern lymphatic mapping. Studying penile cancer patients with lymphography (performed via cut-down and canalization of the dorsal lymphatic of the penis), he found that a sentinel lymph node was always located among the superficial inguinal nodes. He also noted that the sentinel node was involved with disease in all patients who had metastases and that it was the only node positive in a proportion of patients (12 of 80 cases). He suggested that only those patients with a positive sentinel node required complete lymphadenectomy. These findings have been corroborated in other solid tumors including malignant melanoma and breast and vulvar carcinomas.

MAPPING TECHNIQUES

Blue Dye

Developmental steps in refining the lymphatic mapping technique have been promulgated by a need to simplify the procedure and to develop an effective intraoperative strategy enabling precise nodal identification and treatment triage in one step. The first compounds used in this progression were selective lymphotrophic dyes. Wong et al. (1991) experimented with isosulfan blue, methylene blue, and cyalumede in a feline model and found that isosulfan blue associated better with lymphatic vessel uptake and sentinel node identification

(Fig. 3). Alternative mapping materials that have been successful include flourescein and patent blue-V; however, the former requires a dark room and is associated with tissue extravasation (Bostick and Givliano 2000). Typically, 2 to 5 ml of dye is injected via a small gauge needle (e.g., 25 gauge) into the dermis of the normal tissue surrounding the primary tumor. Intradermal injection is important in lesions of the vulva in order to access the superficial dermal lymphatics that communicate with the groin (Fig. 4). Deep subcutaneous injection will result in uptake into the deep lymphatics accompanying the named vessels of the vulva and perineum to the pelvis. In the cervix and other solid organs, such as the uterus and ovaries, the injection is made deep enough to access the stromal lymphatic elements. These are generally located within 5 mm of the overlying epithelium. In some organs, such as the uterine corpus and the vagina, the anastomotic plexus is well developed and intercommunication throughout the entire

organ can be accomplished with a single injection. Preferred routes of lymphatic drainage were thought to exist even among these situations, best illustrated in the vagina where distal lesions were thought to drain into the inguinal femoral system and proximal lesion into the low pelvic lymphatics mirroring cervical drainage (Plentl and Friedman 1971). However, more recent mapping studies of the vagina show that these traditional anatomic routes do not always hold true and lower vaginal lesions may drain into the pelvis while tumors at the apex may preferentially drain to the groins (Fig. 5) (Frumovitz et al. 2008). Once the dye is deposited, uptake is rapid and can be observed in real-time for some sites. Localization into the sentinel node occurs between 5 and 15 minutes and may remain in the node for up to 60 minutes before dissipating. Procedures that require time to identify "at-risk" nodal basins should take into account these temporal constraints prior to dye delivery. For instance, in cases of cervical cancer mapping where laparotomy is planned, it is preferable to have the abdominal field exposed at the time of dye deposition, given the large number of potential lymphatic basins to be evaluated and the rapidity of the dye uptake in the vessel-rich parametrium. Although these dyes are largely lymphotropic and weakly bound to serum proteins, side effects and complications have been observed. Fortunately, these are infrequent, occurring in approximately 1% to 2% of patients (Leong et al. 2000). Primary excretion of isosulfan blue is biliary and thus, patients with hepatic insufficiency may be at increased risk for complications. The most common effect seen with dye administration is a transient cohort change (gray or blue hue) in the skin with discoloration of the urine. In some cases it may be quite dramatic, albeit of limited duration. Allergic reaction and anaphylaxis have been rarely reported and manifest in classic manner with cardiovascular collapse, erythema, angioedema, bronchospasm, urticaria, gastrointestinal symptoms, and pulmonary edema (Sadiq et al. 2001). While these effects are generally observed within 10 minutes of intravenous injection, most mapping procedures are performed by intradermal injection and thus, could be delayed as much as 30 minutes. Treatment is supportive. Occasionally, a pseudo-anaphylaxis

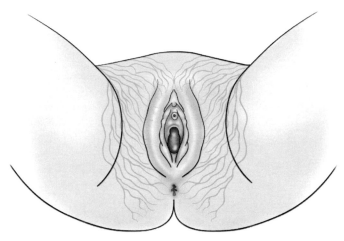

Figure 1 Vulvar and perineal lymphatics as depicted by Sappey in 1874. Use of mercurial dyes in cadaveric tissue led to the erroneous depiction of lymphatic vessels in the vulva and perineum draining across the labiocrural folds two regional lymph nodes sentinel node first site of metastases Peri-lesion injection of blue dye or radiocolloid lymphatic mapping concept lymphatic channel Tumor.

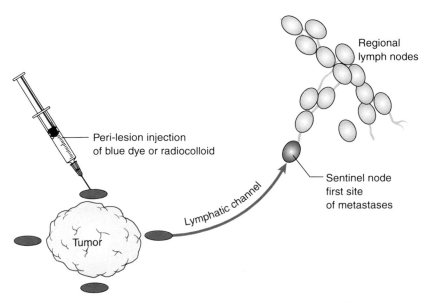

Figure 2 Schematic of the concept of lymphatic mapping. A preferred pathway from the tumor primary to the regional basin drains into the sentinel node.

clinical picture may present, usually first indicated by progressive loss of oxygen saturation. Compounded by gray skin coloring the condition is of concern but lacks features of cardiovascular collapse. Coleman et al. (1999) described this condition and hypothesized its etiology as related to dye interference with non-invasive pulse oximetry saturation algorithms. Peak absorbance of isosulfan blue is 646 nm which is very near that of oxyhemoglobin (660 nm), one of two hemoglobin species measured by non-invasive pulse oximetry. The short-lived condition may be confirmed by a simple arterial blood gas determination. Many hospital operating rooms now have standard protocols for the administration of H2-blockers,

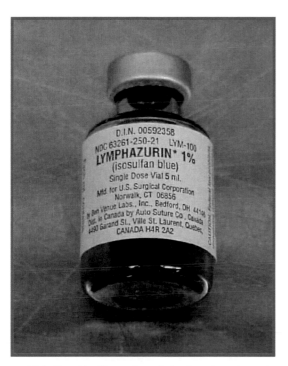

Figure 3 Vial of isosulfan blue trademarked as Lymphazurin 1% (5 cm³).

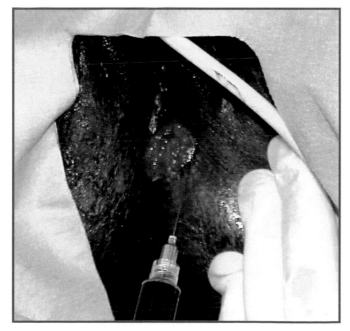

Figure 4 Intradermal injection around a vulvar carcinoma. Deeper injections will drain along the deep lymphatics that line the vascular supply to the vulva.

antihistamines and/or steroids prior to injection of mapping dyes in order to reduce anaphylactic reactions.

Radiocolloid, Lymphoscintigraphy, and Intraoperative Gamma Counters

The blue staining of a node with identification of at least one blue-stained afferent lymphatic channel entering the node remains the gold standard for assessment of whether a lymph node is or is not a true sentinel node. However, introduction of techniques, such as radioactive colloid injections and lymphoscintigraphy, have enhanced the accuracy of detecting the sentinel node. These have been particularly useful in identifying nodes outside of their routine anatomical landmarks of dissection and in aiding the surgeon intraoperatively via a hand-held gamma probe to identify sentinel nodes which have stained poorly or ambiguously. Historically, injection of radionuclides into human subjects to localize regional lymph nodes was first reported by Sherman and Ter-Pogossian in 1953. Numerous radiolabeled compounds have since been used for this purpose. The first gynecologic application of lymphoscintigraphy was in 1982, when Iversen and Aas (1983) studied lymphatic drainage in 24 patients with stage IB cervical cancer. While they were unable to distinguish metastatic from nonmetastatic nodes by radiocolloid uptake, they did remark that radioactivity was higher in certain nodes compared to the background—possibly an early representation of a sentinel node. However, it was

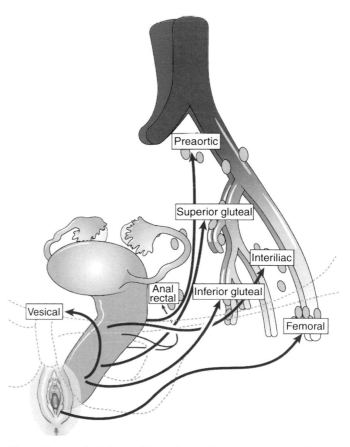

Figure 5 Lymphatic drainage of the vagina. A rich anastomotic network exists that allows intercommunication of lymph throughout the organ. However, specific locales of the vagina will preferentially drain to regional basins from the inguinofemoral nodes to the external iliac nodes.

Table 1 Characteristic of Radionuclides

	^{99m}Tc-SC	^{99m}Tc-HCA	^{99m}Tc-HSA
Particle size (nm)	100–400 (Filtered: 15–50 nm)	5–80	2–3
Transit time to SN (min)	11	10	5
Range (min)	(1–60)	(1–65)	(1–75)
Injection dose at site (3 hr)	76%	83%	–
Visible nodes (30 min) ± SD	2.1 ± 1.9	2.1 ± 1.3	2.2 ± 0.9
Washout $t_{1/2}$ ± SD (hr)	14 ± 12.7	7.5 ± 6.4	4.3 ± 1.4

^{99m}Tc-SC, Technetium-99 Sulfur Colloid; ^{99m}Tc-HCA, Technetium-99 Human Colloidal Albumin; ^{99m}Tc-HAS, Technetium-99 Human Serum Albumin.
Source: Adapted from Wilhelm et al. 1999.

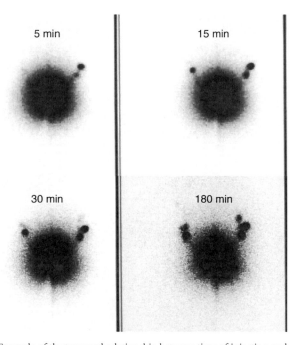

Figure 6 Example of the temporal relationship between time of injection and visualization of the regional basins. This example is from a woman with a stage II vulvar cancer. The time between scans is listed. It is debated as to whether the lateral and newly visualized nodes at 180 minutes represent secondary basins or 'second echelon' nodes.

Morton et al. in 1992, who brought this modality to the clinical arena by demonstrating its utility in identifying "at risk" node basins among 223 cutaneous melanoma patients. Since this report, validation of the strategy has occurred in a number of solid tumors including, head and neck, endocrine, gastrointestinal, genitourinary, breast, and reproductive tract cancers. The ideal radiocolloid must gain access to the lumen of the initial lymphatic channel in sufficient quantity for the lymph vessels to be seen on the dynamic scans. It should combine a rapid and predictable transport toward the sentinel node with persistent retention. The particle size of the radiocolloid is a critical factor in the ease with which these tracers enter the lymphatic system (Table 1). Large particles (500–2000 nm) remain trapped at the injection site and small particles (4–5 nm) will penetrate the capillary membranes and will not be available to migrate through the lymphatic channels (Ege 1976, Henze et al. 1982). In the United States, the most commonly used radiopharmaceutical is filtered technetium-99 m sulfur colloid. This agent has a small particle size (<100 nm), it is uniformly dispersed, highly stable, and has a short half-life (gamma-emitter). Injection flow rate of a radiocolloid is important in the success of sentinel node identification. Once the particles enter the lumen of the lymphatic capillaries, they will move freely and uniformly toward

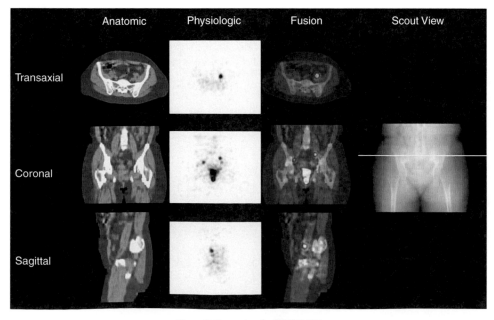

Figure 7 Example of a SPECT-CT.

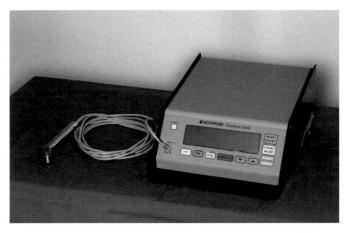

Figure 8 Portable gamma probe for use in vulvar and laparotomy facilitates intraoperative lymphatic mapping.

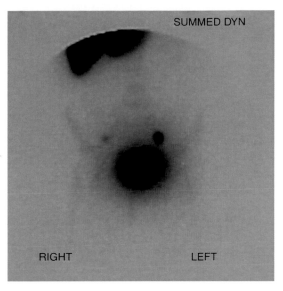

Figure 9 Local injection of radiocolloid may concentrate so highly as to obscure potential identification of proximally situated sentinel nodes. In this example of cervical injection it is easy to appreciate the difficulty of identifying a parametrial node.

the draining lymph nodes. The valves in the lymphatic vessels will generally not allow retrograde flow. Lymphatic flow is fastest in the leg and foot and slowest in the head and neck. The study is performed by injection of 2 to 4 cm³ (1–2.5 mCi) intradermally and perilesionally as with blue dye. A lymphoscintigram is then made to visualize localized uptake (Fig. 6). Dynamic images are usually acquired for a total of 20 minutes. The lymphatic channels are best appreciated by summing the individual dynamic frames to produce a composite dynamic image. Delayed scans are then performed at 2.5 to 3 hours following injection of the radiocolloid tracer. These delayed scans should include all node fields that can possibly receive drainage from the injection site. Each static acquisition should be 5 to 10 minutes in length to ensure that even very faint sentinel nodes are detected (Uren and Howman-Giles 2002). Newer radiologic technologies such as SPECT-CT (Fig. 7) are becoming more routinely used. This exam combines traditional planar lymphoscintigraphy with computed topography (CT) to locate the sentinel node in a three-dimensional image as opposed to the traditional two dimensions seen on lymphoscintograms. The intraoperative detection of the sentinel node relies not only on the visual inspection of the lymphatic basin, but also on the assessment of the radioactive colloid in the sentinel node through the aid of a gamma detection device. This hand-held sensor contains a gamma-sensitive crystal with a preamplifier, and a reading unit (Fig. 8). There are several gamma probes for intraoperative use including laparoscopic devices that can be used in a large spectrum of clinical scenarios. Specificity and accuracy of these devices can be augmented with the use of collimation which will help to reduce background and "bleed-through" radioactivity, frequently encountered in sites where the primary tumor is near its drainage lymphatic basin (Fig. 9). The parametrial nodes in uterine cervical primary and the medial inguino-femoral nodes in an anterior vulvar cancer are good examples of challenging mapping areas. Use of these radiopharmaceuticals appears to be safe given their low dose energy, particle size, and rapid washout rate. Extensive testing has been conducted to determine node safety to health care workers. The amount of radiation exposure from the technique is very small and the cumulative effect is still well within acceptable levels (Eshima et al. 2000).

SENTINEL NODES: PATHOLOGIC EXAMINATION

Traditionally, pathologic assessment of a lymphadenectomy specimen entails teasing out individual lymph nodes from the surrounding fat pad, bisecting each, and embedding them in paraffin for H&E staining. Typically, one slide from each side of the nodes is evaluated. From the pathologist's point of view, each slide has an equal chance of containing metastatic disease. While standardized, the technique evaluates only an estimated 0.1% of the total nodal volume raising the possibility of a false-negative diagnosis. Sentinel node retrieval provides the opportunity for improved precision since the pathologist can focus his/her search for metastatic disease. In this manner, the sentinel node larger than 1 cm can be step-sectioned at 2 to 5 mm intervals and slides developed from each cut surface (Fig. 10). Nodes smaller than this may be totally imbedded or bivalved for evaluation. In breast cancer patients, step-section processing has revealed underestimation of micrometastatic disease in 9% to 33% of node-negative cases (International (Ludwig) Breast Cancer Study Group 1990). In our experience, 20% of patients with metastatic cervical cancer to the lymph nodes will have false-negative findings without ultrastaging of the sentinel nodes (Euscher et al. 2008). The expansion and availability of immunohistochemical techniques during the 1990s has afforded an additional measure of accuracy by allowing pathologists to evaluate the sentinel node tissue sections for specific markers (Table 1).

In the case of gynecologic epithelial tumors such as cervical and vulvar cancer, specific cytokeratins (AE1/AE3 and DF3) are made from pairs of stepsectioned nodal tissue and evaluated for micrometastatic deposits (Fig. 11). The technique has been adapted to be available intraoperatively (Eudy et al. 2003, Munakata et al. 2003, Nahrig et al. 2003). The value immunohistochemistry adds to serial sectioning is debated, but individual series from gynecological lymphatic mapping procedures has reported unidentified micrometastatic disease in up to 4% of negative nodes (de Hullu et al. 2000). An increasingly important question will be how to manage patients with

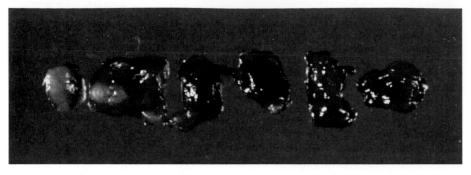

Figure 10 Harvested sentinel nodes are serially sectioned (bread-loafed) to provide additional material for hematoxylin and eosin staining as well as immunohistochemistry.

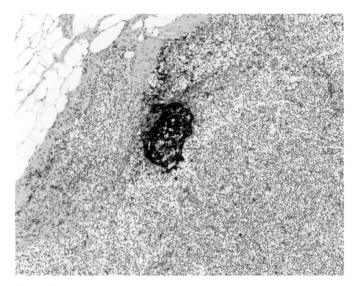

Figure 11 Micrometastasis of squamous cell carcinoma in an inguinofemoral sentinel lymph node. Small tumor deposits may be difficult to distinguish by hematoxylin and eosin staining in the background nodal architecture. In this example, cytokeratin AE1/AE3 is highlighted through immunohistochemistry. (Courtesy of Ate van der Zee).

negative sentinel nodes on traditional H&E staining but positive by immunohistochemisty or other biochemical marker. Van Trappen et al. (2001) used rapid polymerase chain reaction (PCR) testing for cytokeratin 19 in the lymph nodes of radical hysterectomy patients. Lymphatic mapping was not performed, however, it appears that the highest concentration of CK-19-positive nodes was found at the common sites of sentinel nodes. CK-19 was found in only one lymph node from nine patients with benign disease whereas 44% of the H&E-negative lymph nodes in the cervical cancer patients had CK-19 detected. A clearer understanding of micrometastatic disease and how the regional lymphatic process of these cells could form the basis of future molecular work.

CLINICAL EXPERIENCE
Vulvar Cancer

Important contributions dating back to the mid 20th century have identified functional anatomic features, which particularly suit vulvar carcinoma patients with the lymphatic mapping concept. The most important are the clear identification of an ordered pathway from the vulva to the regional inguinofemoral lymphatics and the infrequency of "in-flight" metastatic deposits in the skin bridge between the primary lesion

and the regional basin. Parry-Jones (1963) demonstrated that the vulvar lymphatics did not cross the labiocrural folds as had been previously suggested. He demonstrated by lymphography, that vulvar lymphatic flow drained predictably to the inguinofemoral basin. In the late 1970s, DiSaia et al. (1979) first attempted to apply these concepts in a treatment strategy directed to reducing the morbidity associated with standard radical vulvectomy and inguinofemoral lymphadenectomy. In a manner similar to that of Gould in 1960, these investigators designated the 8 to 10 anatomically situated superficial inguinal lymph nodes as the *sentinel nodes* of the vulva. They reasoned that if these nodes were histologically negative then the femoral nodes would be negative and one could forego deep inguinal dissection resulting in, among others, reduced wound breakdown. Unlike Cabanas (1977), there was no attempt to identify a solitary node directly draining the primary tumor. Several other groups have investigated the sentinel node concept proposed by DiSaia with mixed results. While Berman et al. (1989) reported no groin relapses in a group of 50 early-stage vulvar cancer patients undergoing superficial inguinal lymphadenectomy, Stehman et al. (1992) documented groin recurrences in 7.3% of the 121 patients with negative superficial inguinal nodes. This compared with a recurrence rate of less than 1% following formal inguinofemoral lymphadenectomy with negative nodes in a group of more than 300 patients participating in a Gynecologic Oncology Group (GOG) protocol (Homesley et al. 1986). On the basis of the GOG results, most gynecologic oncologists have abandoned superficial inguinal lymphadenectomy as it was initially purported. It is noteworthy, though, that despite even this manner of limited groin dissection, wound complications and chronic lymphedema were observed in 29% and 19%, respectively, highlighting the true "carrot" of selective node evaluation, if validated. The first report to utilize blue dye to identify a single sentinel node in vulvar carcinoma appeared in 1994 by Levenback et al. (1994). This group, following the growing experience of similar mapping techniques in malignant melanoma, identified sentinel nodes in 7 of 9 patients and in 7 of 12 groins. These authors concluded that the technique was feasible. Subsequent reports have vastly expanded and largely confirmed this experience. Table 2 presents the available data from clinical trials evaluating one, either or both node-localizing techniques (blue dye, lymphoscintigraphy) in patients with operable vulvar carcinoma (Fig. 12). Due to a well-recognized learning curve and technique failures early in a surgeon's experience, the table includes only those published reports that have >20

Table 2 Literature Summary of Vulvar Sentinel Node Trials

Author	Number of patients	Blue dye	Tracer	Scintigraphy	ID rate	False negative SLN
Sideri	44	No	Yes	Yes	100%	0
Ansink	51	Yes	No	No	56%	2 (4%)
De Cicco	37	No	Yes	Yes	100%	0
De Hullu	59	Yes	Yes	Yes	100%	0
Levenback	52	Yes	No	No	88%	2 (4%)
Sliutz	26	Yes	Yes	Yes	100%	0
Moore	21	Yes	Yes	Yes	100%	0
Rob	16	Yes	No	No	69%	1 (6%)
	43	Yes	Yes	Yes	100	0
Vidal-Sicart	50	Yes	Yes	Yes	98	0
Nyberg	47	Yes	Yes	Yes	98	1 (2%)
Hampl	127	Yes	Yes	Yes	98%	3 (8%)

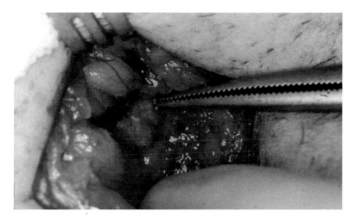

Figure 12 A potential evolution of vulvar lymphatic mapping is limited and selective node sampling through a biopsy incision of 3 cm or less. A blue node with radiocolloid activity is depicted in this photograph.

patients. Although the individual experiences is small compared to the melanoma and breast literature, interest is expanding and has attracted an international investigative audience. Currently, the GOG is evaluating the feasibility of lymphatic mapping in a multi-institutional setting and final results are due to be published shortly. The GOG study was designed as a validation study where all patients will undergo lymphatic mapping and sentinel node biopsy followed by complete inguinofemoral lymphadenectomy to determine the sensitivity, specificity, negative and positive predictive values of sentinel node biopsy in women with vulvar cancer. Another validation study was reported by Hampl et al. (2008). This study enrolled 127 women with T1 to T3 vulvar cancers at seven centers in Germany. The investigators identified at least one sentinel node in 125 (98%) of the 127 women enrolled. Three women had negative sentinel nodes with positive metastatic disease found on complete lymphadenectomy specimens (false-negative rate 7.7%). In two of these three patients, however, primary tumor size was ≥4 cm when sentinel nodes are often difficult to visualize. In addition, none of the three had combined blue dye and radiocolloid used in the mapping procedure (two had radiocolloid only, one had blue dye only). In contrast, the GROningen INternational *Study* on *Sentinel nodes* in Vulvar cancer(GROINSS-V) study was a multi-institutional observational study that performed sentinel node biopsy only then following patients with negative sentinel

nodes with observation only (Van der Zee et al. 2008). In the 259 patients with unifocal disease and negative sentinel nodes, only 6 (2.3%) groin recurrences were observed. They also noted that the wound breakdown and cellulitis of the groin incisions were significantly less than in those who had undergone complete inguinofemoral lymph node dissection. Moore et al. (2008) also performed an observational study in 35 patients with vulvar cancer who underwent sentinel node biopsy only. In their cohort, four women had metastatic disease in the sentinel node. In the remaining 31 women with negative sentinel nodes, two women were noted to have groin recurrences (recurrence rate 6.4%) at a median follow-up of 29 months. Other than these three large, multi-institutional studies, of which there currently exists published data from one, the remainder of the literature's experience is from single institution validation studies that performed the sentinel node procedure followed by complete inguinofemoral lymphadenectomy to evaluate for accuracy of mapping techniques. Levenback et al. (2001) updated their collective experience on 52 patients undergoing blue dye localization. A sentinel node was identified in 46 (88%) patients and in 57 of 76 (75%) dissected groins. Independent effects hampering sentinel node identification were prior excisional biopsy, midline tumor location, and operator experience. A median of one sentinel node was identified in each groin. The sentinel node was not found in 2 of the 12 groins that ultimately proved to have metastatic disease. Both events occurred in the first two years of the study. There were no false negative identified sentinel nodes. The authors demonstrated that following a short learning curve and limiting the procedure to patients with clinically non-suspicious nodes and T1 or T2 squamous cell carcinoma lesions, virtually all patients (95%) were found with sentinel nodes. A similar study by Ansink et al. (1999) had different results. In this multicenter study involving 51 patients undergoing blue dye lymphatic mapping, sentinel nodes were detected in just 56% of the 93 groins dissected. All tumors were squamous cell histology and had clinically non-suspicious groins. Nine groins were found with metastatic disease, six (66%) of which the sentinel node was the only metastatic node. However, in two cases, a sentinel (blue) node was found and was histologically negative, yet metastatic disease was identified in non-sentinel nodes. The low sentinel identification rate and false-negative cases led these authors to conclude that the blue dye alone technique was not feasible and that combination with lymphoscintigraphy should be further studied. Feasibility concerns notwithstanding, the recommendation is of merit given the relative rarity of this tumor and the ability for lymphoscintigraphy to shorten learning curve proficiency. As seen in Table 2, sentinel node localization using lymphoscintigraphy alone or combined with blue dye is highly successful. De Cicco et al. (1998) studied 37 squamous T1 and T2 patients with preoperative and intraoperative lymphoscintigraphy alone. Bilateral groin dissection was performed if the primary lesion was within 2 cm of a midline structure. At least one sentinel lymph node was identified in each patient. Eight patients were identified with metastatic disease, including five (63%) patients where the sentinel node was the only positive node. All 29 cases with negative sentinel nodes had negative groin histology. If lymphoscintigraphy did not identify a sentinel node in a groin, no metastases were found at surgery. Sideri et al. (2000) updated this group's experience with 44 similarly staged and studied patients. A sentinel node was identified in each case. In 77 dissected groins, 13 cases demonstrated metastatic disease—all in sentinel nodes. In 10 cases, the sentinel node was the only positive node. These authors addressing the negative predictive value of an identified sentinel node concluded that if the technique was validated, less aggressive dissection of the groin could be entertained if the sentinel was histologically negative. De Hullu et al. (2000) studied preoperative and intraoperative lymphoscintigraphy in combination with blue dye localization. In this study of 59 patients with T1 and T2 epidermoid cancers, sentinel nodes were identified in all patients with at least one of the techniques. Bilateral groin dissection was performed if the primary lesion was within 1 cm of a midline structure. Of the 107 groin dissections performed, a sentinel node was found in 95 (89%). The literature summary of vulvar sentinel node trials authors noted that they relied primarily on the gamma probe to isolate sentinel lymph nodes, as blue sentinel nodes were observed in just 60% of cases (Table 2). Metastatic disease was found in 20 (34%) patients and in 27 (25%) groins. In 15 (54%) groins, the sentinel node was the only positive node. In this study, immunohistochemical ultrastaging with cytokeratin staining was additionally performed. In 102 histologically negative sentinel nodes, four (4%) were found with micrometastatic disease. The authors concluded that lymphatic mapping was feasible in this manner and that ultrastaging by step-sectioning and staining with immunohistochemical methodology may identify micrometastatic disease in some cases. A similar experience was reported by Moore et al. (2003) in 21 clinically node-negative stage I to IV vulvar cancer patients. Using a combined technique, all nine patients with metastatic disease were identified by lymphoscintigraphy compared to just three of nine patients with blue dye alone. However, in 2 of 31 dissected groins the sentinel node was described as blue only, not containing radiocolloid; similarly, just 29 of 89 (33%) sentinel nodes retained characteristics of both tracers. The importance of using both radiocolloid and blue dye was best shown by Rob et al. (2007). In their prospective study, the first 16 patients underwent mapping with blue dye only with a sentinel node identification rate of only 69% and a false negative rate of 6% (1 one 16 patients). In the remaining 43 patients, the investigators used both blue dye and radiocolloid and sentinel nodes were identified in 100%

of cases with no false negatives. Although some of the improvement may be attributed to surgeon experience with the techniques, we believe the combined technique significantly improves sentinel node detection. It is not known which tumoral features impact the uptake of these individual components, thus making it prudent to use both. Overall, false-negative rates among series using radiotracers, in combination with blue dye, have been very low but may reflect the single institution experience of skilled surgeons. Future directions Lymphatic mapping and sentinel node identification appear at this point to be clinically enticing for patients with vulvar carcinoma. Prior to universal adoption, surgeons need to familiarize themselves with the techniques, as there exists a significant learning curve to performing lymphatic mapping and sentinel node detection consistently. We recommend "practicing" these techniques on 5 to 10 patients with lymphatic mapping and identification of sentinel nodes followed by complete lymphadenectomy to assure no false negative results. The reproducibility of the above clinical experience in the multi-institutional setting is currently underway and if validated, patients will have new options based on triage programs that could offer them improved precision of their disease status and reduced morbidity.

Cervical Cancer
Cervical cancer is an excellent target for the lymphatic mapping strategy. First, most patients undergoing primary surgical treatment will not have metastatic disease. Second, the cervix is a midline structure with numerous potential drainage basins, although, as demonstrated by Leveuf and Godard (1923), the preferred sites are generally at the obturator and external iliac locales. Third, the cervix is easily visible and accessible for injection both prior to and during surgery. Finally, since fertility-sparing and minimally invasive options are now being described in highly selected, low-risk patients, developing a strategy to easily identify the patients in these groups with lymphatic metastases would be of benefit.

Clinical Experience and Data Review
In 2008, the AGO Study Group published the results from their multicenter prospective trial evaluating the sensitivity and specificity of sentinel node biopsy in women with cervical cancer. They enrolled 590 women in this study who underwent lymphatic mapping with blue dye, radiocolloid or both and sentinel node biopsy followed by complete pelvic and, if indicated, para-aortic lymphadenectomies. For all patients in the study, at least one sentinel node was detected in 89% of cases but when combination blue dye and radiocolloid were used, the detection rate rose to 94%. Overall the sensitivity was disappointing at only 77% (Altgassen et al. 2008). However, when subgroup analysis limited analysis to women with tumors ≤2 cm in size, the sensitivity was 91%. The AGO Study Group reported a negative predictive value of 94% but again saw a significantly improved NPV when limiting the analysis to tumors ≤2 cm in size (99%). Other authors have also reported higher sentinel node detection rate in tumors ≤2 cm as compared to larger lesions (Darlin et al. 2010). Limited, single institution clinical trials (summarized in Table 3, studies with >20 patients only) exploring the sentinel node concept in cervical cancer have typically

reported more promising results than the AGO Study. Although mixed in early trials, the experience has generally supported the hypothesis that an identifiable, preferred lymphatic pathway from the cervix to the regional nodal basin exists. However, mapping in this disease site faces special challenges relating to the tumoral injection, high vascularity of the uterus and large number of potential pelvic and para-aortic lymphatic basins (Fig. 13).

Blue Dye

Echt et al. (1999) from the Moffitt Cancer Center were first to report an experience in attempting sentinel node identification among cervical cancer patients. In this 1999 series, 13 patients underwent peritumoral injection with lymphazurin 1% blue dye followed by laparotomy. In 12 of 13 patients, radical hysterectomy was completed; one was aborted following identification of a metastatic para-aortic node (Table 3). Collectively, just two (15%) patients were found

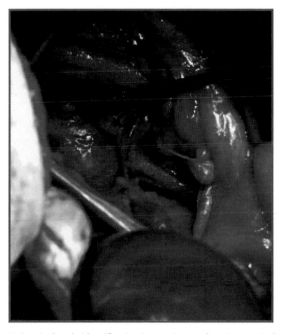

Figure 13 Sentinel node identification in a patient undergoing cervical cancer lymphatic mapping. In this example, the sentinel node, afferent and efferent lymph vasculature are visualized coming from the cervix.

with blue sentinel nodes. In these two cases, the sentinel nodes were found to contain metastatic disease along with positive undyed, non-sentinel nodes. The patient with metastatic para-aortic disease (a solitary node) and the remaining 10 patients did not have an identifiable sentinel node. It is not known if the quantity of dye used (2 ml in this series) or the timing for laparotomy contributed to the low rate of identification. The authors concluded that modification of their technique would be required for future study to accurately assess the concept. In a similar report, Medl et al. (2000) reported on three stage IB to IIA patients they identified with metastatic nodal disease using blue dye alone. These patients underwent laparotomy following dye injection, which was delivered, into the lateral vaginal fornices, rather than cervical stroma. Although the authors voice support for the adaptation of this technology it is not stated what the total number of patients being studied was or if there were any false negative determinations. Technical and clinicopathologic features influencing sentinel node mapping success were detailed in a pilot project from O'Boyle et al. (2000). This group, injecting 5 ml of 1% lymphazurin dye intrastromally, reported sentinel node identification in 12 of 20 (60%) patients undergoing laparotomy for early-stage cervical cancer (stage IB1–IIA). Tumor size (>4 cm) and prior conization were features associated with lack of sentinel node localization. The authors commented that temporal sequence of injection and laparotomy might be important, given the rapidity that blue dye is cleared from nodal tissues in the vascular pelvic basin. While the interiliac and external iliac nodal chains were the common location of the 23 sentinel nodes identified, four nodes were found in the common iliac basin and four were identified in parametrial tissues. Microscopic nodal metastases were found in four (20%) patients, three of whom had disease in identified sentinel nodes. A fourth patient did not have an identifiable sentinel node. In addition, two of these four patients had bilateral nodal metastases, both of whom had only unilateral sentinel nodes (positive) found. Nonetheless, if patients were identified with a sentinel node, its histopathology reflected the nodal basin in each case. Dargent et al. (2000) argued that this technology would be most important for patients undergoing minimally invasive procedures since its validation would limit the nodal dissection necessary and pave the way for total vaginal resection or even fertility-sparing procedures, such as

Table 3 Literature Summary of Cervical Sentinel Node Trials

Author	No of cases	Dye	Tracer	Lymphoscintigraphy	Success	False negative
Echt	33	Yes	No	No	15%	0
O'Boyle	20	Yes	No	No	60%	0
Dargent	23	Yes	No	No	86%	0
Levenback	39	Yes	Yes	Yes	1 (3%)[a]	
Rob	65	Yes	Yes	Yes	77%	0
Malur	50	Yes	Yes	Yes*	78	
Buist	25	Yes	Yes	Yes	88%	1 (4%)[a]
Bats	71	Yes	Yes	Yes	91%	2 (3%)
Kara	32	Yes	Yes	Yes	100%	0
Fader	38	Yes	Yes	Yes	92%	1 (3%)
Ogawa	82	No	Yes	Yes	88%	0

[a]False negative cases in these trials were parametrial nodes identified within the radical hysterectomy specimens.
*Lymphoscintigraphy in first 18 patients only.

radical trachelectomy. In their report, 35 patients underwent laparoscopic mapping procedures and lymphadenectomy. Defining "success" as identifying a sentinel node on each pelvic side-wall, the authors reported that location (fornicies vs. stroma) and volume of dye (4 ml vs. less) were significant factors of a successful study. Overall, they identified sentinel nodes in 59 of 69 (86%) lymphatic dissections (pelvic side-walls). Of these instances, 51 were associated with a single dyed node. Interestingly, blue dyed nodes were identified a median 52 minutes following injection with a range of 20 to 150 minutes. It is tempting to speculate that intra-abdominal pressure during laparoscopic procedures may reduce the rapid clearance of dye seen in laparotomy studies. Metastatic disease was seen in 11 nodes from six patients—all sentinels. No studies without false-negative results have been reported, although one patient had a metastatic node in a basin without a sentinel node identified. Details of sentinel node location in this study confirmed the importance of the lateral lymphatic trunks in cervical drainage. The interiliac, obturator, and external iliac basins (so-called "Leveuf et Godard" area) were the location of 53 sentinel nodes. Rob and colleagues presented their experience of patent blue dye lymphatic mapping in 65 patients undergoing laparoscopy ($n = 12$) and laparotomy ($n = 53$) for early cervical cancer. Unique in this trial was the inclusion of 20 patients undergoing radical hysterectomy following neoadjuvant chemotherapy. Table 4 details the findings from this report. Three patients in the laparoscopy cohort were found with metastatic disease, all within identified nodes sent for intraoperative frozen section. There were no false negative studies. The authors concluded that the technique was feasible in smaller tumors by both laparoscopy and laparotomy but limited in patients with larger tumors following neoadjuvant chemotherapy. They further emphasized the importance of timing the dye infusion to follow port placement or laparotomy incision.

Radiocolloid
In an attempt to bolster the success of finding a sentinel node and to reduce the learning curve for these procedures, many investigators have turned to or added lymphoscintigraphy to their mapping technique. Verheijen et al. (2000) reported their experience with radiocolloid mapping in 10 women with cervical cancer. Focal uptake ("hot") was seen in 6 of 10 patients. Blue dye injection was also used in this study, showing localization in four patients and all within nodes previously identified as hot. A total of 18 sentinel nodes were detected at laparotomy, including the one patient with metastatic disease. Nodal localization was preferentially in the external and

interiliac chains but sentinel nodes in the common iliac basin were seen in three cases. Bilateral sentinel nodes were seen in four cases. Lantzsch et al. (2001) detailed their experience of sentinel node identification in 14 stage IB patients using preoperative and intraoperative lymphoscintigraphy alone. This group performed intraoperative localization with a hand-held gamma probe and then completed radical hysterectomy and pelvic lymph node dissection. Focal uptake of filtered radiocolloid was seen in 13 (93%) patients and it identified 26 sentinel nodes (Table 4). Five patients were found with bilateral sentinel nodes and eight patients had one or more unilateral sentinels retrieved. One patient was found with histologically positive sentinel nodes. There were no false-negative studies. A larger, multi-institutional experience was published by Levenback et al. (2002), in which the combined technique was studied at laparotomy. In this series, 39 patients underwent either preoperative ($n = 23$) or perioperative ($n = 16$) radiocolloid cervical stromal injection. Localized uptake was seen in 33 patients from the lymphoscintigrams. All patients had at least one sentinel node identified and bilateral sentinel nodes were found in 37 of 39 patients. In contrast to other reports, sentinel nodes in this trial retained either or both characteristic of blue and hot. Table 5 demonstrates the relationship seen in this trial. Further, size and preoperative cervical conization did not negatively affect identification of a sentinel node. Metastatic disease was found in 25 nodes from eight patients. In seven of these patients at least one positive sentinel node was retrieved and in five, the only positive node was the sentinel node. In one patient with negative bilateral sentinel nodes a positive parametrial node was identified in the hysterectomy specimen. The relatively high radioactivity observed near the cervix following injection limits precise localization of nodes in the parametrium (unless blue). The clinical relevance of these nodes to survival has been recently called into question (Winter et al. 2002). Although most investigators agree that the combination of patent blue dyes and radiocolloid significantly improves intraoperative sentinel node detection rate, the necessity of preoperative lymphoscintigraphy is likely unnecessary. Frumovitz et al. (2006) reviewed the correlation of preoperative lymphoscintigraphy and intraoperative detection of sentinel nodes and found that the additional preoperative imaging did little to improve intraoperative identification. In fact, there was very poor concordance between the lymphoscinitgraphy and the intraoperative findings while the imaging added to patient cost, time, and discomfort. Fotiou et al. (2010) reported similar findings when they reviewed their experience of preoperative and intraoperative identification of sentinel lymph nodes in women with cervical cancer. Combined technique and laparoscopy as illustrated by Dargent et al. (2000), laparoscopic sentinel node mapping may provide the greatest measure of benefit for patients with early-stage disease. There has been limited experience reported utilizing the intraoperative gamma probe but the early reports would support its feasibility and importance in sentinel node localization. Kamprath et al. (2000), in a letter to the editor, in the *American Journal of Obstetrics and Gynecology*, presented data on 18 patients undergoing laparoscopic lymphadenectomy following preoperative radiocolloid injection. Laparoscopic radical hysterectomy was performed in 15 patients and radical trachelectomy in three

Table 4 Treatment Cohorts in Rob et al. 2004

Cohort	N	Technique	Stage	Detection %
A	12	Laparoscopy	IA2:2 IB1:10	11/12 (92)
B$_1$	13	Laparotomy	IB$_1$ (<2 cm)	11/13 (85)
B$_2$	20	Laparotomy	IB$_1$ (2–4 cm)	16/20 (80)
B$_3$	20	NACT/ Laparotomy	IB$_2$	12/20 (60)

Abbreviation: NACT, neoadjuvant chemotherapy.

patients. Since no blue dye was used in this trial, resected nodes were secondarily scanned ex vivo for activity. "Hot" nodes were labeled sentinel and were found in 16 of 18 (89%) patients. Interestingly, a median 2.1 pelvic sentinel nodes were found, with a median 1.4 para-aortic sentinel nodes found among five patients. Their two non-diagnostic studies included the first two patients given one-fifth and one-half of the radiocolloid dose, respectively. One patient was found with metastatic disease. This patient had one sentinel and three non-sentinel positive nodes. Similarly, Malur et al. (2001), from the same institution, later reported their experience with patent blue dye alone ($n = 9$), radiocolloid alone ($n = 21$), and the combination ($n = 20$) in early-stage cervical cancer patients undergoing pelvic and para-aortic lymphadenectomy via laparoscopy ($n = 45$) or laparotomy ($n = 5$). Table 6 outlines the success of sentinel node identification and representation by technique. Detection rate was similar between laparotomy and laparoscopy (about 78%), although six patients in this series had stage IV disease and were undergoing extirpation by pelvic exenteration. Metastatic disease was documented in 10 (20%) patients, six of whom had identifiable sentinel nodes. In all but one of these cases, the sentinel node had metastatic disease. In two, the sentinel node was the only positive node. One patient identified with blue-dyed, histologically negative sentinel nodes was found with a single, positive metastatic non-sentinel node—a false-negative study. This patient was evaluated by blue dye alone, prompting the authors to recommend the combined technique for further study. In this latter cohort, 18 of 20 patients were identified with sentinel nodes; four with metastatic disease and all within sentinel nodes (Table 5). Barranger et al. (2003) discussed their experience with laparoscopic sentinel node mapping following the combination of patent blue dye and radiocolloid cervical injection. In this limited series of 13 patients, one to three sentinel nodes were identified in 12 patients. No patients were found with metastatic disease on routine H&E staining. However, micrometastatic lesions were found in four sentinel nodes from two patients by immunohistochemical analysis. None of these patients received adjuvant therapy. Interestingly, one patient was found with a sentinel node in the common iliac area. The authors concluded that sentinel node mapping could have a role in minimally invasive surgical procedures for patients with early-stage cervical cancer. Buist et al. (2003) reported on 25 early-stage cervical cancer patients undergoing laparoscopic sentinel node assessment as a triage technique for subsequent abdominal radical hysterectomy. If metastatic disease was detected in the sentinel node, complete lymphadenectomy was performed laparoscopically and the uterus was left in situ.

If no metastatic disease was identified, a laparoscopic pelvic lymphadenectomy was performed followed by an abdominal radical hysterectomy. One or more sentinel nodes were detected in all patients and bilateral sentinel nodes were found in 22 of 25 (88%) patients. Metastatic disease was detected in 40% of the cohort. One patient with two negative obturator sentinel nodes was later found to have a metastatic parametrial node removed with the primary tumor. This represented the only false-negative study. Two additional patients were later identified by immunohistochemistry to have micrometastatic disease. Importantly, six patients underwent only laparoscopic lymphadenectomy and ovarian transposition following sentinel node identification averting exploration for radical hysterectomy. The authors concluded the procedure was feasible and triage in this manner could avert additional morbidity from transperitoneal exploration.

Future Development
Surgical validity of this technology requires prospective investigation in more diverse cohorts, the multi-institutional environment, and with adaptation of newer and more specific pathologic/molecular techniques of nodal evaluation. Further, validation is required for the development of prospective, randomized trials where individual treatment triage is specified on the basis of the sentinel node. Such trials are currently under development. In this regard, it would seem that patients eligible for laparoscopic dissection would be ideal candidates for this technology, as focused dissection and potentially fertility-sparing operations (such as radical trachelectomy) could be offered (Covens et al. 1999). In addition, sparing of potential antigen-recognizing lymphoid cells could be critical to the successful adaptation of vaccine therapies. HPV-L1 virus-like particle (VLP) vaccine therapy is currently under phase I clinical development. The importance of such strategies on the prevention of viral infection has been documented in a randomized double-blind multicenter controlled clinical trial of a HPV-L1 VLP on healthy volunteers (Koutsky et al. 2002) (Table 6). At a median of 17.9 months follow-up the rate of persistent HPV infection was 3.9/100 woman-years

Table 6 Characteristics and Probability Estimates for 50 Patients Undergoing Lymphatic Mapping

Variable	Blue dye	Radiocolloid	Combined	Overall
Number of patients	9	21	20	50
Detection rate %	56	76	90	78
Sensitivity %	50	0	100	83
Specificity %	100	100	100	100
Positive predictive value %	100	0	100	100
Negative predictive value %	75	100	100	97
Accuracy %	80	100	100	97
False negative %	50	0	0	17

Source: From Malur et al. 2001.

Table 5 Relationship of Dye and Radioactivity in 132 Sentinel Nodes

Dye	Radioactivity		Total
	Hot	Not hot	
Blue	65	32	100
Not blue	32	0	32
Total	97	35	132

Source: From Levenback et al. 2002.

in the control group compared to 0/100 woman-years in those receiving vaccine ($p < 0.001$). All cases of HPV-16-related dysplasia occurred in the placebo cohort. Overall, however, more information of the clinical relationship between the primary tumor and its lymphatic basin is required to gain a deeper understanding of tumor biology and unravel the mysteries of clinical behavior.

Uterine Cancer

Endometrial cancer is a difficult target for the mapping strategy. The primary tumor cannot be seen, imaged or palpated with standard clinical tools. However, endometrial cancer is an attractive disease site for lymphatic mapping given the complexity of the lymphatic drainage of the uterus. Sentinel nodes could, theoretically, be found anywhere from the obturator space to the renal vessels (Fig. 14). In this largely experimental cohort, few clinical trials have been reported. Lymphatic mapping studies Echt et al. (1999) described their attempts at sentinel node identification in patients with endometrial cancer. Patent V blue dye was injected into the uterine fundus at a depth of approximately half the thickness of the myometrium. The authors could not identify any sentinel nodes in eight patients. Burke et al. (1996) described intraoperative injection of isosulfan blue into the subserosal myometrium into three midline sites at the fundus, 2 cm anterior and 2 cm posterior to this site. These sites were chosen to mimic a fundal endometrial cancer. Dye uptake was seen in the lymphatic channels and lymph nodes within 10 minutes (Fig. 15). Blue-stained nodes were identified and the location recorded and the nodes were sent to pathology as separate specimens. A selective pelvic and para-aortic lymphadenectomy was then performed. Blue dye was deposited in lymph nodes in 10 of 15 patients and blue nodes were found in the pelvic and para-aortic areas. No stained nodes were found between the bifurcation of the aorta and the origin of the inferior mesenteric artery. This confirms the observations of many anatomists that the lymphatic drainage of the uterus follows two paths, along the uterine vessels to the pelvis and the gonadal vessels to the para-aortics at the level of the renal vessels. Four patients had positive lymph nodes; two in sentinel nodes. One patient with bulky nodes had no dye uptake and one patient had a micrometastases to an unstained node in the obturator space. A follow-up study of fundal injection of radionucleotide and patent blue dye by the same group enrolled an additional 18 women. In this second cohort of women, sentinel nodes were identified in only eight (45%) patients (Frumovitz et al. 2007). Furthermore, seven (88%) of the eight women with a sentinel node identified had only unilateral drainage noted. As the uterus is a midline organ with presumably bilateral drainage, the absence of sentinel nodes on both sides of the pelvis is seemingly troublesome and a potential problem with the technique Holub et al. (2001) described a laparoscopic-assisted technique for lymphatic mapping in patients with endometrial cancer. In this series, eight patients underwent intraoperative injection of blue dye using the same locations as described by Burke et al. using a 5-mm laparoscopic puncture needle. Blue nodes were found in the obturator, internal iliac, and common iliac sites in 11 lymph nodes among five patients. Holub et al. expanded on their experience and reported two techniques for lymphatic mapping in endometrial cancer in 2002. In this study, 13 patients underwent subserosal injection as described in the first report and 12 patients underwent subserosal and cervical injections. The combined injection technique increased the rate of observation of blue-stained lymph nodes from 61.5% in the first group to 83.3% in the current report. The authors suggest that the combined approach is superior. Other authors have focused on the cervical injections only for sentinel node

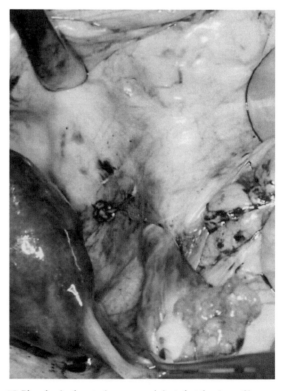

Figure 15 Blue dye in the uterine corpus, injected at the time of laparotomy, is seen traversing the gonadal lymphatics into the low para-aortic region (seen transperitoneally). Although lymphatic mapping in this fashion may not accurately reflect the primary tumor's specific drainage, one can appreciate the vast intrauterine lymphatic anastamotic network.

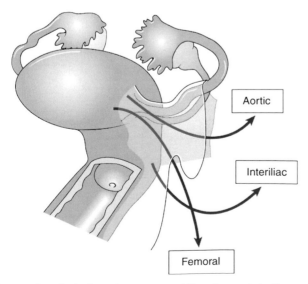

Figure 14 Lymphatics from the uterus may follow the vessels leading to the pelvic nodes or through the gonadal vessels to the para-aortic nodes. Rarely, they may follow the round ligament draining in the inguinofemoral basin.

detection in women with uterine cancer. There are many potential advantages of this approach. First, many investigators are comfortable with this technique having used it in their patients with primary cervical cancer. Second, the cervix is readily accessible preoperatively for injection of radiocolloid in the nuclear medicine suite. This allows for preoperative imaging of sentinel nodes and better surgical planning. Pandit-Taskar et al. (2010) reported on 40 patients with endometrial cancer who underwent SPECT-CT after cervical injection of technecium-99. In their cohort, a sentinel node was identified preoperatively 100% of the time. This allowed for precise anatomic localization of sentinel nodes helping the surgeon detect them intraoperatively. The major disadvantage to this technique is that it essentially ignores the fundal route of drainage of the primary lesion. In the Pandit-Taskar report described above, none of the 40 patients had lymphatic drainage outside the pelvis (i.e., to the aortacaval region). Pelosi et al. (2002) was the first to describe this approach using a combination of radioactive tracer and blue dye in 11 patients with early endometrial cancer during laparoscopic-assisted vaginal hysterectomy and bilateral salpingoophorectomy. The tracer and blue dye were injected into the cervix. Three sentinel nodes were identified that proved to be positive for micrometastases. Similarly, Gargiulo et al. (2003) reported on 11 patients with stage IB to IIA endometrial cancer who underwent preoperative cervical injection of radiocolloid and intraoperative cervical injection of blue dye prior to planned laparoscopic assisted vaginal hysterectomy, bilateral salpingoophorectomy and pelvic and para-aortic lymphadenectomy. Seventeen sentinel lymph nodes were identified, predominantly in the external iliac area—three with micrometastases. No para-aortic nodes were identified. More recently, larger series have been published. Bats et al. (2008a,b) performed cervical injection of both blue dye and radiocolloid in 43 patients with clinical stage I uterine cancer. Sentinel nodes were identified in 30 patients (69.8%). Eight patients had metastatic disease to the pelvic nodes and all were found by lymphatic mapping (no false negatives). However, as expected, none of the 30 patients with sentinel nodes detected had drainage to nodes along the aorta or vena cava. Likewise, Ballester et al. (2008) used the cervical injection technique in 46 patients with uterine cancer and were able to detect a sentinel node in 40 of them (87%). In their 10 patients with metastatic disease to lymph nodes, there were also no false-negatives with the mapping technique. In their series, only 1 of 101 sentinel nodes detected in the 40 patients was found along the aorta. The remaining 100 sentinel nodes were again limited to the pelvis. In an effort to accurately map the lymphatic drainage of the tumor and not the organ, multiple investigators have attempted to inject the tumor directly using hysteroscopic visualization and injection. Most used office hysteroscopy to inject radiocolloid and/or blue dye prior to going to the operating arena for hysterectomy, salpingoophorectomy and staging. This allowed for nuclear imaging prior to incision. Niikura et al. (2004) injected radiocolloid only into 28 consecutive patients with endometrial cancer. At surgery, they were able to find at least one sentinel node in 23 (82%) patients. As expected and in stark contrast to cervical injection techniques, 81% of patients had at least one sentinel node located above the bifurcation of the aorta including 14% with

sentinel nodes only along the aorta (i.e., no pelvic sentinel nodes identified). Maccauro et al. (2005) used combined radiocolloid and blue dye in their hysteroscopic injection of 26 women with uterine cancer. In their study, they were able to identify at least one sentinel node in all 26 women injected. Furthermore, of the 53 sentinel lymph nodes removed surgically, 14 (26%) were found along the aorta and/or vena cava. Both these two early studies had no false negatives in the combined 49 patients. Delaloye et al. (2007), however, did have one false negative (11%) in the nine women with positive metastatic disease in their cohort of 60 patients. In their study, hysteroscopic injection of both blue dye and radiocolloid led to a sentinel node detection rate of 82% (49 of 60 patients). One-third of patients had at least one sentinel node along the aorta/vena cava. Other authors have had more difficulty identifying sentinel nodes using the hysteroscopic technique. Perrone et al (2008) were only able to identify a sentinel node in 65% of patients who underwent hysteroscopic injection while Robova et al. (2009) and Clement et al. (2008) were only able to identify a sentinel node in 50% and 40% of patients, respectively. In our experience, the hysteroscopic technique is quite difficult with good visualization of the entire uterine lesion often impossible. In addition, bleeding at the first puncture sight and leakage of blue dye into the uterine cavity during hysteroscopic injection obscures much of the field. Also, the endometrium is rich in blood supply and much of the radiocolloid and blue dye may be taken up into the vasculature as opposed to the lymphatics. Overall, however, the use of this technique is an improvement over techniques that rely on injection into the uterine fundus or cervix without visualization of the actual tumor as it more likely approximates the lymphatic drainage of the tumor as opposed to the uterus. In addition, this technique provides a preoperative lymphoscintigram that can help plan the operative procedure. The most cephalad sentinel node can be identified and perhaps a determination made about how long an incision it will take to reach it. Conversely, it requires another procedure and a two-day sequence. And, as it is most often done as an office procedure, the hysteroscopic injection can be quite uncomfortable for patients. In the only study to evaluate patient tolerance of preoperative hysteroscopic injection of mapping substances, Clement et al. (2008) reported very high pain scores (visual analog scale score 8 out of 10) for women undergoing the procedure. It remains to be seen if other groups can replicate these results.

Summary

Endometrial cancer is an excellent disease site for lymphatic mapping and sentinel node identification. Many technical challenges remain and the best method for sentinel node identification has not yet been described.

FUTURE DIRECTIONS OF LYMPHATIC MAPPING

Continuing work to validate the concept of lymphatic mapping in gynecologic tumors is being conducted through multi-institutional clinical trials within the international community. Departure from "standard-of-care" lymphatic resection paradigms in cancer management requires prudent and propitious decision making through careful review of clinical outcomes in properly conducted and controlled clinical studies. Many challenges remain, not the least of which lie in the relative rarity of the diseases being studies. However, clear definition of the learning curve and establishment of an acceptable false-negative rate will need to accompany equally important advances in our understanding of the tumor physiology of the regional lymphatics. While selective resection of affected tissues remains the "holy grail" of cancer surgery, treatment success defines the benchmark—a line which the pursuit of minimization cannot compromise. It is anticipated that better tracers and localizing agents, improved pathological processing, and standardized operative techniques will measurably add to this growing body of challenging study.

REFERENCES

Altgassen C, Hertel H, Brandstädt A, et al.; AGO Study Group (2008). Multicenter validation study of the sentinel lymph node concept in cervical cancer: AGO Study Group. *J Clin Oncol* **26**(18):2943–51.

Ansink AC, Sie-Go DM, van der Velden J, et al. (1999) Identification of sentinel lymph nodes in vulvar carcinoma patients with the aid of a patent blue V injection: a multicenter study. *Cancer* **86**:652–6.

Ballester M, Dubernard G, Rouzier R, et al. (2008) Use of the sentinel node procedure to stage endometrial cancer. *Ann Surg Oncol* **15**:1523–9.

Barranger E, Grahek D, Cortez A, et al. (2003) Laparoscopic sentinel lymph node procedure using a combination of patent blue and radioisotope in women with cervical carcinoma. *Cancer* **97**:3003–9.

Bats AS, Clément D, Larousserie F, et al. (2008a) Does sentinel node biopsy improve the management of endometrial cancer? Data from 43 patients. *J Surg Oncol* **97**:141–5.

Bats AS, Lavoué V, Rouzier R, et al. (2008b) Limits of day-before lymphoscintigraphy to localize sentinel nodes in women with cervical cancer. *Ann Surg Oncol* **15**:2173–9.

Berman ML, Soper JT, Creasman WT, et al. (1989) Conservative surgical management of superficially invasive stage I vulvar carcinoma. *Gynecol Oncol* **35**:352–7.

Bostick PJ, Giuliano AE (2000) Vital dyes in sentinel node localization. *Semin Nucl Med* **30**:18–24.

Buist MR, Pijpers RJ, van Lingen A, et al. (2003) Laparoscopic detection of sentinel lymph nodes followed by lymph node dissection in patients with early stage cervical cancer. *Gynecol Oncol* **90**:290–6.

Burke TW, Levenback C, Tornos C, et al. (1996) Intraabdominal lymphatic mapping to direct selective pelvic and para-aortic lymphadenectomy in women with high-risk endometrial cancer: results of a pilot study. *Gynecol Oncol* **62**:169–73.

Cabanas RM (1977) An approach for the treatment of penile carcinoma. *Cancer* **39**:456–66.

Clement D, Bats AS, Ghazzar-Pierquet N, et al. (2008) Sentinel lymph nodes in endometrial cancer: is hysteroscopic injection valid? *Eur J Gynaecol Oncol* **29**:239–41.

Coleman RL, Whitten CW, O'Boyle J, et al. (1999) Unexplained decrease in measured oxygen saturation by pulse oximetry following injection of Lymphazurin 1% (isosulfan blue) during a lymphatic mapping procedure. *J Surg Oncol* **70**:126–9.

Covens A, Shaw P, Murphy J, et al. (1999) Is radical trachelectomy a safe alternative to radical hysterectomy for patients with stage IA-B carcinoma of the cervix? *Cancer* **86**:2273–9.

Dargent D, Martin X, Mathevet P (2000) Laparoscopic assessment of the sentinel lymph node in early stage cervical cancer. *Gynecol Oncol* **79**:411–5.

Darlin L, Persson J, Bossmar T, et al. (2010) The sentinel node concept in early cervical cancer performs well in tumors smaller than 2 cm. *Gynecol Oncol* **117**(2):266–9.

De Cicco C, Sideri M, Bartolomei M, Grana C, Cremonesi M, Fiorenza M, Maggioni A, Bocciolone L, Mangioni C, Colombo N, Paganelli G. Sentinel node biopsy in early vulvar cancer. *Br J Cancer* 2000; **82**(2):295–9.

De Cicco C, Cremonesi M, Luini A, et al. (1998) Lymphoscintigraphy and radioguided biopsy of the sentinel axillary node in breast cancer. *J Nucl Med* **39**:2080–4.

de Hullu JA, Doting E, Piers DA, et al. (1998) Sentinel lymph node identification with technetium-99m-labeled nanocolloid in squamous cell cancer of the vulva. *J Nucl Med* **39**:1381–5.

de Hullu JA, Hollema H, Piers DA, et al. (2000) Sentinel lymph node procedure is highly accurate in squamous cell carcinoma of the vulva. *J Clin Oncol* **18**:2811–6.

Delaloye JF, Pampallona S, Chardonnens E, et al. (2007) Intraoperative lymphatic mapping and sentinel node biopsy using hysteroscopy in patients with endometrial cancer. *Gynecol Oncol* **106**:89–93.

DiSaia PJ, Creasman WT, Rich WM (1979) An alternate approach to early cancer of the vulva. *Am J Obstet Gynecol* **133**:825–32.

Echt ML, Finan MA, Hoffman MS, et al. (1999) Detection of sentinel lymph nodes with lymphazurin in cervical, uterine, and vulvar malignancies. *South Med J* **92**:204–8.

Ege GN (1976) Internal mammary lymphoscintigraphy. The rationale, technique, interpretation and clinical application: a review based on 848 cases. *Radiology* **118**:101–7.

Eshima D, Fauconnier T, Eshima L, et al. (2000) Radiopharmaceuticals for lymphoscintigraphy: including dosimetry and radiation considerations. *Semin Nucl Med* **30**:25–32.

Eudy GE, Carlson GW, Murray DR, et al. (2003) Rapid immunohistochemistry of sentinel lymph nodes for metastatic melanoma. *Hum Pathol* **34**:797–802.

Euscher ED, Malpica A, Atkinson EN, et al. (2008) Ultrastaging improves detection of metastases in sentinel lymph nodes of uterine cervix squamous cell carcinoma. *Am J Surg Pathol* **9**:1336–43.

Fader AN, Edwards RP, Cost M, et al. (2008) Sentinel lymph node biopsy in early-stage cervical cancer: utility of intraoperative versus postoperative assessment. *Gynecol Oncol* **111**:13–7.

Fotiou S, Zarganis P, Vorgias G, et al. (2010) Clinical value of preoperative lymphoscintigraphy in patients with early cervical cancer considered for intraoperative lymphatic mapping. *Anticancer Res* **30**:183–8.

Frumovitz M, Bodurka DC, Broaddus RR, et al. (2007) Lymphatic mapping and sentinel node biopsy in women with high-risk endometrial cancer. *Gynecol Oncol* **104**:100–3.

Frumovitz M, Coleman RL, Gayed IW, et al. (2006) Usefulness of preoperative lymphoscintigraphy in patients who undergo radical hysterectomy and pelvic lymphadenectomy for cervical cancer. *Am J Obstet Gynecol* **194**:1186–93.

Frumovitz M, Gayed IW, Jhingran A, et al. (2008) Lymphatic mapping and sentinel lymph node detection in women with vaginal cancer. *Gynecol Oncol* **108**:478–81.

Gargiulo T, Giusti M, Bottero A, et al. (2003) Sentinel Lymph Node (SLN) laparoscopic assessment early stage in endometrial cancer. *Minerva Gynecol* **55**:259–62.

Gould EA, Philbin WT, Hyland PH, et al. (1960) Observations on a 'sentinel node' in cancer of the parotid. *Cancer* **13**:77–8.

Halsted W (1997) The results of radical operations for the cure of carcinoma of the breast. *Ann Surg* **46**:1.

Hampl M, Hantschmann P, Michels W, et al.; German Multicenter Study Group. (2008) Validation of the accuracy of the sentinel lymph node procedure in patients with vulvar cancer: results of a multicenter study in Germany. *Gynecol Oncol* **111**:282–8.

Henze E, Schelbert HR, Collins JD, et al. (1982) Lymphoscintigraphy with Tc-99m-labeled dextran. *J Nucl Med* **23**:923–9.

Holub Z, Jabor A, Kliment L (2002) Comparison of two procedures for sentinel lymph node detection in patients with endometrial cancer: a pilot study. *Eur J Gynaecol Oncol* **23**:53–7.

Holub Z, Kliment L, Lukac J, et al. (2001) Laparoscopically-assisted intraoperative lymphatic mapping in endometrial cancer: preliminary results. *Eur J Gynaecol Oncol* **22**:118–21.

Homesley HD, Bundy BN, Sedlis A, et al. (1986) Radiation therapy versus pelvic node resection for carcinoma of the vulva with positive groin nodes. *Obstet Gynecol* **68**:733–40.

International (Ludwig) Breast Cancer Study Group (1990) Prognostic importance of occult axillary lymph node micrometastases from breast cancers. *Lancet* **335**:1565–8.

Iversen T, Aas M (1983) Lymph drainage from the vulva. *Gynecol Oncol* **16**:179–89.

Kamprath S, Possover M, Schneider A (2000) Laparoscopic sentinel lymph node detection in patients with cervical cancer. *Am J Obstet Gynecol* **182**:1648.

Kara PP, Ayhan A, Caner B, et al. (2008) Sentinel lymph node detection in early stage cervical cancer: a prospective study comparing preoperative lymphoscintigraphy, intraoperative gamma probe, and blue dye. *Ann Nucl Med* 22:487–94.

Koutsky LA, Ault KA, Wheeler CM, et al. (2002) A controlled trial of a human papillomavirus type 16 vaccine. *N Engl J Med* 347:1645–51.

Lantzsch T, Wolters M, Grimm J, et al. (2001) Sentinel node procedure in Ib cervical cancer: a preliminary series. *Br J Cancer* 85:791–4.

Leong SP, Donegan E, Heffernon W, et al. (2000) Adverse reactions to isosulfan blue during selective sentinel lymph node dissection in melanoma. *Ann Surg Oncol* 7:361–6.

Leveuf J, Godard H (1923) Les lymphatiques de l'uterus. *Revue de Chirurgie* 61:219–48.

Levenback C, Burke TW, Gershenson DM, et al. (1994) Intraoperative lymphatic mapping for vulvar cancer. *Obstet Gynecol* 84:163–7.

Levenback C, Coleman RL, Burke TW, et al. (2001) Intraoperative lymphatic mapping and sentinel node identification with blue dye in patients with vulvar cancer. *Gynecol Oncol* 83:276–81.

Levenback C, Coleman RL, Burke TW, et al. (2002) Lymphatic mapping and sentinel node identification in patients with cervix cancer undergoing radical hysterectomy and pelvic lymphadenectomy. *J Clin Oncol* 20:688–93.

Maccauro M, Lucignani G, Aliberti G, et al. (2005) Sentinel lymph node detection following the hysteroscopic peritumoural injection of 99mTc-labelled albumin nanocolloid in endometrial cancer. *Eur J Nucl Med Mol Imag* 32:569–74.

Malur S, Krause N, Kohler C, et al. (2001) Sentinel lymph node detection in patients with cervical cancer. *Gynecol Oncol* 80:254–7.

Medl M, Peters-Engl C, Schutz P, et al. (2000) First report of lymphatic mapping with isosulfan blue dye and sentinel node biopsy in cervical cancer. *Anticancer Res* 20:1133–4.

Moore RG, DePasquale SE, Steinhoff MM, et al. (2003) Sentinel node identification and the ability to detect metastatic tumor to inguinal lymph nodes in squamous cell cancer of the vulva. *Gynecol Oncol* 89:475–9.

Moore RG, Robison K, Brown AK, et al. (2008) Isolated sentinel lymph node dissection with conservative management in patients with squamous cell carcinoma of the vulva: a prospective trial. *Gynecol Oncol* 109:65–70.

Morton DL, Wen DR, Wong JH, et al. (1992) Technical details of intraoperative lymphatic mapping for early stage melanoma. *Arch Surg* 127:392–9.

Munakata S, Aihara T, Morino H, et al. (2003) Application of immunofluorescence for intraoperative evaluation of sentinel lymph nodes in patients with breast carcinoma. *Cancer* 98:1562–8.

Nahrig JM, Richter T, Kuhn W, et al. (2003) Intraoperative examination of sentinel lymph nodes by ultrarapid immunohistochemistry. *Breast J* 9: 277–81.

Niikura H, Okamura C, Utsunomiya H, et al. (2004) Sentinel lymph node detection in patients with endometrial cancer. *Gynecol Oncol* 92:669–74.

Nyberg RH, Iivonen M, Parkkinen J, et al. (2007) Sentinel node and vulvar cancer: a series of 47 patients. *Acta Obstet Gynecol Scand* 86:615–9.

O'Boyle JD, Coleman RL, Bernstein SG, et al. (2000) Intraoperative lymphatic mapping in cervix cancer patients undergoing radical hysterectomy: a pilot study. *Gynecol Oncol* 79:238–43.

Ogawa S, Kobayashi H, Amada S, et al. (2010) Sentinel node detection with (99m)Tc phytate alone is satisfactory for cervical cancer patients undergoing radical hysterectomy and pelvic lymphadenectomy. *Int J Clin Oncol* 15:52–8.

Pandit-Taskar N, Gemignani ML, Lyall A, et al. (2010) Single photon emission computed tomography SPECT-CT improves sentinel node detection and localization in cervical and uterine malignancy. *Gynecol Oncol* 117:59–64.

Parry-Jones E (1963) Lymphatics of the vulva. *J Obstet Gynaecol Br Commonw* 70:751–65.

Pelosi E, Arena V, Baudino B, et al. (2002) Preliminary study of sentinel node identification with 99mTc colloid and blue dye in patients with endometrial cancer. *Tumori* 88:S9–S10.

Perrone AM, Casadio P, Formelli G, et al. (2008) Cervical and hysteroscopic injection for identification of sentinel lymph node in endometrial cancer. *Gynecol Oncol* 111:62–7.

Plentl A, Friedman E (1971) *Lymphatic System of the Female Genitalia*. Philadelphia: WB Saunders.

Rob L, Charvat M, Robova H, et al. (2004) Sentinel lymph node mapping in early-stage cervical cancer. *Ceska Gynekol* 69: 273–7.

Rob L, Robova H, Pluta M, et al. (2007) Further data on sentinel lymph node mapping in vulvar cancer by blue dye and radiocolloid Tc99. *Int J Gynecol Cancer* 17:147–53.

Robova H, Charvat M, Strnad P, Hrehorcak M, Taborska K, Skapa P, Rob L. Lymphatic mapping in endometrial cancer: comparison of hysteroscopic and subserosal injection and the distribution of sentinel lymph nodes. *Int J Gynecol Cancer* 2009; 19(3):391–4.

Sadiq TS, Burns WW, 3rd, Taber DJ, et al. (2001) Blue urticaria: a previously unreported adverse event associated with isosulfan blue. *Arch Surg* 136:1433–5.

Sherman A, Ter-Pogossian M (1953) Lymph node concentration of radioactive colloidal gold following interstitial injection. *Cancer* 6:1238–40.

Sideri M, De Cicco C, Maggioni A, et al. (2000) Detection of sentinel nodes by lymphoscintigraphy and gamma probe guided surgery in vulvar neoplasia. *Tumori* 86:359–63.

Sliutz G, Reinthaller A, Lantzsch T, et al. (2002) Lymphatic mapping of sentinel nodes in early vulvar cancer. *Gynecol Oncol* 84:449–52.

Stehman FB, Bundy BN, Thomas G, et al. (1992) Groin dissection versus groin radiation in carcinoma of the vulva: a Gynecologic Oncology Group study. *Int J Radiat Oncol Biol Phys* 24:389–96.

Uren RF, Howman-Giles R (2002) The role of nuclear medicine. In: Cody HS, ed. *Sentinel Lymph Node Biopsy*. London: Martin Dunitz, pp. 19–43.

Van der Zee AG, Oonk MH, De Hullu JA, et al. (2008) Sentinel node dissection is safe in the treatment of early-stage vulvar cancer. *J Clin Oncol* 26:884–9.

Van Trappen PO, Gyselman VG, Lowe DG, et al. (2001) Molecular quantification and mapping of lymph-node micrometastases in cervical cancer. *Lancet* 357:15–20.

Verheijen RH, Pijpers R, van Diest PJ, et al. (2000) Sentinel node detection in cervical cancer. *Obstet Gynecol* 96:135–8.

Vidal-Sicart S, Puig-Tintoré LM, Lejárcegui JA, et al. (2007) Validation and application of the sentinel lymph node concept in malignant vulvar tumours. *Eur J Nucl Med Mol Imag* 34:384–91.

Way S (1951) Carcinoma of the vulva. *Malignant Disease of the Female Genital Tract*. Philadelphia: The Blakiston Co.

Wilhelm AJ, Mijnhout GS, Franssen EJ (1999) Radiopharmaceuticals in sentinel lymph-node detection—an overview. *Eur J Nucl Med* 26:S36–S42.

Winter R, Haas J, Reich O, et al. (2002) Parametrial spread of cervical cancer in patients with negative pelvic lymph nodes. *Gynecol Oncol* 84:252–7.

Wong JH, Cagle LA, Morton DL (1991) Lymphatic drainage of skin to a sentinel lymph node in a feline model. *Ann Surg* 214:637–41.

19 Ovarian tissue cryopreservation and transplantation techniques
Erkan Buyuk and Kutluk H. Oktay

INTRODUCTION

Modern improvements in cancer treatment regimens using aggressive chemotherapy, radiotherapy as well as bone-marrow transplantation can result in cure rates exceeding 90% for many cancers (Ries et al. 1999). However, this success has been accompanied by loss of fertility and premature menopause in many women cured of their disease. Ovarian cryopreservation and transplantation is one of the options aimed to preserve fertility in women who face a threat to their fertility. Discovery of modern cryoprotectants and progress in cryopreservation techniques led to successful cryopreservation of gametes, embryos, and ovarian tissue. However, there is significant room to improve revascularization of tissues after auto transplantation, as nearly two-thirds of the ovarian reserve is lost during the initial ischemic state after grafting (Newton et al. 1998, Demirci et al. 2001, Baird et al. 1999).

OVARIAN TISSUE CRYOPRESERVATION

Ovarian tissue cryopreservation for future transplantation can be done in cancer patients as well as for other benign conditions where chemotherapy-, radiotherapy-, or surgically induced ovarian failure is anticipated. Table 1 summarizes the indications for ovarian tissue banking.

Tissue Harvesting

As long as there is no contraindication, ovarian tissue is collected via laparoscopy. In adult patients, we generally remove one ovary to obtain a large reserve of primordial follicles. However, in pediatric age group, a large cortical biopsy may be enough since their ovaries harbor a larger number of follicles than the adult ovary (Richardson et al. 1987). The whole ovary or ovarian cortical pieces are removed by a laparoscopic approach using a 5 mm scope inserted in the umbilicus and 5 and 12 mm trocars in the lower quadrants. Use of electrocautery is not recommended to minimize damage to ovarian cortex containing the follicles. The ipsilateral fallopian tube is left intact to allow a spontaneous pregnancy to occur in case an orthotopic transplantation is performed in the future. An endoscopic specimen bag is used to remove the ovary through the 12 mm trocar; the trocar is pulled out and the specimen is delivered through the 12-mm incision. This incision may need to be widened to extract a large ovary.

Processing of the Ovarian Tissue

The aim of the processing of ovarian tissue before cryopreservation is to obtain ovarian pieces small and thin enough for the cryoprotectants to easily permeate. The sample is transported to the laboratory on ice in Leibovitz L-15 medium. In the case of whole ovary, it is bivalved through its hilum, and the cortex is separated from the medullary portion using a number 10 blade. This step is undertaken because the primordial follicles are contained in the cortical portion, and the medullary portion may decrease tissue permeation of cryoprotectants. The cortex is then divided into $5 \times 5 \times 1$ mm pieces using a number 10 or 11 blade. The preparation is performed under a laminar flow hood, and the tissue is kept in the medium throughout the process. The cortical pieces are then put in cryovials containing 1.5 ml of an ovarian freeze solution (1.5 M 1,2-propanediol, 20% patient's own serum and 0.1 M sucrose in Leibovitz L-15 medium).

Cryopreservation and Thawing

The cryovials are kept in ice for 30 minutes for the equilibration of the cryoprotectants. Cryopreservation is performed using a slow freeze protocol in a programmable freezer. The pieces are cooled to $-7°C$ and seeded at this temperature. They are then cooled to $-140°C$ and plunged into liquid nitrogen (Oktay 2001).

Thawing is done by a rapid thaw protocol in 30°C water bath, followed by washing the tissues in decreasing gradients of cryoprotectant (Oktay 2001).

Ovarian Transplantation Techniques

Before performing ovarian transplantation, the risk of reseeding occult cancer cells should be kept in mind, and the decision to perform ovarian transplantation should be made accordingly. Table 2 summarizes the risk of ovarian involvement in different cancers. For instance, risk of ovarian involvement is higher in leukemia and neuroblastoma patients, compared to lymphoma or Wilm's tumor patients.

Transplantation can be done using an orthotopic or heterotopic approach. In orthotopic transplantation, the tissue is placed in the ovarian fossa (Oktay et al. 2001). Although spontaneous pregnancy can in theory be achieved using this technique, the procedure is technically more challenging, and when there is a higher likelihood of ovarian involvement with cancer, it may be less desirable to graft ovarian tissue retroperitoneally. In heterotopic transplantation, the tissue is grafted into a place other than the ovarian fossa. The operation is done under local anesthesia and follow-up is easier with heterotopic transplantation. However, patients will always need an IVF procedure in order to conceive (Oktay et al. 2001, 2003). In the case of cancer recurrence, tissue sampling and removal will also be easily accomplished. The risk and significance of recurrent cancer at the transplant site is unknown.

Pelvic Orthotopic Transplantation

Following thawing and washing, the ovarian pieces are placed in a petri dish containing transport medium, and transported on ice to operating room. In the operating room, 6-0 Vicryl is used to string the pieces by passing the needle between the cortex and the stroma of each piece under a microsurgical

Table 1 Indications for Ovarian Cryopreservation and Transplantation

I—Cancer patients
  Breast cancer (stage 0–3)
  Cervical cancer
  Non-genital rhabdomyosarcoma
  Childhood cancers
    Hodgkin's lymphoma
    Non-Hodgkin lymphoma (except Burkitt lymphoma)
    Osteosarcoma
    Ewing's sarcoma
    Wilm's tumor
II—Bone-marrow transplant patients
  Aplastic anemia
  Sickle cell anemia
  Autoimmune and immune-deficiency diseases
  (e.g., rheumatoid arthritis)
III—Autoimmune diseases
  Collagen vascular diseases (e.g., SLE)
  Acute glomerulonephritis
  Behcet's disease
IV—Adjunctive oopherectomy
  Recurrent breast cancer
  Endometriosis
V—Benign ovarian tumors
  Recurrent cysts
  Endometriosis
VI—Prophylactic oopherectomy
  BRCA-1 or -2 mutation carriers

Table 2 Risk of Metastases to Ovaries in Various Cancers

High risk
  Leukemia
  Neuroblastoma
  Burkitt lymphoma
  Genital rhabdomyosarcoma
Moderate risk
  Breast cancer
    Stage IV
    Infiltrative lobular histological subtype
  Adenocarcinoma/adenosqamous carcinoma of the cervix
  Colon cancer
Low risk
  Breast cancer
    Stage I–III
    Infiltrative ductal histological subtype
  Squamous cell carcinoma of the cervix
  Non-Hodgkin's lymphoma
  Hodgkin's lymphoma
  Wilm's tumor
  Ewing's sarcoma
  Non-genital rhabdomyosarcoma
  Osteogenic sarcoma

microscope. Several strings are formed depending on the number of the pieces, and they are then anchored to a Surgicel frame (Ethicon, Somerville, New Jersey, USA). A 1-0 Vicryl suture is used on the sides to further strengthen this frame. Some 0 Vicryl sutures are then tagged to the apex and the base. Synchronously, the patient is anesthetized, and three trocars are inserted: an 11-mm one in the umbilicus, a 5-mm one in the right lower quadrant, and a 13-mm one (with fascia anchor) suprapubically. Using sharp and blunt dissection, a pocket is created in the ovarian fossa, posterior to the broad ligament, superior to ureters, and inferior to iliac vessels in the supine position. The graft is then loaded retrogradely, into a 13-mm trocar that is reinserted in the fascia anchor suprapubically. Pulling on the leading suture, the graft is dropped in the pelvis. The leading suture is then placed in the most dependent portion of the pocket, approximately 1 cm above the ureter, and the needle is passed through the peritoneum into the pelvic cavity. By pulling on this suture, the graft is wedged in the pelvic pocket. Next, the base suture is passed through the upper edge of the peritoneal pocket. The graft is stretched and flattened against the pelvic sidewall by pulling this suture from the intra-peritoneal site. With too many pieces, a second graft may be prepared and placed superior and caudal to the first one. Then, using an extracorporeal knot placement technique, the peritoneum is approximated with interrupted sutures. The base of the Surgicel frame is also included into the suture while closing the peritoneum to further secure the graft in place.

The patient is given 150 IU/day of follicle stimulating hormone (FSH) systemically for seven days (Oktay and Buyuk 2002), because of its beneficial effects on graft survival based on the evidence from animal studies (Imthurn et al. 2000). Patient is also given 80 mg of aspirin for seven days, and started on hormone replacement therapy within 48 hours of the transplant, as it is presumed that these treatments may enhance angiogenesis (Morales et al. 1995).

Heterotopic Transplantation

Forearm

After thawing and washing as described previously, ovarian cortical strips are placed in phenol red-free Minimum Essential Medium Alpha Medium (with L-glutamine, ribonucleosides and deoxyribonucleosides, Invitrogen, cat. no. 41061-029), supplemented with 20% patient's own serum and 10 µg/ml cefotetan, and kept on ice. Then, each strip is tagged with 4-0 Vicryl as described previously. The needle is cut, and the cortical pieces are left in the medium until the surgical site is ready for transplantation. To create a pocket for the graft under the skin of the forearm, a 1 cm transverse incision is made over the brachioradialis muscle, 5 cm below the antecubital fossa. If there is a cosmetic concern, the incision and the transplantation may be made more medially. A pocket is created between the fascia and the subcutaneous tissues using blunt dissection. Since this area is relatively vascular, attention must be given to avoid major bleeding. As the ovarian tissue will acquire its blood supply from these vessels, extensive cauterization should be avoided.

Following the creation of the pocket, the free-end of the suture is threaded onto a reusable needle. A ½-circle cutting needle with a chord length of 25 to 38 mm (depending on the size of the strips) is inserted into the subcutaneous pocket as far as possible. It is then passed through the skin, and the cortical piece is wedged into the pocket by pulling on this suture. Care must be taken to place the pieces with their cortical side facing up. The needle is removed, and the free end of the suture is held with a Mosquito clamp. The main purpose of this suture pull through technique is to guide the tissue placement and to avoid overlapping the strips, rather than securing them in place. Depending on the patient's forearm size, 5 to 15 cortical pieces can be placed beneath the forearm skin. Following the placement of the last piece, the sutures are cut. Then the skin is closed subcuticularly and a non-pressure dressing is applied in order not to reduce the blood flow to the area. Seventy-five IU/day of FSH is injected directly in the grafts for seven days starting the day of the surgery. The patient's forearm is splinted for 72 hours to prevent dislodgment of the graft due to muscle movement. In addition, 80 mg of aspirin is administered for seven days, and hormone replacement is started within 48 hours of the surgery as in the case of orthotopic transplantation. The latter is stopped with the first sign of graft function. The ovarian function usually returns within three months.

Abdomen

In patients for whom the use of the forearms is contraindicated, abdominal wall may be used as the transplantation site. For example, forearms are not suitable for transplantation for breast cancer patients who had bilateral axillary dissection, due to risk of lymphedema formation. In that case, we prefer to implant the cortical pieces in the subcutaneous tissue of the abdominal wall (Oktay et al. 2004). The preferred location is the lower abdominal wall, above the waistline of the underwear, but, depending on the previous surgical scars or any other condition of the abdomen, the transplantation site may be adjusted. The technique is the same as forearm transplantation as well as the postsurgical follow-up.

REFERENCES

Baird DT, Webb R, Campbell BK, et al. (1999) Long-term ovarian function in sheep after ovariectomy and transplantation of autografts stored at -196°C. *Endocrinology* **140**(1):462–71.

Demirci B, Lornage J, Salle B, et al. (2001) Follicular viability and morphology of sheep ovaries after exposure to cryoprotectant and cryopreservation with different freezing protocols. *Fertil Steril* **75**(4):754–62.

Imthurn B, Cox SL, Jenkin G, et al. (2000) Gonadotrophin administration can benefit ovarian tissue grafted to the body wall: implications for human ovarian grafting. *Mol Cell Endocrinol* **163**(1–2):141–6.

Morales DE, McGowan KA, Grant DS, et al. (1995) Estrogen promotes angiogenic activity in human umbilical vein endothelial cells in vitro and in a murine model. *Circulation* **91**(3):755–63.

Newton H, Fisher J, Arnold JR, et al. (1998) Permeation of human ovarian tissue with cryoprotective agents in preparation for cryopreservation. *Hum Reprod* **13**(2):376–80.

Oktay K (2001) Ovarian tissue cryopreservation and transplantation: preliminary findings and implications for cancer patients. *Hum Reprod* **7**:526–34.

Oktay K, Aydin BA, Karlikaya G (2001) A technique for laparoscopic transplantation of frozen-banked ovarian tissue. *Fertil Steril* **75**(6):1212–16.

Oktay K, Buyuk E, Rosenwaks Z, et al. (2003) A technique for transplantation of ovarian cortical strips to the forearm. *Fertil Steril* **80**:193–8.

Oktay K, Buyuk E, Veeck L, et al. (2004) Embryo development after heterotopic transplantation of cryopreserved ovarian tissue. *Lancet* **363**:837–40.

Oktay K, Buyuk E. The potential of ovarian tissue transplant to preserve fertility. *Expert Opin Biol Ther* **2**(4):361–70.

Oktay K, Economos K, Kan M, et al. (2001) Endocrine function and oocyte retrieval after autologous transplantation of ovarian cortical strips to the forearm. *JAMA* **286**:1490–3.

Richardson SJ, Senikas V, Nelson JF (1987) Follicular depletion during the menopausal transition: evidence for accelerated loss and ultimate exhaustion. *J Clin Endocrinol Metab* **65**(6):1231–7.

Ries LAG, Percy CL, Bunun GR (1999) Introduction. In: Ries LAG, Smith MA, Gurney JG, et al. eds. *Cancer Incidence and Survival among Children and Adolescents: United States SEER Program 1975–95, National Cancer Institute, SEER program.* Bethesda, MD: NIH Pub. No. 99-4649, pp. 1–15.

20 Lessons from transplant surgery

Giuseppe Del Priore and J. Richard Smith

Transplant medicine, including surgery and medical management, has improved dramatically over its relatively short existence. Transplant medicine in a sense has a unique opportunity to study surgical and perioperative interventions in two systems, that is, the donor and the recipient. Donors and their family, already generous almost beyond imagination, can provide still more benefit to the living through investigations on the donor. For instance, it is possible to provide unequalled surgical experience through the retrieval process. In the opinion of some, it is more acceptable ethically, to perform surgical procedures, for example, hysterectomy, in a donor, than to have residents assist in living patient surgeries. It is also possible to randomize donors in ways that are not possible to randomize recipients. For instance if an intervention is hypothesized to improve perioperative outcomes, donors can be a reasonable first group to experience the innovation prior to introduction into the general surgery population.

Randomized trials using donors have already been reported. These are often medical interventions that have little obvious application in non-transplant settings, for example, immune-suppression trials. However, even these trials can potentially influence common disease states in large groups of non-transplant patients. For instance, transplant and its associated immune-suppression have been reported to change a recipient's allergic reaction profile. In other words, a recipient who is allergic to certain items, say peanuts, may no longer be allergic after receiving a transplanted organ and its immune-suppressive drugs. Theoretically, a child with a peanut allergy could be treated with a very short course of immune-suppressants, then over days, exposed to the allergen continuously. By slowly weaning the immune-suppressant regimen, the allergic patients would in fact become tolerant as he emerged from the induced immunosuppression. This is possible given current encouraging results in solid organ transplant, induced immune-tolerance.

Surgical techniques are perhaps the most obvious choice for research in donors and even recipients. For instance, donors' renal function could be studied in recipients after randomization to liberal versus conservative IV fluid administration. The graft's renal function could be compared in different recipients and the optimal peri-operative care for preserving renal function could be determined. Recently a randomized clinical trial did just that (Schnuelle et al. 2009).

In this trial, investigators randomized 264 deceased heart-beating donors in a multicenter, parallel-group trial. Donors were randomized to receive low-dose dopamine or placebo. Low-dose dopamine significantly reduced renal failure in recipients grafts.

Also in renal transplant recipient patients, stenting may be unnecessary for most ureteral re-implantations. Transplant surgeons have successfully performed ureteral surgery without stents in large numbers of recipients. Although no study in any specifically defined study sample can ever be reliably extrapolated to other patient populations, the transplant lesson does allow for the stenting benefit hypothesis to be re-considered.

Hemorrhage is often encountered in surgical oncology and equally, if not more so, in transplantation of the liver. From these patients, traditional replacement guidelines appear to be questionable. For instance, liberal fluid replacement may further dilute consumed coagulation factors. As example, in a 100-kg patient undergoing a procedure, their approximate whole blood may be estimated around 5 L. If this volume of distribution (Vd) is used to represent 100% of circulating coagulation factors, it can be obvious when a coagulopathy can be anticipated and worsened by IV fluids. In this example, a patient who had estimated blood loss (EBL) of 2L (not unreasonable amount in a pelvic exenteration procedure), the Vd would only contain about 60% of the presurgical coagulation factors (2L/5L). If this blood loss was replaced 1:1 with crystalloid, one would expect a measured reduction in existing coagulation factors approaching a dilution where a coagulopathy might be seen. However, if the replacement were greater, say 3:1 (a ratio commonly used but based on unsubstantiated tradition), the coagulopathy would be far greater. Further, the rate of the crystalloid replacement will factor in transiently and is important as the volume.

In liver transplantation, less crystalloid and more fresh frozen plasma is replaced compared to general surgery situations (Mangus et al. 2007). Conservative crystalloid replacement has been associated with better outcomes compared with traditional replacement strategies (Fischer et al. 2010). In this latter RCT, patients received over 2 L more fluid intraoperatively compared with standard patients. Patients receiving more cystalloids showed a trend toward more grade-3 complications, and complications related to the anastomosis (leak/fistula/abscess) were significantly higher in the excess fluid group (21.5% vs. 7.7%, $P = 0.045$). The intraoperative fluid volume was higher for all patients with anastomotic complications, regardless of randomization arm ($P < 0.042$). The authors concluded that complications were likely related to greater intraoperative fluid administration.

Combining all the advances in transplant medicine and applying it to surgical oncology has led to an exciting option for formerly unresectable masses. In a process yet to be named with a universally agreed upon title, organs from a cancer patient are removed to allow complete resection of tumor masses. Sometimes referred to as an "auto-transplant" a cancer patient would have an organ removed, perfused, chilled, and preserved for a short intra-operative period to allow for the resection of an adjacent tumor (Fig. 1). For instance, if a low-grade borderline ovarian cancer recurred around the celiac

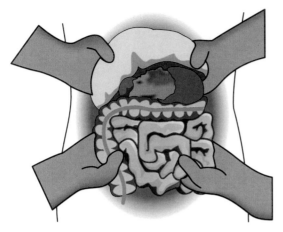
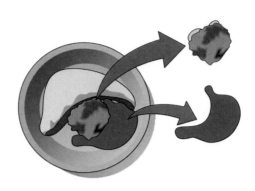

Figure 1 Tumor and organs affected are removed from body. Alternatively, if the organs are removed giving access to the tumor, the tumor can be resected in vivo. Tumor is resected from removed organs. The organs are chilled and perfused with transplant solution that minimizes warm ischemia time and tissue damage. The removed organs are re-implanted, "auto-transplanted" back into the patient.

artery or the hepatobiliary trunk, this tumor could be removed enblock and the affected vital vessels or biliary ducts reconstructed using donor or autologous vessels.

At our institution, approximately 30 cancer patients with declared unresectable tumors have undergone attempts at resection by the transplant service. Some have even been referred from hospice and undergone complete curative resection. The morbidity is significant but appropriate given the circumstances. The indications for such resections are relatively rare in gynecologic oncology. However, there are a few patients each year evaluated by the gynecologic oncology division with transplant surgery, for auto-transplant assisted resection of "unresectable" tumors. Transplant surgery is also consulted in patients with severe radiation enteritis, typically after three or more laparotomies for obstruction, and malabsorption leading to debilitating malnutrition.

Transplant medicine has much to offer cancer patients through direct application of surgical, medical, and laboratory advances. Transplant services are similar to gynecologic oncology services in a number of important parameters. For instance both provide comprehensive and coordinated surgical and medical interventions. Both specialties form lifelong relationships with critically ill patients. Both specialties have demanding but rewarding training and lifestyle.

We have sought to collaborate with our transplant colleagues in all areas of medicine including training. We described the educational value of participation in the organ donor network for residents and fellows in a preliminary report (Del Priore et al. 2007). The gynecologic oncology team enrolled as members of the local organ donor network for an IRB-approved research project. We included residents and fellows as part of the organ procurement team whenever possible. We coordinated lectures and animal surgery with the organ procurement experience. Residents and fellows received lectures on surgical anatomy focused on the pelvis but included urologic, hepatobiliary, vascular, thoracic, and gastrointestinal systems. Animal labs were used to demonstrate related practical skills. During a representative six-month period, 1800 potential donors were identified. Organ procurement surgery eventually took place in 150 of these, that is, 20 to 30 laparatomies per month. Most were multi-organ including every possible combination of heart, lung, liver, kidney, pancreas, and intestines. Uterus procurement was performed as part of the surgery without interference with the retrieval of the other organ. Surgery teams participated in preoperative critical care of donors. Gynecologic oncology members were able to participate in approximately 10 of these surgeries based on our schedule limitations but not duty hour restrictions. Each retrieval process consisted of approximately 18 hours of surgery although the range was 6 to 24 hours depending on the acceptability of the donor organs. Gyn onc team members typically participated in 8 to 12 hours of multi-visceral surgery including cardiac and thoracic areas. Participation in an organ donor network can provide valuable surgical and critical care experience for trainees. Importantly, voluntary participation does not affect resident work hour limitations.

Transplant medicine has much to offer its patients through significant improvements in all areas of research. It may also have much to offer general surgery patients and students. Gynecologic oncologist would be well advised to collaborate with their local transplant community on a variety of shared interests.

REFERENCES

Del Priore G, Fernandez IM, Smith JR, et al. (2007) Educational value of organ retrieval network participation in an integrated comprehensive surgical training curriculum. *Gynecol Oncol* **104**(3)S:52.

Fischer M, Matsuo K, Gonen M, et al. (2010) Relationship between intraoperative fluid administration and perioperative outcome after pancreaticoduodenectomy: results of a prospective randomized trial of acute normovolemic hemodilution compared with standard intraoperative management. *Ann Surg* **252**(6):952–8.

Mangus RS, Kinsella SB, Nobari MM, et al. (2007) Predictors of blood product use in orthotopic liver transplantation using the piggyback hepatectomy technique. *Transplant Proc* **39**(10):3207–13.

Schnuelle P, Gottmann U, Hoeger S, et al. (2009) Effects of donor pretreatment with dopamine on graft function after kidney transplantation: a randomized controlled trial. *JAMA* **302**(10):1067–75.

21 Epithelial ovarian cancer

Jane Bridges and David Oram

PREOPERATIVE ASSESSMENT

Ovarian cancer continues to frustrate. Clinicians are disadvantaged by the characteristics of unreliable, inconsistent symptomatology, which accounts for late presentation and poorly associated survival figures. Even when the patient does present early, the preoperative diagnosis of ovarian cancer is frequently a difficult one to make. This is borne out by the fact that 50% of patients with this disease are initially referred to general physicians or general surgeons for investigation of symptomatology or ascites. The development by Jacobs et al. (1990) of a scoring system, the risk of malignancy index (RMI), which incorporates the use of the serum CA125 level, pelvic ultrasound features, and the menopausal status of the patient, has greatly eased this preoperative difficulty. The details of the calculation are shown in Figure 1, and the RMI has now been validated in clinical practice. Using this calculation to assess the nature of an abdominopelvic mass helps to confirm the diagnosis of malignancy with >95% accuracy. This in turn allows for an appropriate referral to a cancer center to be made, or at least prevents the initial surgery being inappropriately performed by an inexperienced surgeon. The importance of this has been demonstrated in data from the west of Scotland, which confirm improved survival of patients with ovarian cancer if they are managed in a cancer center using a multidisciplinary team approach. Furthermore, accurate preoperative diagnosis enables appropriate counseling to be given to the patient and her family. Appropriate investigation and management planning can be embarked upon in a proactive manner, and by no means the least important consideration is that the patient's initial surgery and exploration can be performed through the correct surgical incision.

PREOPERATIVE INVESTIGATIONS

Investigations should include an assessment of the patient, including her performance and nutritional status; if necessary, parenteral feeding through central lines can be instituted preoperatively. This should not, however, delay the initial surgery. A thorough hematological and biochemical assessment should be undertaken. A chest X-ray or thoracic CT scan is required: If a pleural effusion is present, this should be aspirated and the fluid examined cytologically for malignant cells. Pelvic ultrasonography is usually performed as part of the initial assessment and is complemented by specialist imaging such as computed tomography (CT) and magnetic resonance imaging (MRI) in assessing the extent of the disease spread, including intra- and extra-abdominal metastatic deposits (Fig. 2). Preoperatively the patient requires a bowel preparatory agent, and in selected more advanced cases stoma counseling may be instituted.

The majority of patients will undergo primary laparotomy. However, a small proportion will be deemed unlikely to achieve optimal debulking (<1 cm nodules of residual disease) and may have a radiologically guided biopsy of the omentum or other sites of disease. If confirmed as primary ovarian cancer, the patient may have three cycles of chemotherapy followed by interval debulking surgery. Gynecological oncologists are usually very good at achieving optimal debulking in the pelvis. Results are less good in the presence of pleural and extensive diaphragmatic disease (see chapter 22) but not insurmountable. Much work has been done to try to determine methods of predicting the patient in whom an inadequate debulking procedure (>1 cm deposits) will result. Inadequate debulking is currently regarded as a poorer outcome than interval debulking. Prognostic CA125 levels have been used in many studies but have low sensitivity and specificity. Clearly surgical ability will also be variable and so the extent and frequency of adequate debulking will vary by center.

PRIMARY LAPAROTOMY

The correct staging of ovarian cancer is of paramount importance because it has implications for adjuvant therapy and also for appropriate counseling concerning prognosis. It is unfortunate that under-staging is commonplace in this disease, in spite of attention being drawn to this problem by various authors since the 1970s (Piver and Barlow 1976, Young et al. 1983, McGowan et al. 1985). The surgical procedure should be performed through a midline incision extending from the symphysis pubis to above the umbilicus if necessary. Any ascites present on opening the peritoneal cavity should be aspirated and sent for cytological assessment; otherwise, the pelvis and paracolic gutters should be thoroughly irrigated with saline and the washings aspirated and sent for cytological assessment. Diaphragmatic swabs for cytology may also be taken. Thereafter thorough exploration and assessment of the extent of disease spread are crucial. Particular note should be taken of the tumor deposits in the upper abdomen: the hemidiaphragm should be palpated and inspected; the surface and parenchyma of the liver, the omentum, appendix, and small and large bowel should be assessed, and thereafter all peritoneal surfaces including the paracolic gutters and the pelvic peritoneum. Attention is then turned to the extent of disease in the pelvis: The pelvic and para-aortic lymph nodes should, in the first instance, be palpated. In selected cases adherent

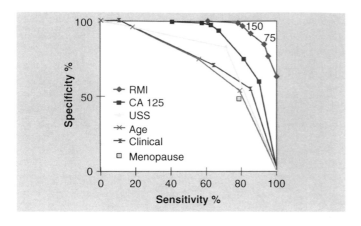

RMI = U x M x serum CA125

where U and M are the ultrasound and menopausal scores.
Ultrasound was assessed for the following features suggestive
of malignancy:

- multiloculated cysts
- evidence of solid areas
- evidence of metastases
- presence of ascites
- bilateral lesions.

A score of 0 was given where none of these was present;
1 if one was present; and a score of 3 for two or more.

A score of 1 or 3 was given to pre- or postmenopausal
patients respectively.

An RMI of 200 had a sensitivity of 85% and a specificity
of 97% for diagnosing ovarian cancer.

Figure 1 Risk of malignancy index (RMI).

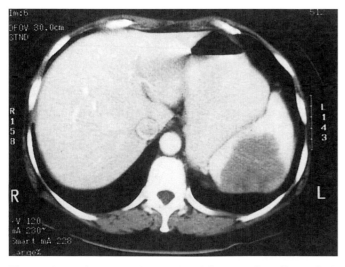

Figure 2 Magnetic resonance imaging (MRI) demonstrating solitary splenic metastasis.

tissue and adhesions should be sampled for biopsy and if it is felt to be helpful by the operating surgeon, frozen section of suspicious areas can be utilized. Where no obvious peritoneal disease is present, random biopsies can be taken from areas at high risk. Biopsy of the subdiaphragmatic peritoneum may be facilitated by the use of long-handled punch biopsy forceps.

Depending on the stage of the disease the surgical problems differ. In advanced disease, the stage is usually obvious and the surgical challenge centers on cytoreductive surgery. In apparent early-stage disease, however, tumor resection is usually easy, but accurate surgical staging is a major consideration. In such cases pelvic and para-aortic lymph node assessment is indicated.

SURGICAL TECHNIQUES FOR ADVANCED DISEASE

Following the completion of the staging procedure, optimal cytoreduction becomes the goal. The surgical approach in ovarian cancer differs from that for other solid tumors where the aim is to remove the tumor with a wide area of normal tissue clearance. In epithelial ovarian cancer, the priority is to remove as much of the bulk disease as possible, but if complete tumor clearance is not achievable then reduction of the tumor burden to minimal residual disease becomes the goal. Tumor debulking was advocated initially in the early part of the 20th century by Meigs (1934) and Bonney (1912) and further developed by Brunschwig (1961). Munnell in the 1950s coined the phrase "maximum surgical effort" and Griffiths quantified this in the 1970s in his seminal paper, which has dictated subsequent surgical practice (Munnell 1952, Griffiths 1975). Griffiths demonstrated an improved survival in patients who had their disease reduced to residual nodules of <1.5 cm. The surgery for advanced-stage disease is often difficult and, unlike other forms of cancer surgery, there are no set moves. It often requires persistence and a flexible approach by the operating surgeon, depending on available tissue planes. At the very least the procedure should incorporate total or subtotal hysterectomy, bilateral salpingo-oophorectomy, omentectomy, and removal of all bulk tumor deposits where possible. In most circumstances the retroperitoneal en bloc approach as described below should be used to clear all pelvic disease. Other surgical procedures that occasionally require to be undertaken include biopsy and excision of parenchymal liver deposits. If the spleen is involved in the omental cake of tumor a splenectomy can be undertaken. Bowel resection (chapter 28) is only indicated in two clinical situations: The first is if there is bowel tumor causing impending obstruction, and the second is if resecting a segment of bowel will help to achieve complete tumor clearance. Prior to concluding the initial surgical procedure it is worth considering whether the patient might be suitable for intraperitoneal adjuvant chemotherapy: if so, an intraperitoneal catheter can then be inserted.

En bloc Resection of Advanced Pelvic Disease

The technique of en bloc resection was first described by Hudson (1968) in the management of patients with advanced pelvic disease where spread to the pelvic peritoneum, rectosigmoid, and/or bladder had occurred. It facilitates resection of locally advanced tumors in one contiguous sample. First the round and infundibulopelvic ligaments are divided and ligated. The pelvic peritoneum is then opened circumferentially from the symphysis pubis anteriorly to the rectosigmoid posteriorly. The peritoneum is dissected free in a lateral-to-medial direction, including that covering the dome of the bladder and the pelvic side walls. The uterine arteries are then divided and ligated in a lateral position close to their origin at the internal iliac artery, allowing the ureters to be mobilized laterally (Fig. 3).The anterior vaginal fornix is exposed by further dissection of the bladder anteriorly and opened

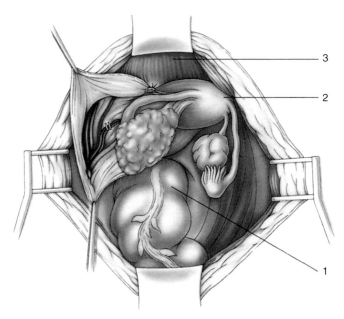

Figure 3 Extraperitoneal dissection. 1 Rectum, 2 Uterus, 3 Bladder.

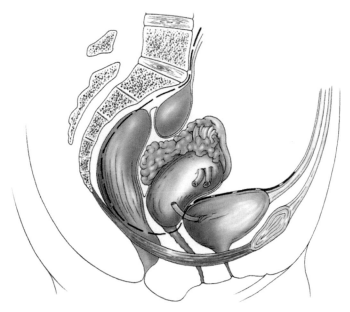

Figure 5 Resection outline.

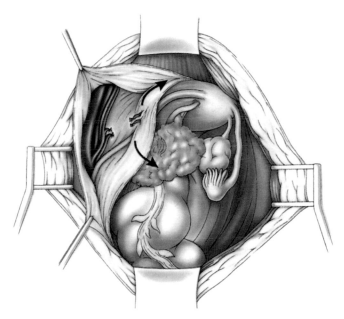

Figure 4 Development of the retrorectal space.

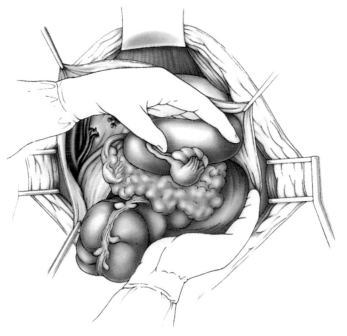

Figure 6 Resection.

transversely. The hysterectomy can then be performed in a retrograde fashion, dividing and ligating the uterosacral and cardinal ligaments. Development of the retrorectal space at this stage will allow elevation of the rectum, uterus, and tumor from the sacral hollow, and an assessment of the need for rectosigmoid resection—depending on the tumor mobility and invasion—can be made (Fig. 4). Where superficial invasion of the sigmoid serosa only has occurred, the tumor may be dissected free by stripping the outer muscular layer from the underlying circular muscular layer and the mucosa. In patients with a small area of deep invasion, local resection of the anterior wall of the sigmoid may be performed and the bowel defect closed in the anterior plane. Resection will include the lateral pelvic and sigmoid peritoneum within the specimen (Figs. 5 and 6). Where there is more extensive rectosigmoid involvement, resection of this segment of the colon can be

performed with a primary anastomosis. Initially the superior hemorrhoidal vessels are identified and ligated at the level of the sacral promontory. The sigmoid mesentery is then divided allowing margins for adequate tumor clearance, facilitated by division of the peritoneum and mobilization of the descending colon if necessary. The sigmoid is then divided, generally with a stapling device, and the proximal end of the sigmoid is placed in the left paracolic gutter while the final dissection of the tumor specimen is performed. Blunt dissection and traction on the distal rectosigmoid portion are used to mobilize the bowel, allowing the specimen to be drawn out of the pelvis and the resection margin of the rectum to be identified. At this stage the posterior anastomosis of the sigmoid to the rectal stump may be performed prior to the final division of the tumor en bloc specimen just above the anastomosis. The anastomosis can then be completed by hand or by a stapling device inserted through the anus. The anastomosis may be covered by a loop colostomy, but as the majority of women will not have received preoperative radiotherapy and will have had adequate bowel preparation, this may not always be necessary. Adequate drainage at the site of the anastomosis should be allowed at the end of the laparotomy, however, in the form of a large-bore tube drain.

The laparotomy should be completed with an omentectomy, with or without appendectomy and assessment of the para-aortic nodes. If these are bulky they should ideally be removed as part of the optimal debulk. If normal in size there is dispute as whether to leave or remove them.

Appendectomy

The appendix is a common site for metastatic disease but should only be removed when clearly involved by tumor (Fawzi et al. 1997) or in the case of mucinous ovarian tumors. The appendix can be easily delivered through the midline incision. The mesoappendix is divided either following a single transfix suture if it is minimal, or by serial clipping section by section (Fig. 7). A clip is then used to crush the base of the appendix, first close to the cecal wall and then immediately above it (Fig. 8). A polyglactin tie is used to ligate the crushed area, and the suture ends are cut short. A purse-string suture is next inserted approximately 1 cm from the appendix, picking up only the seromuscular coat. The appendix is divided close to the clamp (Fig. 9), the stump is invaginated and the purse-string suture tied (Fig. 10).

Splenectomy

Splenectomy is rarely necessary or indicated. However, at the time of surgical staging, disease spread to the spleen may be apparent as an extension of the omental plaque or as implants of more focal disease on the capsule and/or hilum. Occasionally it may appear as an isolated site of recurrence.

First the spleen should be mobilized to allow exposure and division of its ligamentous attachments. Traction in an inferior and medial direction will expose the filamentous attachments to the diaphragm (splenophrenic) and colon (splenocolic), and these may then be divided and ligated. Entry into the lesser sac then allows exposure of the pancreas and the gastrosplenic ligament,

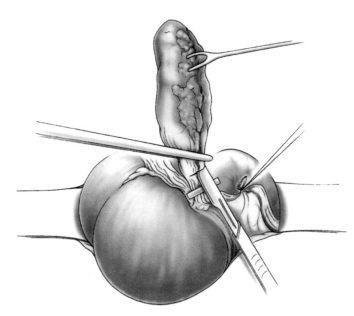

Figure 8 The base of the appendix is crushed.

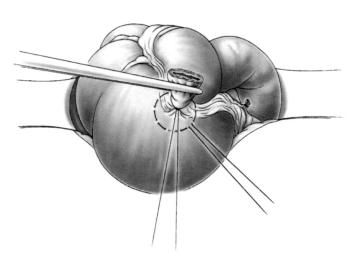

Figure 9 The appendix is divided.

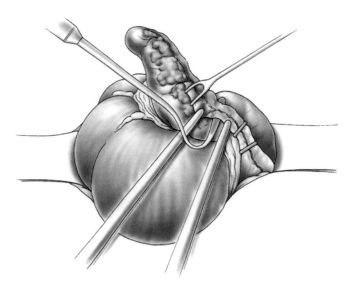

Figure 7 The mesoappendix is clipped.

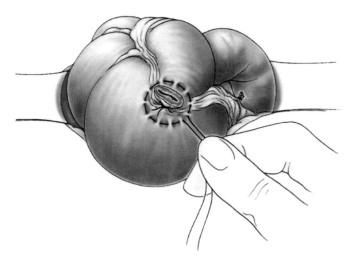

Figure 10 Purse-string suture.

which contains the short gastric arteries (Fig. 11). Division of the short gastric vessels leaves only the splenorenal ligament intact, containing the splenic vessels and the tail of the pancreas. Holding the splenic hilum between the fingers, the operator identifies and protects the tail of the pancreas while the peritoneum over the ligament is taken and the splenic artery identified and divided (Fig. 12). Finally the large splenic vein is identified, ligated, and divided, and the spleen is delivered. Occasionally the tail of the pancreas is sacrificed and requires sutured in two layers to prevent leakage. A drain is mandatory.

Omentectomy

The omentum is frequently the site of massive metastatic deposits of disease and may cause the presenting symptoms at the time of diagnosis. An omental "cake", as it is commonly referred to, may be found at the junction of the greater omentum and the transverse colon. Although initial assessment may give the appearance of gross involvement of the transverse colon, this is usually not the case, and the tumor mass can be carefully mobilized and resected without the need for a transverse colectomy. Care should be taken to assess whether the omentum is adherent to the anterior abdominal wall peritoneum, as this peritoneal layer can be stripped in continuity with the omentum if necessary.

Initially the omentum should be elevated to expose the transverse colon. The posterior leaf of the omentum is then divided, beginning to the left of the hepatic flexure. Gradual mobilization of this layer allows the transverse colon to be rolled in a caudal direction to expose the gastrocolic ligament. Care must be taken to avoid damage to the spleen when dissecting free the left lateral section of the omentum at the level of the splenic flexure. The vessels in the gastrocolic ligament can then be ligated with a series of clips (Fig. 13).

Excision of Liver Nodules

Attempts at resection of large volume disease are sometimes appropriate as part of the tumour reductive surgical process if optimal debulking may be achieved. The deposits may be shelled out digitally after incising the liver capsule. Alternatively, they may be aspirated using a Cavitron ultrasonic aspirator (Cavitron Corporation, USA). Following resection hemostasis may be achieved using diathermy with a roller-ball handpiece (Fig. 14).

SURGERY FOR APPARENT EARLY STAGE DISEASE

At the time of initial laparotomy a proportion of women will have apparent early-stage disease. It is imperative that a meticulous surgical staging procedure is performed to allow counseling regarding prognosis, the place of adjuvant therapy and, where appropriate, fertility options. In women who have completed their family, a total or subtotal abdominal hysterectomy, bilateral salpingo-oophorectomy, together with omentectomy, para-aortic node sampling, and peritoneal biopsies should be performed. More conservative surgery should only be considered in women desiring to maintain fertility options with stage IA disease and well-differentiated or borderline tumors; in these cases the uterus may be conserved and a simple oophorectomy with inspection and biopsy of the contralateral ovary are performed (Fig. 15). The remainder of the staging laparotomy should then be undertaken. Full counseling about risks, completion surgery after childbirth, and the concept of cryopreservation of ova, embryos or ovarian tissue should be undertaken.

INTERVAL DEBULKING SURGERY

The concept of interval debulking has been assessed in two centers. Initially a Birmingham (UK) study failed to demonstrate a survival benefit (Lawton et al. 1990), but a later EORTC study, despite its critics, has suggested that interval debulking of tumor following three courses of initial chemotherapy did confer survival benefits of the order of six months if the patient underwent resection of visible disease (van der Burg et al. 1995). Further validation of this work is in progress, but it remains perhaps the first convincing evidence that interval surgery does have a significant role in management.

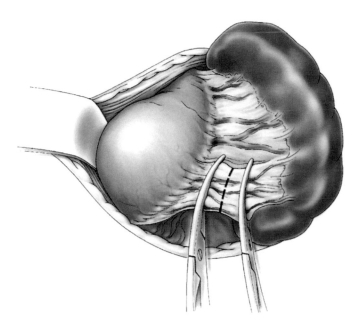

Figure 11 Exposure of the pancreas and gastrosplenic ligament.

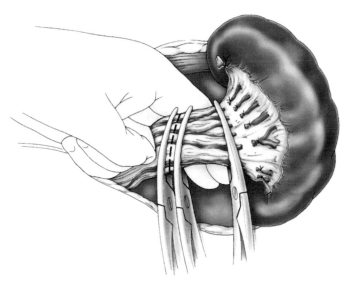

Figure 12 Division of the splenic artery.

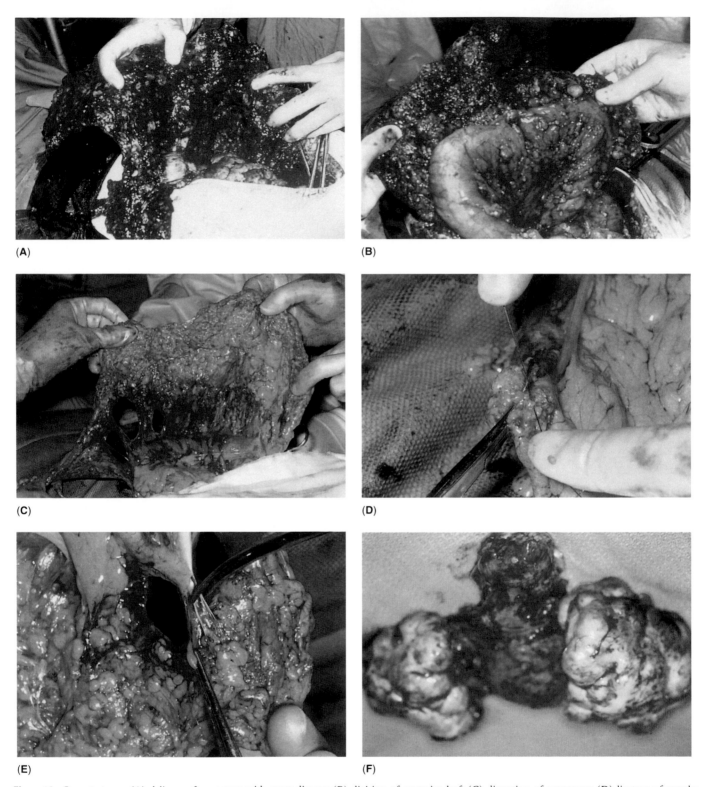

Figure 13 Omentectomy: (**A**) delivery of omentum with gross disease; (**B**) division of posterior leaf; (**C**) dissection of omentum; (**D**) ligature of vessels; (**E**) removal of omentum from bowel; and (**F**) bilateral primary tumor.

SECOND-LOOK SURGERY

Second-look procedures, either laparoscopy or laparotomy following the completion of chemotherapy, in order to test tumor response and establish the need for secondary debulking procedures, have not proved to be helpful in treatment decisions, nor in terms of patient benefit and improved survival. It is now broadly agreed that these should be only undertaken as part of defined research protocols.

PALLIATIVE SURGERY

Palliative procedures often have an important part to play in the management of the pre-terminal stages of this disease and are usually concerned with relieving the effects of intestinal obstruction. The most common of these procedures is the bypass of obstructive loops of small bowel, in which circumstance an ileocolic bypass anastomosis is to be favored over heroic attempts at mass resection (see chapter 28).

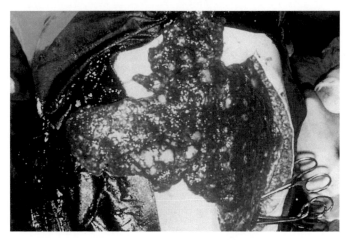

Figure 14 Excision of liver nodules.

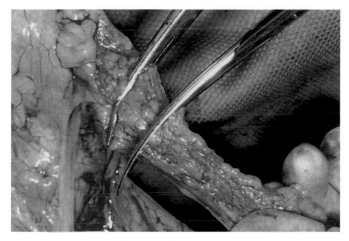

Figure 15 Oophorectomy.

The use of such palliative surgery can provide a great degree of symptomatic relief for patients with bowel obstruction, but it is to be stressed that fine judgment needs to be exercised to ensure that the patient will benefit in her final weeks from such a surgical approach rather than merely have her discomfort increased by the pain of a laparotomy.

GERM CELL AND STROMAL TUMORS OF THE OVARY

Germ cell and stromal tumors occur predominantly in younger women and adolescents. Preoperative diagnosis of these tumors may be facilitated by the use of tumor markers, and conservative surgery should be considered in all cases where fertility preservation is desired. Unilateral adnexectomy with biopsy of the contralateral ovary is sufficient as the pelvic surgical component in the majority of young women since the advent of successful adjuvant chemothcrapy (Gershenson 1988).

REFERENCES

Bonney V (1912) The female genital tract. In: Choice CC, ed. *A System of Surgery*, vol. 2. New York: Funk & Wagnalls.

Brunschwig A (1961) Attempted palliation by radical surgery for pelvic and abdominal carcinomatosis primary in the ovaries. *Cancer* **14**:384–8.

Fawzi HW, Robertshaw JK, Bolger BS, et al. (1997) Role of appendicectomy in the surgical management of ovarian cancer. *Eur J Gynaec Oncol* **18**:34–5.

Gershenson DM (1988) Menstrual and reproductive function after treatment with combination chemotherapy for malignant ovarian germ cell tumours. *J Clin Oncol* **6**:270–5.

Griffiths CT (1975) Surgical resection of tumour bulk in the primary treatment of ovarian carcinoma. Symposium on ovarian cancer. *Nat Cancer Inst Monog* **42**:101–4.

Hudson CN (1968) A radical operation for fixed ovarian tumours. *J Obst Gynaec Br Cwlth* **75**:1155–60.

Jacobs I, Oram D, Fairbanks J, et al. (1990) A risk of malignancy index incorporating CA125, ultrasound and menopausal status for the accurate preoperative diagnosis of ovarian cancer. *Br J Obstet Gynecol* **97**:922–9.

Lawton F, Luesley D, Redman C, et al. (1990) Feasibility and outcome of complete tumor resection in patients with advanced ovarian cancer. *J Surg Oncol* **45**:14–19.

McGowan L, Lesher LP, Norris HJ, et al. (1985) Misstaging of ovarian cancer. *Obstet Gynec* **65**:568–72.

Meigs JV (1934) *Tumours of the Female Pelvic Organs*. New York: Macmillan.

Munnell EW (1952) Ovarian carcinoma. Predisposing factors, diagnosis and management. *Cancer* **5**:1128–33.

Piver MS, Barlow JJ (1976) Preoperative and intraoperative evaluation in ovarian malignancy. *Obstet Gynec* **48**:312–15.

van der Burg ME, van Lent M, Buyse M, et al. (1995) The effect of debulking surgery after induction chemotherapy on the prognosis in advanced epithelial ovarian cancer. *N Engl J Med* **332**:629–34.

Young RC, Decker DG, Wharton JT, et al. (1983) Staging laparotomy in early ovarian cancer. *JAMA* **250**:3072–6.

22 Upper abdominal cytoreduction: including diaphragm resection, splenectomy, distal pancreatectomy, and thoracoscopy

Nick M. Spirtos, Christina L. Kushnir, and Scott M. Eisenkop

Cytoreduction of all visible disease for patients with advanced stage epithelial ovarian cancer (EOC) before adjuvant chemotherapy is associated with maximum survival and is well documented to increase five-year, and even 10-year survival when compared to patients left with visible disease measuring 5 mm to 1 cm and even more so, for those left with residual disease measuring more than 1 cm. Those patients in this last group benefit little from surgery, except for palliative relief of specific symptoms. However, until recently there was controversy about the relative influences of tumor biology and surgical effort on survival and there may still remain some. In a series from 1990 to 2002, Eisenkop et al. prospectively investigated the relative importance of biologic aggressiveness versus completeness of surgery using a ranking system (0–3) to quantify the extent of disease involved in anatomic sections of the abdomen and compared ranks at each section and sum of ranks with completeness of cytoreduction on survival to reflect biologic aggressiveness versus completeness of surgery. Survival was independently (stepwise Cox model) influenced by the sum of rankings ($p = 0.05$) but far more by completeness of cytoreduction ($p = 0.001$), indicating a visibly disease-free outcome has a more significant influence on survival than the extent of disease before surgery (Eisenkop et al. 2003). In a series from 1994 to 1998, Aletti et al. analyzed whether survival was influenced by need for specific operations to accomplish optimal cytoreduction for 194 patients with stage IIIC EOC before chemotherapy. Optimal cytoreduction was accomplished in 67.5% of patients and no specific procedure impacted upon survival (Aletti et al. 2006a, b). Eisenhauer et al. defined optimal as <1 cm of residual disease and stratified 262 stage IIIC/IV EOC patients based on the extent of upper abdominal surgery (group 1) such as diaphragm resection (DR), liver resection, porta hepatis, spleen ± distal pancreas, standard surgery (group 2) which included TAH/BSO, omentectomy, bowel resection, etc., and suboptimal (group 3). The median survival was not reached for group 1 by 68 months, was 84 months for group 2, and 38 months for group 3, indicating patients requiring maximal upper abdominal cytoreduction benefited significantly (Eisenhauer et al. 2006).

It is much more difficult to define the benefit of a maximal cytoreductive effort when residual disease measures more than 1 cm. It is incumbent upon the surgeon to identify disease that is unresectable as early in the procedure as possible, for this determination should result in the termination of surgery, saving the patient unnecessary morbidity and possible mortality. Undertaking surgical procedures, while leaving residual disease of more than 1 cm, should only be done to relieve specific symptoms such as bowel obstruction. It is only in this context that such a maximal surgical effort be pursued.

As virtually all pelvic disease is resectable if the surgeon is willing to approach the disease from a retroperitoneal approach and remove the disease en bloc; exploration of the upper abdomen and under specific settings, the thoracic cavity is most critical in determining if there is unresectable disease. Additionally, removing the upper abdominal disease often provides exposure, opens retroperitoneal spaces that facilitates access to structures that must be dissected during the pelvic phase of surgery, and prevents ongoing production of ascites, etc.; all of which makes the pelvic resection more feasible and timely. Hence, a midline incision extending from the symphysis pubis to the xyphoid process is used for exposure. Upon entering the peritoneal cavity exploration should be done immediately to identify the extent of disease. Once this is accomplished, a complete supra- and infra-colic omentectomy should be performed by transecting the short gastric vessels across the greater curvature of the stomach. This can be accomplished with traditional clamps and ties. Alternatively LDS stapling devices, endo-GIA stapling devices with vascular loads (30 mm staples); or a variety of currently availably pulsed bipolar energy devices such as the Gyrus PK device (Gyrus ACMI, Southeborough, Massachusetts, USA) or the Ligasure device (Covidien Inc., Mansfield, Massachusetts, USA) may be used to decrease anesthesia time. There are several advantages of removing the omentum first. Its removal decreases fluid losses, provides exposure to the remainder of the upper abdomen, and importantly allows for exploration of the lesser sac and the pancreas; both to remove small amounts of metastatic disease and identify a primary pancreatic lesion if present. If a primary pancreatic cancer is identified no further debulking efforts are indicated and surgery should be aborted. Primary pancreatic lesions are distinct in that the disease typically either encases or replaces the pancreas, or there is a solitary parenchymal lesion. In contrast, metastatic disease from an ovarian, tubal, or primary peritoneal primary is typically confluent with the tail and splenic hilum. In order to facilitate complete resection of the omentum and recognizing that 15% to 20% of patients will require splenectomy to achieve optimal cytoreduction, the left colon and splenic flexure should be mobilized. This is best accomplished by incising the left parietal peritoneum from the pelvic brim to the splenic flexure where the phrenico-colic ligament can be transected. Hydro-dissection in this plane can be used to facilitate the elevation of the parietal peritoneum and descending colon anterior to the left kidney. The distal pancreas and spleen can easily be elevated into the operative field permitting en bloc resection of the omentum, spleen, and distal pancreas if necessary. By mobilizing the splenic flexure and mobilizing the mesocolon and descending colon medially the renal vein at the point the ovarian vein drains into it can be easily identified and the lymph nodes in this area can be fully assessed. To assess the lymph nodes involving the celiac plexus all, one must do is transect the lieno-splenic and gastro-splenic ligaments and sweep both the spleen and the pancreas over the midline providing excellent exposure to the great vessels and the associated lymph nodes. Beginning the dissection in this manner, not only is the omentum and possibly the spleen easily removed but an evaluation of two areas that might harbor unresectable disease (the para renal and celiac lymph nodes) can be evaluated and if so determined, minimize the need of further debulking. In the event that the spleen must be removed any remaining attachments of gastro-colic ligament and stomach transected with bipolar instruments and the splenic vessels palpated. Depending on the amount exposure as well as adjacent adipose tissue, inflammation, and proximity to pancreas determines whether the vessels are clamped, cut, and tied or whether they are transected with an endoscopic-GIA and then clipped as well. In the event that confluent disease involves the pancreatic tail adjacent to the spleen the already mobilized pancreas is further mobilized with bipolar cautery and/or the endo-GIA and then stapled across using a GIA stapler with white vascular loads. Tisseel (Baxter Inc., Deerfield, Illinois, USA) can then be applied over the staple line and a retroperitoneal drain placed to minimize and or treat a possible pancreatic leak.

As surgical efforts to remove all visible disease have increased, splenectomy has become an integral part of achieving complete cytoreduction. Splenic metastases have been reported in 20% of patients with advanced ovarian cancer (Rose et al. 1989). Splenic involvement can be classified as parenchymal, hilar, and/or capsular. Numerous authors have reported undertaking splenectomy in the context of both primary and secondary cytoreductive surgery for EOC.

Eisenkop et al. analyzed splenectomy in 49/356 patients with stage IIIC EOC (13.8%) and found that it was associated with longer operative times; increased blood loss and prolonged hospitalization. Patients undergoing splenectomy more often required en bloc resection of the rectosigmoid and the reproductive organs; diaphragm stripping or resection; and the resection of macroscopically involved retroperitoneal lymph nodes. The need for splenectomy to achieve complete cytoreduction is clearly a reflection of advanced disease and as long as complete cytoreduction was achieved survival was not influenced by the need to perform splenectomy. Major complications included hemorrhage requiring reoperation (1–2%); coagulopathy (9%); sepsis (9%); deep venous thrombosis (2%); pneumonia (3%); pulmonary embolism (1–2%), and postoperative death (1–2%). For patients who have splenectomy with the hilum resected adjacent to the pancreas where there is concern about risk of pancreatic injury should have efforts made to minimize the risk of pancreatic leaks. These can be addressed by using intravenous Sandostatin (50 mcg IVPB q8h day 1, 75 mcg IVPB day 2–3, 100 mcg IVBP day 4–10, taper day 11–12) along with total parental nutrition. In addition, the retroperitoneal space in the left upper quadrant should be drained. In this series patients requiring splenectomy had a statistically insignificant trend toward diminished survival (56.8 vs. 76.8 months $p = 0.4$),

but as a group were older, had poorer performance status and more extensive disease as indicated by the additional surgical procedures required to achieve complete cytoreduction (Eisenkop et al. 2006).

Although not identified by Eisenkop et al. (2006) as a factor of prognostic significance, other authors identified parenchymal involvement of the spleen as a poor prognostic factor.

Nicklin et al. (1995) reviewed splenectomy in cytoreductive surgery in 18 patients from The Ohio State University. Three patients (17%) were found to have parenchymal involvement and all died of disease within 21 months. However, two of these patients had stage IV disease so the clinical course described is not so surprising. Sixteen (89%) patients were left with residual disease <2 cm and complications incurred secondary to splenectomy included five cases of pancreatic tail injury or pseudocyst and eight cases of left-sided atelectasis or pleural effusion. Median survival in their series was 12 months. Ayhan et al. (2004) also found that parenchymal involvement was associated with poorer, but not statistically significant decrease in median survival. Forty-one patients with stage IIIC EOC underwent splenectomy for cytoreduction: 34 underwent splenectomy during primary optimal cytoreduction (residual, 1 cm), while seven for secondary cytoreduction. All patients except for those that died within the first month received platinum-based chemotherapy. Estimated five-year survival, and mean survival rates were 37.4 and 36.7 months, respectively, and overall median survival was 24 months.

Specific procedure-related complications appear to be unrelated to whether it is performed during primary or secondary cytoreduction. These include transient leukocytosis and thrombocytosis, pleural effusion, pneumonia, and pancreatic duct injury. Morris et al. (1991) analyzed the indications and complications associated with splenectomy in 45 patients from the M.D. Anderson Cancer Center. In their study, 24 (53%) patients underwent splenectomy during ovarian cancer cytoreduction, 15 of whom as secondary cytoreduction. Postoperative morbidity was seen in 13 (29%) patients, including six patients with left lower lobe atelectasis. Optimal cytoreduction to <2 cm of disease was achieved in 62.5% of patients. Follow-up information was not provided to determine the impact of tumor cytoreduction on survival.

Scarabelli et al. (1998) reported 14 and 26 patients undergoing splenectomy during primary and secondary cytoreductive surgery, respectively. Splenectomy was performed as part of the cytoreductive effort in 34 patients (85%). All patients had <2 cm of residual disease. Left-sided pleural effusions were noted in 10 (25%) patients, and one patient sustained a pancreatic tail injury. Patients undergoing splenectomy and complete secondary cytoreduction were found to have a two-year survival of 78%, compared with only 24% of patients with macroscopic residual disease. Median survival in these two groups was 27 and 16 months, respectively.

Chen et al. (2000) in a similar group of 35 patients (13 primary and 22 secondary surgery) with all but 3 (91%) undergoing optimal cytoreduction (residual <1 cm), found surgical time, estimated blood loss, and units of packed red blood cell transfusions to be comparable between primary and secondary surgeries. However, more patients undergoing primary cytoreduction were transferred to the ICU postoperatively compared to those patients undergoing secondary cytoreduction (84.6% vs. 31.8%). Correspondingly hospital stay was prolonged when comparing primary and secondary cytoreduction (16 vs. 12 days). Postoperative complications noted included pneumonia (five patients) and pancreatitis, (two patients). There was one postoperative death (3%) in a patient who refused all supportive treatments. Postoperative therapy was not specified and median follow-up time among all patients was 17 months. Median progression free interval for primary and secondary cytoreduction groups was 24 and 14 months, respectively.

In reporting a series of 24 patients undergoing splenectomy during secondary cytoreductive surgery. Manci et al. (2006) found that intraparenchymal lesions (9 patients) were always isolated sites of recurrence whereas hilar and superficial metastases were associated with multiple-site recurrence (15 patients). Similar to Eisenkop et al. (2006) surgical procedures reported as part of the cytoreductive effort included small and large bowel resection, diaphragm stripping, distal pancreatectomy, lymphadenectomy, partial hepatectomy, and partial gastrectomy. Survival was significantly related to complete cytoreduction, disease-free interval (>12 months), consolidation intraperitoneal paclitaxel, and platinum-based chemotherapy after splenectomy. Splenectomy was performed at the end of the surgical procedure after having assessed the possibility of achieving optimal cytoreduction. Sixteen patients (67%) had no macroscopic residual disease. Of the 24 patients, 13 patients were still alive at 33 months without evidence of disease, 4 patients were alive at 32 months with evidence of disease, and 7 patients were dead at 21 months. Median progression free survival and overall survival (OS) after secondary surgery were 34 and 56 months, respectively. Mean operative time and mean blood loss were 108 ± 40 minutes and 526 ± 184 ml, respectively, and median postoperative stay was six days.

Splenectomy in five patients undergoing secondary cytoreduction was undertaken by Chi et al. (2006) using hand-assisted laparoscopy or laparoscopy in three and two cases, respectively. Mean operative time was 258 ± 64 minutes and blood loss of 150 ± 117 ml. One patient received a blood transfusion. Four of five patients achieved optimal cytoreduction. The patients were discharged from the hospital at a median time of four days postoperatively. Despite the prolonged operative times the patients were discharged on average in four days.

The benefit of splenectomy in both the primary and secondary cytoreductive settings is clear from reviewing the literature. Associated operative times, morbidity, and mortality are acceptable and when complete cytoreduction is accomplished median survival is prolonged. Some surgical techniques and postoperative management issues remain to be discussed. After completing the splenectomy the superior and lateral aspects of the pancreas should be inspected under magnification and if a duct is seen, it should be clipped with a small hemoclip, after which the pancreas is reinforced with continuous 2-0 prolene. Recently we have been applying Tisseel (Baxter Inc., USA) to the cut surfaces of the pancreas. Postoperatively, patients who undergo distal pancreatectomy or in whom there is a question of pancreatic injury in the context of splenectomy are treated with intravenous Sandostatin (50 mcg IVPB q8h day 1, 75 mcg IVPB day 2–3, 100 mcg IVBP day 4–10, taper day 11–12) along with total parental nutrition. If a drain is placed the fluid collected can be checked for pancreatic enzymes to determine if Sandostatin is necessary. Additionally patients having undergone splenectomy are at increased risk to infection secondary to encapsulated bacteria. Based on this, it is recommended that patients be given polyvalent pneumococcal vaccine as well as *Neisseria meningitidis* vaccine and *Hemophilus influenza* vaccine. The first vaccine should be given either preoperatively or immediately postoperatively. The latter two are best given 7 to 10 days preoperatively.

Although the tail of the pancreas is sometimes involved superficially by disease also involving the spleen and requiring distal pancreatectomy, pancreatic metastasis of ovarian caner is extremely rare. The incidence is difficult to quantitate, and a therapeutic approach to this problem, not well documented. Few studies address pancreatic resection as a component of extensive cytoreductive surgery in EOC. Nakamura et al. (2001) investigated metastatic tumors to the pancreas in 103 Japanese patients: 67 men and 36 women. The incidence of non-primary pancreatic tumors was 15% in the autopsy cases of malignant tumors, and the majority of the secondary tumors were carcinomas. Three patients (3%) were of ovarian origin. In the event that small surface implants are encountered while performing the omentectomy in the lesser sac or on the tail after the splenectomy, these may be either ablated with the argon beam coagulator (ABC) using a lower wattage (60 W) or aspirated with the Cavitron ultrasonic surgical aspirator (CUSA) if the water content is higher.

Others, including Reddy et al. (2008) have undertaken large retrospective reviews including both men and women undergoing pancreatic resection. Reporting on 3830 patients having undergone pancreatic resection at The Johns Hopkins University over a 38-year period, 49 of the 3830 (1.3%) patients were found to have a metastatic, non-hematological cancer originating from a nonpancreatic primary. Of the 49 patients, 27 (55%) were female and only four were found to have metastasis from the ovary. It is unclear from the report what type of pancreatic resection the four ovarian cancer patients underwent. Median cumulative survival for the four ovarian cancer patients was 2.8 years. They concluded that even though historically, pancreatic resection was associated with a high perioperative mortality rate of up to 25% (Kassabian et al. 2000), over the past three decades, the mortality rate has steadily decreased, and in this study, the mortality rate was 0% and the associated morbidity acceptable.

Yildirim et al. (2005) described distal pancreatectomy in six patients with advanced EOC. All six patients had extensive splenic metastasis requiring en bloc resection of the spleen along with distal pancreatectomy. Mean operative time was 170 minutes (range 90–400). Transfusion was required in three patients. Mean hospitalization was 12 days (range 6–17). Four patients (66.7%) experienced early postoperative complications including pancreatitis, atelectasis, pneumonia, and bowel obstruction. There was no perioperative mortality (death within the first 30 days after surgery). All patients received platinum-based chemotherapy. Mean follow-up was 27 months, and three (50%) patients were still alive at the end of the study period. Two-year survival rate is 66.7% (four out of six). In EOC, metastasis to the pancreas is rare, but distal pancreatectomy can be carried out with reasonable morbidity and mortality.

Hoffman et al. (2007) reviewed the records all patients undergoing cytoreductive surgery for ovarian cancer at the University of South Florida from 2002 to 2004. Six patients were identified that underwent optimal cytoreduction that included en bloc resection of omentum, colon, gastrocolic ligament, and spleen. Two of the six patients additionally underwent partial pancreatectomy, and partial gastrectomy. Postoperative complications included one bowel leak from a transverse colon anastamosis, one pulmonary embolism, one left upper quadrant abscess, and one gastric leak requiring emergent laparotomy. There were no perioperative mortalities. Hoffman concluded that the sample size was too small to draw any conclusions with regard to oncologic benefit. He did, however, state that optimal cytoreduction including extensive left upper quadrant resection should be attempted in those ovarian cancer patients who can be left with minimal residual disease.

Kehoe et al. (2009) reviewed the incidence of pancreatic leak after splenectomy and distal pancreatectomy during primary cytoreduction for ovarian, primary peritoneal, or fallopian tube cancer. They identified 41 patients who underwent splenectomy, of which 17 (41%) also underwent distal pancreatectomy. Twelve patients (71%) had ovarian cancer, four (24%) patients had peritoneal caner, and one (6%) had fallopian tube cancer. Four (24%) of the seventeen patients developed a postoperative pancreatic leak. Percutaneous drainage was instituted in all cases, and the diagnosis of pancreatic leak was based on elevated amylase levels from the fluid collected. Thirteen of the seventeen patients did not have a pancreatic leak, but did require drainage of an abdominal and/or pelvic collection. The authors concluded that distal pancreatectomy should be performed to resect metastatic gynecologic cancers.

The authors recommend a number of techniques to identify pancreatic duct injury and the management of patients undergoing distal pancreatectomy. These include the use of magnified inspection (loops) and clipping of any duct that has been transected. Additionally Tisseel (Baxter Inc., USA) can be applied to the transected end of the pancreas. The prophylactic use of intravenous Sandostatin (100 mcg q 8 hours) and TPN for 7 to 10 days while draining the retroperitoneal space in the left upper quadrant is also recommended.

Assuming this portion of the procedure is completed and optimal cytoreduction completed, the diaphragm should be evaluated and all disease removed. Diaphragm metastases, especially the right hemidiaphragm, are common, and can be problematic in patients with ovarian cancer. Up to 40% of patients with advanced ovarian cancer will present with metastatic disease to the diaphragm, and diaphragm metastasis have been described as one of the most common factors precluding optimal cytoreduction (Eisenhauer and Chi 2007).

In a survey of the Society of Gynecologic Oncologists (SGO) (Eisenkop and Spirtos 2001a, b), 76.3% of the respondents cited bulky diaphragmatic disease as the number 1 factor contributing to suboptimal cytoreduction. Significantly, only 24% of those surveyed utilized DR, and 30% had no experience with the procedure. Almost half of the respondents cited a lack of evidence supporting the claim that radical procedures improved survival in patients with advanced stage EOC. This philosophy is in contrast to the longstanding belief that

volume of residual disease is one of the most important independent predictors of survival (Griffiths 1975). Regardless of the opinion one holds on this matter, it is indisputable that if maximal cytoreduction with no visible residual disease is the surgical endpoint, then diaphragm stripping and or resection are techniques that must be mastered.

Aletti et al. (2006a, b) reviewed 244 patients with stage IIIC and IV EOC at Mayo Clinic from 1994 to 1998. For the entire cohort, residual disease was the only independent prognostic factor in multivariate analysis ($p < 0.0001$) when compared to other factors. The five-year OS was 31.5%. The authors also looked at a subgroup of patients ($n = 181$) that had tumor involving the diaphragm. Those patients (41 of 181) who underwent diaphragm surgery: stripping, resection, excision, CUSA had an improved five-year OS relative to those patients (140 of 181) that did not undergo diaphragm surgery (53% vs. 15%; $p < 0.0001$). Additionally, in multivariate analysis of patients with diaphragm disease, both residual disease and performance of diaphragm surgery were independent predictors of outcome ($p < 0.001$). Patients with RD <1 cm, there was a strong survival advantage for those patients who underwent diaphragm procedures (five-year OS: 55% vs. 28%; $p = 0.0005$). The authors concluded that diaphragmatic resection to achieve optimal cytoreduction in advanced ovarian cancer improves OS.

Eisenkop and Spirtos (2001a, b) reviewed 213 patients with stage IIIC EOC from 1990 to 2000 undergoing complete cytoreduction before initiation of systemic platinum-based chemotherapy. Of the 213 patients, 94 required diaphragmatic stripping, and 27 required full thickness resection of the diaphragm. If the diaphragm had tumor involvement, it was either stripped or resected, or the implants were ablated. Small, scattered implants were ablated with an ABC. Bulky diaphragm disease was removed by stripping the peritoneum from the muscle. Full thickness resection was utilized for disease that deeply invaded the diaphragmatic muscle. The overall median follow-up was 31 months. Log rank analysis showed a significant difference in survival on the basis of whether a diaphragm stripping was required to attain a visibly disease-free outcome. Median survival for the 94 patients who underwent diaphragm stripping was 41.8 months, and 47.1 months for the 27 patients who underwent DR. They concluded that median survival for patients with advanced stage EOC who are able to have all or virtually all visible disease resected prior to chemotherapy (platinum-based) is superior to survival of patients with both small volume visible disease, and bulky unresectable disease.

Cliby et al. (2004) reviewed 41 patients at Mayo Clinic that underwent DR to achieve optimal cytoreductive surgery in ovarian carcinoma. The majority of DR occurred in patients undergoing surgery for recurrent disease (35 of 41, 85%), and in 13 of these 35 patients, there had been at least one prior recurrence. Lesions were predominately right-sided (80%), but bilateral resection was necessary in two (5%) patients. Pathologic evaluation of resected areas revealed 35 cases (85%) were full-thickness disease. Pleural surface was involved in a minority of cases, 10 of 35. Forty of forty-one women underwent additional procedures for debulking including splenectomy, liver resection, small bowel resection, and intra-abdominal tumor debulking. At the conclusions of the operation, 33 of 41 (80.1%) had no gross residual disease,

4 of 41 (9.8%) had <1 cm of residual disease, 1 of 41 (2.4%) had residual disease between 1 and 2 cm, and 3 of 41 (7.3%) patients had >2 cm of residual disease. Overall, DR allowed for 90% of patients to achieve optimal debulking (no single lesion larger than 1 cm). Ten of the forty-one patients had chest tubes placed at the time of surgery. Of the remaining 31 patients, 3 (9.7%) subsequently required a chest tube. Complications that could possibly be attributed to DR were symptomatic pneumothorax requiring chest tube placement (2/41, 4.9%) and the accumulation of pleural effusions contributing to respiratory compromise requiring percutaneous thoracentesis (4/41, 9.8%). One of 41 developed a subphrenic abscess that required percutaneous drainage, and antibiotic therapy. One of 41 who underwent left DR as well as splenectomy developed a gastropleural fistula late in her hospital course, and eventually died from sepsis. This study was not designed to evaluate diaphragmatic resection and survival, but was designed to address potential complications from DR, and has shown that DR risks are comparable to other debulking procedures.

Devolder et al. (2008) looked at the role of diaphragmatic surgery in a series of patient from 1993 to 2001. A total of 137 patients underwent cytoreductive surgery. Of these, 69 patients underwent diaphragmatic surgery as part of cytoreduction surgery for advanced EOC. The remaining 68 patients did not have DR either due to being free of visible diaphragm involvement, or they were judged to be poor candidates for complete mobilization of the liver medically, due to other bulky disease, or unstated reasons. For diaphragmatic resection or coagulation, mobilization of the liver was needed in order to have adequate visualization. A Rochard retractor was used to retract the ribs for additional exposure. Seventeen of 69 patients underwent stripping, 22 of 69 underwent coagulation, and 30 of 69 underwent stripping and coagulation. Stripping was preferred when lesions of >5 mm, or extensive spread was appreciated. Coagulation was used in the presence of a small number of lesions (<20), small solitary lesions (<5 mm), and thin lesions (<5 mm). In five cases, the diaphragmatic muscle with the outer pleural layer was removed as well. In three of these five cases, the external pleural layer and the diaphragmatic muscle were closed with an interrupted layer of Polyglactin 910. The authors did not use prophylactic thoracic drains. In the remaining two of the five cases, the diaphragmatic defect was too large to be closed primarily, and was left open without the use of a thoracic drain. These two patients did not subsequently need thoracic drainage in their postoperative period. Complications attributed to diaphragmatic resection were pleural effusion (59%), elevation of the diaphragm (48%), and pneumothorax (5%). Only five patients needed a chest drain, and only seven needed pleural puncture. Stripping of the diaphragm caused a slightly higher morbidity than coagulation, but was also performed in the case of larger and thicker lesions. The authors compared the median OS of patients who underwent stripping ($n = 13$) with the median overall survival of patient who underwent coagulation ($n = 12$) in stage IIIC ovarian cancer and found that the median OS in the stripping group was 66 versus 49 months in the coagulation group. This was not found to be statistically significant. They concluded that debulking to no residual disease results in the best survival in advanced ovarian cancer, diaphragmatic surgery to be feasible, and to have an acceptable morbidity.

Kapnick et al. (1990) in reporting their experience with full-thickness DR at the Brigham and Women's Hospital over a two-year period (12 patients) found a lesion size of greater than 5 cm was correlated to the depth of diaphragm penetration and in primary disease depth of penetration was inversely correlated to survival.

In almost all cases of disease involving the diaphragm, metastatic disease can be surgically removed or ablated with the ABC or aspirated with the CUSA (Tyco, Inc., Princeton, New Jersey, USA) if the disease is small volume and scattered (Adelson 1991). In order to systematically address wide-spread disease involving the diaphragm it is our practice to first mobilize the liver by transecting the falciform, right and left triangular ligaments using a LigaSure device (Covidien Inc.), Gyrus bipolar cutting forceps (Gyrus Inc.), or an ABC (Conmed Inc., Utica, New York, USA). Similarly the upper and lower layers of the coronary ligaments are incised using ABC and as the dissection proceeds posteriorly significant care is required to ensure the inferior vena cava is not injured as it penetrates the diaphragm. In the event that the vena cava is injured at the level of the diaphragm the prudent course of action is to tamponade and either request a vascular consultation or suture with interrupted 4-0 or 5-0 Prolene suture as the wall of the vena cava is thicker than in the lower abdomen and relatively easy to control despite limitations of exposure. The liver can now be elevated and mobilized toward the midline allowing for complete visualization and resection of all diaphragmatic disease or resection of the diaphragm as needed. Special care is also required in mobilizing the liver in this manner as the bare area of the liver is easily fractured resulting in a significant amount of blood loss. The use of a surgical sponge soaked in saline and epinephrine 1/100,000 dilution can minimize this problem. The surgeon must be prepared to address bleeding caused by this dissection. Techniques used most frequently by the authors include the use of topical hemostatic agents with the application of direct pressure. These agents include Arista (Medafor, Inc., Minneapolis, Minnesota, USA), Gelfoam (Baxter Inc., Deerfield, Illinois, USA), and Surgicel (Johnson and Johnson, New Brunswick, New Jersey, USA) soaked in thrombin, or Tisseel (Baxter Inc.) applied to the liver surface. In extreme cases, liver sutures are needed to compress large vessels deep to the surface. In the event that there is oozing from disease that infiltrates, a raw surface, or a significant tear that must be sutured and bleeding is significant, the loss can be reduced by first digitally entering the portal area, palpating the portal triad, and placing an atraumatic clamp or penrose (our preference; i.e., Pringle maneuver) for a brief time. If the liver must be sutured, large atraumatic needles with 0-chromic are specifically made for use on the liver. Of note, during this process the portal area is palpated for any nodal disease, which is either resected after hemostasis is achieved, ablated with the ABC if small, or aspirated with a CUSA if high water content is present. An alternative approach to suturing is using radiofrequency ablation (RFA). The Habib probe (varying length) can be inserted into the bleeding site and energy applied until hemostasis is achieved. Once the liver is completely mobilized and hemostasis achieved the diaphragm can be stripped using any variety of techniques. It is our preference to elevate the peritoneum off the underlying muscle using the ABC and hydrodissection. Traditional sharp dissection using

Metzenbaum scissors can also be used but care taken to minimize the associated oozing. If disease is found to penetrate the muscle resection can be accomplished as described by the authors noted above. Usually the muscle can be re-approximated using a running monofilament suture. If so much of the diaphragm is resected and cannot be primarily repaired, it can be patched using a Gore-Tex graft (W.L. Gore and Assoc. Inc., Newark, Delaware, USA).

A more controversial issue is the appropriateness of addressing disease above the diaphragm. Recent reports suggest that approximately 35% to 40% of patients with apparent stage IIIC ovarian cancer have subclinical stage IV disease, although in only a few cases was suboptimal disease (>1 cm) found in the thoracic cavity. Spirtos et al. recently reported at the European Society of Gynecologic Oncology 2007 on 57 patients undergoing transdiaphragmatic thoracoscopy during surgery for apparent stage IIIC EOC with negative chest radiographs or computed tomography (CT) scans. Twenty-three (40%) were found to have disease involving either the parietal or visceral pleurae. All with pleural disease have involvement of the diaphragmatic peritoneum and over 90% of the patient had positive retroperitoneal lymph nodes. Most of the disease (88%) found above the diaphragm was of small caliber (<1 cm) and could be ablated or resected (Spirtos et al. 2007).

Eisenkop (2002) reviewed 30 patients from 1998 to June 2000 who underwent thoracoscopy at the time of primary cytoreductive surgery. Twenty-six patients underwent transdiaphragmatic thoracoscopy by a gynecologic oncologist, and four patients had a thoracic surgeon undertake the ride-sided thoracoscopy just prior to the abdominal procedure. Indications for thoracoscopy included: untapped pleural effusion, positive pleural cytology in the absence of grossly visible or radiographic evidence of extra-abdominal disease, and intentional or inadvertent entry into the chest cavity at the time of a diaphragm stripping or full-thickness DR. Between 1990 and June 2000, 37 patients with stage IV EOC based on positive pleural cytology or other pleural involvement underwent primary cytoreductive surgery, but did not undergo thoracoscopy, served as controls for evaluating impact of thoracoscopy on survival. Transdiaphragmatic thoracoscopy was performed both with a 0° and a 30° 10-mm laparoscope that entered directly through the opening in the diaphragm. After surgery, patients were treated with cisplatin or carboplatin in addition to cyclophosphamide or paclitaxel. Median operative time was 180 (90–380) minutes. The median operative time of the thoracoscopy was 10 minutes (5–65). The median operative time for transdiaphragmatic thoracoscopy was eight minutes (5–40 minutes). The four transthoracic procedures had operative times of 20, 25, 45, and 65 minutes. There was no postoperative mortality among patients that underwent thoracoscopy. One patient required a chest tube postoperatively for an enlarging pneumothorax. Overall median survival for stage IV patients was 28.9 (0–131) months, and the estimated five-year survival was 42%. At the time this study was published, 38 (62.3%) of the group were alive. The median follow-up for the group was 23.3 months. A log-rank analysis showed a statistically significant difference in survival on the basis of whether or not thoracoscopy was performed for patients with stage IV disease.

Chi et al. (2004) reviewed 12 patients that underwent video-assisted thoracoscopic surgery (VATS) for moderate to large pleural effusions before planned abdominal exploration. A 2-cm incision was made in the chest wall in the fifth intercostal space on the side of the effusion and biopsies taken as indicated by intraoperative findings. After VATS, all patients had a chest tube placed. Those patients with malignant effusions underwent talc pleurodesis either intraoperatively or postoperatively. Median operative time was 31 minutes (20–49 minutes). There were no complications attributed to the procedure. Median amount of pleural fluid drained was 1000 ml (500–2000 ml). In six (50%) of the twelve patients, solid pleural-based tumor was found, with lesion >1 cm found in four patients (33%), and lesion <1 cm found in two patients (17%). The six remaining patients had no grossly visible tumor, but the pleural fluid was positive for malignant cell in two patients (17%), and negative in four patients (33%). Final diagnosis of primary disease site was ovary, 9 (75%), fallopian tube, 1 (8%), endometrium, 1 (8%), and lymphoma, 1 (8%). Based on the findings during VATS, cytoreduction was avoided in four patients (33%), and the cytoreductive procedure was modified in one patient (8%).

Chi et al. concluded that VATS should be considered in patients with suspected advanced ovarian cancer and moderate to large pleural effusions, in order to determine the extent of disease, and to decide if the patient remains a candidate for cytoreductive surgery, or if neoadjuvant chemotherapy should be offered.

Juretzka et al. (2007) reviewed all patients with suspected advanced ovarian cancer and moderate to large pleural effusions who underwent VATS at Memorial Sloan-Kettering Cancer Center between 6/01 and 8/05. Twenty-three patients were identified. VATS was performed for right-sided effusions in 17 patients (74%), and left sided in six patients (26%). The median amount of pleural fluid drained was 1350 ml (400–3700 ml). During the VATS procedure, macroscopic disease was found in 15 patients (65%) with nodules >1 cm in 11 of 15 patients (73%), and <1 cm in 4 of 15 (27%). Macroscopic intra-thoracic disease was found in 4 of 10 (40%) of patients with negative cytology. Intra-thoracic cytoreduction was performed in 3 of 11 patients (27%) with intra-thoracic disease >1 cm. After VATS, 12 of 23 patients (52%) underwent primary cytoreduction with residual disease of <1 cm achieved in 11 of 12 patients (92%). The other 11 patients received primary chemotherapy after undergoing diagnostic laparoscopy (4/11) or no further abdominal exploration (7/11). Nine of these eleven patients went on to have interval cytoreduction. Two of the eleven were found to have gastrointestinal and lymphoma primaries at the time of VATS. Overall, findings at VATS altered primary surgical management in 11 of 23 (48%) patients. Juretzka et al. found that 65% of patients with suspected advanced cancer and pleural effusion had gross intra-thoracic disease, with the majority (73%) having >1 cm in diameter. They concluded that the use of VATS might help identify candidates for cytoreductive surgery including intra-thoracic cytoreduction versus neoadjuvant chemotherapy.

If identification of pleural-based disease impacts upon either the proposed cytoreductive effort or the potential use of intra-peritoneal chemotherapy, then there is potential value in undertaking transdiaphragmatic thoracoscopy intraoperatively or VATS preoperatively. Transdiaphragmatic thoracoscopy is best performed while the anesthesiologist halts ventilation so the parietal and visceral pleurae can be adequately visualized. Small volume disease can be ablated using ABC. If disease involves the lung parenchyma and is readily accessible a TA-60 stapling device can be used to resect disease on the edges of the lung. Tisseel (Baxter Inc.) can be applied after stapling and resecting the involved portion of lung. A chest tube can easily be inserted transdiaphragmatically although it is not universally agreed that it is necessary to do so. If a chest tube is not inserted a purse-string suture using monofilament suture (0-Monocryl or Prolene) (Ethicon Inc., Cincinnati, Ohio, USA) should be placed to close the defect in the diaphragm and a large caliber red Robinson catheter placed into the thoracic cavity. As the anesthesiologist hyperinflates the lungs, the catheter with suction applied, is withdrawn and the purse-string suture secured. If the defect in the diaphragm cannot be closed primarily a Gore-Tex graft can be sutured into place using 0-Prolene suture. After completing the diaphragm and pleural resection the right perinephric area is always thoroughly inspected since this is commonly an area beneath the liver in which it is easy to overlook residual disease. Disease in this area is usually either excised or ablated with the ABC.

Another area of controversy involves the role of liver resection as it pertains to a maximal surgical effort in either primary or secondary cytoreduction in patients with EOC. A number of techniques can be used to achieve this end; however, it is our preference to use the Habib RFA device (AngioDynamics, Latham, New York, USA), and the ABC. During the application of radiofrequency energy, a high-frequency alternating current moves from the tip of an electrode into the tissue surrounding that electrode. As the ions within the tissue attempt to follow the change in the direction of the alternating current, their movement results in frictional heating of the tissue. As the temperature within the tissue becomes elevated beyond 60°C, cells begin to die, resulting in regional necrosis surrounding the electrode. A typical RFA treatment produces local tissue temperatures that exceed 100°C, resulting in coagulative necrosis of the tumor and surrounding hepatic parenchyma (Choi et al. 2001). Only tissue through which electrical current passes directly is heated above a cytotoxic temperature. The tissue temperature falls rapidly with increasing distance away from the electrode (radiofrequency power density), and reliable production of cytotoxic temperature can only be expected 5 to 10 mm away from the multiple array hook electrodes (Curley et al. 2003). An RF needle is advanced into the liver tumor either percutaneously, laproscopically, or during laparotomy. Tumor location, size, number of metastasis, and the number of previous surgeries are variables that can affect the modality chosen. Intraoperative ultrasound can be used to help precisely identify metastasis, as well as identify other lesions not seen on preoperative imaging, or easily identifiable on palpation. High-frequency alternating current is delivered to tissue resulting in rapid tissue destruction, and is essentially bloodless, as is any subsequent resection in the ablated area. These are benefits that distinguish RFA from traditional liver resection techniques (Ravikumar et al. 2000). The four-prong design of the RFA probe allows for precise resection of metastatic disease by creating a circumferential area of coagulative necrosis. An additional benefit is that the Habib device is not technically difficult to use, but still

requires an understanding of liver anatomy. RFA is safe to use on most areas of the liver, but the hilar plate should be avoided. The hilar plate, where the portal vein and hepatic arterial branches enter the liver should always be avoided. Although the blood vessels can tolerate the RFA treatment, the large bile ducts coursing with them do not tolerate heat, and biliary fistulae or strictures can occur after RFA (Choi et al. 2001). Additionally, large caliber vessels can act as a "heat sink", decreasing the likelihood of complete ablation and increasing the risk of recurrence or persistence of tumors in that area (McGahan et al. 1992, Ravikumar et al. 2000). Tumors larger than 2.5 cm require more than one deployment of the electrode. For larger tumors, multiple placements, and deployments of the electrode may be necessary to completely destroy the tumor. In addition, there should be overlapping areas of coagulative necrosis to ensure complete tumor destruction.

The needle electrode is used to produce a thermal lesion that incorporates not only the tumor but also nonmalignant hepatic parenchyma. CT scans performed after RFA of liver tumors will initially show a larger cystic lesion than seen preoperatively, but in time, the lesion size will decrease (Ravikumar et al. 2000). Interpretation of CT, magnetic resonance imaging (MRI), or ultrasound after RFA to determine complete destruction of tumor and evaluate for local recurrence can be difficult. In the experience from M.D. Anderson, RFA, MRI or CT findings performed one to two months after RFA may demonstrate a hypervascular rim of inflammatory tissue around the RFA defect which may be asymmetric and impossible to distinguish from residual tumor. But in the studies done at M.D. Anderson, the inflammatory response noted on early scans resolves, and is not evident on images obtained six months or more after RFA (Choi et al. 2001). It is possible that positron emission tomography (PET) scanning can make a contribution in detection of residual tumor after RFA. Ravikumar et al. (2000) reviewed 11 patients with at least six months follow-up after RFA of the liver for colorectal metastasis. PET scan was able to discriminate between completely treated lesions and recurrent disease in six patients: concurrent CT scans done were equivocal. This study suggests further evaluation of PET is warranted as a routine tool to follow-up patients having undergone RFA of the liver.

In 1963, Brunschwig reported 24 cases of hepatic lobectomy for metastatic carcinoma preformed at Memorial Sloan-Kettering Cancer Center. Of the 24 cases, four were of gynecologic origin (uterus corpus, and cervix). The overall surgical mortality rate was 29%. Three of these four patients died perioperatively (75%), and the fourth died of disease 18 months after left lobectomy. Since Brunschwig's paper in 1963, there have been vast improvements in operative techniques, anesthetic management, patient selection, and postoperative care that have led to a decrease in perioperative morbidity and mortality. Most modern series of hepatic resections report perioperative mortality rates of 5% or less (Chi et al. 2002, Langer and Gallinger 1995).

Fleury et al. (2008) reviewed three cases in which patients with recurrent ovarian cancer (stage IIIC/IV), metastatic to the liver were treated with RFA using the Habib (an RFA device) or partial liver resection using RFA. In order to resect hepatic metastasis, the liver was mobilized transecting the falciform ligament, triangular ligaments, and coronary ligaments using the ABC as described previously. The Habib RFA device was then used to cauterize the hepatic lesions, and the cauterized lesions were resected with a no. 10 blade scalpel. Intraoperative ultrasound was used in order to guide placement. If additional hepatic bleeding occurred at the time of resection, the Habib probe was also used as a coagulative device. The perioperative morbidity consisted of subdiaphragmatic abscess (one of three) requiring percutaneous drainage, pulmonary embolism (one of three), re-intubation (one of three), pelvic abscess (one of three) requiring percutaneous drainage, and wound infection (one of three) requiring a vacuum assisted closure device. There were no perioperative mortalities. Patients were subsequently treated with chemotherapy. Two of the three patients are living and disease free, 20 months after surgery. One patient was disease free for nine months, and was then subsequently diagnosed with metastatic disease in the lung, liver, and vertebral bodies. Fleury et al. concluded that RFA alone, or RFA-assisted resection is safe for the management of metastatic disease to the liver.

After completing the left upper quadrant cytoreduction (omentum ± spleen ± pancreas) and right upper quadrant cytoreduction (diaphragm ± chest ± liver ± perinephric) the central abdomen is addressed since exposure is now optimized. The intestine and its mesentery are now systematically inspected. Implants that are not immediately adjacent to intestinal serosa are most expediously ablated with the ABC using a relatively high wattage (100–150 W). Implants that are immediately adjacent to the serosa or on serosa are aspirated with the CUSA if the water content of the tumor is high; alternatively the implants are excised and seromuscular defects are oversewn with interrupted 3-0 silk. One suggestion we offer, when excising implants from serosal surfaces rather than elevating the implant with Debakey pickups and cutting with Metzenbaum scissors as is intuitive and frequently taught, secure the bowel with one hand and just skim with straight suture scissors along the serosa under the metastatic implant. There will often be little or no defect. If there is a resultant serosal defect this can be easily repaired with 3-0 silk or Vicryl suture. Unfortunately, this is the setting that most often prevents complete cytoreduction and requires the coalescence of the surgeons' judgment and technical ability to fully assess the feasibility of achieving complete cytoreduction in the context of the risk/benefit ratio to the patient. If need be, bulky, confluent disease can be resected with bowel resection and anastamosis.

In order to complete the resection of all upper abdominal disease, the left and right aortic lymph nodes should be resected. Extensive bulky nodes, unlike those associated with metastatic squamous cell cervical cancers and some gastrointestinal malignancies, can be safely removed since the surgical planes between nodes and adjacent vessels can be developed digitally or with the use of hydrodissection, thus facilitating their resection. First, using an endo-GIA the left gonadal vessels can be transected and resected along with the lymph nodes overlying the anterior and lateral aspect of the aorta down to the level of the bifurcation of the aorta. The dissection should continue across the midline, removing the lymph nodes in the interspace between the aorta and vena cava. If macroscopically involved lymph nodes are encountered posterior to these vessels, the lumbar vessels must be ligated and divided in order to safely resect lymph nodes in this area.

After completing the pelvic phase of surgery and the lymph node dissection, the full thickness of the abdomen is typically closed using a running monofilament suture.

In summary:

1. Explore through a midline incision that permits access to the entire abdomen.
2. First address the left upper quadrant.
   a. This provides exposure.
   b. This prevents ongoing fluid loss.
   c. This helps to rule-out pancreatic or gastric primary.
3. If the omental disease is severe be open minded about taking the omentum en bloc with a section of transverse colon or spleen or spleen with pancreas, or uncommonly edge of stomach.
4. In the process of mobilizing the omentum and spleen and colon use the opportunity to mobilize for the anticipated lymph node dissection.
5. After finishing the left upper quadrant address the right upper quadrant.
6. When addressing the right upper quadrant ask the question of whether the disease is a few scattered implants or confluent or many scattered.
   a. If a few scattered ablate with an ABC.
   b. If many scattered implants or confluent disease strip the diaphragm.
   c. When finished with the diaphragm evaluate the right perinephric area and portal area separately.
7. When stripping or resecting the diaphragm first mobilize the liver as described.
   a. If there is an effusion or you enter certainly scope with a laparoscope and be prepared to ablate with an ABC.
8. Be familiar with techniques for hemostasis of liver (Pringle, ABC, Habib, topical agents).
9. After the right upper quadrant address the central disease. Never be in the position of deciding between the ABC, CUSA, and excision. Ideally use all three.
   a. ABC for rapid ablation remote from serosa; although it is acceptable to use very briefly at 40 W on serosa.
   b. CUSA for high water content on serosa and other sensitive areas briefly.
   c. Excision with repair using 3-0 silk.
10. Pelvic resection is usually completed after upper abdominal disease as exposure is optimized.
11. Lymph node dissection is usually completed after pelvic resection as exposure is further optimized.

REFERENCES

Adelson MD (1991) Cytoreduction of diaphragmatic metastases using the Cavitron Ultrasonic Surgical Aspirator. *Gynecol Oncol* **41**:220–2.
Aletti GD, Dowdy SC, Gostout BS, et al. (2006a) Aggressive surgical effort and improved survival in advanced-stage ovarian cancer. *Obstet Gynecol* **107**:77–85.
Aletti GD, Dowdy SC, Podratz KC, et al. (2006b) Surgical treatment of diaphragm disease correlates with improved survival in optimally debulked advanced stage ovarian cancer. *Gynecol Oncol* **100**:283–7.
Ayhan A, Al RA, Baykal C, et al. (2004) The influence of splenic metastases on survival in FIGO stage IIIC epithelial ovarian cancer. *Int J Gynecol Cancer* **14**:51–6.

Bachellier P, Ayav A, Pai M, et al. (2007) Laparoscopic live resection assisted with radiofrequency. *Am J Surg* **193**:427–30.

Brunschwig A (1963) Hepatic lobectomy for metastatic cancer. *Cancer* **16**:277–82.

Chen LM, Leuchter RS, Lagasse LD, et al. (2000) Splenectomy and surgical cytoreduction for ovarian cancer. *Gynecol Oncol* **77**:362–8.

Chi DS, Abu-Rustum NR, Sonoda Y, et al. (2004) The benefit of video-assisted thoracoscopic surgery before planned abdominal exploration in patients with suspected advanced ovarian cancer and moderate to large pleural effusions. *Gynecol Oncol* **94**:307–11.

Chi DS, Abu-Rustum NR, Sonoda Y, et al. (2006) Laparoscopic and hand-assisted laparoscopic splenectomy for recurrent and persistent ovarian cancer. *Gynecol Oncol* **101**:224–7.

Chi D, Temkin S, Abu-Rustum N, et al. (2002) Major hepatectomy at interval debulking for stage IV ovarian carcinoma: a case report. *Gynecol Oncol* **87**:140.

Choi H, Loyer EM, Dubrow RA, et al. (2001) Radiofrequency ablation (RFA) of liver tumors: assessment of therapeutic response and complications. *Radiographics* **21**:S41–S54.

Cliby W, Dowdy S, Feitoza SS, et al. (2004) Diaphragm resection for ovarian cancer: technique and short-term complications. *Gynecol Oncol* **94**:655–60.

Curley SA (2003) Radiofrequency ablation of malignant liver tumors. *Ann Surg Oncol* **10**(4):339.

Devolder K, Amant F, Neven P, et al. (2008) Role of diaphragmatic surgery in 69 patients with ovarian carcinoma. *Int J Gynecol Cancer* **18**:363–8.

Eisenhauer EL, Abu-Rustum NR, Sonoda Y, et al. (2006) The addition of extensive upper abdominal surgery to achieve optimal cytoreduction improves survival in patients with stages IIIC–IV epithelial ovarian cancer. *Gynecol Oncol* **103**:1083–90.

Eisenhauer EL, Chi DS (2007) Liver mobilization and diaphragm peritonectomy/resection. *Gynecol Oncol* **104**(2 Suppl 1):25–8.

Eisenkop SM (2002) Thoracoscopy for the management of advanced epithelial ovarian cancer—a preliminary report. *Gynecol Oncol* **84**:315–20.

Eisenkop SM, Spirtos NM (2001a) Procedures required to accomplish complete cytoreduction of ovarian cancer: is there a correlation with "Biological Aggressiveness" and survival? *Gynecol Oncol* **82**:435–41.

Eisenkop SM, Spirtos NM (2001b) What are the current surgical objectives, strategies, and technical capabilities of gynecologic oncologists treating advanced epithelial ovarian cancer? *Gynecol Oncol* **82**:489–97.

Eisenkop SM, Spirtos NM, Friedman RL, et al. (2003) Relative influence of tumor volume before surgery and the cytoreductive outcome on survival for patients with advanced ovarian cancer: a prospective study. *Gynecol Oncol* **90**:390–6.

Eisenkop SM, Spirtos NM, Lin MCM (2006) Splenectomy in the context of primary cytoreductive operations for advanced epithelial ovarian cancer. *Gynecol Oncol* **100**:344–8.

Fleury AC, Spirtos NM, Eisenkop SM, et al. (2008) The use of radiofrequency ablation in advanced ovarian cancer: resection and ablation of liver metastases. *Clin Ovarian Cancer* **1**(2):135–8.

Griffiths CT (1975) Surgical resection of tumor bulk in the primary treatment of ovarian carcinoma. *Natl Cancer Inst Monogr* **42**:101–4.

Hoffman MS, Tebes SJ, Sayer RA, et al. (2007) Extended cytoreduction of intraabdominal metastatic ovarian cancer in the left upper quadrant utilizing en bloc resection. *Am J Obstet Gynecol* **197**:209.e1–209.e5.

Juretzka MM, Abu-Rustum NR, Sonoda Y, et al. (2007) The impact of video-assisted thoracic surgery (VATS) in patients with suspected advanced ovarian malignancies and pleural effusions. *Gynecol Oncol* **104**:670–4.

Kapnick SJ, Griffiths CT, Finkler NJ (1990) Occult pleural involvement in stage III ovarian cancer: role of diaphragm resection. *Gynecol Oncol* **39**:135–8.

Kassabian A, Stein J, Jabbour N, et al. (2000) Renal cell carcinoma metastatic to the pancreas: a single-institution series and review of the literature. *Urology* **56**:211–15.

Kehoe SM, Eisenhauer EL, Abu-Rustum NR, et al. (2009) Incidence and management of pancreatic leaks after splenectomy with distal pancreatectomy performed during primary cytoreductive surgery for advanced ovarian, peritoneal, and fallopian tube cancer. *Gynecol Oncol* **112**:496–500.

Langer B, Gallinger S (1995). The management of metastatic carcinoma in the liver. In: Cameron JL, ed. *Advances in Surgery*, vol. 28. St. Louis, MO: Mosby-Year Book, pp. 113–32.

Manci N, Bellati F, Muzii L, et al. (2006) Splenectomy during secondary cytoreduction for ovarian cancer disease recurrence: surgical and survival data. *Ann Surg Oncol* **13**:1717–23.

McGahan JP, Brock JM, Tesluk H, et al. (1992) Hepatic ablation with use of radio-frequency electrocautery in animal model. *J Vasc Interv Radiol* **3**:296.

Morris M, Gershenson DM, Burke TW, et al. (1991) Splenectomy in gynecologic oncology: indications, complications, and technique. *Gynecol Oncol* **43**:118–22.

Nakamura E, Shimizu M, Itoh T, et al. (2001) Secondary tumors of the pancreas: clinicopathological study of 103 autopsy cases of Japanese patients. *Pathol Int* **51**:686–90.

Nicklin JL, Copeland LJ, O'Toole RV, et al. (1995) Splenectomy as part of cytoreductive surgery for ovarian carcinoma. *Gynecol Oncol* **58**:244–7.

Ravikumar TS, Jones M, Srrano M, et al. (2000) The role of PET scanning in radio frequency ablation of liver metastasis from colorectal cancer. *Caner J* **6**(Suppl 4):S330–S343.

Reddy S, Edil BH, Cameron JL, et al. (2008) Pancreatic resection of isolated metastases from nonpancreatic primary cancers. *Ann Surg Oncol* **15**(11):3199–206.

Rose PG, Piver MS, Tsukada Y, et al. (1989) Metastatic patterns in histologic variants of ovarian cancer. An autopsy study. *Cancer* **64**:1508–13.

Scarabelli C, Gallo A, Campagnutta E, et al. (1998) Splenectomy during primary and secondary cytoreductive surgery for epithelial ovarian carcinoma. *Int J Gynecol Cancer* **8**:215–21.

Spirtos NM, Eisenkop SM, Fleury AC, et al. (2007) *Transdiaphragmatic Thoracoscopy: Impact in Patients with Stage IIIC Epithelial Ovarian Cancer*. Berlin, Germany: European Society of Gynecologic Oncology.

Yildirim Y, Sanci M (2005) The feasibility and morbidity of distal pancreatectomy in extensive cytoreductive surgery for advanced epithelial ovarian caner. *Arch Gynecol Obstet* **272**:31–4.

23 Retroperitoneal infrarenal, inframesenteric, and pelvic lymphadenectomies
Katherine A. O'Hanlan

INTRODUCTION

Pelvic and para-aortic lymphadenectomy is an essential step in staging of pelvic malignancies, is often used to determine primary therapy, helps remove all grossly or occult positive disease, and enables stratification of malignancies for valid comparisons of treatments, all with the purpose of optimizing survival. A transabdominal laparoscopic approach for pelvic (Querleu et al. 1991) and infrarenal aortic (Querleu et al. 1993) lymphadenectomy was first described by Querleu and colleagues for staging cervical, endometrial, and ovarian malignancies. Urologists (Ferzli et al. 1992) and later Gynecologic Oncologists (Vasilev and McGonigle 1995) subsequently developed retroperitoneal approaches for pelvic, infrarenal aortic (Vasilev and McGonigle 1996), and suprarenal aortic (Possover et al. 1998) artery lymphadenectomy. Because the predominant drainage of malignancies of the cervix is to pelvic nodes, and of the endometrium and ovaries is to pelvic and aortic nodes (Matsumoto et al. 2002), this chapter will focus on use of a direct retroperitoneal approach for staging or restaging cervical, uterine, and ovarian carcinomas.

INDICATIONS
Cervical Carcinoma

Resection of bulky nodes prior to combination chemotherapy and radiotherapy has been shown to result in improved overall survival (Cosin et al. 1998). When PET or CT scans show enlarged pelvic nodes, lymphadenectomy and then radiation of the nodal beds and at least one nodal segment higher is indicated. Additionally, it is useful to rule out aortic adenopathy when there are bulky nodes in the pelvis, prior to initiating radiotherapy to the pelvis alone (Tillmanns and Lowe 2007).

Endometrial Carcinoma

The ability to laparoscopically remove pelvic and inframesenteric aortic nodes implicated in endometrial carcinoma was established by the GOG (Childers et al. 1993). However, it has been demonstrated that endometrial carcinoma can metastasize directly along the infundibulopelvic vessels to the infrarenal aortic lymph nodes in as many as two-thirds of the 77% of women with aortic metastases, especially if they have grade 2 or 3 disease, or a deeply invasive grade 1 endometrial carcinoma (Dowdy et al. 2008). A thorough lymphadenectomy may have a therapeutic benefit, because pathologically negative nodes can be found to harbor occult disease when specially stained or step-sectioned (Amezcua et al. 2006).

Ovarian Carcinoma

Staging of ovarian carcinoma included the right and left inframesenteric nodes and pelvic nodes until it was shown, not surprisingly, that lymphatic metastases could follow the ovarian vascular supply to the infrarenal aortics where the infundibulopelvic vessels originated (Onda et al. 1996). Now it is standard to resect bilateral infrarenal aortic nodes in staging ovarian (Takeshima et al. 2005, Morice et al. 2003) and primary peritoneal (Aletti et al. 2009) epithelial malignancies because there is decussation of lymphatics above the inferior mesenteric artery, even though the left side is slightly favored (Morice et al. 2003, Roger et al. 2008). In these aforementioned instances, a retroperitoneal lymphadenectomy can be performed first in the surgical care plan.

METHODS
Preparation

Patients should always be consented for a laparoscopic lymphadenectomy with the knowledge that laparotomy may be necessary. Any node dissection around a major artery indicates reserving two units of packed red blood cells. While bowel preparation is not indicated if retroperitoneal lymphadenectomy is the sole procedure, it can facilitate the rest of the staging procedure if hysterectomy, omentectomy etc., are to be performed.

All patients with cancer should receive at least 30 to 40 mg of low-molecular weight heparin to prophylax against deep vein thrombus formation. The procedure is performed typically in supine position if it is the sole procedure. If hysterectomy and other abdominal procedures will be performed later, then the modified lithotomy position is preferred. Arms are tucked by the patient's side, and shoulder bolsters are carefully positioned. The surgeon is on the patient's left side with monitors on the right, one at the level of the feet, and the other at the level of the diaphragm.

Technique

Because success of a retroperitoneal approach depends on creating and maintaining a pneumoretroperitoneum, this procedure is always performed first. Any leak of carbon dioxide into the peritoneum will preferentially collapse the retroperitoneum due to the weight of the bowel.

There are two methods of entering the retroperitoneum: laparoscopic guidance or direct incision. When a laparoscopic survey of the abdomen is indicated first, then a single direct transumbilical puncture is made. The apex of the umbilicus is gradually everted to form a nipple, with depression of the periumbilical tissue for incision into the apical scar. Pre-emptive anesthesia with 5 cm³ of bupivicaine without epinephrine is given prior to making a 5-mm incision in the scar, grasping the edges and adjacent skin very widely with towel clips to elevate the umbilicus maximally, and directly inserting an atraumatic 5-mm trocar at a 90° angle (O'Hanlan et al. 2007). Abdominal survey is performed. If a washing is needed, a secondary 5-mm trocar can be inserted near the right anterior superior iliac crest.

Next, a 3-cm incision is made at the left MacBurney site, that is, 2 cm medial and 2 cm superior to the anterior superior iliac crest (Fig. 1). Identifying each of the two paper-thin layers of oblique fascia, and open with a spreading technique using a hemostat and finger guidance. Visual guidance laparoscopically is also useful to show proximity to the peritoneal lining so the surgeon is careful to not perforate this thin layer. Entry into the retroperitoneum is heralded by palpating the absence of any fascia layer attached to the ileac crest, allowing the finger to sweep toward the interior of the ileac fossa (Fig. 2).

If no intraperitoneal inspection is desired first, then it is possible to make a left-sided McBurney skin incision without peritoneal insufflation, and using opening of the hemostat before an advancing finger, again identifying that two fascial layers have been penetrated, and that the underside of the iliac crest has been accessed.

After either entry technique, the surgeon's finger is then used to separate the peritoneum off of the muscular wall as far as possible, sweeping in a cephalad, posterior and caudal directions, and postero-medially to palpate the left common iliac

artery. A blunt-tip 5-mm trocar is inserted directly through a separate 5-mm incision in the axillary line about 4 to 6 cm above the level of the first (see diagram) directly onto the surgeon's fingertip to protect the peritoneum from puncture, also under laparoscopic guidance. The carbon dioxide insufflator is now attached to the new 5-mm port, allowing insufflation of the retroperitoneum to about 10 to 12 mm Hg pressure, and then collapse of the intraperitoneal compartment is facilitated by the opened umbilical trocar. The posterior location of this port permits easier mobility of the operating ports after insertion of the 30° 5-mm laparoscope. A 12-mm blunt-tip hernia trocar is then inserted through the left-sided McBurney incision and secured by the inflated balloon, to maintain the pneumo*retro*peritoneum.

Opening the Space

At this point, usually only adventitia is seen, with hints of the muscular red of the psoas muscle on the dorsal aspect (the "floor"), but more careful inspection will reveal the ureter vermiculating anteriorly medially or on the peritoneal "ceiling", and allow for gentle sweeping of the adventitia up and off of the dorsal "floor" until the major vessels are seen, if they are not seen immediately (Fig. 3). The peritoneum is swept off of the muscular abdominal wall laterally and more superiorly along the anterior axillary line so that a third 5-mm blunt-tip trocar can be inserted under direct visualization with care not to inadvertently puncture the peritoneum (Fig. 4). Now the surgeon can use a 5-mm Ligasure or the 5-mm Advance and a blunt dolphin-tip grasper, to lift the peritoneum off the left common iliac artery from the level of the ureter crossing at the bifurcation, cephalad to the renal artery. The ureter is left attached to the "ceiling" having been identified along its entire length. The ovarian artery and vein are seen lateral to the ureter below the level of the inferior mesenteric artery (IMA), but these vessels cross the ureter medially and find their origins on the antero-lateral aspect of the aorta and the left renal vein. They can be ligated above the ureteral crossing and later resected with their nodal bundles when the dissection is performed. The aorta is exposed along its left side to reveal the

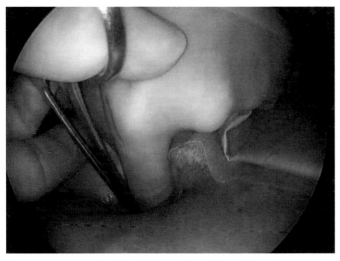

Figure 1 Palpating the two fascial layers while opening with hemostats.

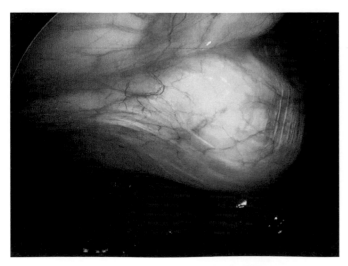

Figure 2 Laparoscopic guidance during dissection through the two abdominal wall fascial layers, careful not to perforate the peritoneum. Using the finger, the peritoneum is swept off of the abdominal wall and the parietal pelvis.

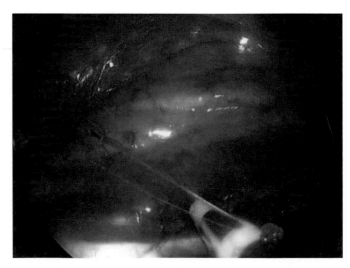

Figure 3 The newly opened adventitial space seen upon insertion of the scope, with the ureter seen crossing the common iliac artery, anterior to the psoas muscle.

origin of the IMA. Above the IMA, the duodenum is identified and lifted up off the aorta up to the level of the left renal vein, typically found crossing anterior to the aorta, often with an azygous branch extending posteriorly and behind the aorta. The tortuous left renal artery is usually posterior and slightly superior to the left renal vein. It is sometimes necessary to sweep the renal capsule superiorly up off the psoas to allow broad access to the left renal vessels. Frequent identification of the vermiculations of the ureter reassure the surgeon of the essential landmarks.

Challenges Establishing Pneumo*retro*peritoneum

When the peritoneum is perforated, the retroperitoneal space will collapse due to the weight of the visceral bowel. Small leaks can sometimes be managed by opening the umbilical trocar a small amount to let the peritoneal compartment vent. Closure of the leak is often possible using hemoclips, suture, or Endoloop. It may, however, be easier to insert an additional 5-mm trocar to allow use of a flexible 5-mm liver retractor, or a 12-mm trocar for use of an Endopaddle (see diagrams) to simply elevate the anterior peritoneal "ceiling" in each area that is being operated on. In fact, this may facilitate all cases in which the anterior peritoneum limits access to the nodal beds with confidence, especially in the obese patients.

Harvesting the Left Aortic Nodes

Nodes are harvested in order of easy access. First the nodes from the IMA down to the crossing of the ureter are resected in a caudal direction (Fig. 5). There is no need to strip the IMA of its own nodal investment, needlessly increasing the risk of chylo*retro*peritoneum. Remove the fibrofatty tissue at the base of the IMA for only 1 cm, and then all the lateral nodal tissue, using bipolar vessel-sealing confidently along the posterior and medial base of the nodal specimen (Lamberton et al. 2008). Remove these nodes using a 10-mm spoon forcep through the 12-mm port.

Next, remove the Infrarenal (IR) nodes starting at the IMA dissecting in a cephalad direction, after confident identification of the ureter and all of the renal vasculature (Fig. 6). The locations of these vessels medial to the ureter must be ascertained with certainty despite distortion of the anatomy caused by the lifting of the anterior peritoneum. There can be significant variability of the left renal vasculature, warranting a cautious technique of spreading, opening and identifying until all of the major vessels and minor variations, including the unusual azygous vein, are exposed (Fig. 7). Use bipolar sealing along the medial base of the aortic specimens to coagulate lumbar vertebral arterial branches and the origins of the left ovarian artery and vein (Fig. 8). The IR nodes should be harvested from the anterior aspect of the aorta over to the left margin of the vena cava, and from the anterior aspect of the renal vein, so that nodes clearly above the ovarian artery origin are thoroughly removed (Fig. 9).

Resecting the Right Aortic Nodes

Next, to obtain the right inframesenteric nodal specimen, cross the bifurcation of the aorta, opening the space below the

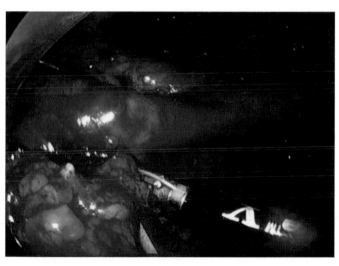

Figure 5 After exposing the length of the left side of the aorta, the nodal bundle sis resected from the inferior mesenteric artery downward to the crossing of the ureter.

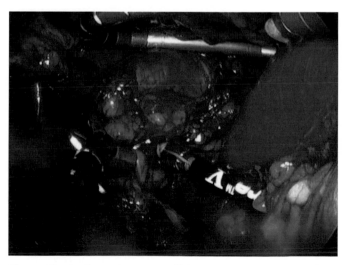

Figure 6 The duodenum is swept up off the nodal bundle above the inferior mesenteric artery using the 5 mm liver retractor. A real hand articulating bullet grasper is used to help resect the nodal bundle working up from the Inferior mesenteric artery.

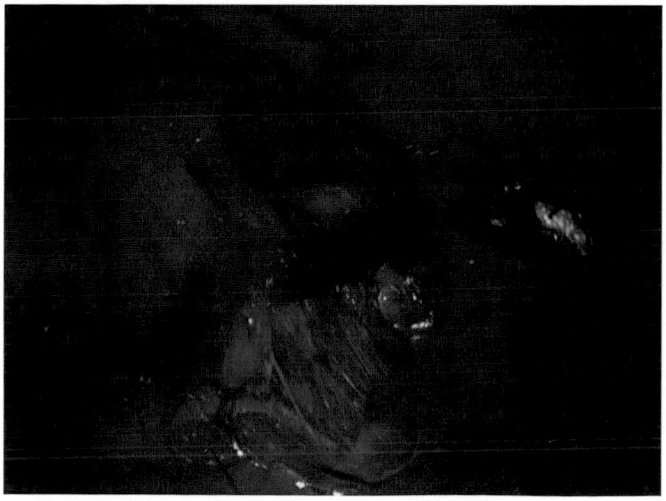

Figure 4 Sweeping the peritoneum away from the abdominal wall, to allow for additionally trocars to be inserted under direct vision.

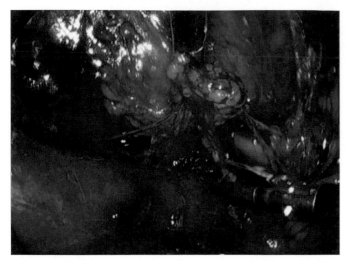

Figure 7 The left renal artery and vein have been identified and the left ovarian artery transected.

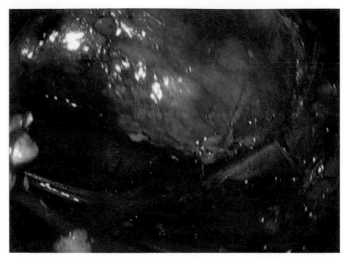

Figure 9 The completed right infrarenal node dissection revealing the right ovarian vein, the left renal vein, and the root of the inferior mesenteric artery.

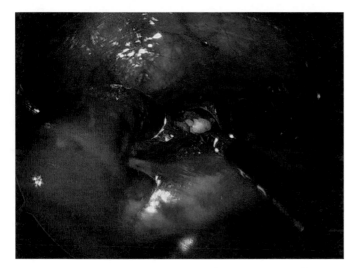

Figure 8 The articulating grasper elevates and facilitates resection of the right infrarenal nodal bundle.

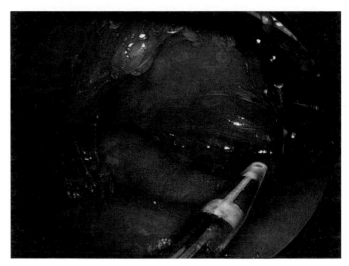

Figure 10 The right common ileac artery has been exposed and the nodal bundle anterior is being resected. Note the ureter, the lateral border of the dissection.

IMA anterior to the right common iliac artery, carefully lifting the peritoneum anticipating the right ureter as the lateral-most border (Fig. 10). Open the space tracing the path of the ureter superiorly, recognizing the crossing of the ovarian vessels, as they course medially to their origins on the right side of the vena cava and aorta, exposing up to the origin of the right renal vein. Be careful not to lift the nodes off the vessels, but to elevate the duodenum off of the nodal bundle.

With the IMA stripped of its most proximal 1 cm, gently open underneath the precaval nodal bundle to expose the bluish vena cava. It is then possible to remove the nodal bundle anterior to the vena cava, starting just above the vessel, transecting confidently with bipolar sealing all the "fellow" veins that arise in this region, stripping all fibro-fatty lymph-bearing tissue off of the right common iliac artery and vein down to the ureter and remove the specimen (Fig. 11). Recall that the rightmost lateral margin of the CIA node dissection is only a filmy avascular web that can be spread and bluntly removed off of the psoas muscle (Fig. 12).

To remove the right IR nodes, again recall that the lateral margin of the upper nodal bundle is also avascular and can be stripped off the vena cava while watching out for the rare additional "fellow" veins, there still being a few above the IMA. It is easiest to start at the right renal vein and work caudally to the IMA.

Harvesting the Pelvic Nodes

To access the pelvic nodes on the right side, sweep the peritoneum off of the anterior sacrum very gently following the aortic bifurcation, using blunt instruments and maintaining broad contact with the membrane so as not to puncture. Expose the external iliac artery down to the level of the crossing of the deep circumflex iliac vein over the external iliac artery going laterally. Strip the superior vesical artery of its lateral attachments and open the paravesical space. Identify the obturator nerve as the posterior margin of resection. Open the posterior aspect to reveal the pararectal space posterior to the internal iliac artery. Identify the genito-femoral nerve and

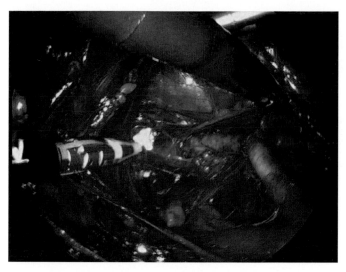

Figure 11 Preparing the right pelvic nodal filed for dissection, the peritoneum is being swept off of the sacrum using the Ligasure.

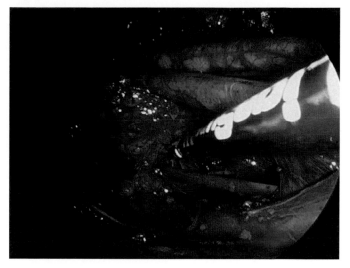

Figure 13 Freeing the obturator nodes from the obturator nerve. These nodes are bulky and solid in this patient with metastatic cervical cancer.

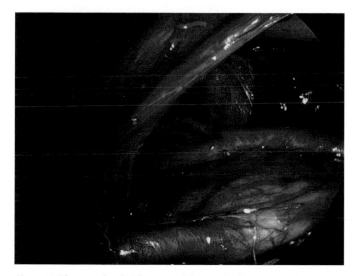

Figure 12 The completed right external ileac node dissection, with presacral nodes exposed.

begin to peel the nodal bundle *en masse* medially off the external iliac artery, then off of the vein, then under the vein off of the sidewall, posteriorly down to the obturator nerve, then medially off of the internal iliac. This large unitary bundle should be removed in a small plastic pouch (Fig. 13).

It is harder to remove the nodes from the left side, but entirely possible, using the same technique. All instruments are torqued inferiorly, and excellent visibility is possible with the 30° scope with the same technique as used for the right side.

After this procedure, the pneumo*retro*peritoneum is collapsed, and at least one fenestration in the peritoneum on each side is made using a transperitoneal view to avoid inadvertent injury to the bowel. No drains are placed. Only the large left inferior site requires closure with suture at the fascial level, and at the skin level. All incisions are treated with Dermabond.

Post-operative Management

Before transferring the patient to a trolley, a stretch binder is placed around the abdomen centered on the incisions, to compress the skin incisions and reduce likelihood of leakage of lymphatic fluid from the abdominal cavity. Discharge is planned for the same day, unless hysterectomy and other procedures are performed.

DISCUSSION

Patients are warned preoperatively that they may experience copious wine-colored fluid leak through the vaginal incision or any of their abdominal incisions for a few days. If a leak develops, they are instructed to place a bundled-up bulky non-sterile washcloth or paper towels in their binder to enhance compression of the leaking port site. It is not clear if this speeds up resolution or only helps manage the significant leakage that some develop, but the leakage always resolves in a few days.

Infectious complications are rare. Chylous retroperitoneum or ascites has been described, with most cases resolving after dietary modification. Vascular complications, while potentially serious, are rare (Querleu et al. 2006). Some surgeons insert a 4 × 4 gauze pad into the retroperitoneum to facilitate visualization and for compression in case of vascular injury. Compression of any vascular injury for five minutes can facilitate laparoscopic suture repair. It is wise to have two units of packed cells prepared, and a 5-mm clip applier available in the room for any emergency. Avulsion of the IMA is not serious, but must be reliably sealed with a clip. Injury to the vena cava or left renal vein by avulsion of the ovarian vein may require multiple clips. Floseal (Baxter) is a 10cc matrix of fibrin-covered collagen gel granules that can be laparoscopically applied to arterial (Aorta included) and venous (fellow veins) bleeders for hemostasis that eludes clips or is not amenable to suture. Ureteral injury should be very rare, due to repeated re-identification, and following the "identify twice, cut once" rule. While obese patients benefit most from this procedure, obesity is also a common cause of converting to laparotomy.

CONCLUSIONS

This report highlights the safe removal of pelvic and aortic lymph nodes by a retroperitoneal approach. Inexperienced surgeons are encouraged to operate with senior surgeons because there is a steep learning curve.

REFERENCES

Aletti GD, Powless C, Bakkum-Gamez J, et al. (2009) Pattern of retroperitoneal dissemination of primary peritoneum cancer: basis for rational use of lymphadenectomy. *Gynecol Oncol* **114**(1):32–6.

Amezcua CA, MacDonald HR, Lum CA, et al. (2006) Endometrial cancer patients have a significant risk of harboring isolated tumor cells in histologically negative lymph nodes. *Int J Gynecol Cancer* **16**(3):1336–41.

Childers JM, Brzechffa PR, Hatch KD, et al. (1993) Laparoscopically assisted surgical staging (LASS) of endometrial cancer. *Gynecol Oncol* **51**(1):33–8.

Cosin JA, Fowler JM, Chen MD, et al. (1998) Pretreatment surgical staging of patients with cervical carcinoma: the case for lymph node debulking. *Cancer* **82**(11):2241–8.

Dowdy SC, Aletti G, Cliby WA, et al. (2008). Extra-peritoneal laparoscopic para-aortic lymphadenectomy–a prospective cohort study of 293 patients with endometrial cancer. *Gynecol Oncol* **111**(3):418–24.

Ferzli G, Raboy A, Kleinerman D, et al. (1992). Extraperitoneal endoscopic pelvic lymph node dissection vs. laparoscopic lymph node dissection in the staging of prostatic and bladder carcinoma. *J Laparoendosc Surg* **2**(5):219–22.

Lamberton GR, Hsi RS, Jin DH, et al. (2008) Prospective comparison of four laparoscopic vessel ligation devices. *J Endourol/Endourol Soc* **22**(10):2307–12.

Matsumoto K, Yoshikawa H, Yasugi T, et al. (2002) Distinct lymphatic spread of endometrial carcinoma in comparison with cervical and ovarian carcinomas. *Cancer Lett* **180**(1):83–9.

Morice P, Joulie F, Camatte S, et al. (2003) Lymph node involvement in epithelial ovarian cancer: analysis of 276 pelvic and paraaortic lymphadenectomies and surgical implications. *J Am Coll Surg* **197**(2):198–205.

O'Hanlan KA, Dibble SL, Garnier AC, et al. (2007) Total laparoscopic hysterectomy: technique and complications of 830 cases. *JSLS* **11**(3):45–53.

Onda T, Yoshikawa H, Yokota H, et al. (1996) Assessment of metastases to aortic and pelvic lymph nodes in epithelial ovarian carcinoma. A proposal for essential sites for lymph node biopsy. *Cancer* **78**(4):803–8.

Possover M, Krause N, Drahonovsky J, et al. (1998) Left-sided suprarenal retrocrural para-aortic lymphadenectomy in advanced cervical cancer by laparoscopy. *Gynecol Oncol* **71**(2):219–22.

Querleu D, Leblanc E, Cartron G, et al. (2006) Audit of preoperative and early complications of laparoscopic lymph node dissection in 1000 gynecologic cancer patients. *Am J Obstet Gynecol* **195**(5):1287–92.

Querleu D, Leblanc E, Castelain B (1991) Laparoscopic pelvic lymphadenectomy in the staging of early carcinoma of the cervix. *Am J Obstet Gynecol* **164**(2):579–81.

Querleu D, Leblanc E, Castelain B, et al. (1993) Celioscopic pelvic and para-aortic lymphadenectomy. *Chirurgie: Memoires de l'Academie de Chirurgie* **119**(4):208–11.

Roger N, Zafrani Y, Uzan C, et al. (2008) Should pelvic and para-aortic lymphadenectomy be different depending on histological subtype in epithelial ovarian cancer? *Ann Surg Oncol* **15**(1):333–8.

Takeshima N, Hirai Y, Umayahara K, et al. (2005) Lymph node metastasis in ovarian cancer: difference between serous and non-serous primary tumors. *Gynecol Oncol* **99**(2):427–31.

Tillmanns T, Lowe MP (2007) Safety, feasibility, and costs of outpatient laparoscopic extraperitoneal aortic nodal dissection for locally advanced cervical carcinoma. *Gynecol Oncol* **106**(2):370–4.

Vasilev SA, McGonigle KF (1995) Extraperitoneal laparoscopic paraaortic lymph node dissection: development of a technique. *J Laparoendosc Surg* **5**(2):85–90.

Vasilev SA, McGonigle KF (1996) Extraperitoneal laparoscopic para-aortic lymph node dissection. *Gynecol Oncol* **61**(3):315–20.

24 Vascular access and implantable vascular and peritoneal access devices
Paniti Sukumvanich and Gary L. Goldberg

INTRODUCTION

Most patients with cancer will undergo multiple courses of chemotherapy and other intravenous infusions as a part of their management. Venous access can become compromised by the intravenous cytotoxic chemotherapies, transfusions, hyperalimentation and other fluids. In 1972, Cole and colleagues reported on the first surgically implanted vascular access device based on a modification of an arteriovenous fistula catheter for renal dialysis (Cole et al. 1972). This was later modified and made popular by Broviac and Hickman (Broviac et al. 1973, Hickman et al. 1979). A decade later, a completely implanted device known as the Port-a-Cath (PAC) was introduced (Ecoff et al. 1983). These devices have become more popular as a greater variety of chemotherapeutic options have become available to patients. The advantage of venous access ports includes fewer access failures with less access-related anxiety and pain (Bow et al. 1999). With the advent of intraperitoneal chemotherapy, PAC devices became a means of obtaining intraperitoneal access. This chapter discusses the indications, techniques of insertion, complications and management of complications for these venous access devices.

INDICATIONS

The main indication for central venous access devices includes the need for venous access in patients undergoing prolonged chemotherapy especially in patients with poor venous access.

PAC devices for use as intraperitoneal access devices are indicated in patients who are expected to undergo intraperitoneal chemotherapy.

CONTRAINDICATIONS

Patients should not undergo venous access catheter placement in the presence of a current infection, such as bacteremia, septicemia, or fungemia. Patients with clinically significant thrombocytopenia or coagulopathy should also not undergo the procedure without special consideration and preparations.

ANATOMIC CONSIDERATIONS

Central venous lines can be accessed through a number of routes. The routes most commonly utilized are the internal jugular vein or the subclavian vein. The internal jugular vein is located within the supraclavicular fossa. The borders of the fossa are the clavicle inferiorly, the sternal and clavicular heads of the sternocleidomastoid muscle anteriorly and posteriorly, respectively. The internal jugular vein empties into the brachocephalic vein which is anterior and lateral to the common carotid artery and posterior to the artery is the apex of the lung. The subclavian vein is a continuation of the axillary vein which runs along the superior border of the pectoralis minor muscle to the level of the first rib. The lateral border of the first rib can be approximated by finding the area on the clavicle where it changes from a convex to a concave curvature (about two-thirds of the distance from the head of the clavicle). It is important to note that there is no major vessel directly posterior to the clavicle lateral to the first rib. Thus, attempts at venous access lateral to this area will usually fail. At the lateral border of the first rib the subclavian vein begins and runs parallel to the first rib, posterior to the clavicle and ends at the medial border of the scalenus anterior muscle. The subclavian vein then merges with the internal jugular vein and forms the brachiocephalic vein. The subclavian artery though it runs parallel with the vein is separated by the scalenus anterior muscle.

TYPES OF PORTS

Venous access catheters can be divided into two types. The first type consists of an externalized Hickman-type catheter. This type of catheter is similar to a central line catheter except that a portion of the catheter is tunneled subcutaneously and has an externalized access site. The second type of venous access catheter is a completely implanted device. The most common example is the PAC. This device has a silicone and titanium reservoir site that is accessed through the skin.

SURGICAL PROCEDURE

Both types of access devices, the externalized Hickman-type and the internalized PAC type, are potential options for central venous access. However, internalized ports are recommended since they are easier to maintain than the externalized devices and they are more "patient-friendly". It was assumed that the Hickman-type catheters had a higher rate of catheter-related infections but a randomized prospective trial did not bear this out (Mueller et al. 1992).

Preoperative Evaluation and Testing

1. Complete blood count, platelet count, and coagulation profile.
2. Prophylactic antibiotics are not recommended. No data exist on the use of prophylactic antibiotics for central venous access device placement. There are limited data regarding the use of antibiotics in central venous catheters. Although possible reductions (Henrickson et al. 2000, Bock et al. 1990, Raad et al. 1998) in infection rates have been reported, the emergence of resistant organisms is of concern and the use of prophylactic antibiotics is currently not recommended (HICPAC 1995).

Surgery

1. Prepare both sides of the neck and chest to the level of the xyphoid process should the attempt on the right side fail.
2. Have the arms tucked on the side of the insertion.
3. In obese patients, a roll of towel can also be placed between the shoulders to allow for easier access in the subclavian approach (Fig. 1).

Venous Access

Venous access can be obtained via either the internal jugular vein or the subclavian vein. The right subclavian vein is usually accessed as the initial choice. The most commonly used approach is the percutaneous technique. However, occasionally, a cutdown procedure is required for access and the cephalic or internal jugular veins can be utilized. Cut-downs have the lowest risk of pnuemothorax.

Percutaneous (Seldinger) Technique
Needle Insertion

1. Local anesthesia using 1% lidocaine (lignocaine) at the site of either the internal jugular vein or the subclavian vein.
2. Set up the 16-gauge needle by lining the bevel of the needle with the numbers on the syringe. This will allow the surgeon to be aware of the direction of the bevel once the needle has been inserted.
3. Insertion into the vein should be done with the bevel pointing inferiorly (Fig. 2).

Subclavian Vein Access
Traditional Method of Insertion

1. Insert the needle directly perpendicular to the skin about 0.5 cm from the edge of the clavicle two-thirds from the head of the clavicle.

2. Once you have gone through the skin, angle the needle toward the subclavian vein underneath the clavicle by aiming for the sternal notch. The needle/syringe should be parallel to the chest wall as negative pressure is applied until there is venous blood return. If there is no blood return on initial insertion, slowly withdraw the syringe.

Alternative Technique

1. Squeeze the clavicle (two-thirds from the head of the clavicle) with the index finger and thumb. Be sure you are grasping the entire clavicle.
2. Insert the needle at the lower edge of the thumb with bevel down. Once through the skin, aim the needle towards the sternal notch while pushing down on the needle with the left thumb. Negative pressure should be applied until there is venous blood return.

Internal Jugular Access
There are two approaches for accessing the internal jugular vein—the anterior and posterior approaches. The anterior or posterior portion of the name refers to whether or not the needle is inserted anterior or posterior to the sternocleidomastoid muscle.

1. *Anterior approach.* Locate the triangle that is formed by two heads of the sternocleidomastoid muscle and clavicle. First, apply 1% lidocaine (lignocaine) to the apex of the triangle in order to anesthetize the skin. Insert the needle at the apex of the triangle, anterior to the muscle, aiming the needle toward the ipsilateral nipple at a 45° to 60° angle until the vein has been accessed. Be careful as to not aim too medially as there is a potential for puncturing the carotid artery.
2. *Posterior approach.* Local anesthesia with 1% lidocaine (lignocaine). Locate the sternocleidomastoid muscle and insert the needle three finger-breadths above the clavicle and posterior to the sternocleidomastoid muscle. Aim the needle towards the suprasternal notch at a 45° angle to the horizontal plane (Fig. 3).

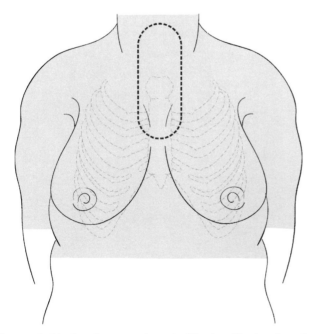

Figure 1 Positioning of patient with towel roll in place. The dotted area indicates where a roll of towel can be placed between the patient's shoulder blades. This can help facilitate access to the subclavian vein in an obese patient.

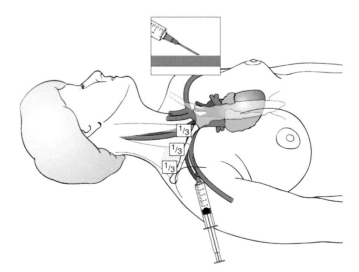

Figure 2 Subclavian venous access with the Seldinger technique. The 16-gauge needle should be inserted in an area that is two-third distal to the head of the clavicle with the bevel of the needle pointing down.

Passing the Guide Wire

1. Once the subclavian vein has been accessed, rotate the bevel of the needle toward the heart (i.e., the numbers on the syringe should be facing the patient's heart). If the internal jugular vein is used, then no rotation of the needle is necessary.

2. Remove the syringe from the needle and gently thread the guide wire through the needle. Remove needle once the guide wire has passed into the vein without resistance. Minimal force should be used as injury to the vein or the heart can occur if undue force is applied. Care should also be taken not to leave the needle hub exposed for a long time as inspiration by the patient can lead to an air embolism.

3. If PVCs are seen on the electrocardiogram (EKG) withdraw the wire until PVCs are no longer seen.

4. Fluoroscopy should be performed at this point to confirm the location of the wire.

5. Estimate the length of the catheter and cut with a pair of mayo scissors. The catheter should be long enough to go from the port site to the superior vena cava (Fig. 4).

Dilating the Skin Incision/passing the Catheter

1. Extend the skin incision with a no. 11 blade on either side of the guide wire. The incision should allow insertion of the port sheath without resistance.

2. Pass the inner dilator sheath over the guide wire. Pull back on the wire at this time to ensure the sheath is patent.

3. Remove the inner dilator sheath leaving the guide wire in place. Connect the inner and outer dilator sheaths and pass this over the guide wire. Again, pull back on the guide wire as the sheath is being inserted. Be sure to not completely pull out the guide wire.

4. Pull out the inner sheath with the guide wire in place.

5. Pass the premeasured catheter over the guide wire and then remove the guide wire.

6. Peel the sheath in half and slowly withdraw the outer sheath, stabilizing the catheter in place at the skin incision with a pair of forceps.

7. Access and flush the catheter with a weak heparinized saline via a blunt Huber needle to confirm venous access (Fig. 5).

Cut-down Technique

Venous Access via the Cephalic Vein

A transverse skin incision is made at the acromial end of the clavicle. Dissect the fascia over the pectoralis muscle and identify the separation between the deltoid muscle and the pectoralis major. Within this groove is the cephalic vein. Retract the vein with a 2-0 silk and make a venotomy on the anterior surface of the vein. Cannulate with the catheter. Check the placement of the catheter by fluoroscopy. Once the position of the catheter tip is confirmed in the superior vena cava, tie the 2-0 silk in order to secure the position of the catheter and to maintain hemostasis (Fig. 6A).

Internal Jugular Cut-down

A transverse skin incision is made 2 cm above the clavicle overlying the supraclavicular triangle. The dissection is performed to the level of the sternocleidomastoid muscle. Separate the muscle to expose the internal jugular vein. A 2-0 silk

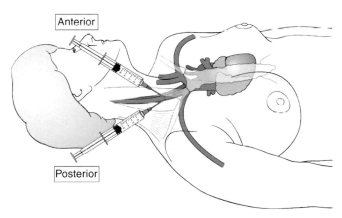

Figure 3 Internal jugular access with the Seldinger technique. The anterior approach involves insertion of a 16-gauge needle at the apex of the triangle that is formed by the two heads of the sternocleidomastoid muscle and the clavicle. In an obese patient where the apex of the triangle is hard to appreciate, the apex is approximately halfway between the sternal notch and the mastoid process.

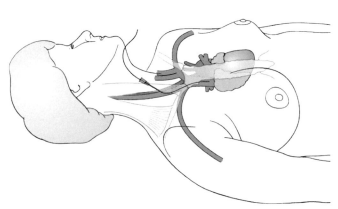

Figure 4 Passing the guide wire. It is important to perform this maneuver with very little force as there should be minimal resistance if the wire is going in the correct direction.

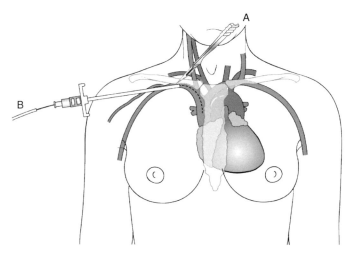

Figure 5 Dilating the skin incision and passing the catheter.

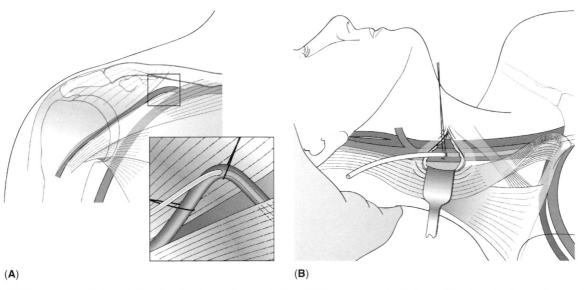

(A)   **(B)**

Figure 6 (**A**) Venous access via the cephalic vein using the cut-down technique. (**B**) Venous access via the internal jugular using the cut-down technique.

purse-string suture is placed in the internal jugular vein, followed by a venotomy. Once vein is cannulated with a catheter and the tip is in the correct position, tie the suture to secure the position of the catheter and to maintain hemostasis (Fig. 6B).

Making the Pocket for the Port
1. The site of the pocket should be lateral enough to prevent kinking of the catheter by the clavicle after the port reservoir and catheter are connected. The site should not be too caudal as the port pocket should be on the anterior chest wall and not the breast tissue.
2. Incise the skin with a knife and dissect posteriorly towards the pectoralis major fascia.
3. Once the fascia has been located, dissect out the pocket for the port inferior to the skin incision. Make the pocket large enough to accommodate the port reservoir without difficulty. Ensure hemostasis in the pocket prior to fixation of the reservoir (Fig. 7).

Creating a Tunnel for the Catheter
1. Tunnel subcutaneously towards the cephalad incision. The tunnel should be under the fat and not directly under the skin. Tunneling too close to the skin will not properly conceal the catheter.
2. Gently pull the catheter through the tunnel, taking care not to twist or kink the catheter at the insertion site.
3. Flush the catheter with weak heparinized saline using a blunt Huber needle to confirm venous return (Fig. 8).

Connecting the Port to the Catheter
1. Make sure the catheter is the appropriate length and trim as necessary.
2. Thread the locking device over the catheter.
3. Connect the catheter to the reservoir and place in the pocket. Care should be taken not to puncture the catheter.

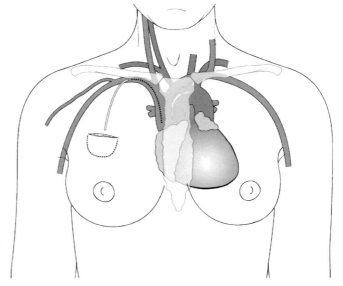

Figure 7 Making a pocket for the port.

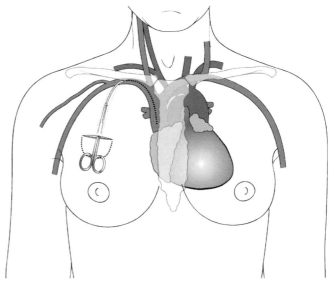

Figure 8 Creating a tunnel for the catheter.

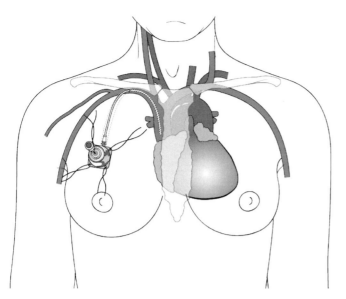

Figure 9 Connecting the port to the catheter.

4. Check the placement of the catheter tip by fluoroscopy. The tip of the catheter should be in the superior vena cava and outside of the heart.
5. Deploy the locking device.
6. Access the port through the skin with a sharp Huber needle. After accessing, flush with 10 cm³ of heparinized saline. Leave the needle in place and suture the port in the pocket (Fig. 9).

Checking Placement of Catheter
   1. A chest X-ray should be obtained after the procedure to confirm position of the catheter and rule out potential complications associated with the placement.
      • Pneumothorax may occur on the same or the contralateral side.
      • The catheter tip should ideally be just outside the heart and parallel with the long-axis of the vein. A good radiologic marker is the carina (Schuster et al. 2000).
      • Hemothorax.

Peritoneal Access Device
   1. Select the site for the peritoneal access device by the 9–10th rib, generally about 2 cm cephalad to the costal margin (Fig. 10).
   2. Once the site has been selected, make a diagonal skin incision 1 cm caudal to the costal margin and enter the peritoneal cavity.
   3. Create a subcutaneous pocket above the rectus fascia and on the rib cage about 3 to 4 cm in size and about 3 to 4 cm away from the incision site.
   4. Trim catheter to about 20–25 cm and insert into peritoneal cavity. Connect non-fenestrated end to the reservoir.
   5. Suture reservoir to the fascia overlying the inferior border of the rib cage.
   6. Close fascial incision around the catheter, with care to make the closure as tight as possible without kinking the catheter.

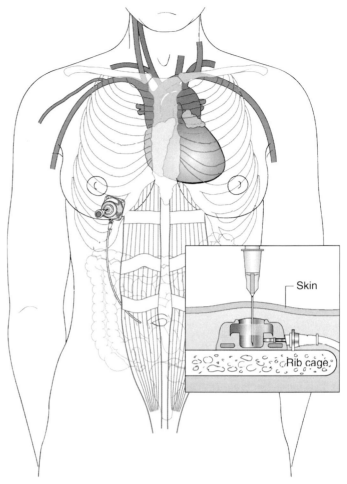

Figure 10 Placement of the peritoneal access device. The reservoir can be rolled up on the rib cage to provide a firm base while trying to access the device.

Maintenance and Access of Catheters

The purpose of routine maintenance of implanted catheters is to ensure venous access return and to prevent infection and thrombotic complications. Upper extremity deep vein thrombosis (DVT) in patients with central venous catheters is associated with pulmonary emboli in about 10% to 15% of cases (Monreal et al. 1994). The risk of upper extremity DVT in patients with implantable venous access devices is quite variable as most are thought to be asymptomatic (Monreal et al. 1996, De Cicco et al. 1997). One strategy to prevent catheter-related thrombosis is to use low-dose coumadin (1 mg/day). Such a low dose has little or no effect on the prothrombin time or activated partial thrombplastin time (Coccheri et al. 1999, Ratcliffe et al. 1999). In a prospective randomized trial, a coumadin dose of 1 mg/day has been shown to decrease the incidence of thrombosis from 37% to 10% without increasing hemorrhagic complications (Bern et al. 1990). However, care should be taken if mini-dose coumadin is given in patients on 5-fluorouracil based chemotherapy as this combination can lead to INR (international normalized ratio) elevation (Masci et al. 2003). Catheter tip occlusion is another frequent complication. One strategy used to reduce this complication is to flush the catheter regularly. In general, Hickman catheters are flushed once a day with heparinized saline (100 U of heparin/1 cm³ of saline). Although PAC devices have usually been

Table 1 Common Complications and Management of Central Venous Catheters

Complications	Incidence	Signs and symptoms	Management
Pneumothorax	0.5–5%	Shortness of breath, hypoxia, chest pain, decreased breath sound on side with pneumothorax	If <–30% pneumothorax seen on initial CXR and patient is relatively asymptomatic, repeat CXR in 4 hr, if no progression of pneumothorax and patient without symptoms, then observe. Repeat CXR in 12–24 hr. If pneumothorax enlarges or if the patient develops symptoms, then place a small pigtail catheter. See protocol below (Laronga et al. 2000). If <–30% pneumothorax with or without hypoxia, then place a small pigtail catheter with a Heimlich valve. Patient may be discharged home after insertion of pigtail. Have patient return in 24–48 hr for a repeat inspiration/expiration CXR with the pigtail clamped. If no pneumothorax seen then pigtail can be removed. Placement of large chest tube is indicated for persistent or worsening pneumothorax.
Hemothorax	Rare	Shortness of breath, decreased breath sounds, chest pain, shoulder pain	If a hemothorax is visible on a CXR, a chest tube must be inserted to prevent a clotted hemothorax and associated restrictive pulmonary function.
Air embolism	Rare	Unstable vital signs, cardiac arrest	Air embolism is fatal only if more than 50–100 ml of air is aspirated. This is less of a risk in intubated patients since there is no negative pressure with inspiration.
Cardiac arrythmia	Common, rarely occurs postop	Palpitations, changes seen on EKG (PVCs, PACs, or right bundle branch block)	If seen during procedure, this is secondary to catheter or guide wire presence in right atrium or ventricle. Right bundle branch blocks are seen with contact of the catheter with the right side of the ventricular septum. Treatment is to pull back on wire or catheter until EKG is normal. If present postop, then catheter should be pulled back and correctly placed and positioned.
Exit site infection	3–20%	Tenderness, erythema, and swelling at port site. Incidence of infection was thought to be higher in Hickman-type catheters, however this was not seen in a randomized trial (Mueller et al. 1992: 11)	The most common cause of infection is Gram-positive organisms such as *Staph. aureus, Staph. epidermidis*, or streptococcal species. Occasionally, Gram-negative organisms, such as *E. coli*, Pseudomonal species, and Klebsiella species, may be the pathogen. Polymicrobial infections with staphyococcal and pseudomonal species can also occur. Fungal infections may occur especially the candidal species. Rarer pathogens, such as Rhodotorula glutinis (a fungal species), *Chyrseobacterium indologenes*, and *Pseudallescheria boydii* have also been reported (Hsueh et al. 2003: 16, Nulens et al. 2001: 15, Perez et al. 1988: 13). Blood cultures (can only be taken from blood!!) should be obtained from the port site and a peripheral site (about 50% of infections will yield a positive culture) (Mueller et al. 1992: 11). It is important to distinguish potentially complicated from uncomplicated patients when treating port infections. Complicated patients are considered to be any patient with endocarditis, artificial heart valves, osteomyelitis, suppurative thrombophlebitis or presence of S. aureus in a patient who is immunocompromise or has active malignancy. In complicated patients, the port should be removed as part of the treatment otherwise port removal is not necessary as initial treatment (Olson et al. 1987: 381, Hiemenz et al. 1986: 37, Mermel et al. 2009: 49). Complete blood count should be obtained to ascertain the patient's granulocyte count. Initial treatment is aimed at Gram-positive species. Non-neutropenic patients should receive vancomycin (40 mg/kg/day) given through the port. Empirical coverage for gram neg bacilli should be based severity of disease (4th generation cephalosporin gentamicin). Neutropenic patients should receive zosyn/gent/vancomycin given through the port. Empirical therapy for suspected catheter-related candidemia should be considered in patients with the following risk factors: total parenteral nutrition, prolonged use of antibiotics or receipt of bone marrow or solid organ transplant. Treatment with the appropriate antibiotics should be given until WBC is normal, patient is afebrile and surveillance cultures are negative. Indications for PAC removal include: (1) unresolved, or worsening symptoms despite adequate antibiotic treatment; (2) persistent bacteremia after 72 hr of appropriate antibiotic therapy; (3) recurrence or persistence of positive blood culture after 14 days of appropriate antibiotic therapy and persistent fungemia.

(Continued)

Table 1 (*Continued*) Common Complications and Management of Central Venous Catheters

Complications	Incidence	Signs and symptoms	Management
Tunnel infection	Not distinguished from above	Induration, erythema, and tenderness over tunneled catheter	See treatment of exit site infection.
Bacteremia	Same as above	Fever, positive blood culture	See treatment of exit site infection.
Catheter tip occlusion	1–22%	Inability to draw back blood or infuse chemotherapeutic agent	Initial strategies include: (1) changing the patient's arm or head position; (2) have patient perform a valsalva maneuver (in case the tip occlusion is secondary to the tip being up against the wall of the vein) (3) flushing with 5–10 ml of normal saline; (4) flushing with 3 ml of heparinized saline (300 U); (5) repeated attempts to aspirate blood. If all the above maneuvers fail then consider thrombolytic therapy. Urokinase can be used in the following manner. 1. 5000 U of reconstituted urokinase can be given through the port. After the urokinase instillation, inject the port with 1–2 ml of heparinized saline 2. Wait 15 min and re-attempt aspiration 3. If this fails, then repeat the above steps twice for a total of the 15 000 U of urokinase instillation 4. If this fails, then instill 40 000 U of urokinase into the port 5. After 12 hr, another aspiration attempt can be performed.
Catheter fracture	Rare	Fairly rare event, most are asymptomatic and seen only on CXR obtained for inability to flush or draw from catheter (36%), pain/swelling by supraclavicular region (29%), shoulder pain (12%), palpitations (7%), pectoral swelling (5%), chest pain (5%), "swishing sound" during fluid infusion (2%)	Catheter fracture is thought to occur to secondary pinch-off syndrome where the catheter has been inserted too medially and is trapped (pinched) between the clavicle and the 1st rib. If the catheter fractures and embolus is suspected, CXR should be obtained. Prompt removal of catheter is necessary. This can be done through a transcutaneous approach via the femoral vein.
Venous thrombosis	1.5–62%	Progressive swelling of the arm or face. Most venous thromboses are asymptomatic, incidence of venous thrombosis in randomized studies where venograms were routinely performed whether or not patient has symptoms reveal an incidence of 38–62%	Anticoagulation should be started with heparin and switched over to coumadin. The duration of antiocoagulation is controversial. Given that these patients are hypercoagulable, a duration of 3–6 mo seems appropriate. Several studies have treated these port-induced thromboses with the port in place without problems. It seems reasonable to leave the port in place while the patient is on anticoagulation therapy.

Abbreviations: CXR, Chest-X-ray; EKG, electrocardiogram; PVC, premature reatricular contractions, PAC, Port-a-Cath; WBC, white blood cell count.

flushed once a month with heparinized saline, more recent data have shown that flushing once every three months is a viable option with a low rate of catheter tip thrombosis (Goldberg, pers. comm.). Routine flushing with heparinized saline has been shown to decrease thrombus formation at the catheter tip as well as catheter-related infection (Rackoff et al. 1995, Randolph et al. 1998). This may be related to the role that thrombus formation plays in facilitating catheter colonization and subsequent infection (Gilon et al. 1998).

Meticulous sterile technique should always be used when ports are accessed. Access of PAC devices should only be done with a none coring needle, such as a Huber needle. After accessing the port and confirming venous access, the port should be flushed with 10 cm³ of normal saline, followed by 5 cm³ of heparinized saline (100 U heparin/1 cm³ of saline).

COMPLICATIONS
Complications secondary to central venous access can be divided into intraoperative complications and postoperative (long-term) complications. Intraoperative complications include pulmonary complications, such as pneumothorax,

hemothorax, and air embolism. Intraoperative cardiovascular complications include cardiac arrhythmia, cardiac tamponade, trauma to a major vessel or the right atrium, and hemorrhage.

Postoperative complications include infections of the exit site, tunnel infection, and bacteremia. Mechanical complications, such as catheter breakage, catheter migration, and catheter tip occlusions, may occur. Upper extremity venous thrombosis occurs in a relatively high number of cases (reported as high as 62%) (Hsueh et al. 2003).

The most common complications of peritoneal ports are infection of the port site and inability to flush or infuse the catheter. Table 1 outlines the more common complications of central venous catheters as well as their management strategies.

REFERENCES

Bern MM, Lokich JJ, Wallach SR, et al. (1990) Very low doses of warfarin can prevent thrombosis in central venous catheters. A randomized prospective trial. *Ann Intern Med* 112(6):423–8.

Bock SN, Lee RE, Fisher B, et al. (1990) A prospective randomized trial evaluating prophylactic antibiotics to prevent triple-lumen catheter-related sepsis in patients treated with immunotherapy. *J Clin Oncol* 8(1):161–9.

Bow EJ, Kilpatrick MG, Clinch JJ (1999) Totally implantable venous access ports systems for patients receiving chemotherapy for solid tissue malignancies: a randomized controlled clinical trial examining the safety, efficacy, costs, and impact on quality of life. *J Clin Oncol* 17(4):1267.

Broviac JW, Cole JJ, Scribner BH (1973) A silicone rubber atrial catheter for prolonged parenteral alimentation. *Surg Gynecol Obstet* 136(4):602–6.

Coccheri S, Palareti G, Cosmi B (1999) Oral anticoagulant therapy: efficacy, safety and the low-dose controversy. *Haemostasis* 29(2–3):150–65.

Cole JJ, Dennis MB, Hickman RO, et al. (1972) Preliminary studies with the fistula catheter—a new vascular access prosthesis. *Trans Am Soc Artif Intern Organs* 18:448–51.

De Cicco M, Matovic M, Balestreri, et al. (1997) Central venous thrombosis: an early and frequent complication in cancer patients bearing long-term silastic catheter. A prospective study. *Thromb Res* 86(2):101–13.

Ecoff L, Barone RM, Simons RM (1983) Implantable infusion port (Port-A-Cath). *Nita* 6:406–8.

Gilon D, Schectes D, Rein AJ, et al. (1998) Right atrial thrombi are related to indwelling central venous catheter position: insights into time course and possible mechanism of formation. *Am Heart J* 135(3):457–62.

Henrickson KJ, Axtell RA, Hoover SM, et al. (2000) Prevention of central venous catheter-related infections and thrombotic events in immunocompromised children by the use of vancomycin/ciprofloxacin/heparin flush solution: a randomized, multicenter, double-blind trial. *J Clin Oncol* 18(6):1269–78.

Hickman RO, Buckner CD, Clift RA, et al. (1979) A modified right atrial catheter for access to the venous system in marrow transplant recipients. *Surg Gynecol Obstet* 148:871–5.

HICPAC (Hospital Infection Control Practices Advisory Committee) (1995) Recommendations for preventing the spread of vancomycin resistance. *Infect Control Hosp Epidemiol* 16:105–13.

Hiemenz J, Skelton J, Pizzo PA (1986) Perspective on the management of catheter-related infections in cancer patients. *Pediatr Infect Dis* 5:6–11.

Hsueh PR, Teng LJ, Ho SW, et al. (2003) Catheter-related sepsis due to *Rhodotorula glutinis*. *J Clin Microbiol* 41(2):857–9.

Laronga C, Meric F, Truong MT et al. (2000) A treatment algorithm for pneumothoraces complicating central venous catheter insertion. *Am J Surg* 180(6):523–6 [discussion 526–7].

Masci G, Magagnoli M, Carnaghi C, et al. (2003) Minidose warfarin prophylaxis for catheter-associated thrombosis in cancer patients: can it be safely associated with fluorouracil-based chemotherapy? *J Clin Oncol* 21(4):736–9.

Mermel LA, Allon M, Bouza E et al. (2009) Clinical practice guidelines for the diagnosis and management of intravascular catheter-related infection: 2009 Update by the Infectious Diseases Society of America. *Clin Infect Dis* 49(1):1–45.

Monreal M, Alastrue A, Rull M, et al. (1996) Upper extremity deep venous thrombosis in cancer patients with venous access devices—prophylaxis with a low molecular weight heparin (Fragmin). *Thromb Haemost* 75(2):251–3.

Monreal M, Raventos A, Lerma R, et al. (1994) Pulmonary embolism in patients with upper extremity DVT associated to venous central lines—a prospective study. *Thromb Haemost* 72(4):548–50.

Mueller BU, Skelton J, Callender DP, et al. (1992) A prospective randomized trial comparing the infectious and noninfectious complications of an externalized catheter versus a subcutaneously implanted device in cancer patients. *J Clin Oncol* 10(12):1943–8.

Nulens E, Bussels B, Bols A, et al. (2001) Recurrent bateremia by *Chryseobacterium indologenes* in an oncology patient with a totally implanted intravascular device. *Clin Microbiol Infect* 7(7):391–3.

Olson TA, Fisher GW, Lupo MC, et al. (1987) Antimicrobial therapy of Broviac catheter infections in pediatric hematology oncology patients. *J Pediatr Surg* 22(9):839–42.

Perez RE, Smith M, McClendon J, et al. (1988) *Pseudallescheria boydii* brain abscess. Complication of an intravenous catheter. *Am J Med* 84(2):359–62.

Raad II, Hachem RY, Abi-Said D, et al. (1998) A prospective crossover randomized trial of novobiocin and rifampin prophylaxis for the prevention of intravascular catheter infections in cancer patients treated with interleukin-2. *Cancer* 82(2):403–11.

Rackoff WR, Weiman M, Jakobowski D, et al. (1995) A randomized, controlled trial of the efficacy of a heparin and vancomycin solution in preventing central venous catheter infections in children. *J Pediatr* 127(1):147–51.

Randolph AG, Cook DJ, Gonzales CA, et al. (1998) Benefit of heparin in central venous and pulmonary artery catheters: a meta-analysis of randomized controlled trials. *Chest* 113(1):165–71.

Ratcliffe M, Broadfoot C, Davidson M, et al. (1999) Thrombosis, markers of thrombotic risk, indwelling central venous catheters and antithrombotic prophylaxis using lowdose warfarin in subjects with malignant disease. *Clin Lab Haematol* 21(5):353–7.

Schuster M, Nave H, Piepenbrock S, et al. (2000) The carina as a landmark in central venous catheter placement. *Br J Anaesth* 85:192–4.

25 Surgical management of trophoblastic disease

Krishen Sieunarine, Deborah C. M. Boyle, Michael J. Seckl, Angus McIndoe, and J. Richard Smith

INTRODUCTION

Management of trophoblastic disease in the first instance involves evacuation of the uterus. This should always be done using a suction curette and preferably with the help of ultrasound guidance. In the presence of persistently elevated human chorionic gonadotrophin (hCG) levels or continuing problems with hemorrhage, further evacuation may be necessary. This should normally be discussed with a gestational trophoblastic disease center because of the high risk of perforation, hemorrhage or infection. Thereafter, if the hCG levels remain elevated, chemotherapy should be instituted. The vast majority of patients will respond to these measures due to the inherent chemosensitivity of gestational trophoblastic disease (GTD). Chemotherapy produces high cure rates while maintaining fertility, allowing women to have further pregnancies.

For the small minority whose hCG levels remain elevated following chemotherapy, more definitive surgical management may be required in the form of a total abdominal hysterectomy. Elevated hCG levels predispose to ovarian cyst formation but this should not encourage bilateral oophorectomy at the time of the hysterectomy unless there is another pre-existing reason. Total abdominal hysterectomy in the presence of choriocarcinoma can prove very taxing. Uterine vascularity may be massively increased, presumably owing to the action of vasoactive peptides, etc., and the uterine arteries may be up to 1 cm in diameter. More troublesome still is the massive enlargement of the uterine venous plexus. This can lead to hemorrhage during ureteric dissection, particularly in cases where the tumor has spread beyond the uterus into the parametrium.

Preoperative assessment should include Doppler flow ultrasonography of the pelvis, CT and/or MRI scans of the chest, abdomen and pelvis, and an MRI of the head, together with hCG, full blood count and blood biochemistry measurements. GTD always produce hCG which allows screening and monitors treatment and follow-up. Four to six units of blood should be cross-matched. The authors have sometimes found it useful in the presence of extrauterine spread to perform ureteric stenting (see chapter 6). The laparotomy is performed, generally via a Pfannenstiel incision, but may require Cherney's muscle cutting or a midline incision depending on the surgeon's preference and the size of the uterus. In the presence of huge vessels, the authors have found it helpful to commence the procedure by opening the broad ligament, identifying the ureter and dissecting it in a cephalad direction as far as the bifurcation of the common iliac artery. Vascular elastic slings can be placed around the internal iliac vessels (Fig. 1). These vessels can be temporarily ligated prophylactically using bulldog surgical clips or the slings left loose until the need arises.

These slings have proved useful to the authors in the face of the torrential hemorrhage which may arise. Dissection of the internal iliac arteries then takes place inferiorly until the origins of the uterine arteries are identified, skeletonized, and ligated using either polyglactin ties or surgical clips. The ureter is identified running under the uterine artery. The multiple uterine vessels are ligated by applying three surgical clips to each vessel and transecting the vessel between them, leaving two proximally (inset in Fig. 1). In general the ureteric canal does not need to be opened; however if the need arises, this should be done as described in chapter 18. If a placental site trophoblastic tumor is suspected, removal of pelvic lymph nodes and para-aortic lymph nodes is advisable for gross lymph node disease involvement.

Excessive uterine manipulation should be avoided during the surgery when possible so as to reduce any possible risk of embolization of trophoblastic tissue. Because these patients may be hemodynamically unstable, it is recommended that these procedures should be carried out by an experienced surgical team at a specialized center providing full medical support, including intensive care.

PLACENTAL SITE TROPHOBLASTIC TUMORS

These are very rare tumors which are characterized by low levels of beta-HCG and can be single-site disease or multiple sites. They most commonly occur within the uterus. If single-site disease is only in the uterus on scanning by CT, MRI, color flow ultrasound, ± CT/PET, then depending upon the position of the tumor it may be possible to attempt a fertility-sparing procedure. Over the last three years, the authors have attempted this on five occasions with, to date, one long-term success. The other four patients have all had completion hysterectomy. Three of the four patients who had completion hysterectomy had it within a fortnight, one had no residual disease in the uterus and the other three did. The standard management for placental site tumors is pelvic lymphadenectomy and a total abdominal hysterectomy/radical hysterectomy depending upon the position of the tumor—those with cervical involvement requiring a more radical approach.

In a 13-yr period from 1993 to 2006, 25 cases were referred to the Chelsea and Westminster hospital and the West London Gynaecological Cancer Centre from Charing Cross hospital (the London center for GTD) for some form of hysterectomy for GTD. These 25 cases who underwent hysterectomy were drawn from 11,213 women who were registered at Charing Cross Centre for Trophoblastic Disease over that period of time. However, in addition to the cases referred to the authors, other cases will have been referred back to referring surgeons, and it is therefore not possible to give the percentage of overall patients who have required surgery. Many centers have

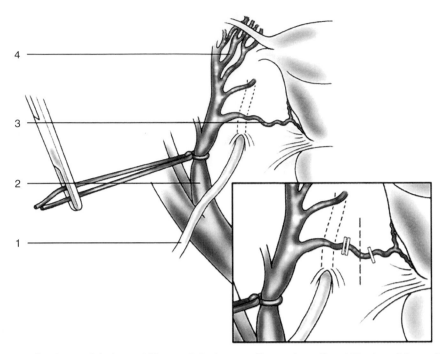

Figure 1 Vascular elastic slings are placed around the internal iliac vessels in the case of hemorrhage. (Inset) Ligation of the uterine artery (incision marked by dotted line). 1 Ureter, 2 Internal iliac vessels, 3 Uterine artery, and 4 Superior vesical arteries.

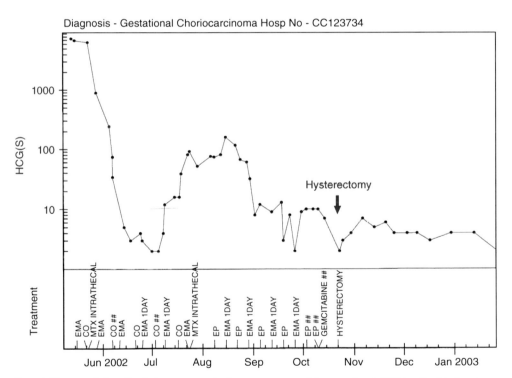

Figure 2 Therapeutic benefit of a hysterectomy in the management of chemoresistant GTD localized to the uterus.

published their experience in the management of GTD by hysterectomy with an incidence ranging from 1.5% to 35%.

In our group of 25 cases, 9 (36%) were choriocarcinomas, 6 (24%) were PSTT, and 10 (40%) were hydatidiform moles. The two main reasons for referral for surgical management were chemo-resistance of the tumor during the initial treatment episode and relapse after treatment. Of the 25, 9 (36%)

women had lymph node sampling. Of the 25, 11 (44%) had bilateral salpingo-oophorectomy concurrently. A radical hysterectomy ± unilateral parametrectomy were required in 3 (12%) out of 25 women.

Despite having a hysterectomy followed by chemotherapy, 3/25 (12%) of these women failed to survive. All were in the high-risk metastatic group. Their poor outcome was unrelated

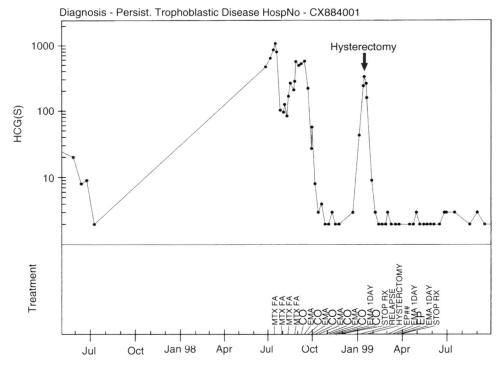

Figure 3 Therapeutic benefit of a hysterectomy during relapse of a GTT.

to the surgery but due to chemoresistant metastatic disease outside the pelvis. The review concluded that surgical management of primary drug resistant and relapse cases of GTD in the form of a hysterectomy is a useful and safe adjunct to chemotherapy and has a satisfactory long-term outcome.

Figure 2 illustrates the therapeutic benefit of a hysterectomy using serum ßhCG levels in the management of chemoresistant GTD which is localized to the uterus. Figure 3 illustrates the therapeutic benefit of a hysterectomy during relapse of a gestational trophoblastic tumor.

In conclusion, total abdominal hysterectomy for trophoblastic disease is rarely required. It may be required for the management of excessive uterine bleeding either at presentation or after the onset of chemotherapy and in the management of chemoresistant disease localized to pelvis. It is the treatment of choice in the management of placental site trophoblastic tumours confined to the uterus. When it is being performed, problems with hemorrhage should be anticipated and the suggested prophylactic measures should make uncontrollable hemorrhage less likely. Management of metastatic

choriocarcinoma outside the area of gynecological competence, for example, in the thorax or brain is beyond the scope of this book, but such tumors may well be amenable to management by the appropriate surgeon.

BIBLIOGRAPHY

Doumplis D, Al-Khatib K, Sieunarine K, et al. (2007) A review of the management by hysterectomy of 25 cases of gestational trophoblastic tumours from March 1993 to January 2006. *BJOG* 114(9):1168–71.

Hancock BW, Newlands ES, Berkowitz RS, et al., eds. (2003) *Gestational Trophoblastic Disease*, 2nd edn. ISSTD website: International Society for the Study of Trophoblastic Diseases.

Ngan HY (2002) The FIGO staging for gestational trophoblastic neoplasia 2000, FIGO Committee Report. *Int J Gynecol Obstet* 77:285–7.

Ngan HYS, Odicino F, Maisonneuve P, et al. (2001) Gestational trophoblastic diseases. *J Epidemiol Biostat* 6(1):175–84.

Pfeffer PE, Sebire N, Lindsay I, et al. (2007) Fertility-sparing partial hysterectomy for placental-site trophoblastic tumour. *Lancet Oncol* 8:744–6.

Sieunarine K, Rees H, Seckl M, et al. (2003) A review of the surgical management of gestational trophoblastic tumours from March 1993 to October 2003. *British Gynaecological Cancer Society Annual meeting*, vol. 22.

Smith JR, Bridges JE, Boyle DCM, et al. (2000) Regarding ligation of the hypogastric artery and blood loss. *Int J Gynecol Cancer* 10:173.

26 Laparoscopy

Farr Nezhat, Carmel Cohen, and Nimesh P. Nagarsheth

INTRODUCTION

This chapter describes the procedures of appendectomy, hysterectomy (both standard and radical), omentectomy, palliative end colostomy, and lymphadenectomy (encompassing both para-aortic and pelvic lymph nodes). Whole textbooks have been devoted to laparoscopic surgery but in line with the "cookbook" approach of this volume, we believe these procedures are more than adequately described in the following text.

APPENDECTOMY

Since the first use of laparoscopy for appendectomy by Kurt Semms in Germany and Nezhat and others in the United States in the 1980s and early 1990s, this procedure has become widely accepted.

Two different techniques have been utilized for laparoscopic appendectomy: one uses sutures, harmonic shears, or bipolar electrodessication for severing the appendiceal blood vessels; the other uses a linear stapling device across the mesoappendix and appendix simultaneously.

Indications

Appendectomy is frequently performed incidentally in association with other pelvic surgical procedures, or whenever pathological changes are identified as in patients with infection, endometriosis or benign or malignant tumors. In the staging and evaluation of certain ovarian tumors (such as mucinous borderline tumor or mucinous cystadenocarcinoma), the appendix is removed due to the high association of mucinous appendiceal tumors.

Anatomic Considerations

The appendix is an elongated vestigial diverticulum of the cecum which is richly endowed with lymphoid tissue. It is normally 7 to 10 cm in length but lengths up to 30 cm have been recorded. It receives blood supply from the appendicular artery, which is a branch of the lower division of the ileocecal artery. An accessory appendicular artery may be present in almost 50% of patients. The major vessels enter the mesoappendix a short distance from the base of the appendix. The location of the appendix is variable; up to 70% will be retrocecal and the remainder present primarily in front of the large bowel. Although it is usually found in the right iliac fossa, in maldescent of the cecum or advanced pregnancy the appendix may be seated in the right hypochondrium. In rare conditions, such as situs inversus, the appendix is in the left iliac fossa.

Surgical Procedure

1. Trocar and cannula placement: the primary trocar is placed infraumbilically for introduction of the video laparoscope. Two 5-mm secondary punctures are made lateral to the inferior epigastric vessels, one on the right and one on the left at the level of the iliac crest, and a 10-mm (or 12 mm if a linear stapling device is being used) puncture is made suprapubically 5 cm above the symphysis pubis.

2. After thorough evaluation of the abdominopelvic cavity any peri-appendiceal adhesions or attachments are lysed and the appendix is mobilized.

3. While the appendix is being elevated and put on traction, bipolar electro-desiccation is applied to the base of the mesoappendix for hemostasis of the appendiceal vessels (Fig. 1). After adequate desiccation, the mesoappendix is cut using sharp or electrosurgical scissors until the base of the appendix is reached. Caution should be exercised to avoid thermal injury to the cecum or the ileum.

4. Next, the base of the appendix is ligated by applying two polydioxal or chromic Endoloop sutures (Ethicon Endosurgery, Somerville, New Jersey, USA). The third Endoloop suture is applied 5 mm distal to the first two sutures. The appendix is cut between the two sets of sutures (Fig. 2). Alternatively, suturing is used for ligation of the appendiceal artery. An opening is made in the mesentery near the base of the appendix and a ligature of polyglactin is introduced into the opening. One ligature is tied around the base of the mesosalpinx and another is tied on the base of the appendix. Similar sutures are placed on the specimen side, and the appendix and mesoappendix are subsequently cut using sharp scissors (Figs. 3 and 4). A linear stapling device can be directly applied across the mesoappendix and the appendix, speeding up the procedure (Fig. 5).

5. After removal of the appendix, the abdominoperitoneal cavity is thoroughly irrigated. The appendix is removed through the 10 or 12 mm suprapubic trocar sleeve using Babcock forceps or by putting the appendix in a laparoscopic bag.

HYSTERECTOMY

Hysterectomy is one of the most frequently performed major surgical procedures in women. Approximately two-thirds of hysterectomies are performed abdominally and one-third vaginally. The purpose of laparoscopic surgery for hysterectomy is to avoid the adverse effects of laparotomy, maintain the principles of oncologic surgery, and offer the advantages of a vaginal approach. Since its introduction in the late 1980s, numerous variants have been developed, described by terms such as "laparoscopically assisted vaginal hysterectomy", "laparoscopic hysterectomy" or "total laparoscopic hysterectomy". While there may be technical differences and different

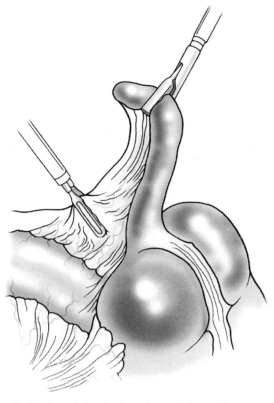

Figure 1 Bipolar electrodesiccation is applied to the base of the mesoappendix.

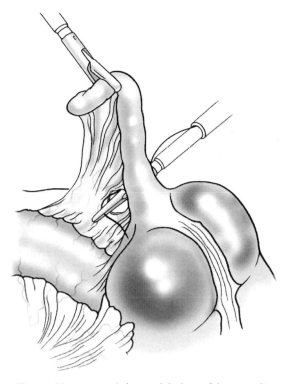

Figure 3 Ligatures are tied around the base of the appendix.

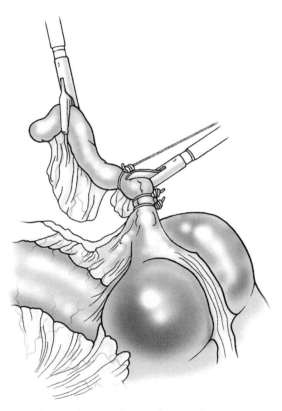

Figure 2 The appendix is cut between the sutures.

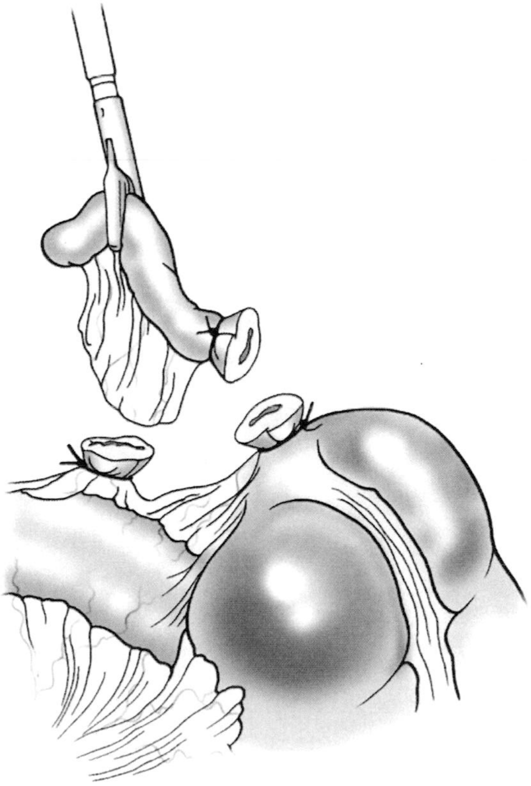

Figure 4 The appendix and mesoappendix are cut.

skill requirements between the various laparoscopic procedures, there is no significant difference in postoperative pain, recovery, complications, or cost. In this chapter, total simple laparoscopic hysterectomy and radical hysterectomy are described.

Indications

In gynecologic oncology, hysterectomy has been performed either as part of the treatment and staging of endometrial, ovarian, or fallopian tube carcinoma, in the form of intra- or

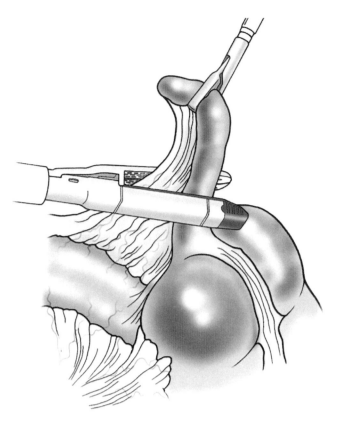

Figure 5 Linear stapling device.

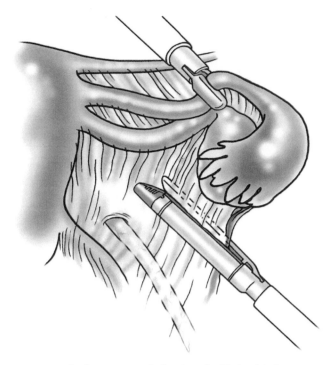

Figure 6 Bipolar forceps are applied to the infundibulopelvic ligaments.

extrafascial hysterectomy, or as radical hysterectomy for treatment of cervical and occasionally vaginal cancer.

Anatomic Considerations

The blood supply of the uterus is from the uterine artery, which anastomoses with the ovarian and vaginal arteries. The nerve supply is from the urogenital plexus.

Surgical Procedure

1. Trocar placement: as well as the primary intraumbilical trocar sleeve which is used for introduction of the video laparoscope, three other low abdominal trocar sleeves are introduced for the passage of the ancillary instruments. For hemostasis, bipolar electrodesiccation, or linear stapling devices are currently favored; suturing or the ultrasonic harmonic scalpel may also be used. For cutting, sharp, or electrosurgical scissors or lasers are commonly used.

2. After the anatomy of the pelvis is evaluated and any associated procedures (such as treatment of pelvic adhesions or endometriosis, or peritoneal biopsy) are performed, hysterectomy, and salpingo-oophorectomy proceed as follows. If oophorectomy is planned, first the infundibulopelvic ligament blood supply is severed using bipolar electro-desiccation, or a stapling device. The direction of the ureter crossing the pelvic brim over the bifurcation of the common iliac artery should be identified. In these patients the ureter can often be visualized, observed for peristalsis and avoided without mobilization. In obese patients, specific dissection may be required to identify and thus avoid injury to the ureter. Retroperitoneal or intraperitoneal ureteral dissection should be performed when there are severe adhesions or tumor involvement between the ovary and the pelvic side-wall. The adnexa should be grasped with the forceps and retracted medially and caudally to stretch and outline the infundibulopelvic ligaments before application of the bipolar forceps or linear stapling device (Fig. 6).

3. The round ligament is transected (Fig. 7) or electrodesiccated approximately 4 to 5 cm lateral to the uterus, and the anterior leaf of the broad ligament is dissected using blunt, sharp or hydrodissection. The bladder is separated from the lower uterine segment and cervix (Figs. 8 and 9). These steps are accomplished bilaterally.

4. While the assistant retracts the uterus to one side using an intrauterine manipulator, the uterine blood supply is skeletonized, and severed, using bipolar electrodesiccation or a linear stapling device (Fig. 10).

5. The direction of the ureters should be further identified and dissected laterally, especially for an extrafascial hysterectomy. The bladder is dissected away completely from the cervix and slightly from the upper vagina. The cardinal and uterosacral ligaments are electrodesiccated and cut or stapled (Fig. 11). For anterior and posterior culdotomy, a folded 10 cm × 10 cm gauze in a sponge forceps, or the tip of a right-angled retractor placed in the vagina, can be used to mark the anterior or posterior vagina cuff (Fig. 12). The vaginal wall is thus clearly demonstrated, allowing horizontal transaction with the cutting instrument. The uterus should be positioned anteriorly for a posterior culdotomy

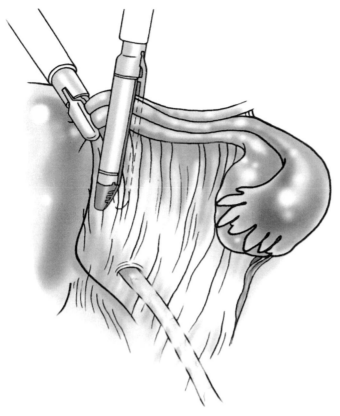

Figure 7 A stapler is used to transect the round ligament, ovarian ligament, and fallopian tube.

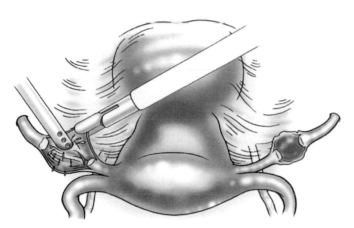

Figure 8 The anterior leaf of the broad ligament is dissected.

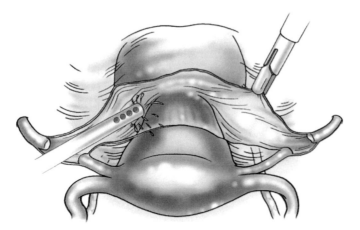

Figure 9 Hydrodessication of the bladder.

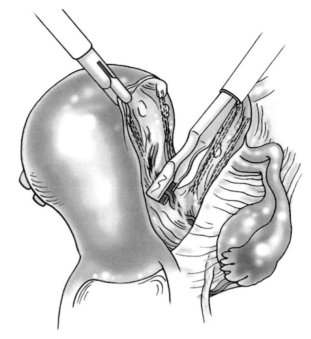

Figure 10 Uterine vessel dessication.

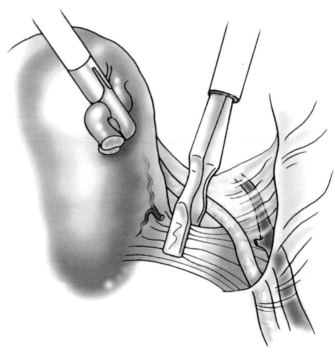

Figure 11 The cardinal and uterosacral ligaments are electrodessicated.

and posteriorly for anterior culdotomy (Figs. 13 and 14). The remaining attachment of the uterus laterally is circumferentially dissected and after the uterus is completely freed it is removed vaginally by introducing a tenaculum through the vaginal vault to grasp the cervix, or to pull the uterus out with the previously attached elevator (Fig. 15).

6. Vaginal vault closure and support: the vaginal vault can be closed either laparoscopically or transvaginally. In a laparoscopic approach to prevent loss of pneumoperitoneum, either the uterus or a

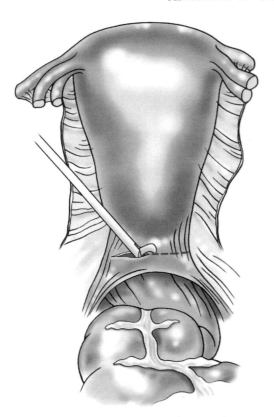

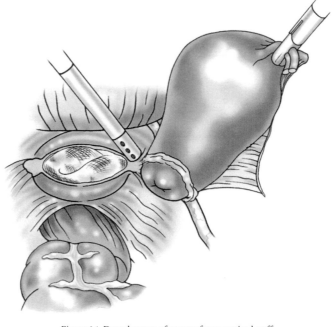

Figure 14 Detachment of uterus from vaginal cuff.

Figure 12 Marking the posterior vaginal cuff and performing posterior culdotomy.

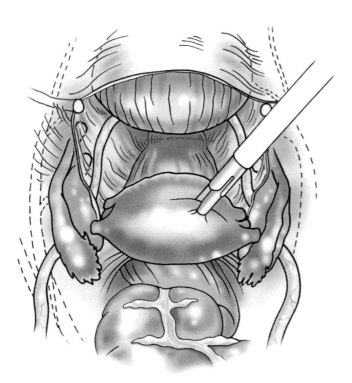

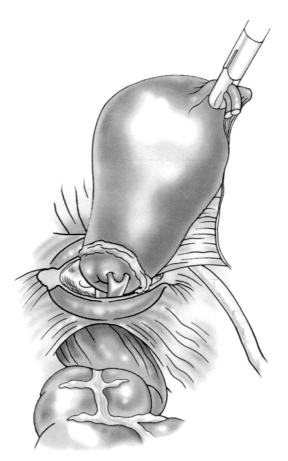

Figure 13 Anterior culdotomy. Anterior vagina is distended by placing sponge forceps attached to a 10 cm × 10 cm gauze transvaginally.

Figure 15 The uterus is removed transvaginally.

partially inflated surgical glove containing a folded wet gauze is left in the vagina. The uterosacral ligament is elevated with a grasping forceps and sutured to the vaginal angle on each side; the knot

tying may be extra- or intracorporeal. The vaginal cuff is closed in the middle using several interrupted sutures, or a single or continuous suture (Figs. 16 and 17).

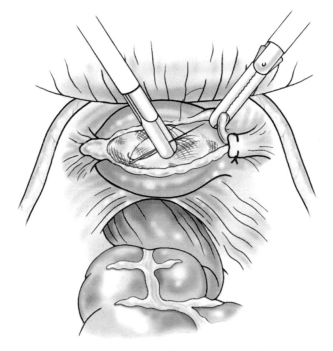

Figure 16 The vaginal cuff is closed in the middle.

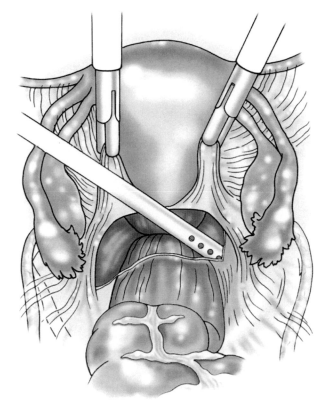

Figure 18 The cul-de-sac peritoneum is incised laparoscopically and the rectovaginal septum is developed.

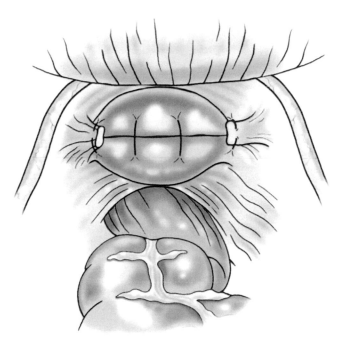

Figure 17 Final appearance.

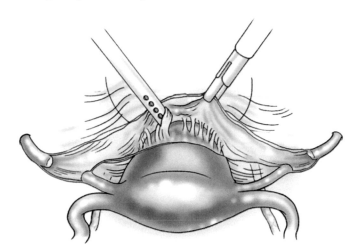

Figure 19 The vesicovaginal space is developed and the vesicocervical uterine ligament is dissected.

RADICAL HYSTERECTOMY

The most common indications for the radical procedure are stage IA2, IB, and IIA carcinoma of the cervix. Less common indications include small centrally recurrent postradiation cervical cancers, adenocarcinoma of the endometrium with clinical involvement of the cervix, and stage I to II carcinoma of the vagina.

Surgical Procedure

1. Development of the rectovaginal space: an assistant elevates the uterus with a uterine manipulator, and with the other hand performs a rectovaginal examination, delineating the rectum and the vagina. The cul-de-sac peritoneum between the attachment to the rectum and to the vagina is incised laparoscopically and the rectum is separated from the posterior vaginal wall using sharp and blunt dissection to a level of 3 to 4 cm below the cervix (Fig. 18). The pneumoperitoneum will help identify the correct plane.

2. Development of the vesicovaginal space: round ligaments are electrodesiccated and cut close to the pelvic side-wall. The peritoneum is incised lateral and parallel to the ovarian vessels. Anterior leaves of broad ligament are incised towards the vesico-uterine peritoneal reflexion. Using hydrodissection, or sharp and blunt dissection, the vesicouterine ligament is divided and the bladder is pushed off the cervix and the upper third of the vagina (Fig. 19).

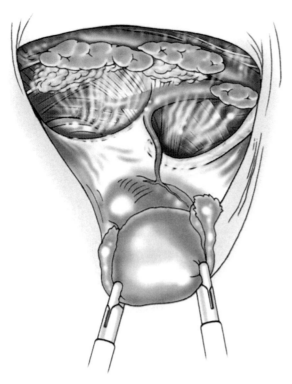

Figure 20 The paravesical and pararectal space is developed.

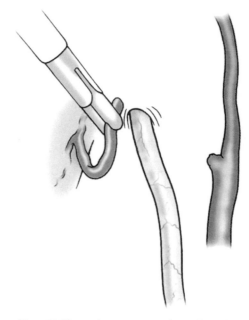

Figure 22 The uterine artery rotated over the ureter.

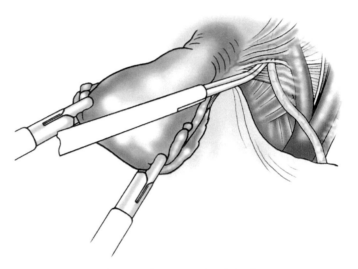

Figure 23 The parametrium is freed.

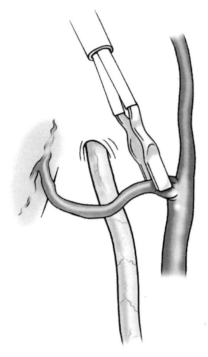

Figure 21 The uterine artery is electrodessicated or clipped at its origin from the hypogastric artery.

3. Development of the paravesical spaces: the obliterated hypogastric artery is identified and is retracted medially with a suction irrigator probe or a grasping forceps. The paravesical space is developed between the obliterated hypogastric artery and the external iliac vein (Fig. 20).

4. Development of the pararectal space: while the infundibulopelvic ligament and adnexa are retracted medially, the obliterated hypogastric artery is traced down until the ureter is identified retroperitoneally

and traced from the pelvic brim towards the bladder. While the ureter is retracted medially, the pararectal space is entered using blunt dissection between the hypogastric artery laterally and the ureter medially and posterior to the uterine artery. Ureteral dissection is performed and the uterine artery is identified at its origin from the hypogastric artery (Fig. 21).

5. Ligation of the uterine artery and unroofing the ureter: the uterine artery is electrodesiccated or clipped just medial to its origin, transected and rotated anterior to the ureter (Fig. 22). An angled tip clamp or the tip of the suction irrigator probe is used to widen the ureteral canal; an incision is made anteriorly, it is opened completely and the ureter mobilized. The ureter is unroofed from the ureteral canal and the parametrium is freed. Bipolar electrodesiccation, staples or surgical clips can be used for achieving hemostasis of the hypogastric venous plexus (Fig. 23). The uterosacral ligaments and the parametrium are stapled or electrodesiccated with bipolar forceps and

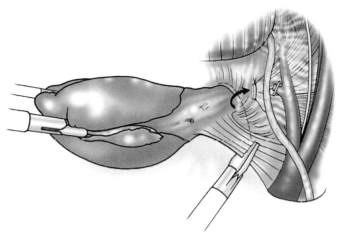

Figure 24 The dissection is taken to 2 to 3 cm below the cervix

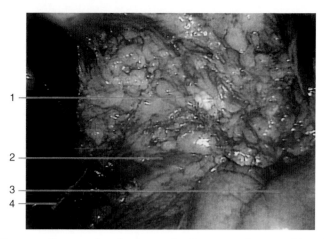

Figure 25 1 Omentum is under the stretch, 2 Transverse colon, 3 Small bowel, 4 Omentectomy is started from the hepatic flexure.

sequentially transected approximately 1.5 to 3 cm lateral to the cervix, based on the type of radical hysterectomy being performed. The dissection is taken to 2 to 3 cm below the cervix (Fig. 24). Anterior and posterior culdotomy are performed as described above. After removal of the uterus the vaginal cuff is closed either laparoscopically or vaginally.

OMENTECTOMY

Omentum frequently is involved with metastatic lesions whenever there is intra-abdominal spread of cancer. Omentectomy is part of the staging of ovarian cancer and is often performed in treating or staging other gynecologic cancers, such as uterine papillary serous adenocarcinoma.

Anatomic Considerations

The greater omentum is a fatty apron attached to the transverse colon and draped over coils of the small intestine. It is attached along the first part of the duodenum; its left border is continuous with the gastrolienal ligament. If it is lifted and turned back over the stomach and liver, it can be seen to adhere to the transverse colon along the latter's whole length across the abdomen.

The omentum receives its blood supply from the gastro-omental arcade which is formed by the anastomosis of the left (a branch of the splenic artery) and right (a branch of the gastroduodenal artery) gastro-omental arteries.

Surgical Procedure

1. Patient position and trocar placement: the patient should be lying flat or in a slightly reversed Trendelenburg position for better access to the omentum. Primary and secondary trocar placement is similar to that described for appendectomy. Although stapling or bipolar electrodesiccation can be used for hemostasis of the omental vasculature, the harmonic scalpel is preferable because of its unique advantages of reducing both tissue damage and smoke plume production.
2. The omentum is elevated using two atraumatic grasping forceps introduced through the 5-mm trocar sleeves. After exposure of the omentum and assessment of its relation to the transverse colon, a

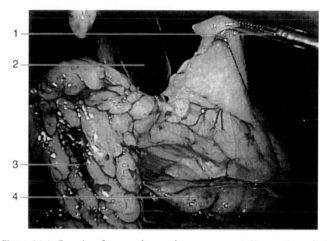

Figure 26 1 Grasping forceps elevate the omentum, 2 Harmonic scalpel, 3 Segment of detached omentum, 4 Transverse colon.

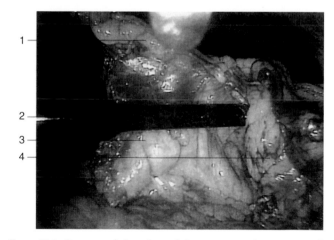

Figure 27 1 Omentum being elevated for exposure of transverse colon, 2 Harmonic scalpel, 3 Transverse colon, 4 Splenic flexure and part of omentum.

harmonic scalpel is introduced through the midline trocar and the omentectomy is started from the middle or the hepatic flexure, proceeding towards the splenic flexure at the line of reflection onto the transverse colon. Attention should be paid to avoiding injury to the colon and its mesentery and the short gastric vascular cascades (Figs. 25–27), especially if the anatomy has been distorted by the tumor deposit or adhesions.

3. After the omentum has been detached it can be extracted from the abdominal cavity in different ways. Following laparoscopic or laparoscopically assisted vaginal hysterectomy, it can be extracted through the vagina either directly or after placing it in a bag. Alternatively, the omentum can be removed through a 12-mm trocar sleeve or an enlarged anterior abdominal trocar site after enclosure in an endoscopic bag. Before termination of the procedure, hemostasis should be assured by decreasing the pneumoperitoneum pressure and evaluating the site of the resection. Individual bleeding sites can be treated with bipolar electrocoagulation, application of clips or suture techniques.

LAPAROSCOPIC BOWEL SURGERY

Laparoscopic bowel surgery is becoming more and more common in the field of gynecologic oncology. When performing laparoscopic bowel surgery, some helpful caveats to keep in mind include the following concepts:

1. In most colon resections, the colon becomes a midline structure and can be removed through a small periumbilical or infraumbilical midline incision.

2. A small bowel resection often does not require extensive mobilization of the bowel. Once the area of disease is identified, the loop of intestine to be resected can be brought out through an expanded port incision. The bowel resection and anastomosis can then be accomplished using traditional extracorporeal techniques. Because in most instances the bowel must be removed through an abdominal incision thereby allowing for the extracorporeal anastomosis, there is often no clear advantage to performing the technically more in depth procedure of intra-corporeal anastomosis.

SMALL OR LARGE BOWEL BYPASS
Indications

In general, indications for laparoscopic bowel bypass are the same as indications for bowel bypass in traditional open surgery in the gynecologic oncology patient. In this context, the most common indication is management of malignant bowel obstruction.

Anatomic Considerations

When performing bypass surgery for bowel obstruction, the surgeon must preoperatively assess the patency of the bowel distal to the planned bypass location to assure that another more distal obstruction is not present. Contrast radiologic studies and/or endoscopic procedures are the most commonly used methods to preoperatively study the bowel in preparation for surgery.

A thorough understanding of the bowel blood supply is imperative when performing laparoscopic bowel surgery. One must be cognizant of the "watershed" areas where blood supply to the bowel can be easily compromised, especially when performing bowel resections and/or anastomosis procedures. As a general rule, if mesentery ligation is required during the procedure, it is best to ligate the bowel mesentery prior to dividing segments of bowel to allow for visualization of demarcation areas (bluish discoloration of the bowel marking areas compromised blood supply). As always, care must be taken to avoid inadvertent ligation of the bowel mesentery when performing anastomosis procedures. This can generally be accomplished by following the classic anti-mesenteric to anti-mesenteric anastomosis techniques.

Surgical Procedure

Because laparoscopic bowel resections are often performed in conjunction with other procedures related to cancer staging and/or cytoreduction, we prefer a standard approach regarding setup and positioning for our patients. First, patients are positioned in the dorsal lithotomy position with adjustable stirrups.

The operating room is arranged with a standard setup of one or two video monitors placed at the foot of the bed. Monitors may be rotated to the patient's right or left side as different quadrants of the abdomen are explored.

In addition to standard laparoscopic equipment, there are three general categories of surgical stapling devices that are particularly useful when performing laparoscopic bowel surgery. These include the thoraco-abdominal linear stapling instruments (extracorporeal stapling), gastrointestinal anastomosis stapling instruments (both intracorporeal and extracorporeal stapling), and the end-to-end anastomosis (EEA) stapling instruments. Although we prefer the use of endoscopic stapling devices when performing intracorporeal bowel division and anastomosis, traditional suture techniques of bowel closure and anastomosis in one or two layers using polyglactin 910 (Vicryl) suture (or other appropriate suture materials) are also appropriate for the skilled laparoscopic surgeon.

1. Trocar placement: after abdominal insufflation via a traditional intraumbilical port, additional working ports are placed. Ports should be placed about a hands breadth apart to allow for adequate range of motion without interfering with other instruments. In most instances we use two lower abdominal ports placed two fingerbreadths medial and superior from the anterior superior iliac spine. Additional ports are placed in the upper abdomen either in the left or right upper quadrant to help triangulate in our operating field. For example, if performing a right lower quadrant bypass, we will use a 10 to 12 mm port in the left lower quadrant for to allow access for bipolar vessel sealing devices and/or endostapling devices. Similarly, if performing a bypass in the left lower quadrant bypass, we will use a 10 to 12 mm port in the right lower quadrant. Alternatively, a 10 to 12 mm midline suprapubic port (instead of in the lateral position) can perform a similar function while allowing access to the deeper pelvis.

2. After careful inspection of the bowel, the two loops of intestine that will be joined during the anastomosis are identified, mobilized, and are lined up side by side. If division of a bowel segment is required, it can be performed using the endoscopic gastrointestinal

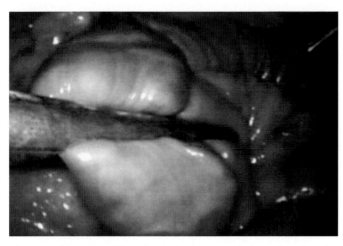

Figure 28 Although small bowel resection is not routinely performed during small bowel bypass, the technique of intracorporeal division is demonstrated here using the endoscopic gastrointestinal stapling device.

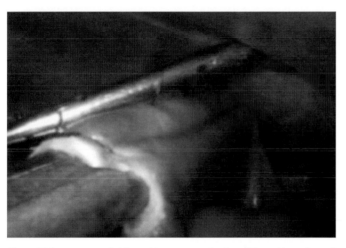

Figure 29 Intracorporeal side to side anastomosis of small bowel is performed using the endoscopic gastrointestinal stapling device. Two fires of the stapling device are performed (one in a proximal direction and one in a distal direction) to ensure an adequate lumen.

stapling device (Fig. 28) and division of the bowel mesentery can be performed using the ultrasonic shears and/or bipolar vessel sealing device. A stay suture (the "crotch stitch") of 3-0 Vicryl is placed via intra or extracorporeal knot-tying techniques allowing for stabilization of these two bowel loops.

3. A small anti-mesenteric enterotomy is made in each bowel loop using the electrocautery or ultrasonic shears device. With the bowel loops stabilized securely in place, an intracorporeal anastomosis is accomplished by firing the endoscopic gastrointestinal stapler one or two times depending on the desired length d the anastomosis creating a classic anti-mesenteric side to side (functional end to end) anastomosis (Fig. 29). As outlined in the anatomic considerations section above, extreme care must be taken to assure that the bowel mesentery is rotated out of the line of fire of the stapling device to avoid inadvertent ligation of blood supply to the anastomosis. The combined enterotomy is then closed using a running two-layer technique via a

laparoscopic suturing technique, or closed by using the endoscopic stapling device.

LOOP ILEOSTOMY

Indications

The most common indications for a laparoscopic loop ileostomy are to create a proximal diversion in the setting of a distal malignant bowel obstruction or bowel perforation, to protect a distal anastomosis, and to manage radiation-related bowel toxicity.

Anatomic Considerations

When performing a loop ileostomy, the surgeon must preoperatively assess the patency of the bowel proximal to the planned ostomy location to assure that a proximal bowel obstruction is not present. Contrast radiologic studies and/or endoscopic procedures are the most commonly used methods to preoperatively study the bowel in this regard.

As with all bowel procedures, a thorough understanding of the bowel blood supply is imperative. Please refer to the anatomic considerations section above on bowel bypass for more detailed information in this regard. For planned ostomy procedures, patients must be counseled and consented preoperatively about the possibility of requiring a temporary or permanent ostomy. An ostomy nurse or other qualified individual should carefully examine the patient in a variety of positions (lying, sitting, and standing) to determine the optimal location for the ostomy. In general, a loop ileostomy will be brought up in the right mid abdomen or right lower quadrant. The ostomy location should be anticipated when considering trocar placement keeping in mind that a trocar site can easily be enlarged into an ostomy site. As a general rule, the ostomy site should be overlying the rectus muscle, be accessible to the patient (both visually and manually), and not fall within the waistline or skin crease (which would make securing of an appliance difficult). Ideally, a patient may wear an appliance preoperatively as a "dry run" to determine the adequacy of the proposed site.

Surgical Procedure

1. Trocar placement: laparoscopic loop ileostomy is performed via three or four ports using a standard placement similar to that as described above for laparoscopic bowel bypass procedures. Ideally, the right mid or lower abdominal port site will also serve as the ostomy site.

2. To facilitate mobilizing the distal ileum, which is often the segment of bowel of interest in this procedure, the small bowel is mobilized by division of peritoneal attachments in the region of the ileocolic junction using a combination of both blunt and sharp dissection using the harmonic shears, bipolar vessel sealing device, or unipolar electrocautery device.

3. At the location of the planned osotomy site, a disc of skin is removed using the unipolar cautery. The dissection is carried down to the fascial layer and a cruciate incision is made approximately two finger breadths in diameter. The rectus muscles are separated bluntly and the posterior sheath and

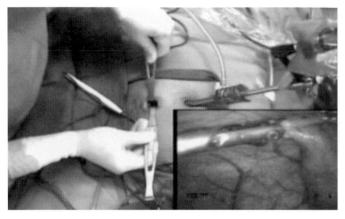

Figure 30 Creation of the abdominal wall defect (stoma site).

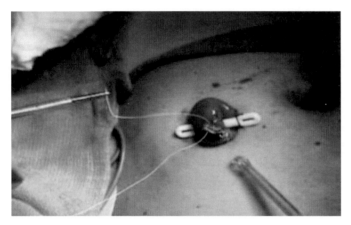

Figure 31 The mucosal edges are everted using a series of 3-0 absorbable sutures in a rose-bud type fashion.

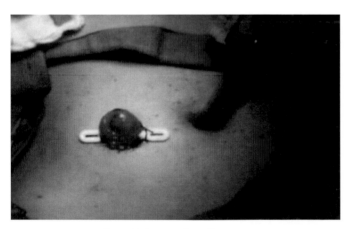

Figure 32 A mature loop ileostomy.

peritoneum are entered sharply (Fig. 30). After creation of the abdominal defect, the small bowel (typically distal ileum) is brought up through the stoma site and a window is made in the bowel mesentery just underneath the bowel wall (between vasa recta). A glass or plastic rod is placed through the window and rested on the skin.

4. The bowel wall is incised via a transverse incision closer to the distal limb and the lumen is entered. The mucosal edges are everted using a series of 3-0 absorbable sutures in a rose-bud type fashion (Fig. 31) and the ostomy is matured (Fig. 32).

RIGHT HEMICOLECTOMY
Indications
In the gynecologic oncology patient, the most common indications for right hemicolectomy are as part of a tumor cytoreduction procedure and/or management of malignant bowel obstruction.

Anatomic Considerations
The right (ascending) colon lies in close proximity to the duodenum, liver, right kidney, and right ureter. The surgeon must be fully aware of the location of the surrounding organs as well as the main blood supply to the right colon including the ileocoloic and right colic arteries, which originate from the superior mesenteric artery. The anastomosis between the main arterial supply from the superior mesenteric artery (right and middle colic arteries) and inferior mesenteric artery (IMA) (left colic artery) marks an important watershed area in the region of the splenic flexure. Whenever possible, resection of the right colon should be performed with preservation of the middle colic artery.

Surgical Procedure
When performing a laparoscopic right hemicolectomy, we follow the standardized techniques as described by Senagore et al. (2004) with slight modifications appropriate for the gynecologic oncology patient.

1. Trocar placement: a standard four port placement is utilized including an intraumbilical 5 mm port, right and left accessory ports (5 to 10 mm), and suprapubic port (12 mm).
2. Elevation of the right colic pedicle and transection of the vessels at an appropriate distance to allow for adequate surgical tumor margins.
3. Elevation of right colon and transverse colon off the retroperitoneum.
4. Entrance of the lesser sac with division of the gastrocolic ligament.
5. Division of the lateral peritoneal reflection.
6. Exteriorization of the specimen through a wound protector.
7. Extracorporeal division and anastomosis.

Following the "medial-to-lateral" approach the vascular pedicles are identified early in the procedure and are separated from vital structures such as the duodenum before division of the lateral peritoneal attachments. The vessels are transected with margins allowing for complete cytoreduction of tumor involving the bowel and mesentery (Fig. 33). Keeping the bowel attached to the lateral abdominal wall during this part of the procedure allows for counter traction and easier mobilization. Once the vessels have been transected, the lesser sac is entered by dividing the gastrocolic ligament and the hepatocolic ligament (Fig. 34). The lateral attachments are divided with sharp dissection using the unipolar cautery device and the bowel is easily mobilized and exteriorized. It is important to note that a lateral to medial approach is equally as effective and preference is based on surgeon expertise and preference. Although no large prospective randomized controlled studies have compared laparoscopic bowel resection versus open bowel resection in the management of gynecologic cancers,

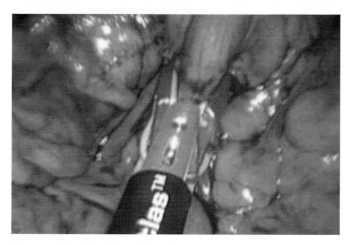

Figure 33 The right-colic and ileo-colic vessels are identified and transected using the bipolar vessel sealing device.

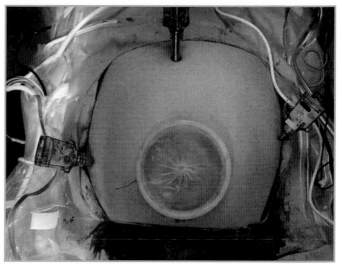

Figure 35 The use of a hand-port can facilitate laparoscopic bowel surgery.

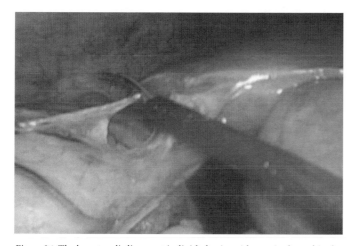

Figure 34 The hepatocolic ligament is divided using either unipolar or bipolar cautery.

extrapolating from the colorectal surgery literature suggests that outcomes would be equivalent.

LEFT HEMICOLECTOMY
Indications
In the gynecologic oncology patient, the most common indications for left hemicolectomy are as part of a tumor cytoreduction procedure and/or management of malignant bowel obstruction.

ANATOMIC CONSIDERATIONS
The left (descending) colon lies in close proximity to the spleen and pancreas, left kidney and left ureter. The surgeon must be fully aware of the surrounding organs as well as the main blood supply to the left colon from the IMA (left colic artery, sigmoid arteries, and superior rectal artery). The anastomosis between the main arterial supply from the superior mesenteric artery (right and middle colic arteries) and IMA (left colic artery) marks an important watershed area in the region of the splenic flexure of the colon. Whenever possible, left colon resection should be performed with preservation of the middle colic artery.

SURGICAL PROCEDURE
1. Trocar placemetnt: as a modification of the standard four port placement as described above, a hand assist device is placed as a suprapubic port through a lower midline incision or "mini" Pfannensteil incision. The incision is made slightly smaller (measured in centimeters) in size than the individuals glove size (Fig. 35).
2. Using a medial to lateral technique, manual retraction of the bowel facilitates mobilization and dissection. Because this procedure is typically performed in conjunction with other gynecologic oncology-related procedures, both the left and right pelvic sidewalls are typically opened and the pararectal spaces are developed allowing for identification of both ureters prior to proceeding with rectosigmoid colon resection. At a minimum, identification of the left ureter is mandatory prior to transection of the sigmoid arteries and superior rectal vessels. For routine rectosigmoid colon resections, it is not our preference to place ureteral stents.
3. Lateral peritoneal attachments to the colon can be divided using the unipolar electrocautery device after mobilization by finger dissection. The dissection is carried proximally with mobilization of the splenic flexure (this includes division of the gastrocolic, phrenocolic, and splenocolic ligaments).
4. Unlike the extracorporeal anastomosis in the right hemicolectomy procedure, the colorectal anastomosis during a rectosigmoid colon resection is routinely performed intracorporeally. After complete mobilization and division of the vessels, the bowel is divided intracorporeally at the distal margin of the specimen with the endostapling device (Fig. 36). The proximal bowel is externalized through the hand port or with a wound protector, and the proximal margin stapled (or divided) extracorporeally. The rectosigmoid colon specimen is sent to pathology and an EEA anvil is placed in the proximal limb and

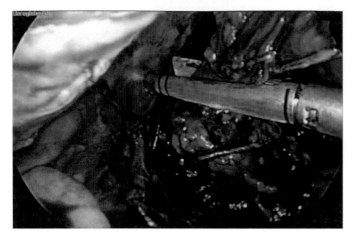

Figure 36 The sigmoid colon is divided using the endoscopic gastrointestinal stapling device.

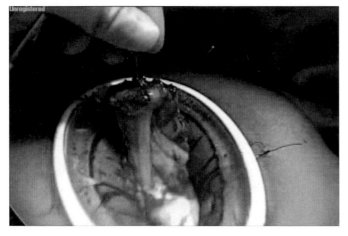

Figure 37 The anvil from the appropriately sized EEA stapling device is placed into the proximal colon and secured in place with a purse-string suture.

secured down using a purse string suture (Fig. 37). The EEA stapling device is then placed into the anus and advanced into the rectosigmoid colon and the spike is deployed through the rectal stump.

5. The anvil is attached to the EEA stapling device and the bowel limbs are fixed in position by tightening the stapling device. An anastomosis is then performed by firing the EEA stapling device.

6. The anastomosis line is visualized using a sigmoidoscope, and is tested for leaks by injecting air (a bubble test) and/or diluted betadine in the rectum. The "donuts" in the EEA stapling device are inspected and any defect found should alert the surgeon about the possibility of a corresponding defect at the anastomosis site.

PALLIATIVE END COLOSTOMY

In palliative end colostomy the fecal stream is diverted above the rectum. End sigmoid colostomy with a Hartmann pouch or distal exteriorization of the distal portion of the sigmoid colon as a fistula in lieu of the Hartmann pouch may be utilized. Palliative end sigmoid colostomy with the Hartmann pouch is most frequently employed in gynecologic oncology when permanent diversion is required.

Indications

Palliative end colostomy in gynecologic oncology is required when the distal bowel has been removed or is permanently unusable, as in the case of non-resectable pelvic tumor causing sigmoid colon obstruction or irreparable fistula caused by tumor or radiation necrosis.

Anatomic Considerations

The blood supply of the entire large intestine comes from the superior and inferior mesenteric arteries, with the former mainly supplying the midgut-derived right and transverse colon whereas the latter supplies the hindgut-derived left colon. The marginal artery of Drummond serves to connect the vascular territories of the two arteries.

The IMA arises from the dorsal side of the aorta often to the left at the level of L3, about 3 to 4 cm proximal to the bifurcation of aorta. After veering to the left it gives off the left colic artery which divides into ascending and descending branches. The sigmoid colon is supplied by two to four arteries. The first one, which is the largest, comes from the left colic artery (30% of cases) or the IMA. From this first sigmoid vessel, second or third vessels may originate, or may arise directly from the IMA. As the IMA enters the pelvis, it becomes the superior rectal (hemorrhoidal) artery.

Venous and lymphatic drainage of the large intestine follows the general pattern of the arterial supply.

Surgical Procedure

1. Patient 3position and trocar placement: the patient is placed in a supine position or slightly turned toward the right side. A principal intraumbilical trocar for video laparoscopy is inserted, with three or four other trocars for introduction of the ancillary instruments (Fig. 38). Two trocars are placed on the left side: one 12-mm trocar between the umbilicus and iliac crest for introduction of a Babcock clamp or linear stapling device, and one 5-mm trocar at the level of the iliac crest for introduction of a grasping forceps. One 12-mm midline trocar is placed 5 cm above the symphysis pubis for introduction of the stapler, clip applier, scissors or harmonic scalpel, and one 5-mm trocar on the right side at the level of the iliac crest for introduction of a grasping forceps (Fig. 38).

2. After thorough evaluation of the abdominal and pelvic cavity, the sigmoid colon is identified and mobilized from its attachment to the pelvic sidewall. By means of a Babcock grasping forceps introduced through the left trocar incision, the sigmoid colon is elevated. Electrosurgery, a harmonic scalpel or a stapling device is used to divide the mesentery of the sigmoid colon and a "window" is made. Vascularity of the proximal end of the bowel should not be compromised. While the bowel is elevated with the Babcock clamp, a laparoscopic linear stapling cutter introduced through the left lower quadrant trocar is passed across the bowel, which is then divided (Figs. 39 and 40).

3. After removal of the left lower quadrant trocar cannula, a disk of the subcutaneous fat at this site is incised and removed in preparation for location of

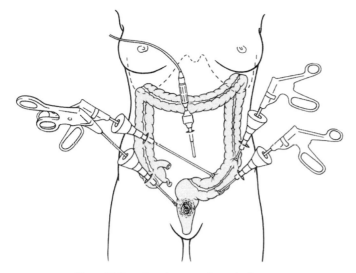

Figure 38 Port sites placement for end colostomy.

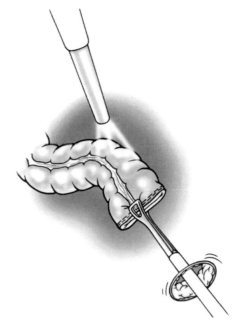

Figure 41 The proximal portion of the sigmoid colon is brought out through the incision.

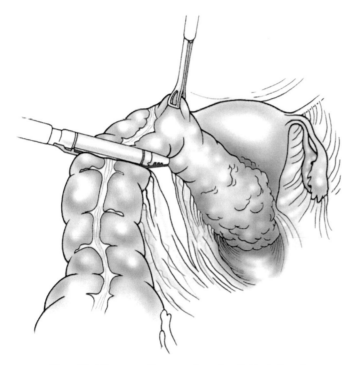

Figure 39 A linear stapling cutter is used to divide the bowel.

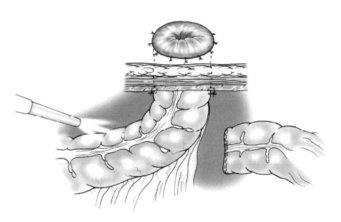

Figure 42 The serosa of the sigmoid colon is sutured to the peritoneum.

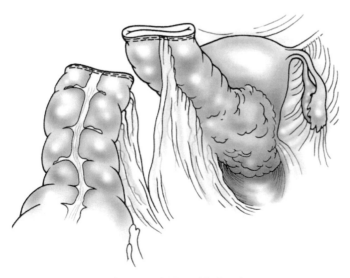

Figure 40 Division of the bowel.

the stoma. The fascia is incised and is enlarged using two fingers. Under direct laparoscopic visualization, a Babcock clamp is introduced through the left quadrant incision and the proximal portion of the sigmoid colon is grabbed and brought out through the incision (Fig. 41).

4. The stapled end of the proximal colon is removed and a "rosebud" stitch is used to evert the colon onto the skin, creating the stoma (Fig. 42). Laparoscopically the serosa of the sigmoid colon is sutured to the peritoneum for prevention of internal hernia, using 2-0 polyglactin.

LYMPHADENECTOMY

Since the initial descriptions of laparoscopic pelvic and para-aortic lymphadenectomy in the late 1980s and early 1990s, numerous reports have verified the feasibility and safety of this technique. Its advocates point to the better magnification, fewer complications and superior visualization of the anatomy of blood vessels and lymph nodes provided by the video laparoscope in comparison with conventional techniques. In the hands of the experienced laparoscopist the efficacy of laparoscopic lymphadenectomy is equal to—if not better than—that achieved during laparotomy, with fewer complications.

Indications

Laparoscopic lymph node resection is performed as part of the treatment of cervical cancer, and node sampling is performed as part of the staging for endometrial or ovarian cancer.

Anatomic Considerations

Para-aortic Nodes

The landmarks which should be kept in mind for para-aortic lymphadenectomies (Fig. 43) are as follows, from right to left:

- psoas muscle;
- right ureter, which is medial to the psoas muscle, lateral to the inferior vena cava and crosses the bifurcation of the common iliac artery;

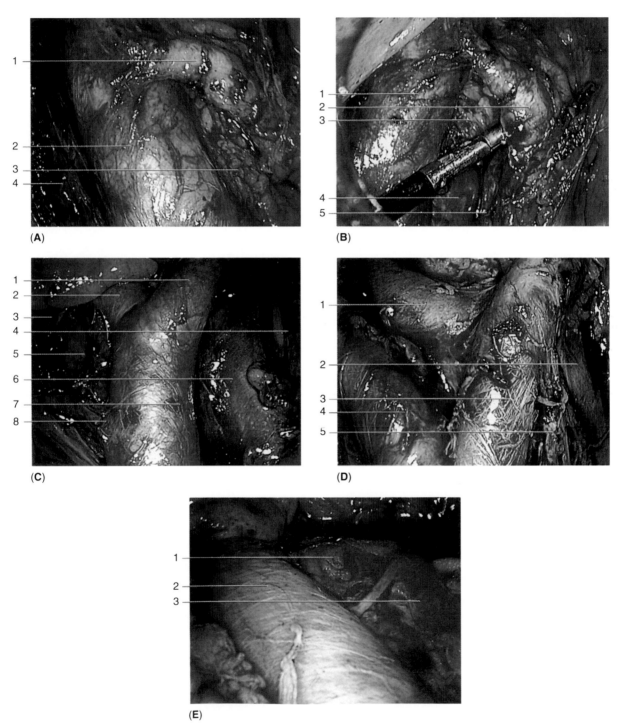

Figure 43 Retroperitoneal anatomy during para-aortic lymphadenectomy. (**A**) 1 Inferior mesenteric artery, 2 Aorta, 3 Left para-aortic nodes, 4 Paracaval nodes. (**B**) Grasping forceps is used to retract inferior mesenteric artery for identification of left ureter. 1 Aorta, 2 Inferior mesenteric artery, 3 Remaining left para-aortic nodes under the inferior mesenteric artery, 4 Left para-aortic area after lymphadenectomy, 5 Left ureter. (**C**) 1 Right common iliac artery, 2 Left common iliac artery, 3 Left ureter, 4 Right ureter, 5 Left para-aortic area after lymphadenectomy, 6 Vena cava, 7 Aorta, 8 Inferior mesenteric artery, (**D**) 1 Left common iliac vein, 2 Vena cava, 3 Right common iliac artery, 4 Left common iliac artery, 5 Remaining vena caval nodes. (**E**) 1 Midsacral vessels, 2 Left common iliac vein after lymphadenectomy, 3 Sacral promontory.

- vena cava (which is lateral to the aorta);
- aorta and both common iliac arteries;
- below the bifurcation of the aorta superficially is the superior hypogastric nerve plexus and beneath it is the left common iliac vein crossing from the left to the right;
- on the left side of the aorta are the IMA, the ureter, sigmoid colon, and its mesentery; the lumbar veins and artery are deep and can be seen after left lymphadenectomy;
- on the far left is the left psoas muscle.

Pelvic Nodes

The important landmarks for pelvic lymphadenectomy (Fig. 44) are as follows:

- laterally, the psoas muscle, the genitofemoral nerve, and the external iliac artery and vein;
- distally, the deep circumflex vein, superior pubic ramus, and obturator internus fascia;
- proximally, the common iliac bifurcation, and bowel;
- anteriorly, paravesical space, obturator nerve, and superior vesical artery;

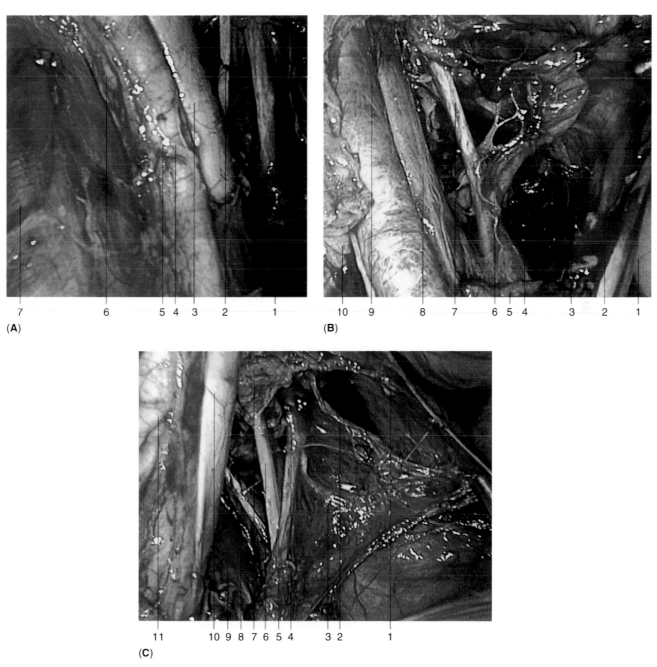

Figure 44 Retroperitoneal pelvic side-wall anatomy dissection during pelvic lymphadenectomy. (**A**) 1 Obliterated hypogastric artery (superior vesical), 2 Obturator nerve, 3 External iliac vein, 4 Left external iliac artery, 5 Genitofemoral nerve, 6 Left external iliac nodes, 7 Left psoas muscle. (**B**) Grasping forceps retracts peritoneum medially. 1 Peritoneum, 2 Left ureter, 3 Pararectal space, 4 Uterine artery branching from hypogastric artery, 5 Remaining hypogastric nodes, 6 Hypogastric artery, 7 Superior vesical artery, 8 External iliac vein, 9 External iliac artery, 10 External iliac nodes. (**C**) Grasping forceps retracts peritoneum medially. 1 Right ureter, 2 Superior vesicle artery, 3 Uterine artery, 4 Obliterated hypogastric artery, 5 Hypogastric artery, 6 Remaining obturator nodes, 7 Obturator nerve, 8 Obturator artery and vein, 9 Right obturator internus muscle, 10 Right external iliac vein, 11 Right external iliac artery.

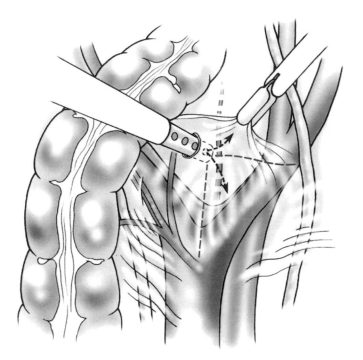

Figure 45 Exposure of aortic caval bifurcation.

- medially, the anterior division of the hypogastric artery and the ureter, and paravesical space;
- inferiorly, the sacral plexus, hypogastric vein, and pararectal space.

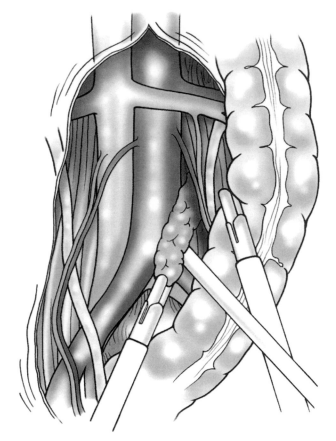

Figure 46 Renal vessel exposure.

Surgical Procedure
Para-aortic Lymphadenectomy

The operating room set-up, the patient's position, and the equipment may require minor variations. These include additional 5 or 10 mm trocars and positioning the video monitor at the head of the operating table, or using two monitors, one on each side of the patient: one for the surgeon's view and the other for the assistants. The surgeon can stand on the right or left side of the patient, although some prefer to stand between the patient's legs. As well as the umbilical port, three to four additional ports are necessary for introduction of the grasping forceps, scissors, and clip applier or bipolar electrocoagulator. The location of the ancillary trocars is adjusted according to the surgeon's preference. The patient is rotated to the left side for better exposure of the para-aortic area.

After insertion of the ancillary instruments and evaluation of the para-aortic area, the aorta is identified under the peritoneum up to the level of the mesenteric root. An incision is made over the posterior peritoneum at the level of the aortic bifurcation and extended towards the right iliac artery. The peritoneal incision is extended to the root of the mesenteric artery and, in the case of ovarian cancer, to the root of the left renal vein. Using two atraumatic grasping forceps, the peritoneum on each side is lifted and retracted laterally. Using blunt and occasionally sharp dissection with the tip of the suction irrigator or scissors, the retroperitoneal fatty tissue is dissected and the retroperitoneal vessels are identified (Fig. 45).

For left para-aortic lymphadenectomy, the rectosigmoid colon is retracted laterally and, after identification of the IMA and ureter, the nodal packet lateral to the aorta and above the left common iliac artery is resected using blunt and occasionally

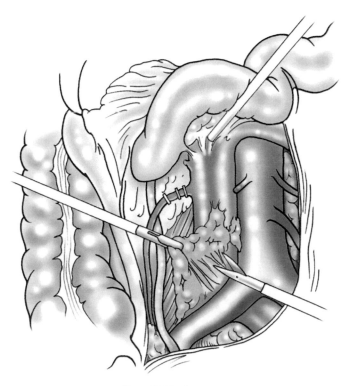

Figure 47 Caval exposure.

sharp dissection. Careful attention should be paid to avoid injury to lumbar vessels, the left common iliac vein, left ureter, and IMA. For ovarian cancer staging, the lymphadenectomy can be extended to the level of the left renal vein (Figs. 46 and 47).

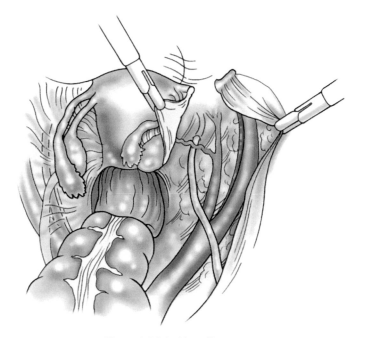

Figure 48 Pelvic side-wall exposure.

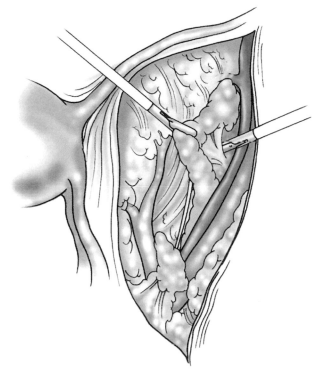

Figure 50 Obturator node removal.

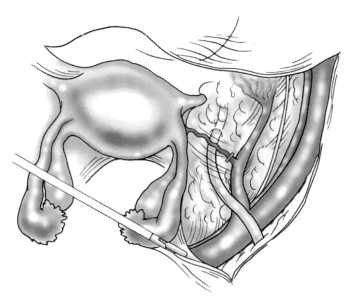

Figure 49 Obturator fossa exposure.

For resection of the paracaval nodes, the right ureter is identified and, while gentle traction is applied using atraumatic grasping forceps, the peritoneum and the ureter are retracted laterally over the psoas muscle. The nodal packet attached to the right common iliac artery is dissected off the vessels using blunt and occasionally sharp dissection. Using a laparoscopic Babcock clamp, the nodal packet is elevated and, using blunt and sharp dissection, the nodal packet is removed from the inferior vena cava. Care must be taken to avoid injury to the perforator veins. Clips or bipolar electrodesiccation can be used for achieving hemostasis. The level of the paracaval lymphadenectomy can be extended to the level of the right ovarian vein and, at times, the ovarian vein can be clipped and dissected for a better approach to the nodal packet in this area (Fig. 47).

Pelvic Lymphadenectomy

In addition to the primary intraumbilical trocar which is used for introduction of the video laparoscope, two ancillary 5-mm ports in the right and the left lower quadrants lateral to the inferior epigastric vessels at the level of the iliac crest and an additional 10-mm port in the midline 5 cm above the symphysis pubis are required. The lymphadenectomy may be performed either before or after hysterectomy. The procedure begins with an incision of the peritoneum between the round and infundibulopelvic ligaments, parallel to the axis of the external iliac vessels (Fig. 48). The round ligament is electrodesiccated and cut, the broad ligament between the round and the infundibulopelvic ligament is opened, and the psoas muscle, genitofemoral nerve, iliac vessels, and ureter are identified. Next the paravesical space is entered and widened by blunt dissection between the umbilical artery medially and external iliac vessels laterally. Caution should be exercised to avoid injuries to the external iliac vein and aberrant obturator veins (Figs. 49 and 50).

The fat and the lymphatic pad between the psoas muscle and external iliac artery are elevated, dissected, and removed distally and proximally toward the circumflex vein and common iliac artery, respectively. The nodal packet below the external iliac vein is grasped medially and, using blunt dissection, separated from the vein. While gentle traction is applied on the nodal packet medially, the obturator nerve is identified inferiorly and the obturator nodal packet is dissected and removed from the obturator nerve up to the level of the bifurcation of the external iliac artery; care is taken to avoid the hypogastric vein which often comes directly up from the pelvic floor. Inferiorly, the nodal packet is removed at the level where the obturator nerve exits from the pelvis. The fatty and nodal tissue between the obturator nerve and the external iliac vein is grasped and thoroughly separated from the pelvic wall by

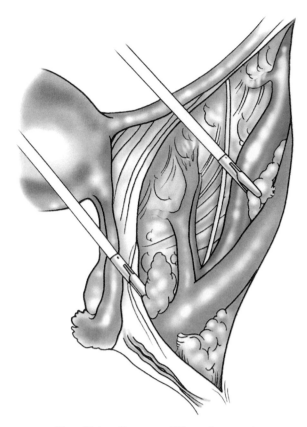

Figure 51 Interiliac-external iliac node removal.

blunt dissection using the suction irrigator or the closed tip of the grasping forceps. Clips can be applied before the removal of the nodal tissue. After removal, the pelvic bone and internal obturator muscle can be seen.

The lymphatic nodal package of the hypogastric artery is grasped and gently separated using blunt dissection from the external and internal iliac artery to the level of the division of the common iliac artery. Interiliac nodes between the external iliac artery and vein are removed (Fig. 51).

At the end of the procedure, the nodal package is removed through the trocar using a Babcock clamp or after placement inside the laparoscopic bag, and the area is thoroughly irrigated. Pneumoperitoneal pressure is decreased for evaluation of hemostasis; the peritoneum is not closed, and no retroperitoneal drain is applied.

BIBLIOGRAPHY

Abu-Rustum NR, Rhee Eh, Chi DS, et al. (2004) Subcutaneous tumor implantation after laparoscopic procedures in women with malignant disease. *Obstet Gynecol* 103:480–7.

Awtrey CS, Cadungog MG, Leitao MM, et al. (2006) Surgical resection of recurrent endometrial carcinoma. *Gynecol Oncol* 102:480–8.

Barakat RR, Goldman NA, Patel DA, et al. (1999) Pelvic exenteration for recurrent endometrial cancer. *Gynecol Oncol* 75:99–102.

Basse L, Hjort Jakobsen D, Billesbolle P, et al. (2000) A clinical pathway to accelerate recovery after colonic resection. *Ann Surg* 232:51–7.

Bradshaw BG, Liu SS, Thirlby RC (1998) Standardized perioperative care protocols and reduced length of stay after colon surgery. *J Am Coll Surg* 186:501–6.

Bristow RE, del Carmen MG, Kaufman HS, et al. (2003) Radical oophorectomy with primary stapled colorectal anastomosis for resection of locally advanced epithelial ovarian cancer. *J Am Coll Surg* 197:565–74.

Bristow RE, Santillan A, Zahurak ML, et al. (2006) Salvage cytoreductive surgery for recurrent endometrial cancer. *Gynecol Oncol* 103:281–7.

Bucher P, Gervas P, Soravia C, et al. (2005) Randomized clinical trial of mechanical bowel preparation versus no preparation before elective left-sided colorectal surgery. *Br J Surg* 48:1509–16.

Bucher P, Mermillod B, Gervas P, et al. (2004) Mechanical bowel preparation for elective colorectal surgery: a meta-analysis. *Arch Surg* 139:1359–64.

Ceraldi CM, Rypins EB, Monahan M, et al. (1993) Comparison of continuous single layer polypropylene anastomosis with double layer and stapled anastomoses in elective colon resections. *Am Surg* 59:168–71.

Chi DS, McCaughty K, Diaz JP, et al. (2006) Guidelines and selection criteria for secondary cytoreductive surgery in patients with recurrent, platinum-sensitive epithelial ovarian carcinoma. *Cancer* 106:1933–9.

Childers J, Surwit E, Tran A, et al. (1993) Laparoscopic para-aortic lymphadenectomy in gynecologic malignancies. *Obstet Gynecol* 82:741–7.

Clarke-Pearson DL, Dodge RK, Synan I, et al. (2003) Venous thromboembolism prophylaxis: patients at high risk to fail intermittent pneumatic compression. *Obstet Gynecol* 101:157–63.

Clinical Outcomes of Surgical Therapy Study Group (2004) A comparison of laparoscopically assisted and open colectomy for colon cancer. *N Engl J Med* 350:2050–9.

Conrad JK, Ferry KM, Foreman ML, et al. (2000) Changing management trends in penetrating colon trauma. *Dis Colon Rectum* 43:466–71.

Curran TJ, Borzotta AP (1999) Complications of primary repair of colon injury: literature review of 2964 cases. *Am J Surg* 177:42–7.

Dargent D, Mathevet P (1992) Hystérectomie élargie laparoscopico-vaginale. *J Gynecol Obstet Biol Reprod* 21:709–10.

Duepree HJ, Senagore AJ, Delaney CP, et al. (2002) Laparoscopic resection of deep pelvic endometriosis with rectosigmoid involvement. *J Am Coll Surg* 195:754–8.

Estes JM, Leath CA, Staughn JM, et al. (2006) Bowel resection at the time of primary debulking for epithelial ovarian carcinoma: outcomes in patients treated with platinum and taxane-based chemotherapy. *J Am Coll Surg* 203:527–32.

Ferron G, Querleu D, Martel P, et al. (2006) Laparoscopy-assisted vaginal pelvic exenteration. *Gynecol Oncol* 100:551–5.

Gillette-Cloven N, Burger RA, Monk BJ, et al. (2001) Bowel resection at the time of primary cytoreduction for epithelial ovarian cancer. *J Am Coll Surg* 193:626–32.

Giuntoli RL, Garrett-Mayer E, Bristow RE, et al. Secondary cytoreduction in the management of recurrent leiomyosarcoma. *Gynecol Oncol* 2007; 106: 82–8.

Goldberg GL, Sukumvanich P, Einstein MH, et al. (2006) Total pelvic exenteration: the Albert Einstein College of Medicine/Montifiore Medical Center Experience (1987 to 2003). *Gynecol Oncol* 101:261–8.

Guillou PJ, Quirke P, Thorpe H, et al. (2005) Short-term endpoints of conventional versus laparoscopic-assisted surgery in patients with colorectal cancer (MRC CLASICC trial): multicenter, randomised controlled trial. *Lancet* 365:1718–26.

Hatch KD, Shingleton HM, Potter ME, et al. (1988) Low rectal resection and anastomosis at the time of pelvic exenteration. *Gynecol Oncol* 32:262–7.

Hoffman MS, Lynch CM, Gleeson NC, et al. (1994) Colorectal anastomosis on a gynecologic oncology service. *Gynecol Oncol* 55:60–5.

Irvin W, Andersen W, Taylor P, et al. Minimizing the risk of neurologic injury in gynecologic surgery. *Obstet Gynecol* 2004; 103:374–82.

Jackson TD, Kaplan GG, Arena G, et al. (2007) Laparoscopic versus open resection for colorectal cancer: a meta-analysis of oncologic outcomes. *J Am Coll Surg* 204:439–46.

Lacy AM, Garcia-Valdecasas JC, Delgado S, et al. (2002) Laparoscopy-assisted colectomy versus open colectomy for treatment of non-metastatic colon cancer: a randomised trial. *Lancet* 359:2224–9.

Leahy PF (1989) Technique of laparoscopic appendectomy. *Br J Surg* 76:616.

Lewis LA, Nezhat C. (2007) Laparoscopic treatment of bowel endometriosis. *Surg Technol Int* 16:137–41.

Maxwell GL, Synan I, Dodge R, et al. (2001) Pneumatic compression versus low molecular weight heparin in gynecologic oncology surgery: a randomized trial. *Obstet Gynecol* 98:989–95.

Morrow CP, Curtin JP (1996) Surgical anatomy. In: Morrow CP, Curtin JP, Osa EL, eds. *Gynecologic cancer surgery*. Edinburgh: Churchill Livingstone. 67–139; 181–268.

Muzii L, Bellati F, Zullo MA, et al. (2006) Mechanical bowel preparation before gynecologic laparoscopy: a randomized, single-blind, controlled trial. *Fertil Steril* 85:689–93.

Nagarsheth NP, Bub DS, Nezhat F (2009) Laparoscopic bowel resection anastomosis, and ileostomy/colostomy. In: Covens Al, Kupet R, eds. *Laparoscopic Surgery for Gynecologic Oncology*, McGraw-Hill, New York, NY, USA, pp. 83–112.

Nagarsheth NP, Rahaman J, Cohen CJ, et al. (2004) The incidence of port-site metastases in gynecologic cancers. *JSLS* 8:133–9.

Nelson R, Edwards S, Tse B (2007) Prophylactic nasogastric decompression after abdominal surgery (review). *Cochrane Review* 2:1–31.

Nezhat C, Nezhat F, Ambroze W, et al. (1993) Laparoscopic repair of small bowel and colon. *Surg Endoscopy* 7:88–9.

Nezhat C, Nezhat F, Gordon S, et al. (1992) Laparoscopic versus abdominal hysterectomy. *J Reprod Med* 37:247–50.

Nezhat C, Nezhat F, Pennington E (1992) Laparoscopic proctectomy for infiltrating endometriosis of the rectum. *Fertil Steril* 57:1129–32.

Nezhat C, Nezhat F, Pennington E (1992) Laparoscopic treatment of infiltrative rectosigmoid colon and rectovaginal septum endometriosis by the technique of videolaserlaparoscopy and the CO_2 laser. *Br J Obstet Gynaecol* 99:664–7.

Nezhat C, Nezhat F, Silfen SL (1990) Laparoscopic hysterectomy and bilateral salpingo-oophorectomy using multifire GIA surgical stapler. *J Gynecol Surg* 6:287.

Nezhat C, Nezhat F (1991) Incidental appendectomy during videolaseroscopy. *Am J Obstet Gynecol* 165:559–64.

Nezhat C, Siegler A, Nezhat F, et al. (2000) The role of laparoscopy in the management of gynecologic malignancy. In: Nezhat C, Nezhat F, Luciano A, eds. *Operative Gynaecologic Laparoscopy Principles and Techniques*, 2nd edn. New York: McGraw-Hill, pp. 301–27.

Noel JK, Fahrback K, Estok R, et al. (2007) Minimally invasive colorectal resection outcomes: short-term comparison with open procedures. *J Am Coll Surg* 204:291–307.

Piver MA, Rutledge FN, Smith JP (1974) Five classes of extended hysterectomy for women with cervical cancer. *Obstet Gynecol* 44:265–70.

Querleu D, Leblanc E. (1991) Laparoscopic pelvic lymphadenectomy in the staging of early carcinoma of the cervix. *Am J Obstet Gynecol* 164:579–81.

Sakorafas GH, Zouros E, Peros G (2006) Applied vascular anatomy of the colon and rectum. clinical implications for the surgical oncologist. *Surgical Oncology* 15:243–55.

Salani R, Santillan A, Zahurak ML, et al. (2007) Secondary cytoreductive surgery for localized recurrent epithelial ovarian cancer. *Cancer* 109:685–91.

Semm K (1983) Endoscopic appendectomy. *Endpscopy* 15:59–64.

Senagore AJ, Delaney CP, Brady KM, et al. (2004) Standardized approach to laparoscopic right colectomy: outcomes in 70 consecutive cases. *J Am Coll Surg* 199:675–9.

The Colon cancer Laparoscopic or Open Resection Study Group (2005) Laparoscopic surgery versus open surgery for colon cancer: short-term outcomes of a randomised trial. *Lancet Oncol* 6:477–84.

Transatlantic Laparoscopically Assisted vs Open Colectomy Trials Study Group (2007) Laparoscopically assisted vs open colectomy for colon cancer. A meta-analysis. *Arch Surg* 142:298–303.

27 Robotic surgery
Rabbie K. Hanna and John F. Boggess

INTRODUCTION

The robotic platform has enhanced the role of minimal invasive surgery (MIS) especially in complex pelvic surgical procedures. In addition to the significant reduction in perioperative morbidity, mortality, and length of hospital stay, as has been proven with conventional laparoscopy, this platform has allowed for less conversions to laparotomy along with better surgical maneuverability while operating in the complex pelvis (Boggess et al. 2008a, b, 2009). The robotic platform, manifested currently as the da Vinci system (Intuitive Surgical, Inc., Sunnyvale, California, USA) has found its path into many of our complex gynecologic oncology procedures.

A description of the operative room setup, anesthesia challenges in addition to patient preparation and positioning will be discussed in this chapter. A brief description of key points of the operative procedures performed with the robotic platform will be presented.

ADVANTAGES AND DISADVANTAGES

The da Vinci robotic system offers the following:

1. A better and stable 3D operative visualization enhanced by the ability of digital zooming.
2. Seven degrees of freedom of articulation offering an improved dexterity coupled with elimination of the fulcrum effect.
3. Computer filtration of physiologic tremor.
4. Better ergonomics for the surgeon with the added benefit of increasing his/her longevity.
5. The learning curve is significantly enhanced as compared to conventional laparoscopy.

The disadvantages are summarized in the bulkiness of the robotic system necessitating dedicated operating rooms. To that note, the new Si Da Vinci system is smaller than the previous versions. The ongoing debate of cost has not been settled as more in-depth analyses of hospital finances is needed to settle this issue. Intuitively, it appears that the platform's advantages in optimizing operative times and minimizing complications translate to improved cost-effectiveness.

OPERATIVE ROOM SETUP

The current size of the robotic platform necessitates a larger operating room than that of a conventional laparoscopy setting. A well thought out operating room setup will optimize the surgical care provided to the patient. The setup should allow for easy communicability among all members of the operative team in addition to easy patient accessibility. Thus, an ergonomic layout of the various components plays a significant role in a smooth perioperative flow of events. We will discuss the setup we currently use for our gynecologic procedures. With this setup, both types of docking

(centrally between the lower limbs and side docking) are applicable.

The robotic platform (Fig. 1) is composed of a surgeon console, a patient side cart that is composed of the surgical cart and the robotic arms; and the vision system that is composed of the video cart that harbors two video control boxes, lights sources, and a synchronizer. The imaging unit is placed in a pivotal point of the surgical theater with the surgical console in the corner as shown in Figure 1. (The surgeon's console and the imaging unit are stationary.) The patient's bed is placed in front of the imaging unit, with the anesthesia team and the surgical cart, cephalad and caudad to the patient respectively. The console is placed in a corner allowing the surgeon to have visual communicability with the primary assistant and the anesthesia team (Fig. 1). Audio communication is enhanced by built in speakers through the console.

An accessory tower is placed to the side of the video cart. This contains the cautery sources, the light source and laparoscopy monitor for conventional laparoscopic equipment, and an insufflator machine. As shown in Figure 1, our operating room is supplemented with two additional monitors allowing both assistants to visualize the procedure from any angle.

PATIENT POSITIONING AND RELATED ANESTHESIA REQUIREMENTS

From an anesthetic standpoint, it is well known that most of our patients are advanced in age with multiple co-morbidities such as hypertension, diabetes, etc. These pose an anesthetic challenge and are managed according to pre-existing guidelines perioperatively which are not within the scope of this chapter. In addition to the preoperative visit and the necessary physical examination performed, all of our patients have their appropriate laboratory data reviewed by the primary surgical team and the anesthesia team as well. Additionally, they are interviewed and examined by the anesthesia team members.

All intravenous (or arterial) lines are to be placed prior to patient positioning. The patient is placed in a lithotomy position with the arms tucked to her sides after wrapping the elbows with a gel pads (to protect the bony prominences). Sponge padding at the level of the hands avoids pressure injury to the stirrup joints. Of note, the patient is placed in dorsal lithotomy position on a torso length gel pad. Shoulder blocks are placed above the acromioclavicular joints after the arms are tucked at the patient's side (Shafer and Boggess 2008). Insufflation of the peritoneal cavity with CO_2 is performed prior to placing her in the desired Trendelenburg position.

Due to this positioning, intravenous accesses need to be secured without kinks and compression. As the patient's accessibility by the anesthesiologists is limited, more than one intravenous access is necessary in addition to a lower threshold of using invasive monitoring which is judged based on the combined experience and comfort level of both the surgical and anesthesia teams. As the surgical cart is placed in between the patient's lower limbs, care should be taken to position the limbs in a manner that will avoid contact with the mobile elements of the cart keeping in mind not to extend the hip joint excessively and cause femoral nerve injury.

The patient is ventilated with pressure control rather than volume control that helps to minimize wide excursion and movement during dissection and reduces the risk of barotrauma. Pressure-controlled anesthesia is mandatory for obese women placed in a steep Trendelenburg position (Shafer and Boggess 2008).

Decompression of the stomach contents via an oro-gastric or naso-gastric tube is necessary. Kinking of the endotracheal tube or its dislodgement is of concern when the robot is docked over the patient's head as advocated by some of our colleagues.

Once the platform is docked, the patient's position cannot be altered; thus, it is essential to place the patient in the desired Trendelenburg position and adjust accordingly before docking the system. Thus complete immobility via muscle relaxation is required and should be monitored for prior to docking the system. All members of the surgical team should be trained in emergency undocking if the situation arises. This requires prompt and clear communication among the surgical and anesthesia team members. As noted in our current operating room setup (Fig. 1), the anesthesiology team and their equipments' position are not in contact with robotic components.

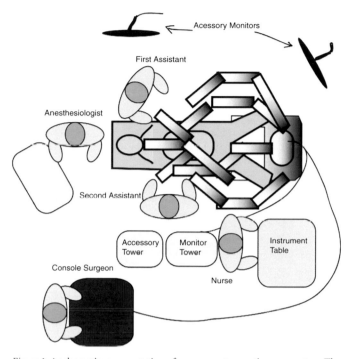

Figure 1 A schematic representation of our current operating room setup. The surgeon is in direct visual communication with the bedside assistant (first assistant) and the anesthesiologist. Two adjustable accessory monitors are available for use by the assistants and observers from different angles of the operating room.

OPERATIVE ENTRY

We start all our robotic procedures in the same fashion from an entry standpoint. After appropriate sterilization and draping of the patient, a incision of 2 to 3 mm is made in Palmar's point and a 2-mm trocar is inserted into the peritoneal cavity followed by insufflation with CO_2 with a goal of 12 to 15 mmHg intra-abdominal pressure. A survey of the abdomen and pelvis is then performed with a 2-mm laparoscope. The patient is then placed in the maximum tolerated Trendelenburg position. The abdomen is marked for the appropriate procedure (Figs. 2 and 3). Any adhesions are taken down using conventional laparoscopic techniques unless they can be done robotically.

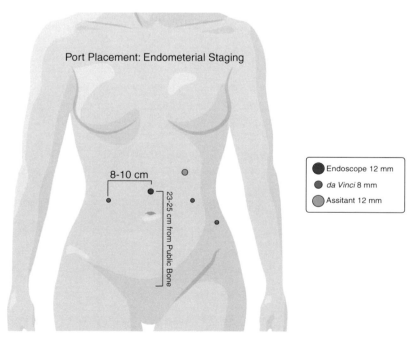

Figure 2 The port placement for robotic-assisted endometrial staging. If the surgeon is not planning on para-aortic lymph node dissection, we recommend using the port placement in Figure 3. *Source:* Photo courtesy of John F. Boggess, 2010.

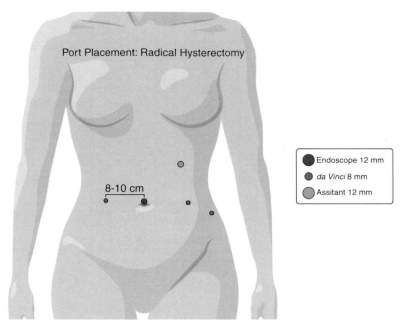

Figure 3 The port placement for robotically assisted radical hysterectomy, radical trachelectomy, and radical parametrectomy. *Source*: Photo courtesy of John F. Boggess, 2010.

SURGICAL PROCEDURES

In this section, we describe port placements for each surgical procedure, discuss the instruments used in addition to tips and challenging points if applicable.

Endometrial Cancer Staging

Robotic-assisted endometrial cancer staging has been a significant application of robotics in gynecologic oncology (Boggess 2007). The port site configuration we advocate in robotic staging of endometrial cancer is shown in Figure 2. After entry via the LUQ and insufflation of the peritoneal cavity, the camera port is marked 23 to 25 cm above the symphysis pubis. The two lateral ports are placed at 15° below and 10 cm away from the camera port. A third port site is marked 10 cm away from the left laterally toward the left anterior–superior iliac spine. A 10 to 12 bladeless trocar is used for the camera site, the 8-mm robotic trocars are placed in their respective ports, and the assistant port is converted to a 10 to 12 port (which allows introduction of Rayteks sponges and introduction of endoscopic pouches).

Instruments

    A zero degree camera.

    Zumi™ Uterine manipulator and Kho™ rings for delineation of the vaginal cuff.

    Hot Shears™ (Monopolar Curved Scissors) used for dissection in addition to cold and hot cutting and monopolar cautery.

    Fenestrated bipolar forceps, which has the capability of coagulating the uterine and ovarian vessels eliminating the need for laparoscopic vascular clips. Another fenestrated forceps is applied to the third arm to assist in intraoperative retraction.

    Suture Cut™ Needle Driver for vaginal cuff closure.

Surgical Tips

    Many endometrial cancer patients are obese; thus, a gradual rather than sudden Trendelenburg positioning illustrates the real capacity of how much can be tolerated by the patient.

    The curved abdomen in obese patients allows for a larger surface area for port placement.

    The procedure begins with the para-aortic lymph node dissection (PA-LND) to avoid accumulation of blood and fluid from the pelvic part of the procedure. During this part of the surgery, we ask the anesthesiologist to run the patient dry to minimize the excursion of the inferior vena cava during the lymph node dissection.

Fold the bowel to uncover the root of the mesentery (Fig. 4) in preparation of PA-LND prior to docking the robotic system but after maintaining Trendelenburg positioning. This is done utilizing a 45-cm bariatric atraumatic laparoscopic grasper. The distal small bowel is folded toward the right (Fig. 4B) whereas the proximal bowel loops are folded to the left side and slightly cephalad (Fig. 4A). Folding the bowel should be performed elegantly without pushing the bowel into the upper abdomen. In some occasions a Raytek sponge may be inserted (Fig. 4C) to prevent some small intestine loops from slipping into the operative field (Fig. 4D). In patients with a short small bowel mesentery, the peritoneal incision over the aortic root will effectively lengthen it and the edge can be tented upward by the assistant using a laparoscopic grasper to create a shield against the small bowel loops cephalad to it (Fig. 5).

On rare occasions, adhesions in the upper abdomen could assist as natural retractors in holding the small

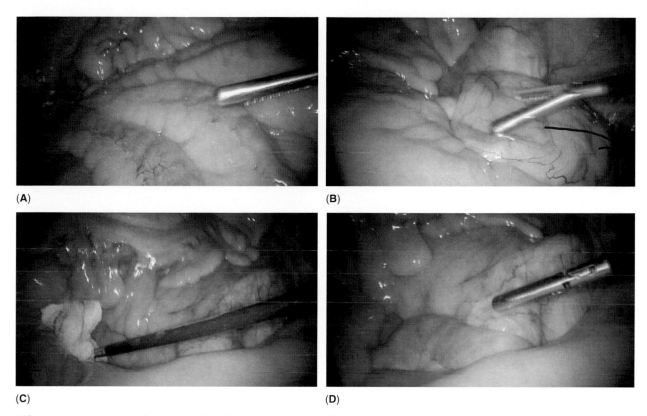

(A)   (B)

(C)   (D)

Figure 4 The appropriate para-aortic lymph node dissection exposure is achieved by folding the small bowel loops systematically using a 45-cm bariatric atraumatic laparoscopic grasper. (**A**) The proximal bowel loops are folded toward the left upper quadrant, loop by loop starting with the most cephalad loops. (**B**) The distal small bowel is folded toward the right. (**C**) A Raytek sponge may be inserted to prevent some small intestine loops from slipping into the operative field as shown in **D**.

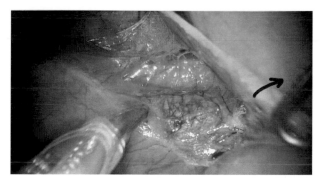

Figure 5 In patients with a short small bowel mesentery, the peritoneal incision over the aortic root will effectively lengthen it, and the edge can be tented upward by the assistant using a laparoscopic grasper to create a shield against the small bowel loops cephalad to it. The site of the arrow is where the grasper will be placed.

bowel in place; thus, lysis of adhesions should be performed in a strategic manner.

In patients with a redundant sigmoid colon that might overlay the root of the aorta, a figure-of-eight suture can be placed through the tenia coli and sutured to the anterior abdominal wall.

While performing the PA-LND, the surgeon can achieve an easier dissection by placing the shears in the second robotic arm to be operated by the surgeon's left hand. Of note, the camera is rotated 90° so that the aorta lies horizontal with its most cephalad end to be located on the right of the surgical field.

We advocate utilizing the robotic equipment rather than foreign apparatuses for vessel coagulation to minimize time without sacrificing technique and outcomes. Bipolar cautery is safe for vessels up to 8 mm in diameter. The cautery's current setting should be set at 45 W.

Utilizing the least amount of cautery while performing the colpotomy minimizes the thermal injury to vaginal cuff and decreases the chance of cuff dehiscence postoperatively. Using a single-blade maneuver during colpotomy will also minimize the thermal injury but increases the possibility of vaginal cuff bleeders that can be controlled with pin-point cautery or while suturing the cuff.

A water seal vaginal cuff closure can be performed by holding the suture tightly by the assistance of the assistant utilizing a laparoscopic needle holder while the console surgeon is suturing the cuff (Fig. 6).

Utilize the third arm as a retractor as much as possible. This allows for better control over the surgical field by the surgeon himself and the assistant will be freed from unnecessary stationary postures.

Radical Hysterectomy, Radical Trachelectomy, and Radical Parametrectomy

The port site configuration we advocate in these procedures is shown in Figure 3. After entry via the LUQ and insufflation of the peritoneal cavity, the camera port is marked at the supraumbilical site. The two lateral ports are placed 10 cm away

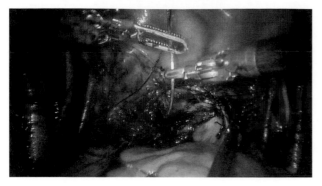

Figure 6 The assistant uses a laparoscopic needle driver to hold the suture on tension while console surgeon is suturing the vaginal cuff. This allows for a secure approximation of the vaginal cuff.

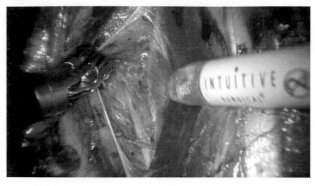

Figure 7 Portion of the right pelvic lymph node dissection depicting an efficient method to locate the obturator nerve and release the most lateral attachments of the lymphatic bundle from the pelvic sidewall muscles, the space is approached lateral to the external iliac vessels.

from the camera port maintaining a straight line across all three port sites. A third port site is marked 10 cm away from the left lateral toward the left anterior superior iliac spine. A 10 to 12 bladeless trocar is used for the camera site, the 8-mm robotic trocars are placed in their respective ports, and the assistant port is converted to a 10 to 12 port (which allows introduction of Rayteks sponges and introduction of endoscopic pouches).

Instruments

A zero degree camera.

An EEA sizer for identification of the vaginal fornices and achieving a good vaginal margin.

Hot Shears™ (Monopolar Curved Scissors) used for dissection in addition to cold and hot cutting and monopolar cautery.

The Maryland forceps' tips are utilized as excellent dissectors at the level of the ureteric tunnels and uterine artery dissection.

Fenestrated forceps is applied to the third arm and assists in retraction intraoperatively.

Suture Cut™ Needle Driver for vaginal cuff closure.

Surgical Tips

In addition to the tips mention in the endometrial staging section (when applicable) the following should be considered in cervical cancer surgery.

Restoration of the normal anatomy by developing all the appropriate surgical spaces allows for a smoother operative procedure.

We advocate for preservation of the uterine arteries when performing a radical trachelectomy.

When dissecting the ureteric tunnels, the ureter is protected from the bipolar cautery thermal effect by deviating it with the tips and body of the scissors.

To perform an optimal pelvic lymph node dissection (P-LND), the following is stressed; after deviating the superior vesical artery medially and releasing the lymphatic and adipose tissue from its lateral side, the space between the obturator lymphatic bundle and the psoas muscle is entered lateral to the external iliac vessels allowing release of the lateral

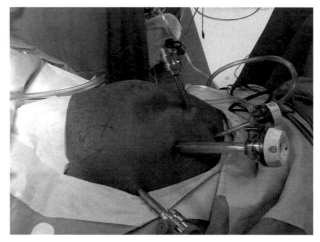

Figure 8 A deviation in port placement is sometimes necessary such as in this patient where the camera port is situated in the left upper quadrant, and the two lateral ports are maintained at a distance of 10 cm from each side.

attachments of the obturator lymphatic bundle (Fig. 7). Additionally, removal of all lymphatic tissue in between the external iliac artery and vein should be performed.

Separation of the neural bundle parallel and lateral to the uterosacral ligament can be achieved by gently separating it from the ligament without unnecessary dissecting the lateral aspect of the ligament. This minimizes nerve damage and avoids bladder dysfunction.

Closure of the vaginal cuff is performed with two separate sutures, one on each half of the vaginal cuff.

Pelvic Masses in Pregnancy

To date, we have performed close to 25 robotic-assisted ovarian cystectomies or adnexectomies in pregnancy. The advantages of the robotic platform are improving the success rate of the intended procedure minimizing the chances of laparotomy during pregnancy. All of our patients had the desired procedure performed successfully without any complications. We attempt to schedule the procedure in the 16 to 20 week gestation period. The challenge such patients pose is related to the size of the ovarian pathology. Any suspicious ovarian cysts or masses should be dealt with carefully to avoid intraperitoneal rupture. An endoscopic pouch is inserted to contain them as they are removed and safely morcellated through one of the ports.

Port placement is not universal, and the following tips are followed:

Entry through the left upper quadrant as mentioned earlier.

Placement of the camera port above the umbilicus by 3 to 7 cm, depending on the gestational age, to avoid the gravid uterus and provide a better view of the pelvic organs.

The two lateral ports must maintain the universal distance of 8 to 10 cm from the camera port.

Utilization of two robotic arms rather than three with the bipolar fenestrated grasper on the left arm and the monopolar shears on the right.

On rare occasions where the uterus is larger than 20 to 22 weeks, a deviation in the port placement plan is allowed. In such situations, the potential space in the left upper quadrant is utilized for the camera port with placement of the other two robotic ports 8 to 10 cm on either sides (Fig. 8).

Other Uses of the Robotic Platform

Management of urinary system complications such as ureteric reanastomosis or ureteroneocystotomy formation.

Bulky lymph node dissection.

Staging ovarian cancer in its early stages, which requires careful laparoscopic evaluation of the bowel loops and the upper abdomen to role out the presence of metastatic implants.

Localized recurrence of pelvic malignancies and pelvic exenterative procedures.

REFERENCES

Boggess J (2007) Robotic surgery in gynecologic onology: evolution of a new surgical paradigm. *J Robotic Surg* 1:31–7.

Boggess JF, Gehrig PA, Cantrell L, et al. (2008a) A comparative study of 3 surgical methods for hysterectomy with staging for endometrial cancer: robotic assistance, laparoscopy, laparotomy. *Am J Obstet Gynecol* 199:360.e1–9.

Boggess JF, Gehrig PA, Cantrell L, et al. (2008b) A case-control study of robot-assisted type III radical hysterectomy with pelvic lymph node dissection compared with open radical hysterectomy. *Am J Obstet Gynecol* 199:357.e1–7.

Boggess JF, Gehrig PA, Cantrell L, et al. (2009) Perioperative outcomes of robotically assisted hysterectomy for benign cases with complex pathology. *Obstet Gynecol* 114:585–93.

Shafer A, Boggess JF (2008). Robotic-assisted endometrial cancer staging and radical hysterectomy with the da Vinci surgical system. *Gynecol Oncol* 111:S18–23.

28 Gastrointestinal surgery in gynecologic oncology
Eileen M. Segreti and Charles M. Levenback

INTRODUCTION

The gastrointestinal tract is often secondarily involved by gynecologic malignancies. Extirpation of gynecologic tumors may require gastrointestinal surgical procedures. Additionally, the gastrointestinal tract may be injured during the course of treatment requiring subsequent surgical intervention during the follow-up period, particularly after exposure to ionizing radiation. Finally, gastrointestinal symptoms may dominate the end of life circumstances requiring palliative gastrointestinal procedures. This chapter will focus on common surgical procedures performed on the gastrointestinal tract during the management of gynecologic malignancies.

STOMACH
Indications

The most common procedure on the stomach performed in the management of gynecologic malignancy is the tube gastrostomy. Gastrostomy tubes are useful for decompression of the stomach and the small bowel. In the postoperative setting, gastrostomy tubes may also be used for enteral nutrition. A prolonged ileus may occur after small bowel resection and enterolysis for radiation complications. Most commonly in gynecologic patients, gastrostomy tubes are used to palliate women with end-stage ovarian cancer who suffer with vomiting secondary to carcinomatosis and multiple areas of partial small bowel obstruction.

Anatomic Considerations

The blood supply to the stomach is derived from the celiac trunk. The greater curvature of the stomach is supplied by the right and left gastroepiploic arteries. The lesser curvature is supplied by the right and left gastric arteries. The right gastric artery and the right gastroepiploic artery are branches of the common hepatic artery and gastroduodenal artery, respectively. The left gastric artery is a branch of the celiac trunk, and the left gastroepiploic artery is a branch of the splenic artery. Routes of veinous drainage include the gastric and gastroepiploic veins as well as small tributaries of the esophageal veins.

Surgical Procedures

Gastrostomy tubes may be placed percutaneously with endoscopic guidance or may be placed at the time of laparotomy. The stomach should be mobile enough to reach the anterior abdominal wall. Multiple tubes can be utilized for this purpose including a specialized gastrostomy tube or a self-retaining flanged Malecot urologic tube or even a Foley catheter can placed into the stomach via a left upper quadrant incision. Two concentric purse strings sutures of absorbable suture are placed in the anterior stomach seromuscular wall approximately 1 cm apart. The electrosurgical instrument is used to create an opening in the stomach through which the tube is

placed. The inner pursestring is tied first, then the outer pursestring, creating an inverted tunnel. Three to four interrupted 2-0 nonabsorbable sutures are placed to approximate the stomach to the anterior abdominal wall. After the abdomen is closed, the tube is secured to the skin with a nonabsorbable suture (Fig. 1). If the tube is subsequently dislodged, it can often be immediately replaced through the gastrocutaneous fistula.

SMALL BOWEL
Introduction

Small bowel resection is often necessary to remove strictured, perforated, or tumor-infiltrated intestine. Resection of small bowel is preferred over bypassing a damaged segment. However, a bypass procedure may be preferable when damaged small bowel is densely adherent to a fibrotic and heavily irradiated pelvis. If the stomach is not accessible for a safe tube gastrostomy, a small bowel bypass may be considered to palliate an intestinal obstruction in a woman with advanced gynecologic cancer.

Anatomic Considerations

The small bowel begins at the pylorus and ends at the ileocecal valve. The duodenum and jejunum are separated by the ligament of Trietz. The duodenum is almost entirely retroperitoneal. The distinction between the jejunum and the ileum is gradual. The small bowel is perfused by straight vessels that disperse into the anterior and posterior surfaces of the bowel. The straight vessels emerge from the arcades of the superior mesenteric artery. In the ileum the straight vessels are surrounded by fat, and the fat encroaches upon the bowel wall. In the jejunum, the vasa recta are more easily seen, as the mesenteric fat ends prior to reaching the jejunal serosa. The venous drainage of the small bowel is to the superior mesenteric vein which is a tributary of the portal vein. The autonomic nervous system, in conjunction with the gastrointestinal hormonal system, regulates peristalsis and bowel secretory action. The parasympathetic ganglia lie within the bowel wall, whereas the sympathetic ganglia lie close to the origin of the superior mesenteric artery.

The small intestine has four layers. They are the mucosa, the submucosa, the muscularis, and the serosa. The mucosa contains villi and crypts, which greatly increase the absorptive surface area. The submucosa is a strong connective tissue layer important for structural integrity. It is essential to include this layer during bowel anastomosis. The muscularis consists of an inner circular layer and an outer longitudinal layer. The serosa is the outermost layer and is a continuation of the mesothelium that lines the peritoneal cavity (Fig. 2).

The terminal ileum is the site of absorption of the fat soluble vitamins, A, D, E, and K, as well as Vitamin B12. Extensive resection of the terminal ileum will require vitamin supplementation.

Surgical Procedures

To be successful, a small bowel resection must completely remove the damaged or involved intestinal segment. Intestinal continuity must then be re-established using healthy ends of bowel with good blood supply that are re-approximated without tension. Tissues should be handled gently, and a watertight anastomosis should be achieved. There should be no downstream areas of obstruction that could adversely affect healing. The submucosal layer of the bowel wall is the most critical layer to incorporate into the anastomosis. There are several different means to affect a small bowel anastomosis. Staplers are fast but incur increased cost. A handsewn anastomosis takes more time, but requires no special devices. It is important to be familiar with both methods of bowel anastomosis.

The damaged or obstructed portion of the small bowel is identified. The vascular arcades are visualized by transillumination. Either a linear cutting stapler or Kocher clamps are used to isolate the abnormal section of small intestine. The stapler or clamps are oriented obliquely to maximize the mesenteric side of the bowel and minimize the anti-mesenteric side (Fig. 3). This maneuver will also create a larger lumen thereby decreasing the chance of a subsequent stricture. The mesentery is scored with scissors or with an electrosurgery device, and the vessels are isolated between small clamps. The vessels are cut and secured with 2-0 suture. Alternatively, a vascular stapler or an electrothermal bipolar tissue fusing device can be used to secure the mesenteric vessels.

Commonly, staplers are used to create a side-to-side, functional end-to-end, anastomosis. The ends of the small bowel are juxtaposed and inspected for viability. If there is any doubt as to bowel viability, the bowel is excised further until there is no question as to the quality of the bowel. The anastomosis

must be tension-free. The bowel loops are mobilized as necessary to relieve any tension. The anti-mesenteric borders are lined up in parallel. Stay sutures are placed 5 to 8 cm from the closed bowel ends along the anti-mesenteric border to facilitate proper alignment. The corners of the anti-mesenteric staple line are then excised (Fig. 4). One arm of the stapler is then placed along the anti-mesenteric border of each limb of bowel and the stapler closed (Figs. 5 and 6). Firing the stapler places two double rows of titanium staples, between which a knife cuts. Typically, staples used for small bowel anastomosis are 4 mm in width when open and 3.5 mm in depth, with a closed depth of 1.5 mm, contained often in a blue colored cartridge. The staple line is then inspected for bleeding. Any bleeding area should be reinforced with an interrupted absorbable suture. The remaining luminal opening is grasped with Allis clamps, and a TA (thoracoabdominal) stapler is set and fired to close the remaining enterotomy. The staple lines should overlap to prevent leakage at the anastomosis (Fig. 7). Excess tissue above the TA device can be excised.

The small bowel can also be anastomosed end to end with a single or double layer of sutures. If the bowel lumens are of disparate sizes, to equalize them a Cheatle slit can be made on the anti-mesenteric border of the smaller lumen (Fig. 8). After the bowel is anastomosed, the mesenteric defect is then closed to prevent an internal hernia and subsequent bowel strangulation.

A meta-analysis in 2006 of six trials and 670 patients did not demonstrate superiority of the two-layer versus the single-layer closure (Shikata et al. 2006). The double-layer closure consists of a continuous inverting layer of absorbable suture and an outer layer of interrupted silk seromuscular sutures. Both continuous and interrupted single-layer closures have been described. In the Gambee interrupted inverted seromucosal technique, 3-0 sutures are placed from the mucosa through the bowel wall to the serosa and back through, serosa to mucosa. The knots are tied on the mucosal side, and the interrupted sutures are placed 3 mm apart (Gambee et al. 1956) (Fig. 9). More recently described is a continuous over and over seromuscular running suture. Theoretical concerns

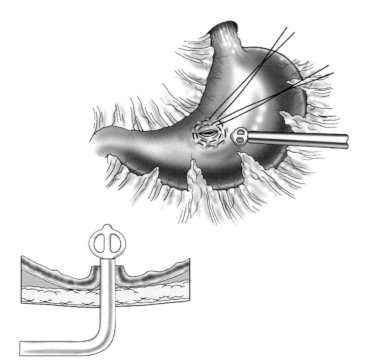

Figure 1 Gastrostomy tube with Malecot urologic catheter.

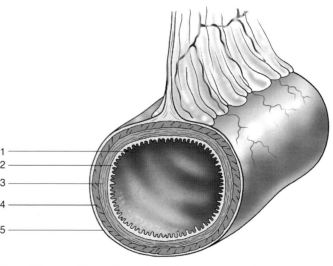

Figure 2 Layers of the small intestine wall. 1 Mucosa; 2 Submucosa; 3 Inner circular muscle; 4 Outer longitudinal muscle; 5 Serosa.

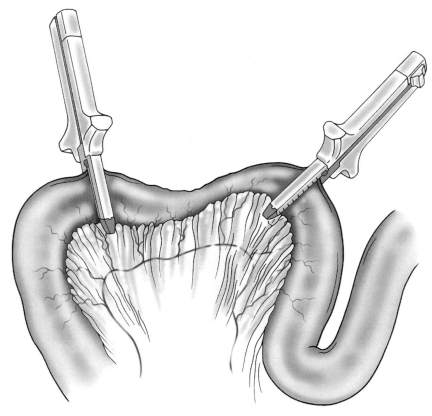

Figure 3 Positioning of clamps.

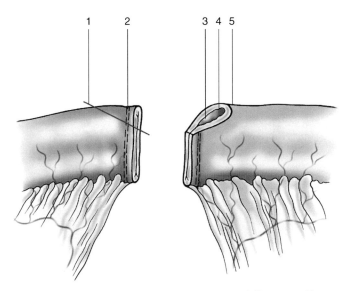

Figure 4 Preparation for anastomosis. 1 Incision; 2 Staple line; 3 Bowel lumen; 4 Mucosa; 5 Serosa.

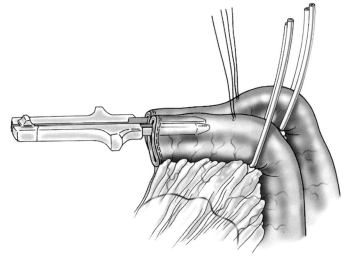

Figure 5 Positioning of stapler.

regarding a single-layer running closure include an increased risk of luminal narrowing and a potentially increased risk of anastomotic leak compared to a double-layer technique; however, this has not been born out in randomized trials (Burch et al. 2000).

An alternative to small bowel resection is small bowel bypass, whereby an abnormal area of bowel is bypassed, and a bowel anastomosis is created proximal to the abnormal area. This will allow intestinal contents to progress beyond an area of obstruction. A side-to-side enteroenterostomy is created, either with staplers or a double- or single-layer suture technique.

Alternatively, the bowel is divided proximally and distally to the damaged segment, and the damaged bowel is completely excluded from the intestinal stream. One end of the bypassed limb is brought up to the skin as a mucous fistula. A third option is to divide the bowel proximal to the damaged area and create an anastomosis distally. The mucous fistula may be incorporated into the inferior aspect of the incision. A disadvantage of bowel bypass is that it may subsequently foster a blind-loop syndrome. The blind-loop syndrome is characterized by bacterial overgrowth with subsequent cramps, diarrhea, anemia, and weight loss (Schlegel and Maglinte 1982). If a small bowel fistula is being bypassed, it is important to completely isolate this bowel from the intestinal stream.

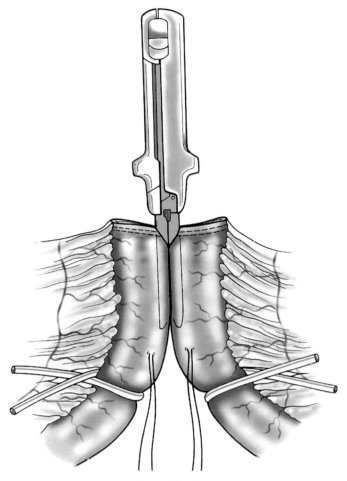

Figure 6 Stapling.

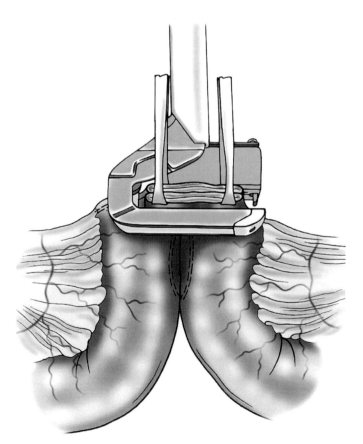

Figure 7 Positioning of TA Stapler.

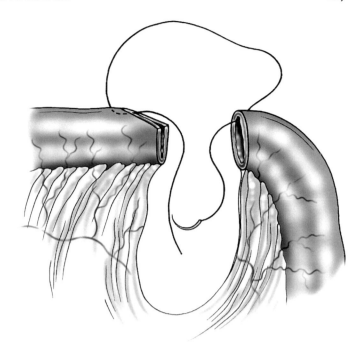

Figure 8 Cheatle slit on small bowel.

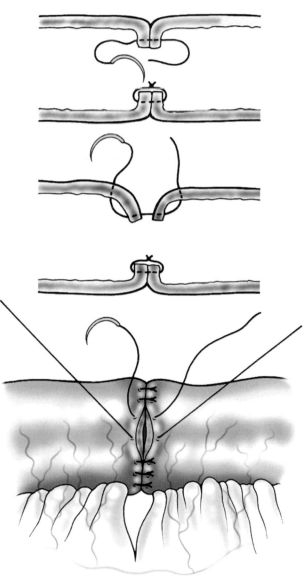

Figure 9 The Gambee technique.

Laparoscopic treatment of small bowel obstruction secondary to adhesive disease is possible in a subset of patients with two or fewer prior surgeries. There is a high conversion rate to open surgical repair as perforation as well as poor visualization have been reported (Wullstein and Gross 2003).

LARGE INTESTINE SURGERY
Indications
Partial colectomy, rectosigmoid resection, and abdominal perineal resection are all utilized to treat gynecologic malignancies. These procedures may be integral to ovarian cancer debulking, treatment of radiation complications, or a component of pelvic exenteration for cervical, endometrial, vaginal, or vulvar cancer. If the sphincter or distal rectum is damaged or involved with tumor, colostomy may be required to provide fecal continence. Stoma formation is required for either permanent or temporary fecal diversion. End colostomies are typically preferred for permanent stomas, as they are smaller and are less prone to complications (Segreti et al. 1996). Loop colostomies are preferred when stomal closure in the future is anticipated or bowel obstruction occurs as a result of advanced, refractory ovarian cancer, and anticipated life expectancy is short. After a colostomy has served its purpose, allowing a distal anastomosis to heal or a fistula to be repaired, intestinal continuity is restored by closing the colostomy. Lastly, removal of the appendix may facilitate ovarian cancer debulking, urinary conduit construction, or serve as a prophylactic maneuver against future infectious or neoplastic complications.

Anatomic Considerations
The blood supply to the colon and rectum is derived from branches of the superior mesenteric, inferior mesenteric, and the internal iliac arteries. The right colon is supplied by the ileocolic artery, the right colic artery, and a branch of the middle colic artery. The transverse colon is chiefly supplied by the middle colic artery, but there is a communication with the inferior mesenteric arterial system via the marginal artery of Drummond. The inferior mesenteric artery supplies the colon from the splenic flexure to the proximal rectum. The inferior mesenteric artery branches into the superior rectal artery, the sigmoid arteries, and the left colic artery. The distal rectum receives its blood supply from the paired middle and inferior rectal arteries which originate from the internal iliac artery system (Fig. 10).

The appendix is the embryologic continuation of the cecum. Its location is identified by the confluence of the three taenia of the cecum. The position of the tip of the appendix relative to the cecum may vary. The tip may be found lateral, medial, or behind the cecum. The mesentery of the appendix passes behind the terminal ileum. The blood supply to the appendix is derived from the appendiceal artery, which is a branch of the ileocolic artery.

The nerves to the colon parallel the blood supply and consist of sensory afferent nerves, and the motor nerves from the autonomic system. The anal sphincter is under voluntary motor control. The colonic wall is more muscular than that of the small bowel. In addition, the longitudinal muscles are gathered in three places to form the taenia coli. The colon also has numerous fatty epiploica that hang from the taenia.

Surgical Procedures
Mechanical bowel preparation prior to elective colorectal surgery, once thought to be mandatory, is now under scrutiny and may not be necessary. A recent updated Cochrane database review of 13 randomized controlled studies that included 4777 participants undergoing elective colorectal surgery did not demonstrate any advantage to mechanical bowel preparation verses no prep in regard to the rate of anastomotic leakage or wound infection (Guenaga et al. 2009). Regardless of whether mechanical bowel preparation is used, administration of preoperative intravenous antibiotics, with or without preoperative oral antibiotics, remains an important step prior to colorectal surgery (Nelson et al. 2009).

Factors that may impair anastomotic healing are frequently encountered in gynecologic oncology patients, including hypoalbuminemia in ovarian cancer patients, smoking in cervical cancer patients, prior irradiation in cervical or endometrial cancer patients and prior chemotherapy, radiation, and diabetes mellitus in many gynecologic oncology patients. Efforts should be made to optimize all reversible adverse factors if possible, that is, preoperative and postoperative nutritional support, avoid smoking, achieve euglycemia, etc.

The principles of large bowel resection and anastomosis are similar to those for small bowel anastomosis and are based on

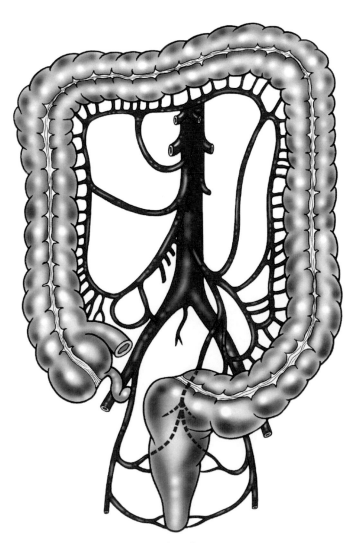

Figure 10 Blood supply to the colon and rectum.

the blood supply and the location of the pathologic segment. Resection and anastomosis of the colon and proximal rectum are performed equally well with either a handsewn or stapled technique. The Cochrane Colorectal Group performed an updated review of randomized trials in 2008 which confirmed earlier conclusions of non-superiority of either stapled or handsewn technique used for colorectal anastamosis. However, they did note an increased risk of anastomotic stricture with staplers and a longer time to perform the anastomosis with a handsewn technique (Matos et al. 2001). However, for ileocolic anastomoses, this group found an advantage to the stapled technique versus the handsewn technique with fewer leaks noted in the stapled group (1.4% vs. 6%) (Choy et al. 2007). Important to both methods is the adequate clearance of fat and vessels away from the colonic ends to be connected. The cardinal rules for a successful anastomosis remain a tension free, well vascularized, and watertight anastomosis.

Hand-sutured colonic anastomoses have classically been two layers in the tradition of Lembert and Halsted. Popular and commonly used by many surgeons for years is the double-layer closure. This method incorporates successive interrupted inverting seromuscular Lembert sutures (far–near–near–far), mucosa sparing sutures placed in the posterior wall until half of the circumference is approximated (Fig. 11). The bowel lumens are then exposed by excising excess tissue adjacent to the Kocher clamps or excising the staple line. The mucosal layer is closed with 4-0 or 5-0 running over and over absorbable suture. A Connell stitch is used on the anterior surface to complete the entire circumference of mucosal apposition. A Connell stitch varies from a running stitch in that advancement occurs on the same side of the bowel, for example, the suture goes through the wall from the serosa to the mucosa, then back from the mucosa to the serosa on the same side. The stitch then crosses the incision to the serosa on the other side and then repeats (Fig. 12). Finally, the anterior surface is closed with an outer layer of Lembert sutures (Fig. 13). Several investigators have reported using a one-layer inverting colonic closure with satisfactory results (Curley et al. 1988, Max et al. 1991, Ceraldi et al. 1993). One-layer closures are faster and less expensive than the two-layer closure. The single-layer closure is performed with 3-0 or 4-0 polypropylene or polyglyconate suture using a double-armed needle. The suture is started at the mesenteric border of the bowel (Fig. 14). The sutures are placed from outside in, including a larger amount of serosa, muscularis, and submucosa (approximately 5 mm) than mucosa (minimal) to affect mucosal inversion. The knot is secured outside the bowel lumen. Each end of the suture is then continued around to the anti-mesenteric border, spacing the stitches 3 to 4 mm apart. The sutures are then tied together.

The TA instrument can also be used to create an end-to-end anastomosis by triangulation (Figs. 15–20). Three stay sutures are placed equidistantly on each limb of the bowel.

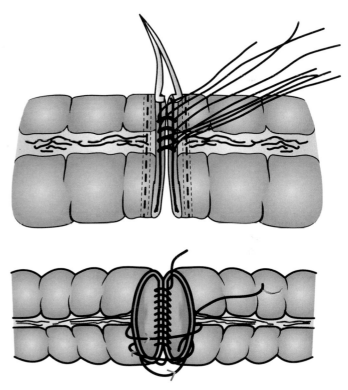

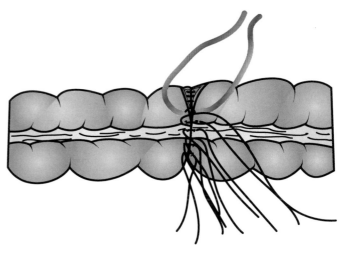

Figure 12 Anterior running closure using Connell stitch (lower).

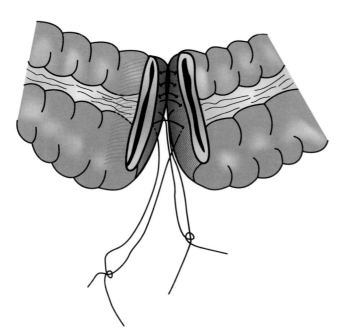

Figure 11 Back row of Lembert sutures (upper).

Figure 13 Front row of Lembert sutures.

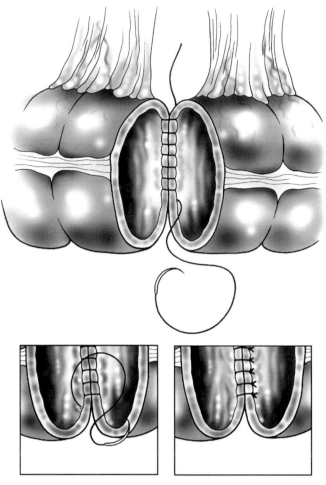

One stay suture should be located at the level of the mesentery, and the other two stay sutures should be placed to form an equilateral triangle. The back wall is stapled first, and the mucosa is inverted. The second row of staples is placed to overlap the first row. The last row of staples is placed, and the mucosa is everted. The diameter of the lumen is palpated to ensure adequate size.

For the distal rectum, the automatic end-to-end circular stapling device (EEA) has provided the ability to perform successful low and very low rectal anastomoses. Adequate mobility of the sigmoid must be achieved by incision along the lateral peritoneal reflection. The two ends of the bowel to be anastomosed must be mobile enough to lie adjacent to each other without tension. The largest EEA device that fits comfortably

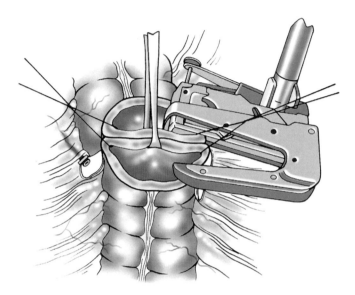

Figure 14 Single-layer anastomosis, (inset left) continuous sutures and (inset right) interrupted sutures.

Figure 16 The posterior wall is stapled first.

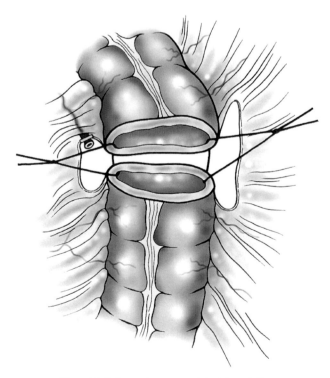

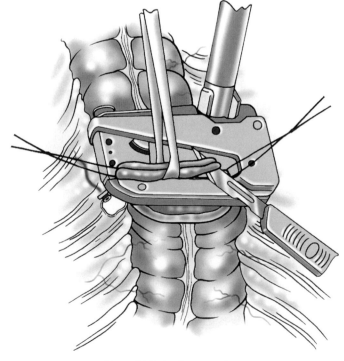

Figure 15 End to end anastomosis by triangulation.

Figure 17 Excise the excess tissue.

should be used. Sizers are available to measure the lumen. After resection of the diseased large bowel, a pursestring is placed around the proximal lumen. This is easily performed with the pursestring instrument and a straight needle. The pursestring suture is then secured tightly around the anvil of the EEA instrument (Fig. 21). The rectal stump can similarly be circumscribed with a pursestring suture. Alternatively, a stapler can be used to close the rectal pouch. A trocar attached to the EEA is then used to puncture the closed rectal pouch at the site of the future anastomosis. The trocar is then removed, and the anvil shaft can be inserted into the EEA instrument. By

turning the wing nut on the EEA handle, the two lumens are approximated. After releasing the safety, the handle is squeezed and two circular rows of staples are placed. A circular knife cuts the excess inverted tissue, and two donuts are created. The wing nut is then turned in the opposite direction to open the instrument which is then withdrawn gently through the

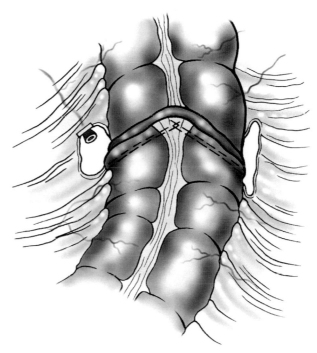

Figure 20 Completed anastomosis.

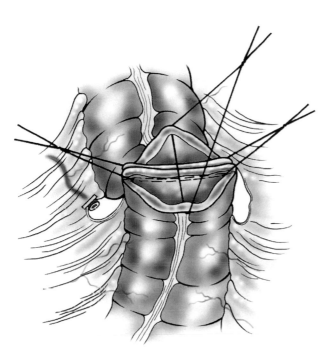

Figure 18 Place traction suture midway.

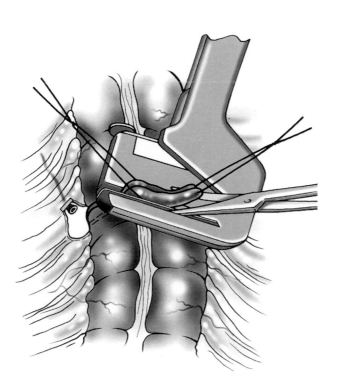

Figure 19 Excise redundant tissue after stapling.

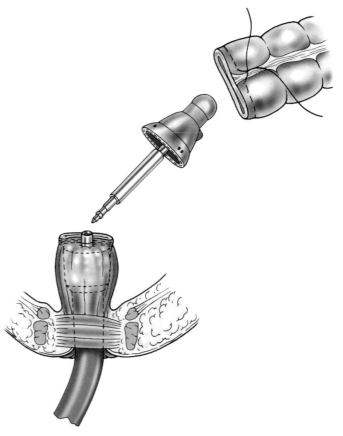

Figure 21 Positioning of purse-string suture.

anorectum. The two donuts should be inspected and be intact (Fig. 22). A defect in one of the donuts is the reason to redo or repair the anastomosis. The seal of the anastomosis can be tested by filling the pelvis with saline and injecting air into the rectum. Bubbles indicate an air leak that should be oversewn. One can also visually inspect the anastomosis with a sigmoidoscope.

When colostomy formation is considered, the patient should meet with an enterostomal therapist for preoperative teaching and evaluation of the abdominal wall for stomal placement. Stomas should ideally pass through the rectus muscles and avoid abdominal wall folds or creases (Fig. 23). The patient should be examined in both the sitting and standing position. Stoma placement in the waistline should be avoided. The skin is then marked for ideal stomal placement. A laparoscopic or open technique can may used. Prior to dividing the colon, the bowel is mobilized by dividing the lateral peritoneal attachments. Adequate mobility must be achieved to provide a tension-free stoma. The distal bowel is resected or oversewn as a pouch. A 3-cm circular skin button is removed at the previously marked site. The subcutaneous tissues are bluntly separated. The anterior rectus sheath is incised in a cruciate fashion. The rectus muscles are split longitudinally with care taken to avoid the deep epigastric vessels. The peritoneum is then incised, and two fingers are passed through the abdominal wall. The stapled bowel end is grasped with a Babcock clamp

and brought through the stomal aperture. Care is taken to not twist the mesentery. Excess fat and mesentery are trimmed from the stoma. The stoma is secured to the parietal peritoneum with absorbable suture, and the mesentery can be fixed to the lateral peritoneum to prevent internal hernia. The abdominal incision is then closed. The staple line on the bowel is excised. The stoma is matured in a rosebud fashion by inserting the needle into the skin 1 cm from the stomal edge, then running it up the bowel serosa and muscularis for one or two stitches, exiting on the mucosal side and securing the knot over the mucocutaneous junction (Fig. 24).

A loop colostomy may be situated at either the transverse or the sigmoid colon depending on site of obstruction and length of mesentery relative to body habitus. If a loop colostomy is performed for palliation of a sigmoid obstruction secondary to advanced, refractory ovarian cancer, the distal transverse colon is usually easy to identify through a small left upper quadrant incision. However if the purpose is to create a temporary diverting colostomy while an anastomosis heals, the proximal transverse colon or terminal ileum are usually preferred. To relieve obstruction, a transverse skin incision of 10 to 12 cm is made in the right or left upper quadrant. The fascia is incised transversely, and the rectus muscles are separated longitudinally. The peritoneal cavity is entered sharply. The transverse colon is easily identified due to its dilatation, when a large bowel obstruction is present. The adjacent

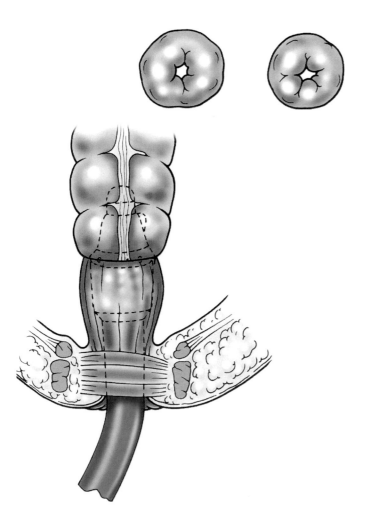

Figure 22 Closure of the EEA stapler and donuts.

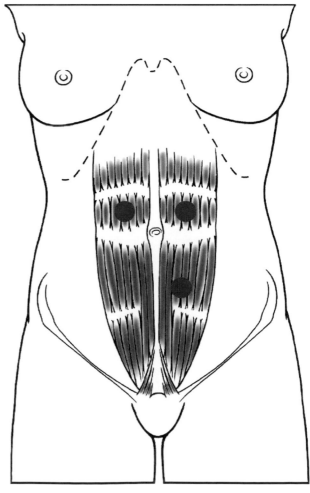

Figure 23 Ideal sites for stomas.

omentum is dissected off of the loop of colon. A defect is created in the mesentery to allow passage of a penrose drain with which to lift and manipulate the colon. The fascia is then partially closed. A flat plastic bridge may be passed through the mesenteric defect and secured to the skin with monofilament suture. Instead of a plastic bridge, a skin bridge can be created from skin flaps to elevate the loop colostomy. The skin incision, if larger than needed for the stoma, may be partially closed with skin staples or absorbable sutures. The colon is then opened either longitudinally along the taenia, or at a transversely oriented angle. If a plastic bridge is used, it may be removed in 7 to 10 days.

A loop stoma may be closed by incising the skin adjacent to the mucocutaneous junction, elevating the stoma with Allis clamps, and dividing the filmy attachments to the subcutaneous tissues. The edge of the fascia is then identified, and the plane sharply developed between the stoma and the fascia. The peritoneal adhesions are then lysed. The stomal edge can then be excised, and an extraperitoneal one- or two-layer closure can be performed. The loop is then dropped back into the peritoneal cavity, and the fascia closed with delayed absorbable suture. The skin defect can be packed open and left to close secondarily, or alternatively staples can be used for immediate skin closure (Hoffman et al. 1993).

A faster option to close a loop colostomy is to use the TA stapler. After incising the mucocutaneous junction, the edges of the stoma are grasped with Allis clamps. The colostomy edges are held together to form a line perpendicular to the long axis of the bowel. This will allow maximal lumen diameter. The stapler is fired, and the excess tissue is excised.

To close an end stoma, an exploratory laparotomy is usually required to identify the distal limb and create a large bowel anastomosis. Laparoscopy may alternatively be used and an extraperitoneal closure affected, if the distal limb is nearby and can be mobilized adequately. The end stoma is excised in a similar manner to that described for a loop stoma. The mucocutaneous junction of the distal end is excised. A large bowel anastomosis is performed similarly to that described in the previous section. Mesenteric defects are closed to prevent internal hernias.

Another option to palliate a large bowel obstruction is a colonoscopically placed endoluminal stent to acutely alleviate the obstruction. This may serve as a bridge prior to a definitive resection or as a pure palliate step in a poor operative candidate (Carter et al. 2002).

Appendectomy is often performed during debulking surgery for ovarian cancer. Appendectomy is accomplished by isolating and ligating the blood supply to the appendix and closing or burying the stump of the appendix to prevent fecal spillage. If present, filmy adhesions from the appendix to the peritoneal surfaces are lysed. If the appendix is retrocecal, the cecum is mobilized by incising the peritoneum along the peritoneal reflection. The appendiceal artery is isolated, doubly clamped, cut and secured with 2-0 suture. The base of the appendix is

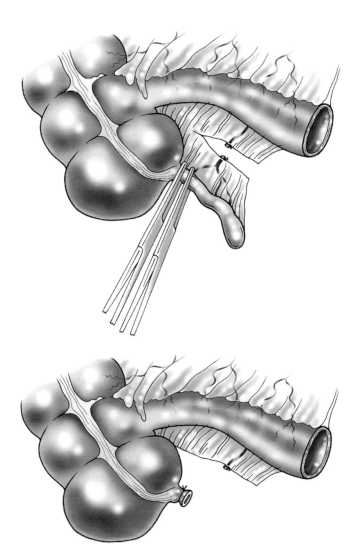

Figure 25 Appendectomy.

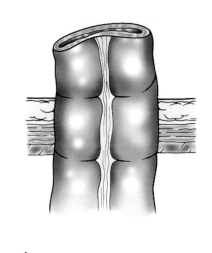

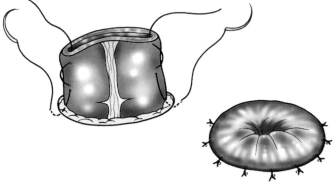

Figure 24 Maturation of the stoma in a "rosebud" fashion.

then crushed between two straight hemostats. The specimen is excised between the hemostats, and the stump tied off with 2-0 suture (Fig. 25). Alternatively, the unligated stump can be buried into the cecum with a Z stitch or pursestring suture. Ligation of the stump, prior to burial into the cecum, may promote a mucocele or an abscess. Another approach after dividing and securing the appendiceal artery is to remove the appendix using the GIA or the TA stapling device.

REFERENCES

Burch JM, Franciose RJ, Moore EE, et al. (2000) Single-layer continuous versus two-layer interrupted intestinal anastomosis: a prospective randomized trial. *Ann Surg* **231**:832–7.

Carter J, Valmadre S, Dalrymple C, et al. (2002) Management of large bowel obstruction in advanced ovarian cancer with intraluminal stents. *Gynecol Oncol* **84**:176–9.

Ceraldi CM, Rypins EB, Monahan M, et al. (1993) Comparison of continuous single layer polypropylene anastomosis with double layer and stapled anastomoses in elective colon resections. *Am Surg* **59**:168–71.

Choy P, Bissett I, Docherty J, et al. (2007) Stapled versus handsewn methods for ileocolic anastomoses. *Cochrane Database Syst Rev* (**3**):CD004320.

Curley SA, Allison DC, Smith DE, et al. (1988) Analysis of techniques and results in 347 consecutive colon anastomoses. *Ann Surg* **155**:597–601.

Gambee LP, Garnjobst W, Hardwick CE (1956) Ten years' experience with a single layer anastomosis in colon surgery. *Am J Surg* **92**:222–7.

Guenaga KKFG, Matos D, Wille-Jørgensen P (2009) Mechanical bowel preparation for elective colorectal surgery. *Cochrane Database Syst Rev* (**1**):CD001544.

Hoffman MS, Gleeson N, Diebel D, et al. (1993) Colostomy closure on a gynecologic oncology service. *Gynecol Oncol* **49**:299–302.

Matos D, Atallah ÁN, Castro AA, et al. (2001) Stapled versus handsewn methods for colorectal anastomosis surgery. *Cochrane Database Syst Rev* (**3**):CD003144.

Max E, Sweeney WB, Bailey HR, et al. (1991) Results of 1,000 single-layer continuous polypropylene intestinal anastomoses. *Am J Surg* **162**:461–7.

Nelson RL, Glenny AM, Song F (2009) Antimicrobial prophylaxis for colorectal surgery. *Cochrane Database Syst Rev* (**1**):CD001181.

Schlegel DM, Maglinte DDT (1982) The blind pouch syndrome. *Surg Gynecol Obstet* **155**:541–4.

Segreti EM, Levenback C, Morris M (1996) A comparison of end and loop colostomy for fecal diversion in gynecologic patients with colonic fistulas. *Gynecol Oncol* **60**:49–53.

Shikata S, Yamagishi H, Taji Y, et al. (2006) Single versus two layer intestinal anastomosis: a meta-analysis of randomized controlled trials *BMC Surg* **6**:2.

Wullstein C, Gross E (2003) Laparoscopic compared with conventional treatment of acute adhesive small bowel obstruction. *Br J Surg* **90**(9):1147–51.

29 Urologic procedures
Jonathan A. Cosin, Jeffrey M. Fowler, and Kathleen Connell

REPAIR OF URETERAL INJURIES
Introduction
Ureteral injury occurs in 1% to 2% of all major gynecologic procedures. Pelvic irradiation, large pelvic tumors, endometriosis, and the radicality of the procedures all increase the risk of damage. Ureteral obstruction can also occur as a result of any of the above processes, necessitating reimplantation. The underlying principles to be adhered to in repairing any postoperative ureteral obstruction are as follows:

1. Adequate vascular supply.
2. Adequate surgical exposure.
3. Gentle tissue handling.
4. Tension-free suturing.
5. Placing the minimum number of sutures.
6. Stenting to allow the repair to heal.

Indications
The nature and extent of the injury, the overall health of the patient and the underlying disease process must all be considered when deciding upon the type of procedure to be performed.

Ureteroneocystotomy is the procedure of choice for injuries or obstruction within the pelvis at or below the level of the common iliac vessels. Bladder mobilization with a psoas hitch and/or bladder flap (Demel or Boari) may be required in order to yield a tension-free anastomosis. Ureteroneocystotomy is the preferred procedure where possible as the complication rate is lower than with ureteroureterostomy.

Ureteroureterostomy is required for injuries to the abdominal portion of the ureter when the proximal portion will not reach the bladder directly.

Anatomic Considerations
Vascular Supply
Bladder
The bladder receives its blood supply mainly from the superior and inferior vesical arteries, both of which are branches of the anterior division of the hypogastric artery. The obturator, uterine, and vaginal arteries may all also send branches to the bladder.

Ureter
The ureter takes its blood supply from branches of major vessels which it courses near. This includes the aorta as well as the renal, ovarian, iliac (common and internal), vesical, and uterine vessels.

Nerve Supply
Bladder
The bladder is innervated by the vesical plexus which carries efferent and afferent autonomic fibers, both sympathetic and parasympathetic. The plexus arises from T11 to L2 and courses through the base of the cardinal ligament.

The renal (T9–T12), aortic (L1), and superior and inferior hypogastric (S2–S4) plexuses all contribute to the innervation of the ureter with autonomic fibers.

Muscles
Psoas
The psoas muscle originates from the anterior surface and lower borders of the transverse processes of the lumbar vertebral bodies and joins the iliac muscle to insert on the lesser trochanter of the femur. The muscle acts to flex the hip. It is innervated by fibers from L1 to L3. Several important nerves are closely related anatomically to the psoas muscle. The iliohypogastric, ilioinguinal, lateral femoral cutaneous, and femoral nerves all emerge from the lateral border of the muscle. The genitofemoral nerve arises anterolaterally, and the obturator, accessory obturator, and upper roots of the lumbosacral trunk all arise medially.

Operative Procedure
Ureteroureterostomy
In cases of crush or similar injury, the injured ends of the damaged ureter are trimmed if necessary to reach viable bleeding tissues. This is generally not necessary for transection injuries. Each end is partially spatulated by making an incision of approximately 3 to 5 mm longitudinally in each ureter. These incisions should be 180° apart (Fig. 1).

The ureter can be stented either by passing a stent through the injured ends toward both the bladder and the renal pelvis or by performing a cystotomy and passing a stent up through the ureter to the renal pelvis. This should be done before suturing the ureter. A closed suction drain should be placed in the operative field (Fig. 2).

Interrupted 4-0 absorbable sutures (polyglycolic acid) are used to create the anastomosis. Care should be exercised to avoid tying the sutures too tightly or putting in too many sutures. Generally, four to six sutures are sufficient (Fig. 3).

Ureteroneocystotomy With or Without Psoas Hitch and Bladder Flap
In cases of crush injury or obstruction, ligate and divide the ureter as distally as possible, being mindful of the presence of

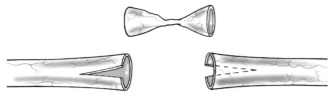

Figure 1 The injured segment is excised, ensuring that the ends to be approximated are well vascularized. Both ends are then spatulated to aid in preventing stenosis at the anastomosis site.

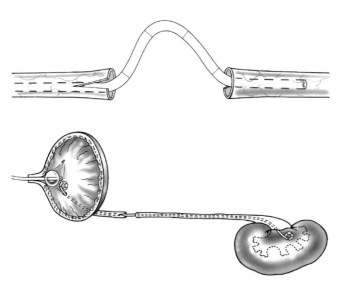

Figure 2 Repair should be stented for at least two to three weeks. An intravenous pyelogram or pull-back ureterogram is recommended prior to stent removal to ensure patency of ureter.

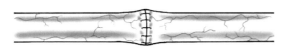

Figure 3 Ureteral repair is accomplished with four to six interrupted absorbable sutures.

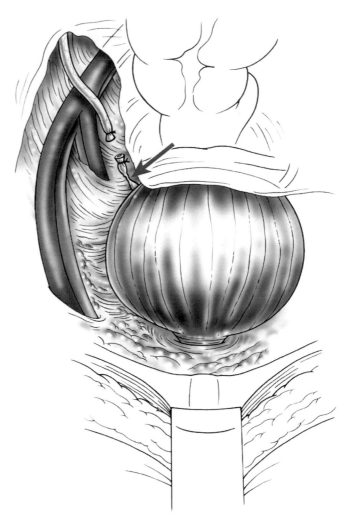

Figure 4 For ureteral injuries occurring in the pelvis, the ureter is divided and the distal end permanently ligated with non-absorbable suture.

fibrosis such as from radiation therapy. The distal stump is ligated with a permanent suture, such as 2-0 silk. If the ureter has been transected, the distal end should still be identified and ligated with a permanent suture. The proximal end is trimmed as necessary to ensure that the terminal ureter has adequate vascular supply to allow healing of the anastomosis. The ureter is also partially freed from its peritoneal attachments to provide mobility of the most distal segment. Care is taken to avoid disruption of the adventitial layer which carries the blood and nerve supply to the ureter (Fig. 4).

If the ureter and the bladder can be placed in approximation without tension, then the surgeon may proceed with the anastomosis. Otherwise, an extending bladder flap may be necessary (see below).

A longitudinal extraperitoneal incision is made in the dome of the bladder. At the conclusion of the repair, this is closed transversely to take further tension off the anastomosis. A finger or a long, curved instrument is then placed in the bladder to indicate the posterolateral position on the bladder that most

closely approximates to the ureter, and a cystotomy is made at this point. The ureter is then brought through the incision (Fig. 5).

The ureter is spatulated by making two 5 mm longitudinal incisions 180° apart (Fig. 6). The angles of the incisions are sutured using 4-0 absorbable sutures (polyglycolic-acid) which are tagged with the needles left on. A 28 to 30 cm, 7 or 8 Fr single or double J is then passed up the ureter toward the renal pelvis.

The anastomosis is performed using 4-0 absorbable interrupted sutures which include the full thickness of the ureter, but only the mucosa and submucosa of the bladder (Fig. 7). Generally six sutures are required, including the previously placed angle sutures. The cystotomy is then closed and a closed suction drain is placed in the area of the anastomosis. Closure may be accomplished with a running 2-0 absorbable suture using through-and-through stitches. A second layer of 2-0 absorbable sutures may be placed incorporating the serosa and muscle but not the mucosa (Fig. 8). Retrograde transurethral filling of the bladder should be performed to ensure a watertight seal. The ureteral stents may be removed in two weeks if a cystogram or intravenous pyelogram demonstrates ureteral patency and no leaks. A follow-up intravenous pyelogram is

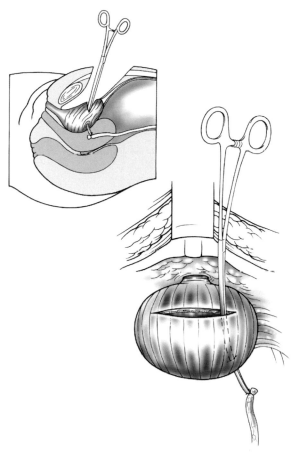

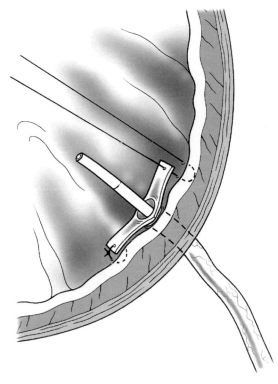

Figure 7 The anastomosis is created with interrupted absorbable sutures, full thickness through the ureter, and partial thickness through the bladder.

Figure 5 Working through an incision in the dome of the bladder, the ureter is brought through the bladder wall at a point that will ensure the most tension-free anastomosis.

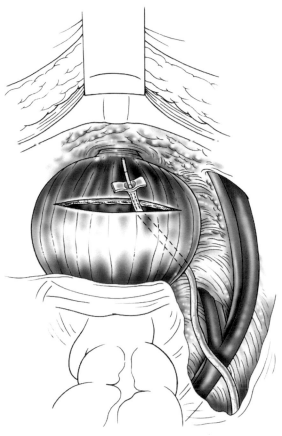

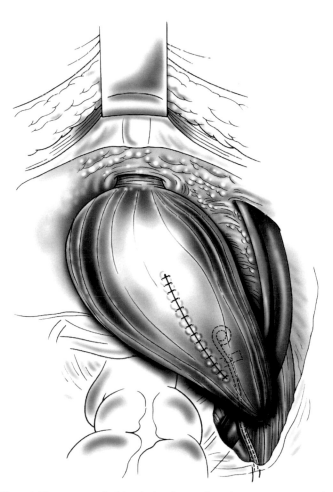

Figure 6 The ureter is spatulated and stented.

Figure 8 The cystotomy incision is closed. By making the incision transversely and closing longitudinally, the site of anastomosis can be brought closer to the ureter, thus relieving tension. A psoas hitch can then be performed (see text).

recommended after one month to confirm patency, especially in patients who have received prior radiotherapy.

If the ureter and bladder do not approximate easily, then additional measures must be taken. Sufficient mobility of the bladder can often be obtained by developing the space of Retzius and dividing the anterior peritoneum and the lateral bladder attachments. The bladder can then be sutured to the psoas muscle to hold it closer to the ureter and to take up the tension that would otherwise be exerted on the repair. Use 2-0 permanent suture, taking care to avoid damage to any of the nerves related to the psoas muscle. In cases where still further mobility is required, an extending bladder flap such as those described by Boari (Figs. 9–11) or Demel (Figs. 12–14) may be used. The incisions are made and sutured as shown, resulting in the "lengthening" of the bladder toward the ureter. Once this step is complete, the anastomosis is performed as described above.

URINARY DIVERSION
Introduction
Urinary diversion was first described in the mid 1800s. Many different tissues and techniques have been employed, each with their own inherent advantages and disadvantages. The major types now in use in gynecological practice are the

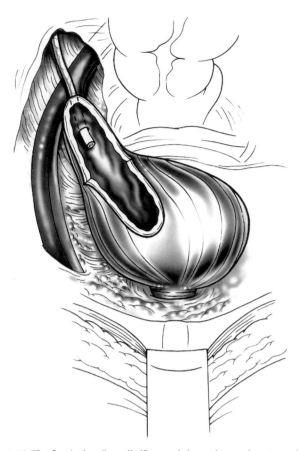

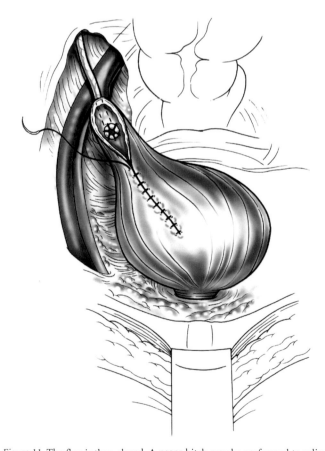

Figure 10 The flap is then "unrolled" toward the undamaged ureter and the anastomosis performed. Care must be exercised not to perform the anastomosis too close to the cut edge of the bladder.

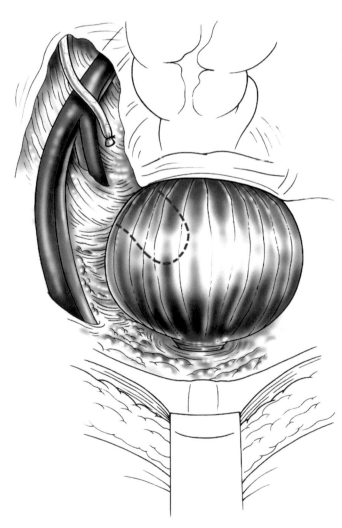

Figure 9 Boari flap: a U-shaped incision is made in the bladder.

Figure 11 The flap is then closed. A psoas hitch may be performed to relieve any excess tension.

intestinal conduits using either small or large bowel, and various versions of the ileocecal continent urinary reservoir.

Indications

In gynecology, most urinary diversions are performed as part of the reconstructive phase of a pelvic exenteration or because of severe irradiation injury to the bladder. The type of diversion employed depends on the surgeon's preference, the patient's overall health, the prognosis, and the patient's ability to perform the tasks necessary to catheterize a continent pouch.

The ileal conduit is the simplest diversion to perform. Care must be exercised in patients who have undergone radiotherapy as the vascular supply to the conduit may be compromised. The patient must also wear an appliance at all times.

Colonic conduits have the benefit that the segment may be taken from anywhere along the length of the colon. Anatomically, the sigmoid is the easiest part as it is ideally located for a urinary conduit. Like the ileum, however, it can be affected by prior radiotherapy. The transverse colon conduit avoids this problem, but because it is located in the upper abdomen, it is more difficult to perform the ureteral anastomoses.

Continent urinary reservoirs have the chief advantage that the patient is not required to wear an appliance continuously. The patient must be able to self-catheterize at least four times a day and irrigate the reservoir as needed. This can be particularly difficult for visually impaired, obese, or elderly patients. The pouch is also more technically difficult and time consuming to construct.

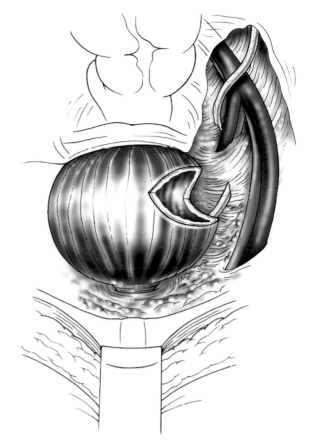

Figure 13 The bladder is opened and the lateral aspect brought into approximation with the injured ureter.

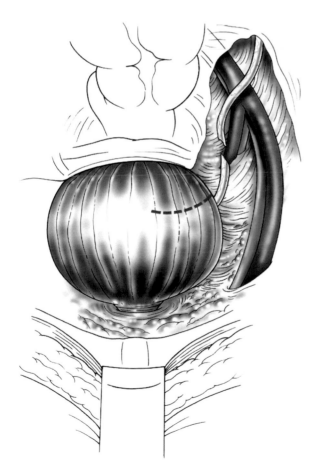

Figure 12 Demel flap: initial incision.

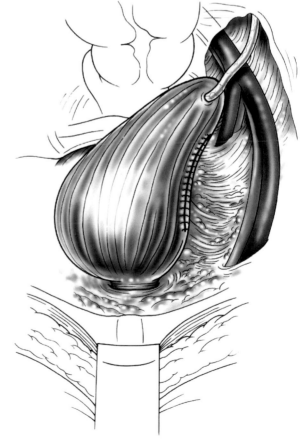

Figure 14 Anastomosis is performed and the bladder closed.

Anatomic Considerations

Vascular Supply

Ileum

The ileum receives its vascular supply from the ileocolic artery, which is a branch of the superior mesenteric artery (SMA). Collateral circulation is from the right colic artery, which is also a branch of the SMA. The terminal ileum is at particular risk of vascular insufficiency owing to the fact that it is supplied by the terminal branches of the ileocolic artery and collateral circulation is poor.

Colon

The colon is supplied by branches of the superior and inferior mesenteric arteries (IMA). The right and middle colic arteries arise from the SMA and supply the right and transverse colons respectively up to the splenic flexure. The left colic and sigmoid arteries are branches of the IMA and supply the left and sigmoid colon, respectively. Collateral circulation to the sigmoid is via the superior rectal artery, a branch of the IMA, which anastomoses with the middle and inferior rectal arteries, both branches of the hypogastric artery.

Nerve Supply

Ileum

The ileum is innervated by the superior mesenteric plexus, which carries autonomic fibers from the vagus and thoracic splanchnic nerves.

Colon

The innervation of the colon is from the superior and inferior mesenteric plexuses, which carry autonomic fibers from the vagus, thoracic, and lumbar splanchnic nerves.

Operative Procedure

General Considerations

Preoperative preparation should include a mechanical and antibiotic bowel preparation using a bowel cleansing solution such as Golytely (Schwarz Pharma, Inc., Milwaukee, Wisconsin, USA), and oral neomycin, erythromycin and an antifungal such as fluconazole. Perioperative antibiotics may also be required. A preoperative renogram should be performed to assess baseline renal function in all patients receiving a continent conduit and in any other patient whose renal function is in question.

Our preference is to stent all ureters prior to performing the anastomosis. This eliminates the risk of sewing the ureter closed or of disrupting the sutures, which can occur when stenting is performed after suturing. Stents are held in place by placing a 5-0 or 6-0 plain gut suture through the ureter and the stent approximately 2 cm from the junction of the ureter and pouch. We also study all stents radiographically prior to removing them. Retrograde "stentograms" can demonstrate leaks if present and strictures can be identified with a pull-back study. We generally study with intent to remove stents two to three weeks postoperatively.

A closed suction drain (e.g., Jackson Pratt) is placed behind the pouch or conduit in the area of the ureteral anastomoses in all patients. The major benefit is in the detection of anastomotic leaks. The drain is removed at the same time as the ureteral stents.

Ileal Conduit

The ileum is carefully inspected for the presence of radiation injury, if applicable. Where injury is present, a colonic conduit is preferred. The conduit can be as short as 4 to 6 cm or as long as 15 cm. Shorter conduits are less prone to electrolyte disturbances, but may make it difficult or impossible to perform tension-free ureteroileal anastomoses. The ileal segment is transected at both ends using an intestinal stapler. The distal end should be at least 10 cm from the ileocecal valve. An ileoileal anastomosis restores bowel continuity. The mesentery is disrupted as little as possible (Fig. 15).

The ureters are divided as far distally as is practical without involving diseased sections. The ureters and the conduit must be behind the ileal mesentery and the left ureter must be tunneled through the retroperitoneum behind the base of the sigmoid mesentery to bring it to the patient's right side (Fig. 16).

The site for the anastomosis should be about 2 cm from the closed end of the conduit (Fig. 17). A small (less than 1 cm) ellipse of tissue is removed from the wall of the ileum at the chosen site for the anastomoses. The ureteral ends are widened by first cutting them at an angle and then making a single longitudinal incision such that the ureteral opening corresponds to that in the bowel wall. Full-thickness sutures of 4-0 polyglycolic acid are used to perform end-to-side ureteroileostomies. Usually four to six sutures are sufficient (Fig. 18). A stoma is then created with the distal end of the ileal segment. The stoma is generally located in the right lower quadrant and is ideally marked preoperatively, taking into consideration the type of appliance to be used, the patient's body habitus and the location of her belt line when standing. A circle of skin is excised, the subcutaneous fat is either spread apart with retractors or excised, and a cruciate incision is made in the fascia. The fibers of the rectus muscle are bluntly separated and the posterior sheath and peritoneum are incised. The stoma should admit one to one and a half fingers if it is of adequate caliber. The stoma is everted into a "rosebud" raised slightly above skin level. The proximal end can then be sutured to the peritoneum overlying the sacral promontory.

An alternative technique is a modification of the Bricker ileal conduit that provides for tension-free ureteral anastomosis while better defining conduit length. Because ureteral anastomosis is performed after the stoma is matured, this technique also reduces post-anastomosis manipulation. While the technique is presented as a modification for ileal conduits, it has been used for colonic conduits as well.

The terminal ileum is transected at about 10 to 15 cm proximal to the ileocecal valve using a stapling device. The proximal portion of ileum is mobilized so that the stapled end can be brought through the anterior abdominal wall to mature the conduit stoma. After maturing the stoma as previously described, the ileum is transected proximally after approximating the conduit to the ureters and assessing the appropriate length. The distal end of the Yankaur suction device is then manually inserted through the stoma and advanced into the proximal end of the conduit. The conduit wall is incised directly over the tip of the suction using an electrosurgical instrument. Gently advancing the Yankaur tip partially through this new aperture exposes the conduit mucosa. A single-J 70 cm ureteral stent of the desired size (7.0–8.5 Fr) is inserted through the Yankaur suction device

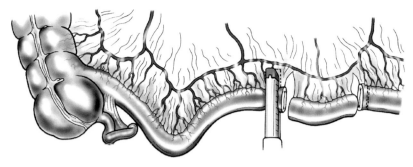

Figure 15 A segment of ileum is isolated sufficiently distant from the ileocecal junction to avoid the "watershed" area.

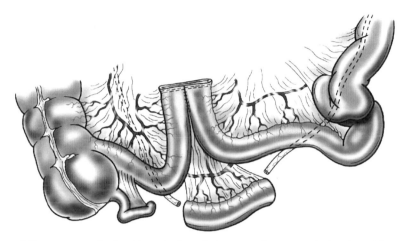

Figure 16 Bowel continuity is restored. The ureters are freed and brought through the retroperitoneum to the location of the conduit (generally, in the area of the sacral promontory).

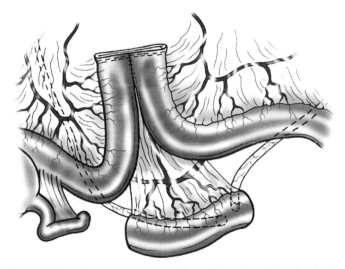

Figure 17 Ureteral anastomoses are performed about 2 cm from the closed end of the conduit.

and advanced into the ureter to the renal pelvis. A mucosa-to-mucosa ureteral anastomosis is performed using four to five interrupted stitches using a 4-0 delayed absorbable suture (Fig. 19).

Colonic Conduit

Colonic conduits are usually 15 to 20 cm in length. Since the colon will contract once isolated, a segment somewhat longer

than desired should be selected. Bowel continuity can then be restored or a colostomy can be created if the distal colon is to be removed as part of an exenterative procedure. The mesenteric incisions should be of sufficient length to allow mobility of the conduit without interfering with the vascular supply to either the conduit or the remaining colon. The colonic anastomosis is performed anterior to the conduit. For a transverse colon conduit, the omentum must be dissected off the colon prior to isolating the conduit. The conduits should be isoperistaltic to prevent stasis, but can be constructed in an antiperistaltic fashion if anatomically necessary with no significant adverse effects.

The ureteral anastomoses are performed with 4-0 interrupted absorbable mucosa-to-mucosa sutures in separate teniae. Again, four to six sutures usually suffice. The right ureter must be brought over to the left side retroperitoneally and behind the sigmoid mesentery (for a sigmoid conduit). The ureters are spatulated as described above for ileal conduits. The ureteral anastomoses should be staggered by 2 to 3 cm so that one is more proximal than the other.

A stoma is created with the distal end of the conduit. The stoma is usually on the left side, but it can be on the right if dictated by anatomical concerns or if the patient has a colostomy as well. The stomal site must be larger than that for an ileal conduit and should admit at least two fingers. Finally, the proximal end is fixed to the psoas muscle with one or two interrupted permanent sutures.

Continent Ileocolic Reservoir
A 10-cm length of distal ileum and 32 cm of ascending and proximal transverse colon are isolated and mobilized. An ileotransverse enterocolostomy is performed in the standard fashion to restore bowel continuity. The appendix is removed at this time if it is present (Fig. 20).

The colon is then folded on itself in a U configuration, bringing the transected end of the transverse colon in

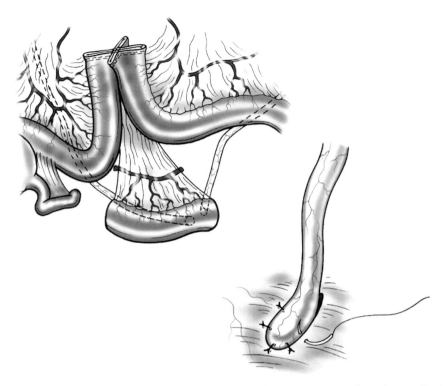

Figure 18 Detail of anastomosis. After removal of a small portion of the wall of the bowel the anastomosis is performed externally with full thickness, interrupted absorbable suture.

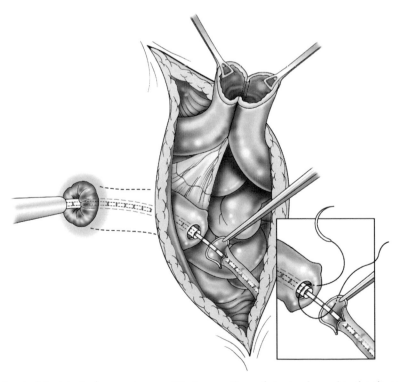

Figure 19 After isolating the distal end of the intestinal segment, a metal Yankaur suction catheter is advanced to the planned anastomotic site. A transmural incision is made over the end of the catheter with the electrosurgical instrument. The ureteral anastomosis is secured with interrupted 4-0 vicryl sutures. The catheter helps incorporate the seromuscular and mucosal layers as the needle is placed against and run along the metal catheter from outside to inside (insert). A 7-Fr 70 cm single-J stent is threaded through the catheter and passed directly into the ureteral lumen (reproduced with permission from *Gynecologic Oncology*, Winter et al., Modified technique for urinary diversion with incontinent conduits).

approximation to the cecum. Two interrupted stay sutures are used to maintain alignment of the colon. Electrocautery is used to make two small colotomies (2–4 cm) in the center of each segment of colon (Fig. 21A and B).

A PolyGIA stapler (US Surgical, Norwalk, Connecticut, USA) is then used to detubularize the colon. Each arm is passed into adjacent colon segments toward one end of the reservoir. Once the stapler is articulated and fired, a common lumen is created with two rows of absorbable staples on each side of the incision line created by the knife within the instrument (Fig. 22A and B). A second instrument is then fired from this same point toward the opposite end of the reservoir, thus completing the detubularization process.

The continence mechanism is constructed by tapering the ileum and reinforcing the ileocecal valve (Fig. 23). A 14-Fr red rubber catheter is placed in the ileum. Allis clamps are placed along the antimesenteric border to create countertension and a gastrointestinal stapler is used to taper the ileal segment so that the inside diameter approaches that of the catheter. More than one firing of the stapler may be required.

Two or three purse-string sutures of 2-0 silk suture are then placed at the level of the ileocecal valve. The sutures are placed through the serosa and muscularis layers, but not through the mucosa (Fig. 24).

Working through the unified colotomy in the center of the pouch, the ureters are then anastomosed to the pouch (Fig. 25). A long, curved instrument is passed through the colotomy into the pouch to the intended location of the anastomosis. A colotomy is made at this point and the ureter is then drawn into the interior of the pouch. The ureters are spatulated and anastomosed from within the pouch with mucosa-to-mucosa

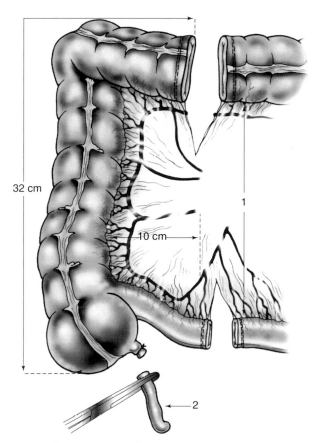

Figure 20 To begin a continent ileocecal reservoir the ileum is divided about 10 cm from the ileocecal valve and the colon is divided 32 cm from the cecum. If possible, this should be proximal to the middle colic artery. The appendix, if present, is removed. 1 Anastomosis performed to restore bowel continuity. 2 Appendectomy performed.

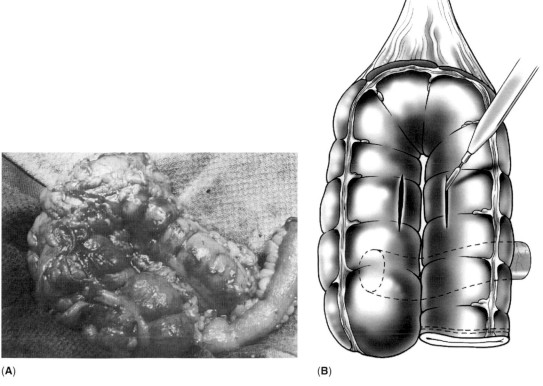

(A) **(B)**

Figure 21 The colon is folded over on itself into a U as A and enterotomies are made.

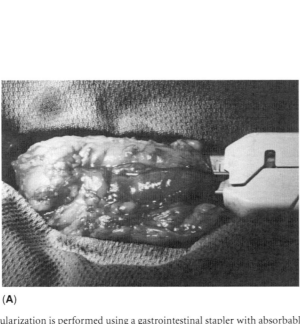
(A)

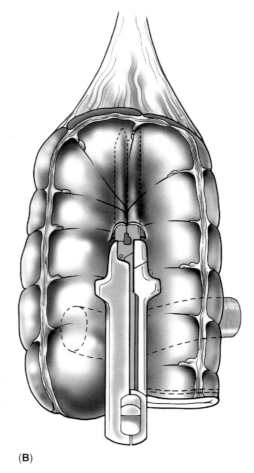
(B)

Figure 22 Detubularization is performed using a gastrointestinal stapler with absorbable staples. Two staplers are required, one toward each end of the conduit, as the staplers are not reloadable.

interrupted 4-0 delayed absorbable sutures, full thickness through the ureter, and partial thickness through the bowel (mucosa and submucosa only). Externally, the serosa of the bowel and the adventitia of the ureters are sutured together in a similar fashion with two or three sutures. The left ureter must be brought to the right side retroperitoneally behind the sigmoid mesentery.

Single J ureteral stents (7 Fr) are placed and fixed in position with a 5-0 or 6-0 plain gut suture which passes through the ureter and the stent approximately 2 cm from the junction of ureter and pouch. The stents are externalized through the anterior wall of the pouch and the abdominal wall, and the pouch is fixed to the anterior abdominal wall with permanent sutures. The external end of the right stent can be cut at a right angle, and the end of the left stent can be cut at a 45° angle for easy differentiation later.

The 14-Fr red rubber catheter is exchanged for a triple-lumen Foley catheter of similar size. The Foley catheter is then left in place for two weeks until radiographic imaging confirms an intact system. At that stage the colotomy can then be closed with sutures or a TA-55 thoracoabdominal intestinal stapler. The ileum is also then externalized in the right lower quadrant. In some patients, the stoma can be placed in the umbilicus, which gives an excellent cosmetic result and makes catheterization easier as this is the thinnest portion of the abdominal wall. The continent stoma should not form a rose-bud, but simply be everted flush with the skin. It is important

that the course of the ileum be relatively straight to ease catheterization. A closed suction drain is placed behind the pouch and is removed with the ureteral stents.

Postoperative pouch drainage via intermittent low pressure wall suction and irrigation can be performed via the Foley catheter. It is essential to monitor input and output of the pouch and to irrigate the pouch gently with 30 to 50 ml of normal saline frequently—as often as every two to four hours—in the immediate postoperative period to prevent mucus build-up. If output is significantly less than input, an ultrasound scan of the pouch can be done to ensure that it has not become overdistended. Urine output is followed separately from the stents which are connected to individual urimeters, carefully marked "left" and "right". The stents can also be irrigated with 10 mL of normal saline if urine output falls off. If there is no response to repeated irrigations, the stent should be studied radiographically to ensure proper placement and function. When the output decreases the pouch can be changed to gravity drainage, but the irrigations should continue at least four times a day with the irrigation fluid removed immediately.

A contrast study of the pouch and the ureters is performed about two weeks postoperatively. If all is normal, the stents are removed and the patient is then taught self-catheterization which initially should be performed every two to four hours. The patient should also continue to irrigate the pouch at least four times a day to prevent mucus build-up.

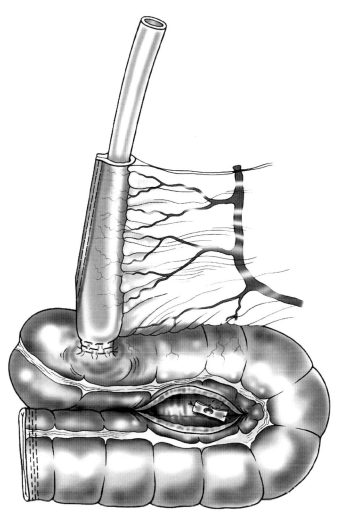

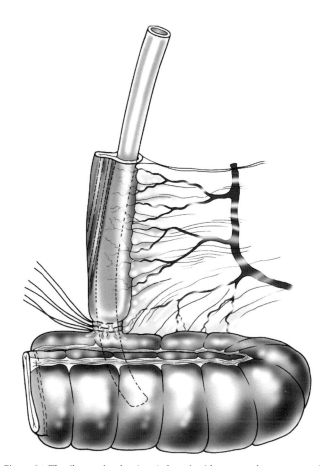

Figure 23 Using a standard gastrointestinal stapler, the ileal section is tapered over a 14-Fr red rubber catheter. 1 Rubber catheter, 2 Allis clamp.

Figure 24 The ileocecal valve is reinforced with two to three purse-string sutures of non-absorbable suture such as silk.

Figure 25 Working through the colotomy, the ureteral anastomosis is performed. After bringing the ureter through the wall of the conduit, the end is spatulated; interrupted absorbable sutures incorporating the full thickness of the ureter, and partial thickness of the colon wall are used to perform the anastomosis.

ORTHOTOPIC NEOBLADDER

Orthotopic reconstruction has played a major role in the evolution of urinary diversion. It was first described in 1888 and later revisited in 1951. Advances in surgical techniques have improved the quality of life in women requiring radical cystectomy by allowing volitional, physiologic voiding. In the past 15 years, orthotopic neobladder surgery has emerged as an appealing alternative to the time-honored conduit for urinary diversion.

Indications

Orthotopic neobladder surgery is selected when radical cystectomy is required for primary and secondary cancer of the bladder. It is often performed in conjunction with pelvic exenteration. Although desirable for its physiologic features described above, the neobladder is contraindicated in several situations. Absolute contraindications include impaired renal function due to longstanding obstruction, chronic renal failure (serum creatinine 150–200 μmol/L), and hepatic dysfunction. Compromised intestinal function may also preclude neobladder surgery, particularly in the case of the presence of inflammatory bowel disease. In addition, the rhabdosphincter must be left intact following cystectomy, and the urethra must be free of tumor.

Previously, it was believed that removing the urethra at the time of cystectomy was necessary to obtain adequate margins. However, studies of cystectomy specimens have suggested that the urethra is free of tumor in the majority of cases where the bladder neck and proximal urethra are free of disease, and that skip lesions are rare. Therefore, intraoperative frozen section analysis of the surgical margin, including the proximal urethra, is necessary to determine candidacy of orthotopic diversion.

Anatomic Considerations
Vascular Supply
Bladder
The main blood supply to the bladder involves the superior and inferior vesical arteries, which are branches of the anterior division of the hypogastric artery. Branches of the obturator, uterine, and vaginal arteries may also be involved.

Urethra
The urethra receives its blood supply from branches of the pudendal and inferior vesical arteries.

Ileum
The ileocolic artery, a branch of the SMA, is the main blood supply to the ileum. The right colic artery (also a branch of the SMA) supplies collateral circulation.

Colon
The colon is supplied by the superior and IMA. Arising from the SMA, the right and middle colic arteries supply the right colon and the transverse colon up to the splenic flexure. The left colic and sigmoid arteries are IMA branches that supply the left and sigmoid colon. The superior rectal artery, another branch of the IMA, anastomoses with the middle and inferior rectal arteries, supplying collateral circulation to the sigmoid colon.

Nerve Supply
Bladder
The bladder is innervated by the vesical plexus, which arises from T11 to L2 and travels through the cardinal ligament. The plexus carries efferent and afferent autonomic fibers, including sympathetic and parasympathetic innervation.

Urethra
The proximal urethra is innervated by the sympathetic fibers of the pelvic plexus which courses through the cardinal ligament. The distal two-thirds of the urethra, including the rhabdosphincter, is innervated by branches of the pudendal nerve which course along the pelvic floor posterior to the levator muscles.

Ileum
The superior mesenteric plexus innervates the ileum. It carries autonomic nerve fibers from the vagus and thoracic splanchnic nerves.

Colon
The colon is innervated by the superior and inferior mesenteric plexuses, carrying autonomic fibers from the vagus, thoracic, and lumbar splanchnic nerves.

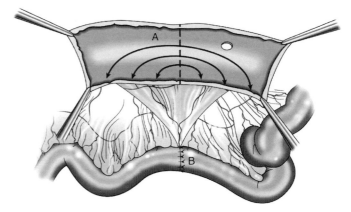

Figure 26 (**A**) Ileal re-anastamosis (**B**) Spatulation of the ileum.

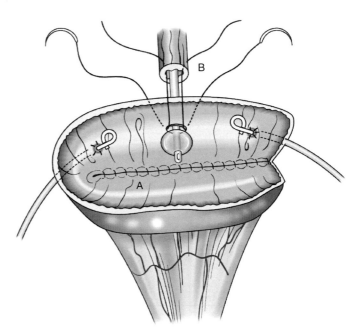

Figure 27 (**A**) U-shaped reservoir (**B**) Urethral attachment.

Surgical Procedure
When performing an orthotopic reconstruction, the radical cystectomy is modified to preserve the urethra and maintain the continence mechanism. This modification includes minimal dissection anteriorly to avoid disruption of the urethral innervation, as well as preserving the pubourethral suspensory ligaments.

Any segment of the gastrointestinal tract may be used for the neobladder, provided it has the ability to reach the graft site without tension. However, the ileum has become a popular choice over the large bowel because it has less contractility and less reabsorption of urinary constituents.

The cystectomy is carried out in an anterograde fashion to the level of the vaginal apex, where a plane is created between the posterior bladder base (trigone) and vagina. The Foley catheter balloon may be palpated and used as an indicator of the urethrovesical junction. Dissection is then continued just distal to this point. Extensive dissection distally along the posterior urethra is avoided in order to prevent the disruption of pudendal innervation of the urethra and its musculofascial support of the anterior vagina.

After completion of the posterior dissection, a Satinski vascular clamp is placed across the bladder neck to prevent any tumor spillage from the bladder. While applying gentle traction, the proximal urethra is transected below the bladder neck and clamped. Frozen-section analysis of the proximal urethra is necessary to exclude the presence of tumor. Eight-to-ten urethral sutures are placed which will later be used to attach the urethra to the neobladder.

When small intestine is chosen for the bladder substitution, a 40 to 60 cm segment of ileum is isolated from the bowel. Ileal reanastomosis is performed to restore the integrity of the main portion of the bowel (Fig. 26A). The isolated ileum is detubularized along the antimesenteric border. At the end, where the ileourethral anastmosis will occur, the incision is curved toward the mesenteric border, spatulating the ileum (Fig. 26B). The spatulated ileum is then folded into a U-, S-, or W-shaped reservoir (Fig. 27A). The limbs of ileum are sutured together with running absorbable material to form a broad plate. An opening is made for the urethral reattachment in the caudal portion of the neobladder (Fig. 26B).

Using the previously placed urethral sutures, the urethra is connected to the reservoir. These sutures, originally placed from inside to outside of the urethra, are sewn through the full thickness of the neobladder at the posterior margin of the ileourethral anastomosis. They are tied so that the knots lie within the lumen of the anastomosis (Fig. 27B).

Two small openings are made in the wall of the neobladder lateral to the urethral implantation site. The ureters are reimplanted in an antirefluxing fashion (described previously in this chapter) with stent placement. The ileal plate is then folded to form a pouch and closed with running absorbable suture. To reduce tension on the anastomosis, the pouch is sutured to the pelvic fascia.

Various techniques to create a neobladder exist. Alternative approaches to the surgery described above use similar techniques using other segments of the bowel. The distal 20 cm of ileum and 15 cm of cecum and ascending colon (MAINZ pouch) or 20 to 30 cm of cecum and ascending colon may also be used. The selection bowel segment should be based on the ability to avoid tension on the completed anastomosis.

ACKNOWLEDGMENT
The authors would like to thank Dr William E. Winter for his contribution to this chapter.

BIBLIOGRAPHY

Camey M (1990) Detubularized U-shaped cystoplasty (Camey 2). *Curr Surg Tech Urol* **3**:1–8.

Cosin JA, Carter JR, Paley PJ, et al. (1997) A simplified method for detubularization in the construction of a continent ileocolic reservoir (Miami pouch). *Gynecol Oncol* **64**:436–41.

Hartenbach EM, Saltzman AK, Carter JR, et al. (1995) Nonsurgical management strategies for the functional complications of ileocolonic continent urinary reservoirs. *Gynecol Oncol* **56**:127–8.

Kock NG, Nilson AE, Nilsson LO, et al. (1982) Urinary diversion via continent ileal reservoir: clinical results in 12 patients. *J Urol* **128**:469–75.

Penalver MA, Darwich EB, Averette HE, et al. (1989) Continent urinary diversion in gynecologic oncology. *Gynecol Oncol* **34**:274–88.

Rowland RG, Mitchell ME, Bihrle R, et al. (1989) Indiana continent urinary reservoir. *J Urol* **137**:1136–9.

Stein JP, Ginsberg DA, Skinner DG (2002) Indications and technique of the orthotopic neobladder in women. *Urol Clin North Am* **29**:725–34.

Symmonds RE (1976) Ureteral injuries associated with gynecologic surgery: prevention and management. *Clin Obstet Gynecol* **19**:623–44.

Thuroff JW, Alken P, Reidmiller H, et al. (1985) The MAINZ pouch (mixed augmentation ileum 'n cecum) for bladder augmentation and continent diversion. *World J Urol* **3**:179–84.

Walsh PC, Retik AB, Starney TA, et al. (1998) *Campbell's Urology*, vol. 3, 7th edn. Philadelphia: WB Saunders, pp. 3201–14.

Wheeless CR, Jr (1992) Recent advances in surgical reconstruction of the gynecologic cancer patient. *Curr Opin Obstet Gynecol* **4**:91–101.

Winter W (2002) Modified technique for urinary diversion with incontinent conduits. *Gynecol Oncol* **86**:351–3.

30 Fistula repair
Paul Hilton

ETIOLOGY AND EPIDEMIOLOGY

Urogenital fistulas may occur congenitally, but are most often acquired from obstetric, surgical, radiation, and malignant causes. The same factors may be responsible for intestino-genital fistulas, although inflammatory bowel disease is an additional important etiological factor here. In most developing countries over 90% of fistulas are of obstetric etiology, whereas in the United Kingdom and United States approximately 70% follow pelvic surgery.

Obstetric Causes

The overwhelming proportions of obstetric fistulas in the developing world are complications of neglected obstructed labor. In the developed world, however, obstetric fistulas are associated with rupture of the uterus following previous cesarean section, or assisted vaginal delivery (Table 1). Obstetric factors leading to ano-vaginal or recto-vaginal fistulas include an unrecognized fourth-degree tear or infection and the breakdown of repair of a third- or fourth-degree tear.

Surgical Causes

Genital fistula may occur following a wide range of surgical procedures within the pelvis (Table 1). It is often supposed that this complication results from direct injury to the lower urinary tract at the time of operation. Certainly on occasions careless, hurried, or rough surgical technique makes injury to the lower urinary tract much more likely. Of the 310 cases of urogenital fistulas referred to the author over the last 10 years, 216 (70%) were associated with pelvic surgery and 150 followed hysterectomy (48% overall, 69% of surgical cases); of these, only 6 (4%) presented with leakage of urine on the first day postoperatively. In other cases, it is presumed that tissue devascularization during dissection, inadvertent suture placement, pelvic hematoma formation, or infection developing postoperatively results in tissue necrosis with leakage developing most usually 5 to 10 days later. It may also be inevitable and unavoidable in some cases. Approximately, 10% to 15% of post-surgical fistulas present late, between 10 and 30 days after the procedure. Overdistension of the bladder postoperatively may be an additional factor in many of these latter cases. It has recently been shown that there is a high incidence of abnormalities of lower urinary tract function in fistula patients; whether these abnormalities antedate the surgery, or develop with or as a consequence of the fistula is unclear. It is likely that patients with a habit of infrequent voiding, or those with inefficient detrusor contractility, may be at increased risk of postoperative urinary retention; if this is not recognized early and managed appropriately, the risk of fistula formation may be increased. Although it is important to remember that the majority of surgical fistulas follow apparently straightforward hysterectomy in skilled hands, several risk factors may make

direct injury more likely (Table 2). Data from the author's own series and from U.K. Hospital Episode Statistics suggest a rate of one urogenital fistula in 700 total (simple) abdominal hysterectomies, one in 2600 vaginal hysterectomies, one in 5000 subtotal hysterectomies, and one in 100 radical hysterectomies (Hilton 2009, unpublished). Ano- and recto-vaginal fistulas may also have a surgical etiology with vaginal hysterectomy, rectocele repair, hemorrhoidectomy, low anterior resection, and panproctocolectomy being commonly associated.

Radiation

Injury to the gastrointestinal tract may arise following therapeutic radiotherapy with the incidence of complications increasing when the radiation dose exceeds 5000 cGy. The obliterative endarteritis associated with ionizing radiation in therapeutic dosage may proceed over many years and may result in fistula formation long after the primary malignancy has been treated. Patients with a vesico-vaginal fistulas often have symptoms of radiation cystitis that improve on appearance of the fistula. Of the 28 radiation fistulas in the author's series, the interval between fistula development and radiotherapy ranged from 1 year to 30 years. The associated devascularization in the adjacent tissues means that ordinary surgical repair has a high likelihood of failure, and modified surgical techniques are required.

Malignancy

Excluding the effects of treatment, malignant disease itself may result in genital tract fistula. Carcinoma of cervix, vagina, and rectum are the most common malignancies to present in this way. It is relatively unusual for urothelial tumors to present with fistula formation, other than following surgery or radiotherapy. The development of a fistula may be a distressing part of the terminal phase of malignant disease; it is nevertheless one deserving not simply compassion, but full consideration of the therapeutic or palliative possibilities. Bilateral permanent nephrostomies may give continence when all else fails.

Inflammatory Bowel Disease

Inflammatory bowel disease is the most significant cause of intestino-genital fistulas in the United Kingdom, although these fistulas rarely present directly to the gynecologist. Diverticular disease can produce colo-vaginal fistulas and rarely colo-uterine or colo-vesical fistulas, with surprisingly few symptoms attributable to the intestinal pathology. It has been estimated that 2% of patients with diverticulosis will develop fistulas arising either through direct extension from a ruptured diverticulum or through erosion from a diverticular abscess. The possibility should not be overlooked if an elderly woman complains of feculent discharge or becomes

Table 1 Etiology of Uro-genital Fistulas in Two Series, from the North of England, and From South-east Nigeria

Etiology	NE England n = 310		SE Nigeria n = 2389[a]	
Obstetric				–
Obstructed labor	2		1918	–
Caesarean section	13		165	–
Ruptured uterus	8		119	–
Forceps/ventouse	5			–
Breech extraction	1			–
Placental abruption	1			–
Caesarean hysterectomy	3			–
Symphysiotomy	2			–
Obstetric subtotal (% of total)	35	11.3%	2202	92.2%
Surgical				–
Abdominal hysterectomy	122		33	–
Radical hysterectomy	16			–
Urethral diverticulectomy	16			–
Colectomy	9			–
Colporrhaphy	10		35	–
Vaginal hysterectomy	5		25	–
Mid-urethral tape procedures	6			–
LAVH	3			–
Cystoplasty and colposuspension	2			–
Colposuspension	2			–
Cervical stumpectomy	2			–
LLETZ	3			–
Nephroureterectomy	2			–
Subtotal hysterectomy	2			–
TAH and colporrhaphy	1			–
Mesh colporrhaphy + tape	1			–
TAH and colposuspension	1			–
Laparoscopic oophorectomy	1			–
Sling	2			–
Partial vaginectomy	2			–
Periurethral bulking agents	1			–
Needle suspension	1			–
Sub-trigonal phenol injection	1			–
Lithoclast	1			–
Partial vaginectomy	1			–
Ileoanal pouch	1			–
Sacrospinous fixation	1			–
Unknown surgery in childhood	1			–
Suture to vaginal laceration			12	–
Surgical subtotal (% of total)	216	69.7%	105	4.4%
Radiation	28	9.0%	0	–
Malignancy	2	0.6%	42	1.8%
Miscellaneous				–
Vaginal pessary	9			–
Infection	5		7	–
Congenital	5			–
Foreign body	4			–
Catheter induced	3			–
Trauma	2		11	–
Coital injury	1		22	–
Miscellaneous subtotal (% of total)	29	9.4%	40	1.7%

[a]2389 patients for whom notes were examined, out of total series of 2484 patients. LAVH - laparoscopically assisted vaginal hysterectomy. LLETZ - large loop excision of Transformation Zone. TAH - Total Abdominal Hysterectomy.

Table 2 Risk Factors for Postoperative Fistula

Risk factor	Pathology	Specific example
Anatomical distortion		Fibroids Ovarian mass
Abnormal tissue adhesion	Inflammation	Infection Endometriosis
	Previous surgery	Cesarean section Cone biopsy Colporrhaphy
	Malignancy	
Impaired vascularity	Ionizing radiation	Preoperative radiotherapy
	Metabolic abnormality	Diabetes mellitus
	Radical surgery	
Compromised healing		Anemia Nutritional deficiency
Abnormality of bladder function		Voiding dysfunction

incontinent without concomitant urinary problems. Pneumaturia and fecaluria are late presenting signs of a colovesical fistula. Crohn's disease appears to be increasing in frequency in the Western world, and a total fistula rate approaching 40% has been reported; in females the involvement of the genital tract may be up to 7%. Ulcerative colitis, unlike Crohn's disease, is not a transmural disease and therefore it is associated with only a small incidence of rectovaginal fistula. In the author's own series of recto-vaginal fistulas, 65% are obstetric in origin, 21% relate to inflammatory bowel disease, 7% follow radiotherapy, and 7% are of uncertain cause.

Miscellaneous
Other miscellaneous causes of fistulas in the genital tract include infection (lymphogranuloma venereum, schistosomiasis, tuberculosis, actinomycosis, measles, noma vaginae), trauma (penetrating trauma, coital injury, neglected pessary, or other foreign bodies) and catheter-related injuries.

CLASSIFICATION
There is no standardized or universally accepted method for describing or classifying fistulas although development of such a system has been recommended by the WHO International Consultation on Incontinence, to include location and size of the fistula; functional impact and quantification of the degree of vaginal scarring. Many different fistula classifications already proposed are based on anatomical site; often sub-classified into simple fistulas (where the tissues are healthy and access good) or complicated fistulas (where there is tissue loss, scarring, impaired access, involvement of the ureteric orifices, or a coexistent recto-vaginal fistula). Urogenital fistulas may be classified into urethral, bladder neck, sub-symphysial (a complex form involving circumferential loss of the urethra with fixation to bone), mid-vaginal, juxta-cervical or vault fistulas, massive fistulas extending from bladder neck to vault, and vesico-uterine or vesico-cervical fistulas. While over 60% of fistulas in the developing world are mid-vaginal, juxta-cervical or massive

(reflecting their obstetric etiology), such cases are relatively rare in Western fistula practice; 50% of the fistulas managed in the United Kingdom are situated in the vaginal vault (reflecting their surgical etiology). Recto-vaginal fistulas are also classified according to anatomical site and relationship to the underlying anal sphincter.

PRESENTATION

Fistulas between the urinary tract and the female genital tract are characteristically said to present with continuous urinary incontinence, with limited sensation of bladder fullness, and with infrequent voiding. Where there is extensive tissue loss, as in obstetric or radiation fistulas, this typical history is usually present, the clinical findings gross, and the diagnosis rarely in doubt. With surgical fistulas, however, the history may be atypical and the orifice small, elusive or occasionally completely invisible. Under these circumstances the diagnosis can be much more difficult, and a high index of clinical suspicion must be maintained.

Ureteric fistulas have similar causes to bladder fistulas, and the mechanism may be one of direct injury by incision, division or excision, or of ischemia from strangulation by suture, crushing by clamp or stripping by dissection; the presentation may therefore be similarly variable. With direct injury leakage is usually apparent from the first postoperative day. Urine output may be physiologically reduced for some hours following surgery, and if there is significant operative or postoperative hypotension oliguria may persist longer. Once renal function is restored, however, leakage will usually be apparent promptly. With other mechanisms obstruction is likely to be present to a greater or lesser degree, and the initial symptoms may be of pyrexia or loin pain, with incontinence occurring only after sloughing of the ischemic tissue, from around five days up to six weeks later.

INVESTIGATIONS

If there is suspicion of a fistula, but its presence is not easily confirmed by clinical examination with a speculum, further investigation will be necessary to confirm or exclude the possibility fully. Even where the diagnosis is clinically obvious, additional investigation may be appropriate for full evaluation prior to deciding upon treatment. The main principles of investigation therefore are as follows:

- to confirm that the discharge is urinary/fecal
- to establish that the leakage is extra-urethral rather than urethral
- to establish the site of leakage
- to exclude other organ involvement.

Biochemistry and Microbiology

Excessive vaginal discharge or drainage of serum from a pelvic hematoma postoperatively may simulate a urinary fistula. If the fluid is in sufficient quantity to be collected, biochemical analysis of its urea content in comparison with that of urine and serum will confirm its origin. Urinary infection is surprisingly uncommon in fistula patients, although urine culture should be undertaken (especially where there have been previous attempts at surgery) and appropriate antibiotic therapy instituted.

Dye Studies

Although other imaging techniques undoubtedly have a role (see below), carefully conducted dye studies remain the investigation of first choice. *Phenazopyridine* may be used orally (no longer available in United Kingdom), or indigo carmine intravenously, to stain the urine and hence confirm the presence of a fistula. The identification of the site of a fistula is best carried out by the instillation of colored dye (methylene blue or indigo carmine) into the bladder through a catheter with the patient in the lithotomy position. The traditional "three swab test" has its limitations and is not recommended; the examination is best carried out with direct inspection, and multiple fistulas may be located in this way. If leakage of clear fluid continues after dye instillation a ureteric fistula is likely, and this is most easily confirmed by a "two dye test", using *phenazopyridine* to stain the renal urine and methylene blue to stain bladder contents.

Dye tests are less useful for intestinal fistulas, although a carmine marker taken orally may confirm their presence. Rectal distension with air via a sigmoidoscope may be of more value; if the patient is kept in a slight head-down position and the vagina filled with saline, the bubbling of any air leaked through a low fistula may be detected.

Imaging

Excretion Urography

Although intravenous urography is a particularly insensitive investigation in the diagnosis of vesico vaginal fistula, knowledge of upper urinary tract status may have a significant influence on treatment measures applied, and should therefore be looked on as an essential investigation for any suspected or confirmed urinary fistula. Compromise to ureteric function is a particularly common finding when a fistula occurs in relation to malignant disease or its treatment (by radiation or surgery).

Dilatation of the ureter is characteristic in ureteric fistula, and its finding in association with a known vesico-vaginal fistula should raise suspicion of a complex uretero-vesico-vaginal lesion (Fig. 1). While essential for the diagnosis of ureteric fistula, intravenous urography is not completely sensitive; the presence of a periureteric flare is, however, highly suggestive of extravasation at this site.

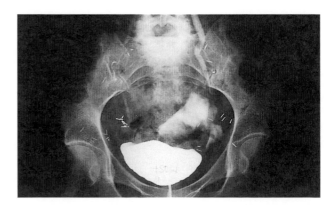

Figure 1 Intravenous urogram (with simultaneous cystogram) demonstrating a complex surgical fistula occurring after radical hysterectomy. After further investigation including cystourethroscopy, sigmoidoscopy, barium enema, and retrograde cannulation of the vaginal vault to perform fistulography, the lesion was defined as a uretero-colo-vesico-vaginal fistula.

Retrograde Pyelography

Retrograde pyelography is a more reliable way of identifying the exact site of a uretero-vaginal fistula, and may be undertaken simultaneously with either retrograde or percutaneous catheterization for therapeutic stenting of the ureter (see chapter 6).

Cystography

Cystography is not particularly helpful in the basic diagnosis of vesico-vaginal fistulas, and a dye test carried out under direct vision is likely to be more sensitive. It may, however, occasionally be useful in achieving a diagnosis in complex fistulas or vesico-uterine fistulas.

Fistulography

Fistulography is a special example of the X-ray technique also referred to as sinography. For small fistulas, a ureteric catheter is suitable, although if the hole is large enough a small Foley catheter may be used to deliver the radio-opaque dye; this is particularly valuable for fistulas for which there is an intervening abscess cavity. If a catheter will pass through a small vaginal aperture into an adjacent loop of bowel its nature may become apparent from the radiological appearance of the lumen and haustrations, although further imaging studies are usually required to demonstrate the underlying pathology.

Barium Enema, Barium Meal and Follow-through

Proctography may be used to identify the site of ano-vaginal or recto-vaginal fistulas, although it has been suggested that vaginography has a higher sensitivity. Barium enema, barium meal, or both may be required when a fistula is present above the ano-rectum. Aside from confirming the presence of a fistula, this allows evaluation of the intestinal condition and malignant or inflammatory disease may be identified.

Ultrasonography, CT, and MRI

Ultrasonography, computerized tomography (CT), and magnetic resonance imaging (MRI) may occasionally be appropriate for the complete assessment of complex fistulas. A water-soluble alternative to barium may be preferred to actual barium as it does not interfere with future imaging. Endoanal ultrasound scans and MRI are particularly useful in the investigation of anorectal and perineal fistulas and have been shown to have positive predictive rates of 100% and 92%.

Examination Under Anesthesia

Careful examination, if necessary under anesthesia, may be required to determine the presence of a fistula, and is deemed by several authorities to be essential for definitive surgical treatment. It is important at the time of examination to assess the available access for repair vaginally, and the mobility of the tissues. The decision between the vaginal and abdominal approaches to surgery is thus made; when the vaginal route is chosen, it may be appropriate to select between the more conventional supine lithotomy, with a head-down tilt, and the prone (reverse) lithotomy position with head-up tilt. This may be particularly useful in allowing the operator to look down onto bladder neck and sub-symphysial fistulas, and is also of advantage in some massive fistulas in encouraging the reduction of the prolapsed bladder mucosa. A recto-vaginal examination may detect a recto-vaginal fistula; probing of a perineal sinus with a fine metallic catheter may identify an ano-perineal tract.

Endoscopy (Please also see other related chapters)

Cystoscopy

Although some authorities suggest that endoscopy has little role in the evaluation of fistulas, it is the author's practice to perform cystourethroscopy in all but the largest defects. Although in some obstetric and radiation fistulas the size of the defect and the extent of tissue loss and scarring may make it difficult to distend the bladder, nevertheless much useful information is obtained. The exact level and position of the fistula should be determined, and its relationships to the ureteric orifices and bladder neck are particularly important. Most post-hysterectomy fistulas are supra-trigonal and located on the posterior bladder wall whilst post-radiation fistulas usually involve the trigone and/or bladder neck. With urethral and bladder neck fistulas the failure to pass a cystoscope or sound may indicate that there has been circumferential loss of the proximal urethra, a circumstance which is of considerable importance in determining the appropriate surgical technique and the likelihood of subsequent urethral incompetence.

The condition of the tissues must be carefully assessed. Persistence of slough means that surgery should be deferred, and this is particularly important in obstetric and post-radiation cases. Biopsy from the edge of a fistula should be taken in radiation fistulas, if persistent or recurrent malignancy is suspected. Malignant change has been reported in a longstanding benign fistula, so where there is any doubt at all about the nature of the tissues, biopsy should be undertaken. In endemic areas, evidence of schistosomiasis, tuberculosis, and lymphogranuloma may become apparent in biopsy material, and again it is important that specific antimicrobial treatment is instituted prior to definitive surgery.

PREOPERATIVE MANAGEMENT

Before epithelialization is complete an abnormal communication between viscera will tend to close spontaneously, provided that the natural outflow is unobstructed. Bypassing the sphincter mechanisms, for example by urinary catheterization or defunctioning colostomy, may encourage closure.

Uro-genital Fistula

The early management is of critical importance, and depends on the etiology and site of the lesion. If surgical trauma is recognized within the first 24 hours postoperatively, immediate repair may be appropriate, provided that extravasation of urine into the tissues has not been great. They most often cannot be recognized intra-operatively even if suspected. The majority of surgical fistulas, however, are recognized between 5 days and 14 days postoperatively, and should be treated with continuous bladder drainage. It is worth persisting with this line of management in vesico-vaginal or urethra-vaginal fistulas for six to eight weeks, since spontaneous closure may occur within this period.

Obstetric fistulas developing after obstructed labor should also be treated by continuous bladder drainage, combined with antibiotics to limit tissue damage from infection. Indeed, if a patient is known to have been in obstructed labor for any significant length of time, or is recognized to have areas of slough on the vaginal walls in the puerperium, prophylactic catheterization should be undertaken.

Immediate management should also include attention to palliation and skin care, nutrition, physiotherapy, rehabilitation, and overall patient morale. In women wishing to avoid surgery and where bladder drainage is unsuccessful other conservative treatments may be indicated when the vesico-vaginal fistula is very small. Small series and case reports have indicated success with fibrin glue, electrofulguration, laser ablation, or combinations of these modalities; no large series however have confirmed their value.

Surgical fistula patients are usually previously healthy individuals who entered hospital for what was expected to be a routine procedure, and end up with symptoms different than their initial complaint. Obstetric fistula patients in the developing world are social outcasts. It is vital that they understand the nature of the problem, why it has arisen, and the plan for management at all stages. Confident but realistic counseling by the surgeon is essential and the involvement of nursing staff or counselors with experience of fistula patients is also highly desirable. The support given by previously treated sufferers can also be of immense value in maintaining patient morale, especially where a delay prior to definitive treatment is required.

Intestino-genital Fistula

In determining the most appropriate management consideration should be given to the underlying etiology of the intestino-vaginal fistula. In patients with obstetric fistula, endoanal ultrasound should be performed to detect anal sphincter damage as the presence or absence of sphincteric injury may alter the choice of procedure. In patients with radiation recto-vaginal fistulas or in those with inflammatory bowel disease preoperative anorectal manometry is necessary to assess rectal compliance. When rectal reservoir function is poor then there is unlikely to be a good response from local repair. For recurrent fistulas, radiation-induced fistulas, for those associated with active inflammatory bowel disease, or for ileo- or colo-vaginal fistulas, a preliminary defunctioning colostomy may be appropriate. However, for the majority of recto-vaginal fistulas, defunctioning of the bowel is not required. Surgeons vary in the extent to which they prepare the bowel prior to recto-vaginal fistula repair, and some would simply administer an enema prior to operation. It is the author's preference to carry out formal preparation in all cases of intestino-genital fistula, whatever the level of the lesion. A low residue diet should be advised for a week prior to admission, followed by a fluid only diet for 48 hours preoperatively. Poly ethylene glycol 3350 (Klean Prep, Norgine Ltd, Harefield, Middlesex, UK) four sachets in 4 L of water over a four-hour period, or alternatively sodium picosulphate (Picolax, Ferring Pharmaceuticals Ltd, Langley, Berks, UK) 10 mg repeated after six hours, is given orally on the day before operation. Bowel wash out should be carried out on the evening before surgery, and if the bowel content is not completely clear this procedure should be repeated on the morning of surgery. For bowel anastomosis, equal or better results have been reported with no bowel preparation. This may or may not be applicable to fistula repair.

GENERAL PRINCIPLES OF SURGICAL TREATMENT
Timing of Repair
Uro-genital Fistula

The timing of surgical repair is perhaps the single most contentious aspect of fistula management. While shortening the waiting period is of both social and psychological benefit to patients who are always very distressed, one must not trade these issues for compromise to surgical success. The benefit of delay is to allow slough to separate and inflammatory change to resolve. In both obstetric and radiation fistulas there is considerable sloughing of tissues, and it is imperative that this should have settled before repair is undertaken. In radiation fistulas it may be necessary to wait 12 mo or more. In obstetric cases most authorities suggest that a minimum of three months should be allowed to elapse, although others have advocated surgery as soon as slough is separated.

With surgical fistulas the same principles should apply, and although the extent of sloughing is limited, extravasation of urine into the pelvic tissues inevitably sets up some inflammatory response. Although early repair is advocated by several authors, others suggest that 10 to 12 weeks postoperatively is the earliest appropriate time for repair.

Pressure from patients to undertake repair at the earliest opportunity is always understandably great, but is never more so than in the case of previous surgical failure. Such pressure must however be resisted, and eight weeks is the minimum time that should be allowed between attempts at closure.

Intestino-genital Fistula

Similarly repair should be delayed until infection has been treated and until inflammation, and induration has resolved to allow improved tissue handling. Some recto-vaginal fistulas will heal spontaneously during this time. After a failed repair, an interval of three months should be allowed before undertaking further repair surgery. When there is a coexisting urogenital fistula then recto-vaginal fistula repair should be undertaken after and separately from urogenital fistula repair. In such cases, transverse colostomy may used to temporarily divert feces away from the urogenital repair site until repair of the recto-vaginal fistula. In patients with inflammatory bowel disease repair should delayed until the disease is quiescent and sepsis treated.

Route of Repair
Uro-genital Fistula

Many urologists advocate an abdominal approach for all fistula repairs, claiming the possibility of earlier intervention and higher success rates in justification. Others suggest that all fistulas can be successfully closed by the vaginal route. Surgeons involved in fistula management must be capable of both approaches, and have the versatility to modify their techniques to select that most appropriate to the individual case. Where access is good and the vaginal tissues sufficiently mobile, the vaginal route is usually most appropriate. If access is poor and the fistula cannot be brought down, the abdominal approach should be used. When the fistula lies close to the ureteric orifices and there is a risk of ureteric injury during repair then ureteric stenting may allow the vaginal approach. Alternatively the need for ureteric re-implantation necessitates an abdominal approach. In the presence of a greatly reduced cystometric capacity as often seen in post-radiation fistulas, the need for concomitant cystoplasty necessitates an abdominal approach. Overall, more surgical fistulas are likely to require an abdominal repair than obstetric fistulas, although in the author's series of cases from the United Kingdom, and those reviewed from Nigeria, two-thirds of cases were satisfactorily treated by the vaginal route regardless of etiology.

Intestino-genital Fistula

This will depend on the anatomical site of the fistula, number of previous repair attempts, surgeon's preference, presence or absence of anal sphincter damage and presence or absence of intestinal, or vaginal stenosis. In cases of colo-vaginal or entero-vaginal fistulas then laparotomy is usually required and recurrence rates are low because of mobilization of healthy tissue. In repairing recto-vaginal fistulas then the current approaches include transperineal, transanal, or transvaginal repair.

Instruments

All operators have their own favored instruments, although those described by Chassar Moir and Lawson are eminently suitable for repair by any route (Fig. 2). The following are particularly useful:

- series of fine scalpel blades on the no. 7 handle, especially the curved no. 12 bistoury blade
- Chassar Moir 30° angled-on-flat and 90° curved-on-flat scissors
- cleft palate forceps
- Judd-Allis, Stiles, and Duval tissue forceps
- Millin's retractor for use in transvesical procedures, and Currie's retractors for vaginal repairs
- Skin hooks to put the tissues on tension during dissection
- Turner-Warwick double curved needle holder, particularly useful in areas of awkward access, has the advantage of allowing needle placement without the operator's hand or the instrument obstructing the view.

Dissection

Great care must be taken over the initial dissection of the fistula, and this stage should probably take as long as the repair

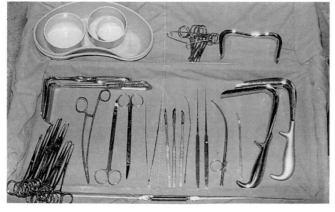

Figure 2 Fistula repair instruments.

itself. The fistula should be circumcized in the most convenient orientation, depending on size and access. All things being equal a longitudinal incision should be made around urethral or mid-vaginal fistulas; conversely, vault fistulas are better handled by a transverse elliptical incision. The tissue planes are often obliterated by scarring, and dissection close to a fistula should therefore be undertaken with a scalpel or scissors. Sharp dissection is easier with counter traction applied by skin hooks, tissue forceps, or retraction sutures. Blunt dissection with small pledgets may be helpful once the planes are established, and provided it takes place away from the fistula edge. Wide mobilization should be performed, so that tension on the repair is minimized. Bleeding is rarely troublesome with vaginal procedures, except occasionally with proximal urethra-vaginal fistulas. Diathermy is best avoided, and pressure or under running sutures are preferred.

Suture Materials

Although a range of suture materials have been advocated over the years, and different opinions still exist, the author's view is that absorbable sutures should be used throughout all urinary fistula repair procedures. Polyglactin (Vicryl, Ethicon, Edinburgh, UK) 2-0 suture on a 25-mm heavy tapercut needle is preferred for both the bladder and vagina, and polydioxanone (PDS, Ethicon, Edinburgh, UK) 4-0 on a 13-mm round-bodied needle is used for the ureter; 3-0 sutures on a 30-mm round-bodied needle are used for bowel surgery, polydioxanone for the small bowel, and either polydioxanone or braided polyamide (Nurolon, Ethicon, Edinburgh, UK) for large bowel re-anastomosis.

OPERATIVE TECHNIQUE
Uro-genital Fistula Repair
Dissection and Repair in Layers

Two main types of closure technique are applied to the repair of urinary fistulas: the classical saucerization technique described by Sims in 1852, and the much more commonly used dissection and repair in layers. Figures 3–8 demonstrate the latter form of repair in a post-hysterectomy vault fistula.

Tissue forceps or traction sutures are applied to bring the fistula more clearly into view, and obtain optimal access for repair. Infiltration with 1 in 200,000 adrenaline/epinephrine helps to reduce bleeding, and may aid dissection by separating tissue planes to some degree. With small lesions it may be helpful to identify the fistula with a probe or Fogerty catheter, so that the track is not "lost" after dissection. The fistula is then circumcized in a transverse elliptical fashion, using a no. 12 scalpel blade (Fig. 3); this should start posteriorly, and be completed on the anterior aspect. The dissection is then extended using scissors; Chassar Moir 30° angled-on-flat and 90° curved-on-flat scissors are particularly useful in this respect (Fig. 4). The vaginal walls should be undermined so that the underlying bladder is mobilized for 1 to 2 cm beyond the fistula edge. The vaginal scar edge may then be trimmed, although most often it is simply inverted within the repair. Sutures must be placed with meticulous accuracy in the bladder wall, care being taken not to penetrate the mucosa which should be inverted as far as possible. The repair should be started at either end, working toward the midline, so that the least accessible aspects are sutured first. Interrupted sutures

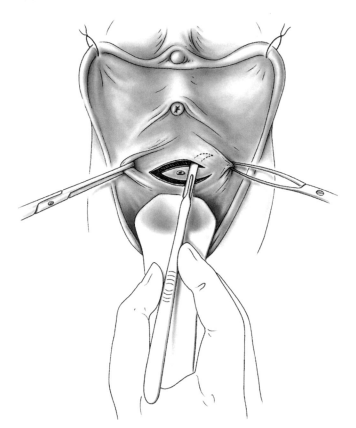

Figure 3 Traction sutures or tissue forceps allow the fistula to be brought into a more accessible position; the fistula is then circumcised in a transverse elliptical fashion, using a no. 12 scalpel blade.

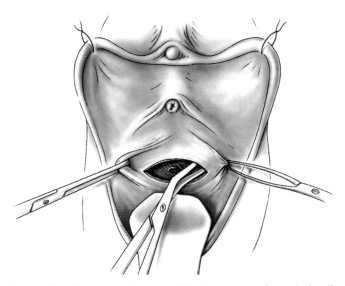

Figure 4 The dissection is then extended using scissors; the vaginal walls should be undermined so that the underlying bladder is mobilized for 1 to 2 cm beyond the fistula edge.

are preferred and should be placed approximately 3 mm apart, taking as large a bite of tissue as feasible. Stitches that are too close together, or the use of continuous or purse-string sutures, tend to impair blood supply and interfere with healing. Knots must be secure with three hitches, so that they can be cut short, leaving the minimum amount of suture material. With dissection and repair in layers the first layer of sutures in the bladder should invert the bladder edges (Figs. 5 and 6); the second adds bulk to the repair by taking a wide bite of bladder wall,

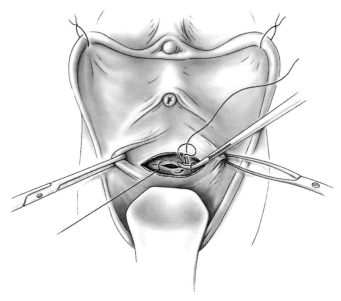

Figure 5 The repair is started at either end, working towards the midline, so that the least accessible aspects are sutured first.

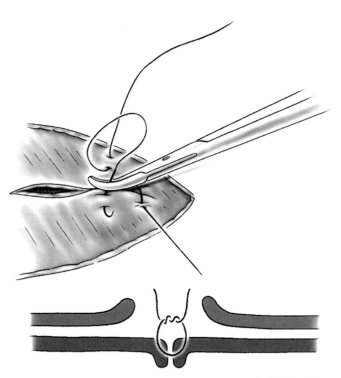

Figure 6 The first layer of sutures in the bladder inverts the bladder edges.

but also closes off dead space by catching the back of the vaginal flaps (Fig. 7). After the repair has been tested, a third layer of interrupted mattress sutures is used to evert and close the vaginal wall, consolidating the repair by picking up the underlying bladder wall (Fig. 8).

Saucerization
The saucerization technique involves converting the track into a shallow crater, which is closed without dissection of bladder from vagina using a single row of interrupted sutures (Fig. 9). The method is only applicable to small fistulas, and perhaps to residual fistulas after closure of a larger defect; in other situations the technique does not allow secure closure without tension.

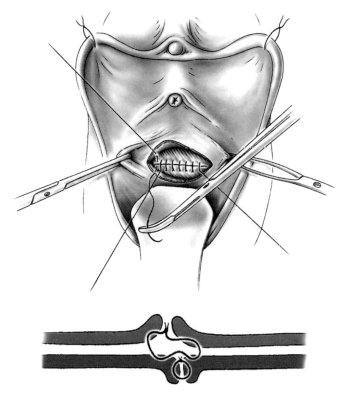

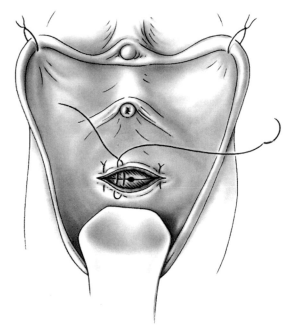

Figure 9 The saucerization technique involves converting the track into a shallow crater, which is closed without dissection of bladder from vagina using a single row of interrupted sutures.

Figure 7 The second layer of sutures adds bulk to the repair by taking a wide bite of bladder wall, and closes off dead space by catching the back of the vaginal flaps.

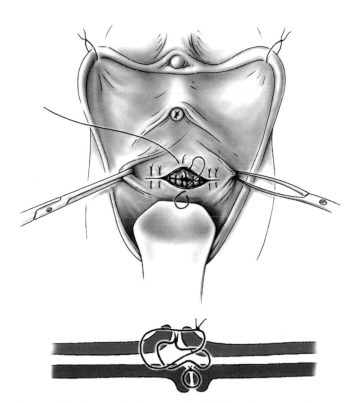

Figure 8 After the repair has been tested, a third layer of interrupted mattress sutures is used to evert and close the vaginal wall, consolidating the repair by picking up the underlying bladder wall.

Vaginal Repair Procedures in Specific Circumstances

The conventional dissection and repair in layers as described above is entirely appropriate for the majority of mid-vaginal fistulas, although modifications may be necessary in specific

circumstances. In juxta-cervical fistulas in the anterior fornix, vaginal repair may be feasible if the cervix can be drawn down to provide access. Dissection should include mobilization of the bladder from the cervix. The repair should be undertaken transversely to reconstruct the underlying trigone and prevent distortion of the ureteric orifices; the second layer of the repair is used to roll the defect onto the intact cervix, for additional support (Fig. 10).

Vault fistulas, particularly those following hysterectomy, can again usually be managed vaginally. The vault is incised transversely and mobilization of the fistula is often aided by deliberate opening of the pouch of Douglas. The peritoneal opening does not need to be closed separately, but is incorporated into the vaginal closure.

With sub-symphysial fistulas involving the bladder neck and proximal urethra as a consequence of obstructed labor, tissue loss may be extensive, and fixity to underlying bone a common problem. The lateral aspects of the fistula require careful mobilization to overcome disproportion between the defect in the bladder and the urethral stump. A racquet-shaped extension of the incision facilitates exposure of the proximal urethra. Although transverse repair is often necessary, longitudinal closure gives better prospects for urethral competence.

Where there is substantial urethral loss, reconstruction may be undertaken using the method described by Chassar Moir or Hamlin and Nicholson. After a U-shaped incision is made on the anterior vaginal wall, extending from the posterior edge of the fistula to the intended position of the external meatus, a strip of anterior vaginal wall is constructed into a tube over a catheter (Fig. 11). Plication of muscle behind the bladder neck is probably important if continence is to be achieved. The interposition of a labial fat or muscle graft not only fills up the potential dead space, but also provides additional bladder neck support and improves continence by reducing scarring between bladder neck and vagina. When intrinsic sphincter

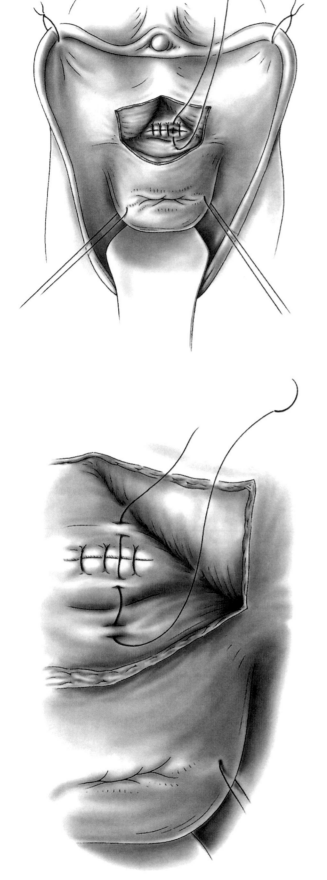

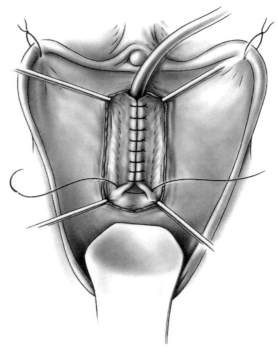

Figure 11 In urethral reconstruction a strip of anterior vaginal wall is constructed into a tube over a catheter.

Figure 10 Vaginal repair of a juxtacervical fistula may be feasible if the cervix can be drawn down to provide access; dissection includes mobilization of the bladder from the cervix, and the repair should be undertaken transversely to reconstruct the underlying trigone and prevent distortion of the ureteric orifices. The lower diagram shows this in greater detail.

deficiency is present, continence has been reported in 87% when a rectus sheath sling is fashioned at the time of the flap repair and where the sling is positioned below the interposition graft separating it from the urethra.

With very large fistulas extending from bladder neck to vault, the extensive dissection required may produce considerable bleeding. The main surgical difficulty is to avoid the ureters. They are usually situated close to the supero-lateral angles of the fistula, and if they can be identified they should be catheterized. Straight ureteric catheters passed transurethrally, or double pigtail catheters, may both be useful in detecting the intramural portion of the ureters internally; nevertheless, great care must be taken during dissection.

Radiation fistulas present particular problems, in that the area of devitalized tissue is usually considerably larger than the fistula itself. Mobilization is often impossible, and if repair in layers is attempted the flaps are likely to slough; closure by colpocleisis is therefore required (Fig. 12). Some have advocated total closure of the vagina although it is preferable to avoid dissection in the devitalized tissue entirely, and to perform a lower partial colpocleisis converting the upper vagina into a diverticulum of the bladder. It is usually necessary to fill the dead space below this with an interposition graft (Figs. 13 and 14).

Abdominal Repairs
Transvesical Repair
Repair by the abdominal route is indicated when high fistulas are fixed in the vault and are therefore inaccessible per vaginam. Transvesical repair has the advantage of being entirely extraperitoneal. It is often helpful to elevate the fistula site by a vaginal pack, and the ureters should be catheterized under direct vision. The technique of closure is similar to that of the transvaginal flap-splitting repair except that for hemostasis the bladder mucosa is also closed, using a continuous suture (Fig. 15).

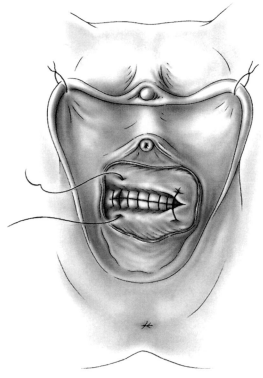

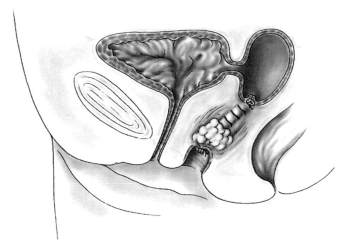

Figure 14 The vaginal or vulval skin is closed with interrupted sutures to cover the fat graft.

Figure 12 In colpocleisis for the treatment of a radiation fistula by the vaginal route, the dissection should be commenced well away from the fistula edge, aiming to be in normally vascularized tissues as far as possible. Several rows of sutures may be required.

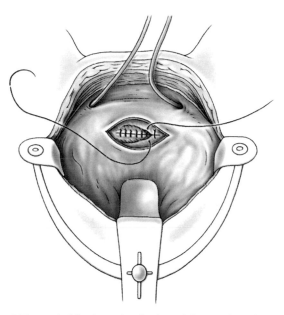

Figure 15 Transvesical fistula repair. After its mobilization from the overlying bladder wall, the vagina has been closed with a single layer of inverting interrupted sutures. The figure shows the bladder being closed with a similar layer of interrupted sutures, picking up the vagina also to close dead space. A continuous suture will be inserted into the urothelium for haemostatic purposes.

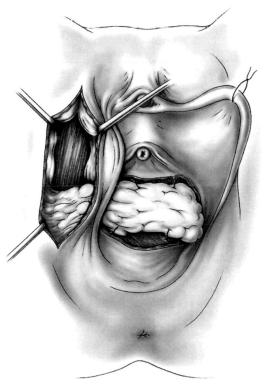

Figure 13 A Martius labial fat graft may often be necessary to fill dead space.

useful for vesico-uterine fistulas following caesarean section. A midline split is made in the vault of the bladder; this is extended downwards in a racquet shape around the fistula (Fig. 16). The fistulous track is excised and the vaginal or cervical defect closed in a single layer (Fig. 17). The bladder is then closed in one or two layers; either continuous or interrupted sutures may be employed. The interposition of an omental graft may also be considered if there is doubt over the integrity of the repair; this is also particularly appropriate when the technique is used for the repair of radiation fistulas.

Transperitoneal Repair

It is often said that there is little place for a simple transperitoneal repair, although a combined transperitoneal and transvesical procedure is favored by urologists and is particularly

Ureteric Re-implantation

For ureteric fistulas not manageable by stenting, re-implantation is considered preferable to re-anastomosis of the ureter itself, which carries a greater risk of stricture. Several techniques are

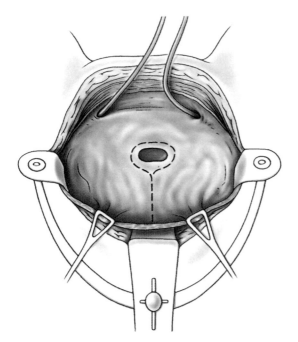

Figure 16 Transperitoneal transvesical repair. A midline split is made in the vault of the bladder, and is extended downward in a racquet shape around the fistula.

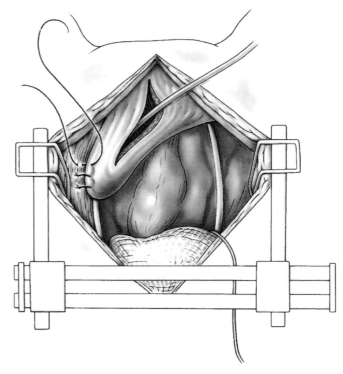

Figure 18 Ureteric re-implantations. Where the bladder cannot easily be mobilized sufficiently, a psoas hitch may allow reimplantation without tension.

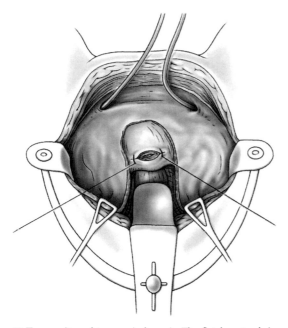

Figure 17 Transperitoneal transvesical repair. The fistulous track is excised and the vaginal or cervical defect closed in a single layer; the bladder is then closed in either one or two layers. An omental interposition graft may also be inserted, particularly when the technique is used for the repair of radiation fistula.

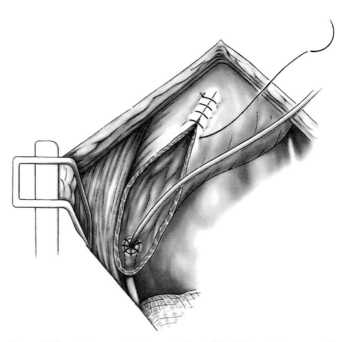

Figure 19 For high ureteric injury the Boari-Ockerblad technique may be appropriate, utilizing a flap of bladder wall to fill the deficiency.

described for ureteroneocystostomy, and the choice will depend on the level of the fistula and the nature of the antecedent pathology. For ureteric lesions within the pelvis, mobilization of the bladder from the opposite pelvic side-wall may be all that is required to allow re-implantation without tension. Otherwise the most widely used techniques are re-implantation using a psoas hitch (Fig. 18), or the creation of a flap of bladder wall, the Boari-Ockerblad technique (Fig. 19) (see further chapter 29). There are few lesions that are too high for these approaches, although where there is significant

deficiency it may be necessary to perform an end-to-side anastomosis between the injured ureter and the good contralateral ureter, that is, a transureteroureterostomy or to interpose a loop of small bowel.

Interposition Grafting

Several techniques have been described to support fistula repair in different sites (see also chapter 29). While there is no high-level evidence to support these techniques, the interposed tissue serves to create an additional layer in the repair, to fill dead space, and to bring new blood supply into the area. The tissues used include the following:

- Martius graft—a vertical incision is made over the labium majus and a graft of labial fat and bulbocavernosus muscle fashioned by antero-superior separation from the deep fascia (Colles fascia) over the urogenital diaphragm. Vascular supply is from the posterior labial branches of the internal pudendal artery. Good results are also seen when inferior separation is undertaken and the external pudendal vessels are preserved. The graft is passed subcutaneously to cover a vaginal repair; this is particularly appropriate to provide additional bulk in a colpocleisis and in urethral and bladder neck fistulas may help to maintain competence of closure mechanisms by reducing scarring (Fig. 13).
- Gracilis muscle passed either via the obturator foramen or subcutaneously is used as above (see chapter 32).
- Omental pedicle grafts may be dissected from the greater curve of the stomach and rotated down into the pelvis on either the right or left gastroepiploic arteries; this may be used at any transperitoneal procedure, but has its greatest advantage in post-radiation fistulas (see chapter 13).
- Peritoneal flap graft is an easier way of providing an additional layer at transperitoneal repair procedures, by taking a flap of peritoneum from any available surface, most usually the paravesical area. The anterior vaginal wall is opened and after the fistula closed as described earlier, a peritoneal flap is created by dissecting posteriorly along the anterior vaginal wall to expose the edge of peritoneum in the anterior cul-de-sac. The peritoneal edge may then be mobilized from the posterior bladder wall and the flap tacked over the site of fistula closure. Cure rates of 97% and 96% are reported when Martius graft and peritoneal flap interposition respectively are used in cases of complex and/or failed vesico-vaginal fistula.

Anal and Recto-vaginal Fistula Repair

Laying Open of Fistula Track

An ano-perineal fistula may be treated by laying open the tract using a diathermy probe and curetting to remove granulation tissue. Where there is an inter-sphincteric tract, it is laid open to the uppermost level by dividing the internal sphincter. If there is trans-sphincteric extension on the under surface of puborectalis, then the perianal skin should be incised at the external opening using fistula scissors and the granulation tissue curetted along the line of the tract.

Rectal Advancement Flap

This is indicated in cases of high trans-sphincteric anal fistulas. An Eisenhammer retractor is placed in the anus. A broad-based inverted U-shaped flap comprising rectal mucosa and muscularis is fashioned and separated from the internal sphincter muscle within the anal canal. The internal opening of the fistula tract is excised within the base of the flap (Fig. 20), and the tract opening into the internal sphincter is

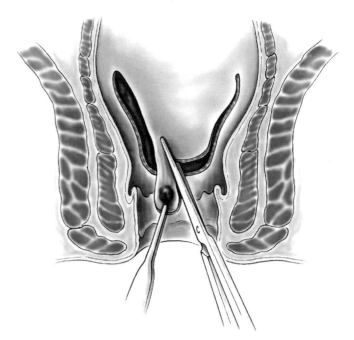

Figure 20 Rectal advancement flap. A flap of the whole thickness of rectal wall is fashioned, the internal opening excised, and the track curetted.

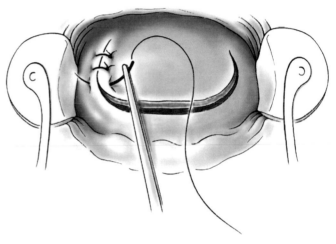

Figure 21 After mobilization of the flap, and closing the defect in the internal sphincter, the flap is sutured in place with interrupted 2/0 polyglactin or polydioxanone sutures.

curetted. The external opening of the tract is laid open and curetted. The internal anal sphincter is repaired with interrupted polyglactin sutures. The flap is then held in the advanced position and beginning at the base and working toward the apex it is sutured around the margins with interrupted polyglactin sutures so that it comes to overlie the sphincter closure and advances to the mucocutaneous margin (Fig. 21). The inter- or trans-sphincteric portion is left open to drain.

Transperineal

Conversion to Third-degree Tear

Although dissection and repair in layers is appropriate for lesions high in the vagina, most gynecologists when repairing fistula low in the vagina use the transperineal route and convert them into a "complete perineal tear" during the course of dissection. This technique is suitable for incompletely healed third or fourth degree obstetric perineal lacerations. The patient is positioned in the lithotomy position and the skin bridge incising with a scalpel. The fistula tract and perineal scar are then excised and the vagina and rectum (close to the fistula) are separated from prerectal fascia sufficiently to allow closure without tension and from the anal sphincters. The cut ends of the external sphincter should be identified and secured with stay sutures; if disrupted, the ends should be sought by dissection into the pararectal tissues. Only when all layers are clearly dissected and identified should the repair commence.

The rectal mucosa is closed with either continuous or interrupted suture using 3-0 polyglactin or polydioxanone, commencing above the limit of the dissection. The second layer comprising muscularis (including the internal sphincter) and submucosa is repaired with a series of Lembert sutures where the sutures do not enter the bowel lumen (Fig. 22). An additional layer of sutures may be placed more superficially into the muscularis to help to create a zone of high pressure within the rectum, although simply reconstructing the prerectal fascia over the rectal repair as an alternative is entirely appropriate.

The external sphincter should then be repaired using 3-0 polydioxanone or prolene sutures. The conventional end-to-end technique with a series of vertical mattress sutures has been found to be unsatisfactory in many cases, and the overlapping repair technique developed by Parks is perhaps particularly appropriate where there is sphincter deficiency in addition to the fistula. The repair is accomplished by a series of interrupted sutures transfixing both layers of muscle, to achieve 2 cm overlap where possible (Fig. 23). The superficial transverse perineal muscles are then reapproximated, and the vaginal wall is closed to the level of the hymenal ring, using continuous 2-0 polyglycolic acid. The perineal body may then be further built up using the medial fibers of the levator ani and bulbocavernosus muscles, before the perineal skin is closed. If interposition grafting is thought to be necessary, the Martius graft is the most appropriate for use in low recto-vaginal fistula repair.

Transverse Transperineal
This is another transperineal method used for low recto-vaginal fistulas when it is important to preserve sphincteric function such as in patients with Crohn's disease where it may be performed without the need for a defunctioning colostomy.

The patient is placed in the dorsal lithotomy position, and the tissues are injected with 1:200,000 adrenaline. A transverse incision is made in the skin across the perineal body above the anal sphincter, and the perineal skin is mobilized in a cephalad direction by sharp dissection and extended laterally and superiorly around the fistula between the anterior rectal wall and posterior vaginal wall. Scar tissue is then excised from the vaginal opening of the fistula and the vaginal mucosa repaired longitudinally in two layers with interrupted sutures. Scar tissue from the fistulous opening at the rectal end is then excised and the rectal wall repaired transversely with interrupted sutures to invert the rectal mucosa followed by a second layer to imbricate and reinforce the first layer. The puborectalis muscle is then approximated in the midline with one or two interrupted sutures and the transverse perineii approximated with interrupted sutures. The skin is closed with interrupted sutures.

Transvaginal
This route offers the advantages of better access than the transanal route and avoidance of transection and repair of the anal sphincters. It does not however allow direct access to repair the rectal opening of the tract, the highest pressure end of the fistula and compared to some of the other procedures it may be complicated by inadequate tissue mobilization; vaginal narrowing and subsequent dyspareunia. The patient is placed in the lithotomy position and the fistula is identified with a

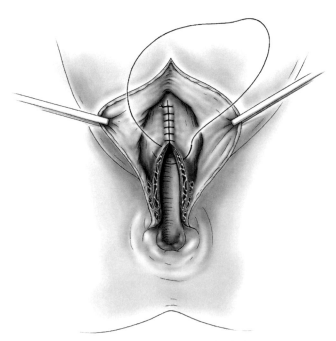

Figure 22 Repair of a low recto-vaginal fistula. After the lesion has been converted into a "complete perineal tear", the tissues are widely mobilized. The rectal wall is closed using a continuous suture.

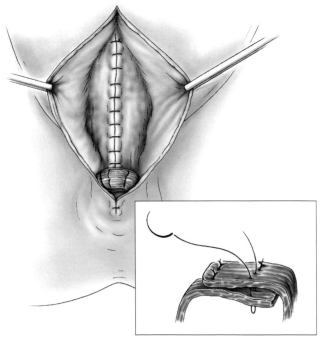

Figure 23 The "overlapping" technique of sphincter repair.

probe. Infiltration with 1:200,000 adrenaline/epinephrine is followed by circumferential incision of the fistula on the posterior vaginal wall and the fistula tract is excised to the rectal mucosa. The vaginal mucosa is then separated from the underlying prerectal fascia with fistula scissors and the rectum closed with a series of interrupted polyglactin sutures to invert the fistulous opening into the rectal wall. The vaginal mucosa is then closed in the usual way. When the tissues are devitalized such as in radiation fistulas the repair may be combined with tissue interposition as described earlier.

Transanal

The transanal approach is favored by coloproctologists and it is suitable for patients with low recto-vaginal fistulas without fecal incontinence and with intact anal sphincters although it may be combined with sphincteroplasty when there is sphincter involvement. It is not a suitable technique for radiation fistulas because of the lack of vascularized tissues. Dissection and repair in layers or rectal advancement flap, as described earlier may be undertaken.

Advancement Rectal Sleeve Procedure

This is a more complex alternative to the transanal advancement flap in which a circumferential incision is made from the mucocutaneous junction and extended circumferentially to the submucosa in a cephalad direction, to beyond the anorectal ring and supralevator space. The flap usually extends 7 cm in to the rectum with the base at least 4 cm cephalad to the fistula and is raised from the apex to the base with dissection commencing laterally and moving distally. The anterior rectal wall is then mobilized if necessary to the level of the peritoneal reflection and separated laterally from the submucosa and internal sphincter muscle so that it may be pulled down to the level of the dentate line without tension. The internal sphincter and submucosa are then approximated in the midline with interrupted polyglactin sutures. The rectal wall flap is advanced over the repaired area and unhealthy anorectal mucosa with the site of the fistula is excised. The flap margins are attached with interrupted 30 polyglactin sutures.

Transabdominal

The transabdominal route is often chosen when the rectum is ulcerated or stenotic following radiation. At laparotomy the splenic flexure, left colon and sigmoid colon and rectum are mobilized to the level of the levator hiatus, and the diseased rectum is resected. A colonic reservoir is fashioned either as a J-pouch or as a coloplasty. In the frail or very elderly colostomy may be the treatment of choice for radiation fistulas.

In patients with Crohn's disease affecting the rectum then proctectomy with colonic pull-through and delayed coloanal anastomosis may be the treatment of choice.

POSTOPERATIVE MANAGEMENT
Fluid Balance

Nursing care of patients who have undergone urogenital fistula repair is of critical importance, and obsessional postoperative management may do much to secure success. As a corollary, however, poor nursing may easily undermine what has been achieved by the surgeon. Strict fluid balance must be kept, and an adequate daily fluid intake should be maintained

until the urine is clear of blood. Hematuria is more persistent following abdominal surgery than vaginal procedures, and intravenous fluid is therefore likely to be required for longer in these patients.

Bladder Drainage

Continuous bladder drainage in the postoperative period is crucial to success, and nursing staff should check catheters hourly throughout each day, to confirm free drainage and check output. Bladder irrigation and suction drainage are not recommended. Views differ as to the ideal type of catheter. The caliber must be sufficient to prevent blockage, although whether the suprapubic or urethral route is used is to a large extent a matter of individual preference. The author's usual practice is to use a "belt and braces (suspenders)" approach of both urethral and suprapubic drainage initially, so that if one becomes blocked free drainage is still maintained. The urethral catheter is removed first, and the suprapubic retained, and used to assess residual volume, until the patient is voiding normally. Bedside ultrasound examination has eliminated the need for intermittent catheterization to assess for urine retention.

The duration of free drainage depends on the fistula type. Following repair of surgical fistulas, 12 days is adequate. With obstetric fistulas up to 21 days' drainage may be appropriate, and following repair of radiation fistulas 21 to 42 days are required. If there is any doubt about the integrity of the repair, it is wise to carry out a dye test prior to catheter removal. Where a persistent leak is identified free drainage should be maintained for six weeks.

Mobility and Thromboprophylaxis

The biggest problem in ensuring free catheter drainage lies in preventing kinking or drag on the catheter. Restricting patient mobility in the postoperative period helps with this, and some advocate continuous bed rest during the period of catheter drainage. If this approach is chosen, patients should be looked on as being at moderate to high risk for thromboembolism, and prophylaxis must be employed (see chapter 1). Most patients can be educated in catheter management to avoid the need for limited mobility.

Antibiotics

Antibiotic cover is advised for all intestino-vaginal fistula repairs. There is no evidence of benefit from prophylactic antibiotics in patients undergoing urogenital fistula repair, and only symptomatic infection need be treated in the catheterized patient.

Bowel Management

If patients are restricted to bed following urogenital fistula repair, a laxative should be administered to prevent excessive straining at stool. Following abdominal repair of an intestino-vaginal fistula patients, tradition often included either a nasogastric tube or nil by mouth until they are passing flatus; the majority prefer the latter approach. Once oral intake is allowed, or following vaginal repair of a recto-vaginal fistula, a low-residue diet should be administered until at least the fifth postoperative day. Some authorities advocate total parenteral nutrition throughout the first week postoperatively for all intestino-vaginal fistulas. Enemas and suppositories should be avoided, although a mild aperient such as dioctyl sodium (docusate sodium) is advised to ease initial bowel movements. Early postoperative feeding has been shown in randomized clinical trials to improve outcomes after other gastro-intestinal surgeries. It is not know if these results are applicable to fistula repair surgery.

Subsequent Management

On removal of catheters most patients will feel the desire to void frequently, since the bladder capacity will be functionally reduced after being relatively empty for so long. In any case it is important that the bladder does not become over distended, and hourly voiding should be encouraged and fluid intake limited. It may also be necessary to wake patients once or twice during the night for the same reason. After discharge from hospital patients should be advised gradually to increase the period between voiding, aiming to achieve a normal pattern by four weeks postoperatively. Tampons, pessaries, douching, and penetrative sex should be avoided until three months postoperatively.

BIBLIOGRAPHY

Bladou F, Houvenaeghel G, Delpero JR, et al. (1995) Incidence and management of major urinary complications after pelvic exenteration for gynecological malignancies. *J Surg Oncol* **58**:91–6.

Blaivas JG, Heritz DM (1996) Vaginal flap reconstruction of the urethra and vesical neck in women: a report of 49 cases. *J Urol* **155**(3):1014–7.

Chassar Moir J (1967) *The Vesico-vaginal Fistula*, 2nd edn. London: Bailliere.

Eilber KS, Kavaler E, Rodriguez LV, et al. (2003) Ten-year experience with transvaginal vesicovaginal fistula repair using tissue interposition. *J Urol* **169**(3):1033–6.

Elkins TE, DeLancey JO, McGuire EJ (1990) The use of modified Martius graft as an adjunctive technique in vesicovaginal and rectovaginal fistula repair. *Obstet Gynecol* **75**(4):727–33.

Emmert C, Köhler U (1996) Management of genital fistulas in patients with cervical cancer. *Arch Gynecol Obstet* **259**:19–24.

Evans LA, Ferguson KH, Foley JP, et al. (2003) Fibrin sealant for the management of genitourinary injuries, fistulas and surgical complications. *J Urol* **169**(4):1360–2.

Hamlin R, Nicholson E (1969) Reconstruction of urethra totally destroyed in labour. *Br Med J* **2**:147–50.

Hawley P, Burke M (1985) Anal sphincter repair. In: Henry M, Swash M, eds. *Coloproctology and the Pelvic Floor. Pathophysiology and Management.* London: Butterworths, pp. 252–8.

Hilton P (1997) Debate: post-operative urogenital fistulae are best managed by Gynaecologists in specialist centres. *Br J Urol* **80**(Suppl 1):35–42.

Hilton P (1998a) The urodynamic findings in patients with urogenital fistulae. *Br J Urol* **81**:539–42.

Hilton P (1998b) Bladder drainage. In: Stanton S, Monga A, eds. *Clinical Gynaecological Urology.* London: Churchill-Livingstone, pp. 541–50.

Hilton P (2002) Urogenital fistulae. In: Maclean A, Cardozo L, eds. *Incontinence in Women – Proceedings of the 42nd RCOG Study Group.* London: RCOG, pp. 163–81.

Hilton P, Ward A (1998) Epidemiological and surgical aspects of urogenital fistulae: a review of 25 years experience in south-east Nigeria. *Int Urogynecol J Pelvic Floor Dysfunct* **9**:189–94.

Huang WC, Zinman LN, Bihrle W 3rd (2002) Surgical repair of vesicovaginal fistulas. *Urol Clin North Am* **29**(3):709–23.

Hudson CN (1968) Malignant change in an obstetric vesicovaginal fistula. *Proc Roy Soc Med* **61**(12):1280–1.

Jonas U, Petri E (1984) Genitourinary fistulae. In: Stanton S, ed. *Clinical Gynecologic Urology.* St Louis: CV Mosby, pp. 238–55.

Kelly J, Kwast B (1993) Epidemiologic study of vesico-vaginal fistula in Ethiopia. *Int Urogynecol J* **4**:278–81.

Kiricuta I, Goldstein A (1972) The repair of extensive vesicovaginal fistulas with pedicled omentum: a review of 27 cases. *J Urol* **108**:724–7.

Kodner IJ, Mazor A, Shemesh EI, et al. (1993) Endorectal advancement flap repair of rectovaginal and other complicated anorectal fistulas. *Surgery* **114**(4):682–9.

Lawson J (1972) Vesical fistulae into the vaginal vault. *Br J Urol* **44**:623–31.

Lawson J (1978) The management of genito-urinary fistulae. *Clin Obstet Gynaecol* **6**:209–36.

Lawson L, Hudson C (1987) The management of vesico-vaginal and urethral fistulae. In: Stanton S, Tanagho E, eds. *Surgery for Female Urinary Incontinence.* Berlin: Springer-Verlag, pp. 193–209.

Lee R, Symmonds R, Williams T (1988) Current status of genitourinary fistula. *Obstet Gynecol* **71**:313–9.

Morita T, Tokue A (1999) Successful endoscopic closure of radiation induced vesicovaginal fistula with fibrin glue and bovine collagen. *J Urol* **162**(5):1689.

Parks A, McPartlin J (1971) Late repair of injuries of the anal sphincter. *Proc Roy Soc Med* **64**:1187–9.

Saclarides TJ (2002) Rectovaginal fistula. *Surg Clin North Am* **82**(6):1261–72.

Smith ARB, Chang D, Dmochowski R, et al. (2009) Surgery for urinary incontinence in women. In: Abrams P, Cardozo L, Khoury S, Wein A, eds. *Incontinence – WHO – ICUD International Consultation on Incontinence,* 4th edn. Portsmouth, UK: Health Publications, pp. 1191–272.

Stoker J, Rociu E, Schouten WR, et al. (2002) Anovaginal and rectovaginal fistulas: endoluminal sonography versus endoluminal MR imaging. *Am J Roentgenol* **178**(3):737–41.

Sultan AH, Kamm MA, Hudson CN, et al. (1994) Third degree obstetric and sphincter tears: Risk factors and outcome of primary repair. *Br Med J* **308**:887–91.

Waaldijk K (1989) *The Surgical Management of Bladder Fistula in 775 Women in Northern Nigeria.* MD Thesis, Amsterdam.

Wiskind AK, Thompson JD (1992) Transverse transperineal repair of rectovaginal fistulas in the lower vagina. *Am J Obstet Gynecol* **167**(3).694–9.

White A, Buchsbaum H, Blythe J, et al. (1982) Use of the bulbocavernosus muscle (Martius procedure) for repair of radiation-induced rectovaginal fistulas. *Obstet Gynecol* **60**(1):114–8.

World Health Organisation (1989) *The Prevention and Treatment of Obstetric Fistulae: A Report of a Technical Working Group.* Geneva: WHO.

Wall L, Arrowsmith S, Briggs N, et al. (2002) Urinary incontinence in the developing world: the obstetric fistula. In: Abrams P, Cardozo L, Khoury S, Wein A, eds. *Incontinence; 2nd WHO International Consultation on Incontinence.* Portsmouth, UK: Health Publications.

Zacharin R (1988) *Obstetric Fistula.* Vienna: Springer-Verlag.

Yeates W (1987) Uretero-vaginal fistulae. In: Stanton S, Tanagho E, eds. *Surgery for Female Urinary Incontinence.* Berlin: Springer-Verlag, pp. 211–7.

31 Treatment of vascular defects and injuries
Karl A. Illig, Kenneth Ouriel, and Sean Hislop

INTRODUCTION

The pelvis and groin contain a complex web of blood vessels. Given the magnitude of resection often needed when treating pelvic malignancies, it is not uncommon to be faced with the need to address major vascular issues. These fall into three general categories: inadvertent injuries requiring repair; planned resection as part of tumor excision, requiring reconstruction; and use of inferior vena cava filters to reduce the risk of fatal pulmonary embolism.

Whenever major vascular hemorrhage is encountered, simple measures to initially control hemorrhage should be employed expeditiously. Initial attempts at repair may result in increasing the risk of further injury at the cost of significant blood loss. In general, apply direct pressure at the site of bleeding to control hemorrhage and consult a surgeon with experience in vascular reconstruction. Preservation of life should always take priority over preservation of blood flow to limbs.

INDICATIONS

The primary indication for vascular repair is, of course, a vascular injury. Major blood vessels may at times need to be resected along with the specimen as part of an en bloc extirpation. Not every defect requires reconstruction, however.

The aorta, common iliac, and external iliac arteries form the blood supply to the legs, and must always be reconstructed if the limb is to remain viable. If direct reconstruction is not possible, an "extra-anatomic" (femoral–femoral or axillary–femoral) bypass may be constructed to preserve limb blood flow. Venous bleeding can be much more serious than arterial bleeding, primarily because the thin walls and prodigious tributaries make control and repair difficult. Collateral drainage, also, is rich. These two concepts suggest that virtually any vein can be ligated if absolutely necessary. At times a venous reconstruction will be required, but urgency is less than after ligation of arterial structures.

ANATOMIC CONSIDERATIONS

The two hypogastric (internal iliac) arteries and the inferior mesenteric artery (IMA) supply blood to the pelvis, including the buttocks, left colon, and terminal spinal cord. It is a near-absolute requirement that at least one of these three vessels be preserved. The IMA is frequently the least important source of pelvic blood flow; every effort should be made, however, to preserve at least one hypogastric artery. Be aware of the impact of vascular disease and previous vascular or colorectal surgery on the vascular patency and anatomy of the colon and pelvis, as these factors may indicate a need for reconstruction. Within these guidelines, essentially any other vessel can be ligated with impunity.

The anatomy of the lower abdomen, pelvis, and groin vasculature is illustrated in Figures 1 and 2. Remember that arteries are thick walled, resistant to tearing, and easier to repair than veins. Veins, by contrast, are thin-walled, do not hold their shape, and tear easily.

The veins tend to lie behind arteries (Fig. 3). This is critically important at the region of the aortic bifurcation and proximal iliac arteries, where dissection behind these arteries (circled area) or within the aortic bifurcation can easily precipitate massive, life-threatening venous hemorrhage.

In general, trying to control an injury directly is counterproductive. For arterial injuries, proximal and distal control at sites remote from the bleeding source are required (Fig. 4). Direct clamping can sometimes be problematic, for example, in the hypogastric arteries or in patients with significant atherosclerotic disease. In these cases, control can be accomplished by intraluminal balloon catheter occlusion. For venous injuries, direct pressure or packing while the situation is sorted out is much more useful that trying to see the injury or control it with a clamp. Direct manipulation with rigid instruments will often extend the tear or worsen the situation.

For vessel repair, autologous tissue is usually preferred (especially in a potentially infected field), although this "rule" must often be violated. An option in unfavorable situations is to route a graft through an unviolated, "extra-anatomic" plane. If vessel resection is planned or possible, include a source of autogenous vein (e.g., a leg, circumferentially prepared) in the surgical field (Fig. 5).

The best procedure to follow in any unplanned vascular injury is first to control the bleeding with direct pressure; this may be accomplished with a finger or by packing with a sponge. Once bleeding is controlled, get help (in terms of both additional staff and specialist advice, when needed) and formulate a plan before anything further is done.

ARTERIAL CONTROL AND REPAIR

When dealing with an arterial injury or planned resection and repair, proximal and distal control are vitally important—this point cannot be overemphasized. In general, circumferential dissection of the aorta and common iliac arteries is counterproductive due to the risk of venous injury; dissection limited to the sides is usually sufficient. If the aorta is to be clamped, dissection should be carried down to the spine. In arterial surgery, a dissection plane directly on the adventitia is easiest and safest (Fig. 6). Systemic heparin (125 units/kg) should be administered before clamping if bleeding is not diffuse; anticoagulation is reversed after arterial blood flow is re-established with protamine sulfate (1 mg per 100 units of heparin administered).

The ureter passes over the iliac bifurcation (Fig. 7), making continuous exposure of the top of the iliac vessels problematic.

Small lacerations of the major vessels, especially if oriented transversely to the vessel axis, can be readily repaired using

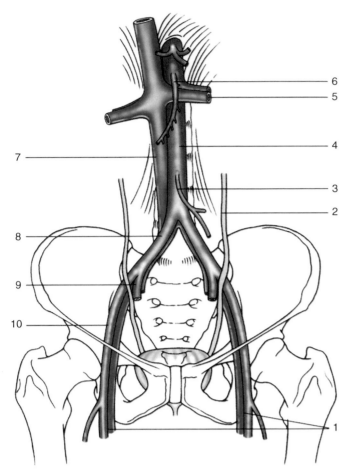

Figure 1 Abdominal and pelvic vasculature. 1 Femoral artery and vein, 2 Ureter artery, 3 Inferior mesenteric artery, 4 Aorta, 5 Renal artery and vein, 6 Superior mesenteric, 7 Inferior vena cava, 8 Common iliac artery and vein, 9 Internal iliac artery and vein, 10 External iliac artery and vein.

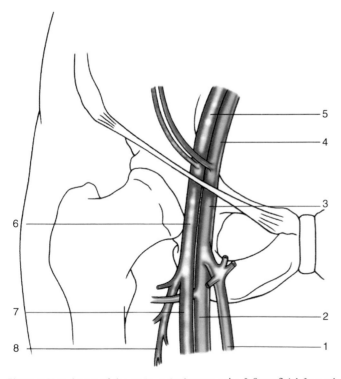

Figure 2 Vasculature of the groin. 1 Saphenous vein, 2 Superficial femoral vein, 3 Common femoral vein, 4 External iliac vein, 5 External iliac artery, 6 Common femoral artery, 7 Superficial femoral artery, 8 Deep femoral artery (profunda).

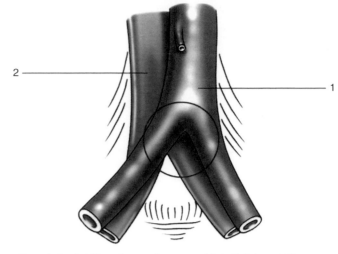

Figure 3 Aortic bifurcation—a danger area (circled). 1 Aorta, 2 Vena cava.

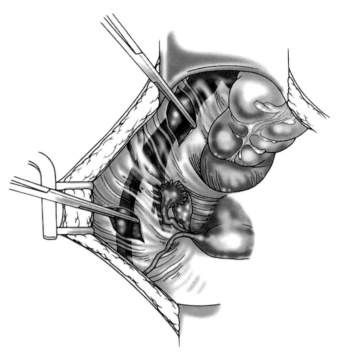

Figure 4 Control at sites remote from the bleeding is essential for arterial injuries.

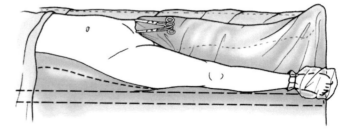

Figure 5 Draping to gain access for saphenous vein harvest.

monofilament, nonabsorbable suture (3-0 or 4-0 for aorta, 5-0 for iliac arteries). When the artery is diseased, the needle should be passed from inside to outside on the distal vessel wall to avoid dislodging intraluminal plaque or raising a distal intraluminal flap that could cause a dissection. All knots

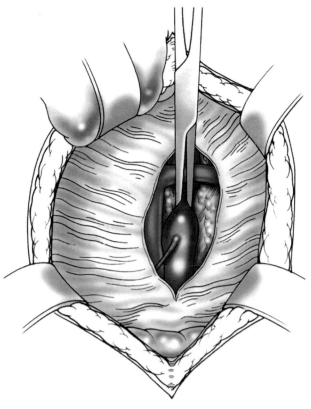

Figure 6 Exposure of the infrarenal aorta (duodenum is retracted laterally and superiorly). Note that the aorta itself is well cleared.

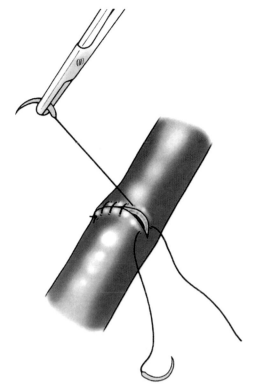

Figure 8 Suture technique for closure of a transverse arteriotomy.

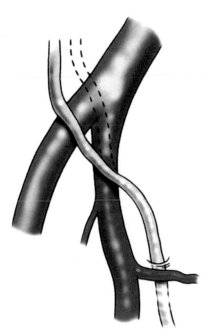

Figure 7 Ureter and the iliac bifurcation.

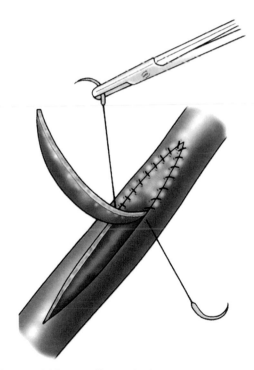

Figure 9 Initial stages of longitudinal arteriotomy: patch closure.

should extraluminal (Fig. 8). Direct repair of longitudinal injuries in the iliac (or smaller) vessels will usually narrow the lumen, so patch repair is preferred (Figs. 9 and 10).

Any defect involving a large amount of tissue loss, especially encompassing the entire circumference of a vessel, will usually require an interposition vein or prosthetic graft. In a minority of these situations a primary repair may be possible, however only in cases where the vessel can be generously mobilized to

provide a tension-free repair. These techniques are beyond the scope of this discussion, and a surgeon familiar with vascular reconstructive techniques should be consulted to assist in the repair of such defects.

VENOUS CONTROL AND REPAIR

Major venous injuries, somewhat paradoxically, can be more life-threatening than arterial defects. Veins are thin-walled, do

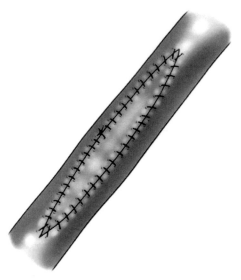

Figure 10 Completed closure.

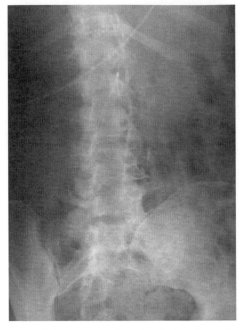

Figure 11 Inferior vena cava filter placed below the renal veins.

not hold their shape, and are often less accessible. When faced with a major venous injury (dark, non-pulsatile bleeding), the first step is to apply gentle pressure. The temptation to control the injury with forceps or a clamp, even if the tear is apparently visible, should be resisted; doing so will often extend the tear and often convert a remediable situation into one that is very serious indeed. Several options are available. First, pressure itself will often solve the problem; if you are fortunate, resist the temptation to fiddle any further! Don't look, don't dissect, just accept your good fortune, and move on. Second, pressure proximally and distally, without any dissection (e.g., digitally or with sponge-sticks) can control the bleeding enough to make the defect visible. Third, blind suturing is sometimes acceptable if no critical structures (such as the ureter) are near. Finally, ligation is usually safe and well tolerated, especially if the patient's life is at risk.

In these situations, obtaining help, in terms of both experienced assistants to provide exposure and vascular surgical assistance, is of utmost importance, as is gaining control of the hemorrhage without any further damage so that a plan may be formulated and carried out.

VASCULAR PATCHES

Most longitudinal defects, even if no tissue is resected, will result in a narrowed lumen if repaired primarily. Thus, patch angioplasty is required for repair of most longitudinal defects in the iliac and smaller vessels.

Autologous tissue is preferred, especially in the presence of a potentially infected field. The greater saphenous vein is an excellent choice, as is the hypogastric artery. It is important that the endothelial surface should be oriented luminally. If, in a clean field, autologous tissue is not available, Dacron or polytetrafluoroethylene (PTFE) can be used. Fine monofilament nonabsorbable double-armed suture material on a noncutting needle is used. Suturing begins at one corner of the defect being careful to drive sutures from the inside to the outside on the native vessel. Exposure is best achieved by starting at one end and placing the first two or three stitches on either side of the corner in a "parachute" fashion before bringing the patch in contact with the vessel (Fig. 9). The first

"heel" suture should be mattressed at the corner so that the needle always passes from inside to outside the native artery (outside to inside on the patch). The suture is then continued around the patch and the knot tied along the long end of the patch (Fig. 10).

INFERIOR VENA CAVA FILTERS

Malignancy is a well-known risk factor for venous thromboembolism (VTE, a collective term for deep venous thrombosis (DVT) and pulmonary embolism (PE)) and occurs in up to 15% of women with cancer. Half of all VTE that occur in surgical patients occur in the operating room. VTE accounts for almost one-half of all postoperative deaths among women undergoing surgery for gynecological malignancy.

IVC filters are placed for the prevention of a fatal pulmonary embolism and work by mechanically preventing the embolism of large lower extremity clots capable of causing hemodynamically significant cardiopulmonary events. They have been shown to decrease the short-term incidence of PE from 5% to 1% in patients with a proximal venous thrombus. Indications for placement of an IVC filter in women with gynecological cancer and a diagnosis of VTE include:

1. Surgery as a primary treatment for cancer.
2. Surgery as a delayed procedure as part of a definitive treatment (i.e., those undergoing neoadjuvant chemotherapy).
3. Contraindication to anticoagulation such as acute hemorrhagic anemia or recent hemorrhagic stroke.
4. VTE despite appropriate therapeutic anticoagulation.
5. Proximal (iliac or IVC) thrombosis in a patient with decreased cardiopulmonary reserve who is unlikely to tolerate an embolic event.
6. Complication of anticoagulation which prevents further anticoagulation such as significant bleeding.

IVC filters come in many shapes and delivery system sizes and have been refined to point where they are smaller (6 French) than the typical introducer sheath (9 French) used for IV resuscitation. They can be placed safely through either the femoral of internal jugular veins and are deployed in the IVC just below the renal veins (Fig. 11). IVC filters are placed under local anesthesia, similar to the placement of a central venous catheter. It takes approximately 10 to 15 min for a vascular surgeon to perform the procedure under fluoroscopic guidance. In patients that are too moribund to be moved, IVC filters can be placed safely by a vascular surgeon at the bedside under intravascular ultrasound guidance.

BIBLIOGRAPHY

Adib T, Belli A, McCall J, et al. (2008) The use of inferior vena caval filters prior to major surgery in women with gynaecological cancer. *BJOG* **115**:902–7.

Ouriel K, Rutherford RB (1998) *Atlas of Vascular Surgery: Operative Procedure.* Philadelphia: WB Saunders Co.

Rutherford RS (1993) *Atlas of Vascular Surgery: Basic Techniques and Exposures.* Philadelphia: WB Saunders Co.

32 Plastic reconstructive procedures
Andrea L. Pusic, Richard R. Barakat, and Peter G. Cordeiro

INTRODUCTION
Surgical cure demands adequate disease-free margins. Since large debulking procedures are often necessary, reconstructive techniques are required to restore anatomy and promote uncomplicated healing. Regional flaps are the most commonly used and effective of procedures. Flap selection is based on the type of defect and patient characteristics. The pudendal thigh flap is relatively simple and has the distinction of being at least partially sensate. The rectus abdominis muscle flap is a very versatile flap, useful in covering many defects. It is highly reliable, with a consistent vascular supply and muscular development. The gracilis flap has been popular for many years for vaginal reconstruction, but it is somewhat less reliable.

ANATOMIC CONSIDERATIONS
Vascular Supply
Skin vascularization may be direct or indirect. Direct vessels travel between muscles and along fascial planes to enter the skin. Indirect vessels arise from named vessels as perforators of the fascia from the underlying muscle. Regional flaps (e.g., gracilis flap) require a well-defined vascular pedicle to support the indirect blood supply to the overlying skin. Certain muscles used for flaps have a single dominant vascular pedicle (e.g., epigastric vessels for the rectus abdominis) or one dominant vascular pedicle with several minor ones (e.g., the medial femoral circumflex or femoral artery for the gracilis muscle). The pudendal thigh flap derives its blood supply mostly from the posterior labial vessels and the anastomotic channels involving the medial femoral circumflex and the obturator arteries. Knowledge of the vascular anatomy will allow better planning of the available territories for covering defects.

Nerve Supply
No major nerve should be encountered during these reconstructive procedures. Although the gracilis muscle is innervated by a branch of the obturator nerve, it is usually not identified as a distinct structure. As with all surgical procedures, some loss of sensation will be encountered in the operative field. Because reconstructive surgery involves the retention of a large skin island after it is severed from its nerve supply (e.g., the rectus flap), the patient may be more aware of this deficiency than after non-reconstructive surgery. With use of either the pudendal thigh flap or gracilis flap, a partially sensate reconstruction may be achieved.

Muscles Involved
The rectus abdominis muscle inserts in the pubic tubercle and arises from the sixth, seventh, and eighth ribs. It plays a role in protecting the abdominal contents, breathing and defecating, and stabilizes the pelvis during walking. The gracilis muscle arises from the pubic tubercle and inserts on to the medial tibia pes anserinus. It helps to stabilize the knee and laterally rotates the thigh. Loss of these muscles is usually compensated for by the remaining muscles in their functional group so that no significant motor defect remains.

Bony Landmarks
A line drawn from the pubic symphysis to the medial epicondyle should approximate the anterior border of the gracilis muscle.

INDICATIONS
Vaginal defects may be classified based on their location and size (Fig. 1). The type of defect determines the most appropriate flap choice. Small defects may be amenable to primary or advancement flap closure while more significant defects will require regional flaps. Defects are either partial (type I) or circumferential (type II). Type I, or partial, defects can be further classified based on whether they involve the anterolateral or posterior walls of the vagina. Type II, or circumferential, defects involve either the upper two-thirds of the vagina or the entire vaginal cylinder (Fig. 2).

Partial defects involving the anterior or lateral vaginal walls (type IA) may be reconstructed with pudendal fasciocutaneous flaps. Unilateral or bilateral flaps can be used. Partial defects involving the posterior wall (type IB) will benefit from use of the rectus flap. This flap will supply bulk to close dead space in the posterior pelvis. It will also provide sufficient skin to resurface the posterior vaginal wall. Circumferential defects of the upper two-thirds of the vagina (type IIA) are also best reconstructed with the rectus flap. The flap may be "tubed" to create a cap that can be sutured to the remaining vaginal cuff. Circumferential total defects (type IIB) are generally reconstructed with bilateral gracilis flaps. Such defects commonly result from total pelvic exenteration. The large surface area of the gracilis flaps facilitate restoration of the vaginal cylinder while also providing sufficient volume to fill the pelvis and promote healing.

SURGICAL PROCEDURE
Full-thickness Cutaneous Advancement Flaps
Cutaneous advancement flaps (V-Y procedure, Z-plasty) are useful for closure of small wounds, where mobilization of adjacent skin and subcutaneous tissue can reduce tension and allow adequate skin approximation. Such flaps should not be

Type I Partial defect

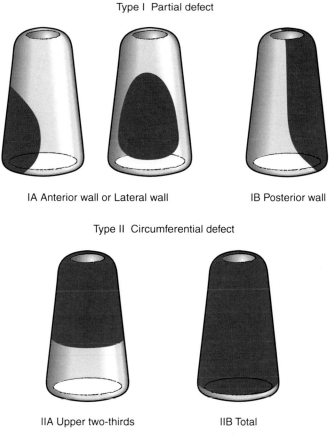

IA Anterior wall or Lateral wall   IB Posterior wall

Type II Circumferential defect

IIA Upper two-thirds   IIB Total

Figure 1 Classification of acquired vaginal defects. Defects are either partial (type I) or circumferential (type II).

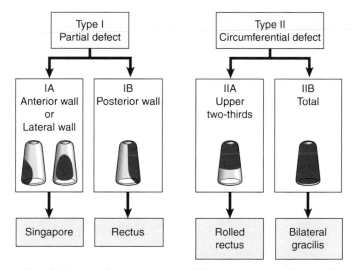

Figure 2 Algorithm for reconstruction of the vagina based on defect type I.

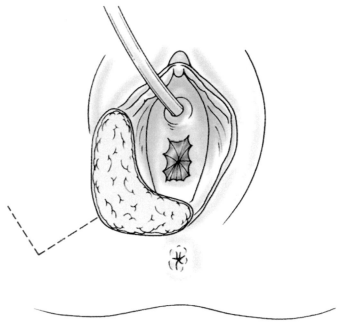

Figure 3 Z-plasty.

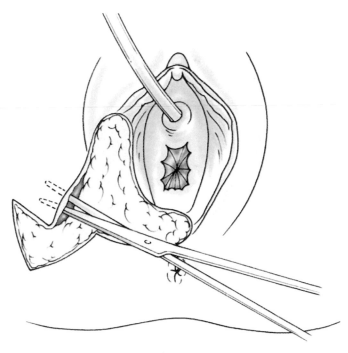

Figure 4 Z-plasty mobilization.

used for larger defects. Skin islands of varying sizes and shapes can be created adjacent to the defect as long as the patient has a good microvasculature (Fig. 3). Advancement flaps should be used with great caution in irradiated tissue. The skin and subcutaneous tissue are mobilized from the underlying fascia of the transverse perineal muscle (Fig. 4). The size of the flap is tailored to the size of the defect. The flap is undermined and in a Z-plasty is rotated through 90° to fill the defect (Fig. 5). Once the flap is rotated, the remaining skin edges are united (Fig. 6).

In a V-Y procedure the initial wedge (Fig. 7) is advanced to fill the gap and then closed as a Y (Fig. 8). Prolene 4-0 sutures should be used for these closures.

The Rectus Abdominis Flap

The flap is dissected with the patient supine or in the lithotomy position. Skin islands may be designed in a wide variety of shapes and orientations as long as a significant portion of the skin and subcutaneous tissues is centered over the muscle.

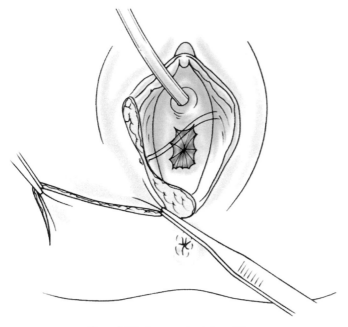

Figure 5 Ninety percent rotation of flap.

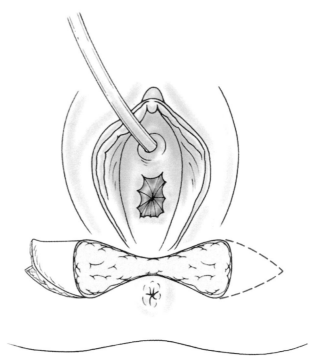

Figure 7 V-Y procedure.

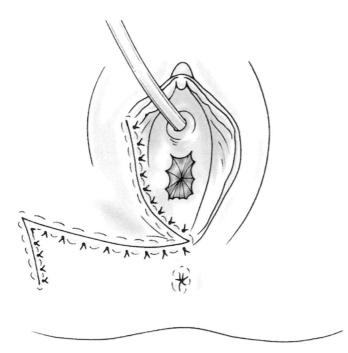

Figure 6 End result.

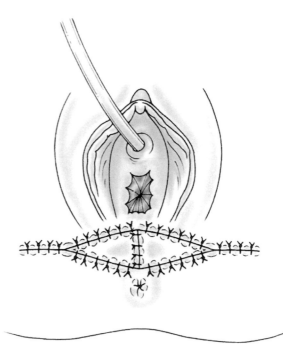

Figure 8 End result.

In most cases, an elliptical skin island is oriented vertically over the muscle (Fig. 9). For vaginal reconstruction, a more transversely oriented skin island may be designed above or below the level of the umbilicus, depending on the placement of ostomy sites. The skin islands should approximate the dimensions of the defect to be covered.

The skin incision is carried down to the level of the anterior rectus sheath; subcutaneous tissue and skin are then elevated off the sheath to allow an incision through the fascia to be made 1 cm from the lateral edge of the muscle. The dissection is then carried around the anterior and lateral surfaces of the muscle to the posterior surface. Care is taken to minimize injury to the tendinous intersections while mobilizing the muscle. The muscle can be divided above the level of the costal margin if needed. The muscle is then dissected away from the abdominal wall in a distal to proximal direction along the posterior rectus sheath toward the inferior epigastric pedicle. Several large intercostal perforators are ligated laterally and the deep inferior epigastric pedicle (artery and two venae comitantes) is then identified and dissected out of its origin from the iliac

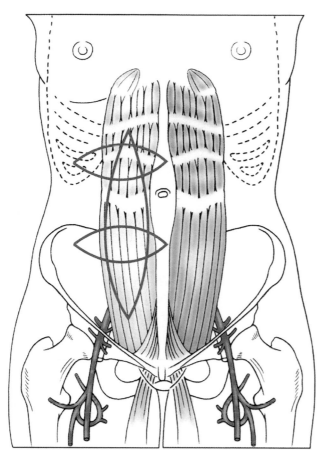

Figure 9 Possible elliptical skin islands.

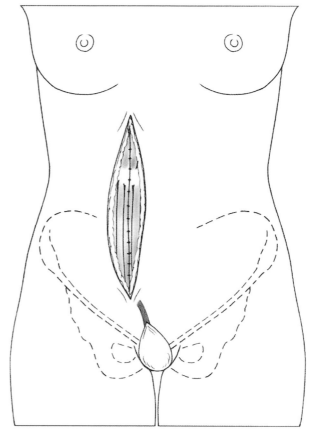

Figure 11 The anterior rectus fascia is approximated.

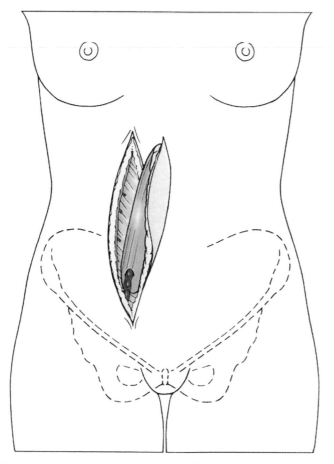

Figure 10 Rectus abdominis myocutaneous flap elevated. Note the inferior epigastric pedicle entering the caudal aspect of the flap.

vessels (Fig. 10). The insertion of the muscle into the pubic symphysis can be left intact or detached, depending on the arc of rotation that is required. For vaginal reconstruction, the skin island can be tubed and shaped into a pouch. It is then sutured to the remaining vaginal cuff from above. If perineal coverage is necessary, the flap can be tunneled in the subcutaneous plane over the inguinal ligament into the perineum or groin as needed (Fig. 11). The donor site is closed primarily by approximating the remaining 1 cm cuff of anterior rectus sheath to itself with a large non-absorbable suture. If necessary, skin and subcutaneous tissue flaps can be mobilized to reapproximate the skin flaps in the abdominal donor site.

The Gracilis Flap
The patient is usually placed in the lithotomy position for resections in this area. The hips are flexed and abducted. The medial thigh is prepared circumferentially down to the knee allowing access to the medial group of muscles. Figure 12 shows the underlying anatomy.

An elliptical skin island measuring up to 6 cm × 20 cm is outlined over the proximal two-thirds of the muscle (Fig. 13). The anterior border of the incision lies on a line drawn between the pubic tubercle and the semitendinosus tendon. A separate, small access incision may be made distally if needed to identify the muscle tendon.

The skin is incised anteriorly down to the medial group of muscles. The sartorius muscle is identified and retracted superiorly. The gracilis tendon can now be identified distally, usually through a separate short distal incision, and the tendinous insertion divided (Fig. 14). The posterior incision is made down to the muscle, taking care not to undermine perforators from the muscle to the skin or to shear the cutaneous aspect of the flap off the muscle. The flap is then elevated from distal to proximal on the thigh. One or two large perforators to the muscle are ligated distally. The main pedicle is identified entering the proximal third of the gracilis muscle in the space between the adductor longus and adductor magnus muscles (Fig. 15), approximately 8 to 10 cm

below the pubic tubercle. Once the pedicle is identified and preserved, the proximal muscle can be dissected and, if necessary, the origin from the pubic symphysis may be divided. The entire myocutaneous flap can then be tunneled through the subcutaneous skin bridge into the vaginal defect (Fig. 16) and exteriorized through the introitus (Fig. 17). The bilateral flaps are sutured to each other in the midline (Fig. 18). The neovagina is shaped into a pouch by approximating the

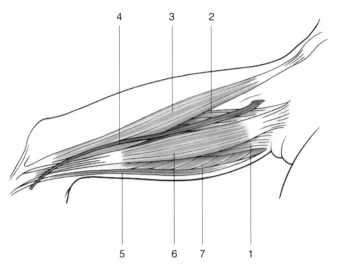

Figure 12 Underlying anatomy of medial thigh. 1 Adductor magnus muscle, 2 Adductor longus muscle, 3 Sartorius muscle, 4 Greater saphenous vein, 5 Semitendinosus muscle, 6 Gracilis muscle, 7 Semimembranosus muscle.

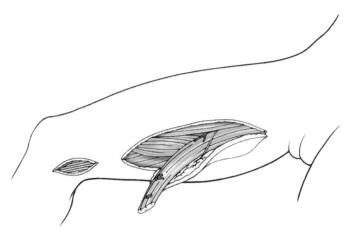

Figure 15 Myocutaneous flap elevated. Note neurovascular pedicle entering into proximal third of muscle.

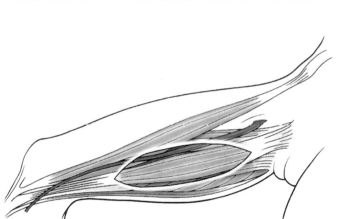

Figure 13 Outline of skin island over proximal two thirds of gracilis muscle.

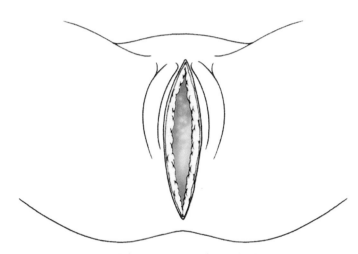

Figure 16 Typical defect in perineum after total pelvic exenteration.

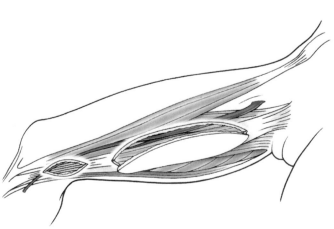

Figure 14 Skin and cutaneous skin island incised and distal gracilis muscle identified near knee.

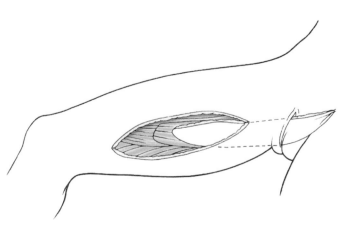

Figure 17 Myocutaneous flap exteriorized through the Introitus.

anterior, posterior, and distal skin edges of the flaps (Fig. 19); this can then be inserted into the pelvic space that is left after the exenteration. The proximal end of the neovagina is sutured to the introitus (Fig. 20).

Fasciocutaneous Neurovascular Pudendal Thigh Flaps

The fasciocutaneous flap is based on the posterior labial arteries, which are a continuation of the perineal artery. The posterior aspect of this flap is innervated by the posterior

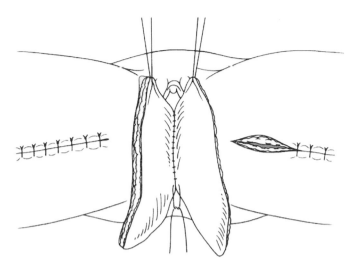

Figure 18 Bilateral gracilis myocutaneous flaps sewn together.

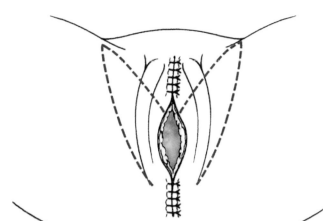

Figure 21 Partial anterior and posterior defect repair.

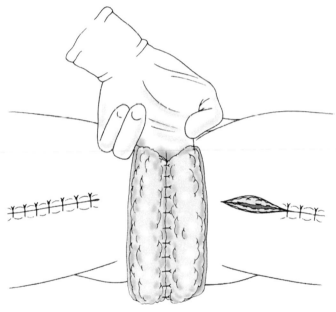

Figure 19 Bilateral flaps shaped into a pouch.

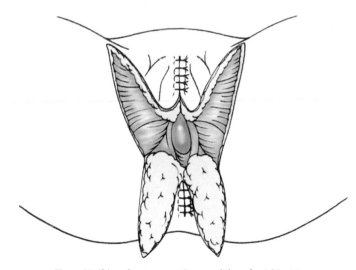

Figure 22 Skin subcutaneous tissue and deep fascial incision.

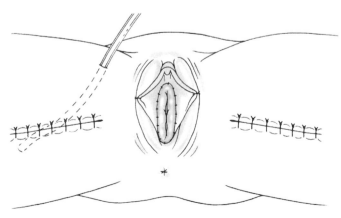

Figure 20 Neovaginal pouch inserted into pelvic space and sutured to the introitus.

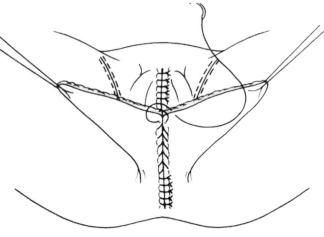

Figure 23 Flap elevation.

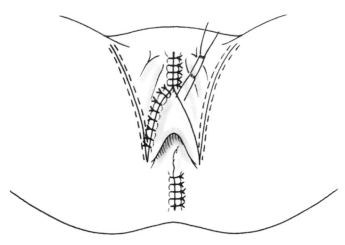

Figure 24 A suture of lateral margins of bilateral flaps to each other.

labial branches of the pudendal nerve and the perineal branches of the posterior cutaneous nerve of the thigh.

The patient is placed in the lithotomy position. A flap 3 to 6 cm wide and 10 to 15 cm long can be designed within the medial groin crease just lateral to the labia majora and the defect. Bilateral flaps can be designed for large posterior wall defects. The perineal defect is partially closed anteriorly and posteriorly leaving an entrance of suitable size into which the neovagina will be inserted (Fig. 21).

The skin and subcutaneous tissues are incised as well as the deep fascia overlying the muscles of the medial thigh compartment as they insert onto the pubis and ischium (Fig. 22).

The flap is then elevated from distal to proximal in the subfascial plane over the adductor muscles in order to avoid injury to the neurovascular pedicle (Fig. 23). The large distal branches of the perineal and pudendal vessels are identified and preserved. Often, the dissection is carried into the fat of the ischiorectal fossa in order to achieve adequate rotation and mobilization of the flap. The flap can then be rotated into the defect. The donor site is closed primarily in layers. A neovaginal pouch can be reconstructed by suturing the lateral margins of bilateral flaps to each other (Fig. 24); the neovagina is then transposed into the rectovesical space and the proximal ends sutured into the new vaginal introitus.

BIBLIOGRAPHY

Cordeiro PG, Pusic AL, Disa JJ (2002) A classification system and reconstructive algorithm for acquired vaginal defects. *Plast Reconstr Surg* **110**(4): 1058–65.

Crowe PJ, Temple WJ, Lopez MJ, et al. (1999) Pelvic extenteration for advanced pelvic malignancy. *Semin Surg Oncol* **17**:152–60 [Review].

Martello JY, Vasconez HC (1995) Vulvar and vaginal reconstruction after surgical treatment for gynecologic cancer. *Clin Plast Surg* **22**:129–40.

McCraw JB, Massey FM, Shanklin KD, et al. (1976) Vaginal reconstruction with gracilis myocutaneous flaps. *Plast Reconstr Surg* **58**:176–83.

Small T, Friedman DJ, Sultan M (2000) Reconstructive surgery of the pelvis after surgery for rectal cancer. *Semin Surg Oncol* **18**:259–65.

Tobin GR, Day TG (1988) Vaginal and pelvic reconstruction with distally based rectus abdominis and myocutaneous flaps. *Plast Reconstr Surg* **83**:62–73.

Tobin GR, Pursell SH, Day TG, Jr (1990) Refinements in vaginal reconstruction using rectus abdominis flaps. *Clin Plast Surg* **17**:705–12.

Wee JT, Joseph VT (1989) A new technique of vaginal reconstruction using neurovascular pudendal thigh flaps. A preliminary report. *Plast Reconstr Surg* **83**:701–9.

33 Objective assessment of technical surgical skill
Isabel Pigem, Thomas Ind, and Jane Bridges

INTRODUCTION
In the last few years, there has been growing interest from bodies involved in surgical education, evaluation and certification, and from the public, press and politicians in the assessment of surgical competence. Surgical competence is dependent on many factors, such as core knowledge, decision-making ability, communication skills, and technical surgical ability. Whereas most of these qualities are already formally assessed in written, oral and clinical examinations, there is as yet no standardized method for assessing technical surgical skill in an objective manner. The area of technical performance has historically been the most problematic in terms of objective assessment. Technical performance has traditionally been appraised in a subjective manner within the operating room environment. New technologies have been developed in the last decade that seem likely to facilitate objective assessment of technical surgical skill. These have been validated for general surgeons in the main rather than gynecologists. The objective of this chapter is to review available methods for the objective assessment of technical surgical skill and their limitations.

SURGICAL COMPETENCE
The objective assessment of technical surgical skill must be seen in the wider context of surgical competence. But what is surgical competence? Darzi and Mackay (2001) propose a simple model of its components (Box 1). In this context we regard technical surgical skill as the dexterity component of technical performance.

METHODS OF ASSESSMENT
Although advances in the objective assessment of technical surgical skill have been made in recent years, different investigators have been using different tests, criteria, validation methods, and even nomenclature. An international workshop of experts, convened in July 2001, reviewed all available methods of assessment of surgical technical skill, and provided a standardization of definitions, measurements, and criteria, and a foundation for communication among educators, researchers, training bodies, and certification boards (Satava et al. 2003).

There are a few essential definitions for objective assessment (Box 2).

There are several validated methods for objective assessment that measure abilities, skills, tasks, and/or procedures (Table 1). Some of these methods will be reviewed in detail later in this chapter. Only a few of the existing methods evaluate fundamental abilities or total procedures; the majority assess the same or similar technical skills and complex tasks, and therefore can be expected to provide a basis for comparison of results. There are a few abilities and skills, such as haptic aptitude or tissue handling, that are considered important, for which there are no validated methods of assessment.

There are some parameters that have been suggested as potential outcome data to measure technical surgical skill (Box 3).

The Good Method of Assessment
Reznick (1993) suggests that a good method of assessment should exhibit three basic components: feasibility, validity, and reliability (Box 4).

CURRENT METHODS OF ASSESSMENT
There are now several methods available for the objective assessment of technical surgical skill. Whereas some of these methods are well established, others are research tools in the process of being evaluated. Broadly speaking, the majority of these methods involve a standardized set of tasks. Although most assessments are carried out in the laboratory setting, there are some methods that are amenable for use in the operating room environment.

Basic Methods
Watts and Feldman (1985) report five basic methods used to assess technical surgical skill with varying degrees of reliability and validity (Table 2).

Procedure Lists with Logs
A common method of assessment of technical surgical skill is the use of procedure lists with logs. It consists of keeping a record of all the procedures carried out by a surgeon without any description of the quality of the performance.

Procedure lists with logs are not a new concept for many trainees. They have traditionally maintained a log of the procedures that they have performed, including a description of the level of supervision received, and have been asked to submit them at the time of annual assessments, examinations, and job interviews. More recently, even accredited surgeons in some countries need to keep such records as part of their revalidation process.

This method of assessment is cheap and easy to evaluate. However, it is a pure numerical account of operative performance and not a reflection of surgical dexterity; it therefore exhibits poor content validity (Reznick 1993, Cuschieri et al. 2001). Assuming that a surgeon is competent after having performed a designated number of procedures is wrong. Although repetition and practice are very important for the acquisition of technical surgical skill, in the absence of feedback a surgeon may learn to be consistently wrong (Kaufman et al. 1987).

Direct Observation without Criteria
Another common method of assessment of technical surgical skill is by direct observation without criteria. It consists of

Box 1 Components of Surgical Competence

Diagnostic ability: Ability to reach a diagnosis or differential diagnoses on the basis of history, physical examination, and investigations (these need to be recommended and explained to the patient, and their results interpreted)

Treatment plan: Ability to establish a plan of treatment (after considering available options, evaluating their pros and cons, and discussing them with the patient), and to change the plan if the clinical situation dictates so

Technical performance: Ability to carry out a surgical or other procedure effectively. This ability is a combination of three components: *Judgment:* Decision making that takes place during a surgical procedure and establishment of a plan to carry it out (e.g., deciding whether or not to perform a bowel resection in the course of an operation for ovarian cancer) *Knowledge:* Knowledge base required to implement the plan (e.g., knowing how to perform the bowel resection) *Dexterity:* Ability required to execute the plan accurately and effectively (e.g., whilst performing the bowel anastomosis tying knots tight enough to prevent fluid leakage but loose enough to prevent tissue damage)

Postoperative care: Ability to deliver routine care, and to diagnose and treat complications at an early stage

Box 2 Essential Definitions for Objective Assessment

Ability: The natural state or condition of being capable, such as psychomotor, visuospatial, perceptual, and haptic (tactile) aptitudes

Skill: A developed proficiency or dexterity in some art, craft, or the like, such as instrument handling, bimanual dexterity, navigation, ligation, suturing, knot tying, incision, exploration, palpation, cannulation, tissue handling, cutting, and blunt dissection

Task: A piece of work to be done, such as anastomosis, excision, closure, tissue extraction, exploration, and camera navigation

Procedure: A series of steps taken to accomplish an end, such as laparoscopic cholecystectomy, tracheostomy, chest tube insertion, diagnostic peritoneal lavage, vein patch, and breast biopsy

Table 1 Validated Methods for Objective Assessment

Method	Abilities	Skills	Tasks	Procedures
ADEPT	X	X		
OSATS		X	X	X
MISTELS		X	X	
MIST VR		X	X	
ICSAD		X	X	X
Rosser drills		X	X	
PicSOr	X	X		
ESSS		X	X	X
FSM		X	X	
LST 2000		X	X	
LapSim		X	X	
BSSC		X	X	X

Abbreviations: ADEPT, advanced Dundee endoscopic psychomotor tester; OSATS, objective structured assessment of technical skill; MISTELS, McGill inanimate system for training and evaluation of laparoscopic skills; MIST VR, minimally invasive surgical trainer, virtual reality; ICSAD, Imperial College surgical assessment device; PicSOr, pictorial surface orientation; ESSS, endoscopic sinus surgery simulator; FSM, fundamental surgical manipulations; LST 2000, laparoscopic surgery trainer, 2000; LapSim, laparoscopic simulator; BSSC, intercollegiate basic surgical skills course.

Box 3 Suggested Outcome Data

- Economy of movement
- Purposefulness of movement
- Absence of movement (indecision)
- Path length
- Time to completion
- Sequence of steps
- State analysis (still/moving)
- Force measurements
- Errors
- Recovery from error
- Repose latency (time to recover from error)
- Final product
- Global assessment of performance

Direct Observation with Criteria

Direct observation with criteria consists of assessing surgical dexterity by direct observation of a surgeon performing a procedure on a patient with explicit criteria against which technical surgical skill can be assessed.

It has been suggested that criteria turn raters into observers, instead of interpreters, of performance and therefore add objectivity to the assessment process (Regehr et al. 1998). This method of assessment satisfies most validity concerns and exhibits high inter-rater reliability (Kopta 1971). The more objective and structured the criteria are, the more reliable is the process. It has been shown that if a group of raters cooperatively identify important items for inclusion in a list of criteria, there is greater reliability than if the list was to be created by one rater alone (Valentino et al. 1998).

Models with Criteria

Another method of assessment of technical surgical skill is the use of models with criteria. It consists of assessing surgical

assessing surgical dexterity by direct observation of a surgeon performing a procedure on a patient with no explicit criteria. Direct observation without criteria is again not a new concept for many trainees, as this form of assessment currently takes place on a regular basis in the operating room.

This method of assessment exhibits poor test–retest reliability, as no explicit criteria are used and the process is therefore influenced by the subjectivity of the observer. It also exhibits poor inter-rater reliability, as two senior surgeons assessing a junior surgeon performing a procedure will have a high level of disagreement in their results (Reznick 1993).

Box 4 Components of a Good Method of Assessment

Feasibility: A method of assessment exhibits feasibility if it is practical and straightforward to administer

Validity: A method of assessment exhibits validity if it gives genuine information about what is being measured

Content validity: Refers to the extent to which the trait we are intending to measure is being measured by the method of assessment

Concurrent validity: Refers to the extent to which the results of the method of assessment correlate with the accepted reference gold standard known to measure the same trait

Construct validity: Refers to the extent to which the method of assessment is capable of discriminating between different levels of experience

Face validity: Refers to the extent to which the method of assessment resembles a situation in real life

Predictive validity: Refers to the extent that the method of assessment is able to predict future performance

Reliability: A method of assessment exhibits reliability if it can be repeated with minimal variation in the results

Inter-rater reliability: Refers to the extent of agreement in the results by independent raters

Test–retest reliability: Refers to the extent of agreement in the results achieved by administering the test to the same individual on separate occasions in the absence of any learning

Table 2 Reliability and Validity of Five Basic Methods of Assessment

Method of assessment	Reliability	Validity
Procedure lists with logs	NA	Poor
Direct observation without criteria	Poor	Modest
Direct observation with criteria	High	High
Models with criteria	High	Proportional to realism
Videotapes	High	Proportional to realism

Abbreviation: NA, not applicable.

dexterity by direct observation of a surgeon performing a procedure on a model. The model can be a live animal (such as an anesthetized pig), animal tissue (such as pigs' trotters or small bowel), or a bench model.

The use of models, when explicit criteria are applied, exhibits high reliability. The validity of this method of assessment is directly proportional to the realism of the process; it is directly proportional to the degree to which it mirrors operations on real patients.

Although anesthetized animal models have been used for education and research, there is growing concern about the moral and ethical issues involved in the use of live animals for this purpose. The legislation in some countries even prohibits the use of live animals for surgical training, although there may be no restriction to the use of animal parts. It is therefore increasingly difficult to justify the use of animals if alternative

methods, such as bench models, are available. It has been shown that the use of live anesthetized animals is equivalent to the use of bench models for evaluating technical surgical skill (Martin et al. 1997). Using bench models instead of patients or animals has the advantage that the former are cheaper, easier to transport, reusable, readily available, and do not create ethical dilemmas.

Videotapes

Another method of assessment of technical surgical skill consists of videotaping a surgeon performing a procedure on patients or models, and then having the tape analyzed by raters using explicit criteria.

Setting up the camera in such a way that the surgeon's face is not visible and eliminating any sound, will preserve anonymity and therefore add objectivity to the assessment process. The use of videotapes exhibits high reliability. Its validity is again proportional to the realism of the process.

This method of assessment is invaluable for providing feedback to a surgeon. However, it is expensive, and reviewing the videotapes can be very time consuming.

Other Methods

Time Taken for a Procedure

The time taken to complete a surgical procedure does not assess the quality of the operative performance. These types of data are an unreliable measure when used during real procedures, due to the influence of other variable factors.

Morbidity and Mortality Data

Morbidity and mortality data are commonly used as a method of assessment of operative performance. These forms of data often attribute the outcome of a patient solely to the operation and skill of the surgeon performing it, without taking into account other factors, such as patients' characteristics, case selection, preoperative morbidity, postoperative care, and local facilities. It is therefore believed that they do not truly reflect surgical competence (Poloniecki et al. 1998, Bridgewater et al. 2003).

RECENT DEVELOPMENTS IN ASSESSMENT

Task-specific Checklists and Global Rating Scales

Research aimed at developing objective methods of assessment of technical surgical skill, such as checklists and rating scales, is promising. Winckel et al. (1994) demonstrate that task-specific checklists and global rating scales exhibit high construct validity and high inter-rater reliability when used to assess surgical dexterity in the operating room. However, consistently valid and reliable assessment in this environment may be difficult to achieve mainly due to lack of standardization.

Objective Structured Assessment of Technical Skill (OSATS)

The objective structured assessment of technical skill (OSATS) is an objective method of assessment of technical surgical skill developed at the University of Toronto (Canada).

It consists of assessing surgical dexterity by direct observation of a surgeon performing a variety of standardized laboratory-based tasks within a time-limited multistation setting with explicit criteria against which technical surgical skill can be assessed. Both live anesthetized animals and bench models have been used in this setting.

Two types of scoring systems are used in the OSATS, a task-specific checklist and a global rating scale.

The task-specific checklist (Table 3) is different for each task. It identifies the steps that are necessary to perform a task effectively. These range between 22 and 32 steps, depending on the particular task that is being assessed. The observer indicates which of these steps are correctly or incorrectly performed. If a new task is included in the assessment, a new task-specific checklist must be developed and validated.

By contrast, the global rating scale (Table 4) is identical for each task. It identifies seven general operative competencies that are necessary to perform a task effectively. The observer rates the level of performance of each competency on a five-point scale that is anchored at the middle and extreme points by behavioral descriptors. The global rating scale assesses surgical skill in a less concrete way than the task-specific checklist, but has broad applicability.

The OSATS evaluates skills (such as cannulation and clamping), tasks (such as sutured and stapled bowel anastomosis, skin lesion excision, abdominal wall closure and major hemorrhage control), and procedures (such as chest tube insertion, and more recently tracheostomy and pyloroplasty).

There are now several studies that demonstrate that the OSATS is a valid and reliable objective method of assessment of technical surgical skill. Faulkner et al. (1996) show that both task-specific checklists and global rating scales correlate well with the independent opinion of senior surgeons regarding the surgical dexterity of more junior surgeons, suggesting that this method of assessment exhibits concurrent validity. Martin et al. (1997) demonstrate that the use of bench models is equivalent to the use of live anesthetized animals in this setting. Also, both task-specific checklists and global rating scales exhibit moderate to high interstation reliabilities, and their correlations are high, both within the live anesthetized animal format and the bench model format, suggesting that both scoring systems are measuring the same quality. Further, the inter-rater reliabilities found indicate that the use of one rater per station is adequate. Reznick et al. (1997) show that the OSATS exhibits high construct validity and high interstation reliability for both scoring systems. Regehr et al. (1998) demonstrate that global rating scales exhibit higher concurrent validity, higher construct validity and higher interstation reliability than task-specific checklists. Further, the use of task-specific checklists in conjunction with global rating scales does not improve the validity or reliability of the global rating scale over that of the global rating scale used in isolation. Also, global rating scales are more useful the more senior the surgeons and the more difficult the tasks are.

Motion Analysis Systems

Motion analysis consists of using markers placed on a surgeon's hands to track their movements during the performance of a standardized surgical task, and then to analyze the data obtained as an alternative method of assessment of technical surgical skill. Motion tracking can be based on electromagnetic, mechanical, or optical systems.

Imperial College Surgical Assessment Device (ICSAD)

The Imperial College Surgical Assessment Device (ICSAD) is an objective method of assessment of technical surgical skill developed at Imperial College of Science Technology and Medicine in London (UK).

The ICSAD (Fig. 1) consists of a commercially available electromagnetic tracking system and bespoke software to assess surgical dexterity by analyzing the hand movements of a surgeon performing a standardized surgical task. The tracking system (Isotrak II, Polhemus, USA) uses electromagnetic fields to determine the position of a remote object, in this case a surgeon's hands. The technology is based on generating magnetic field vectors from a transmitter, and detecting the field vectors with a receiver. The sensed signals are input to a mathematical algorithm that computes the receiver's position relative to the transmitter. A single electromagnetic tracker or receiver is attached by velcro straps to the back of each hand at standardized positions. Three-dimensional information from each tracker is obtained with an update rate of 20 per second. These raw three-dimensional positional data from the tracking system are transferred to a computer and extrapolated by the software into scores of technical surgical skill, such as path length, number, and speed of hand movements, and time to task completion. The software includes a filter to eliminate background noise from sources, such as hand tremor and experimental error in the tracking device, ensuring that only purposeful actions are recorded.

Table 3 Task-specific Checklist for Sutured Bowel Anastomosis Used in the OSATS

Steps	Correctly performed	Incorrectly performed
Bowel orientated mesenteric border to mesenteric border, no twisting		
Stay sutures held with artery forceps		
Selects appropriate instruments		
Selects appropriate suture		
Needle loaded 1/2 to 2/3 from tip		
Use of index finger to stabilize needleholder		
Needle enters bowel at right angles on 80% of bites		
Single attempt at needle passage through bowel on 90% of bites		
Follow-through on curve of needle on entrance on 80% of bites		
Follow-through on curve of needle on exit on 80% of bites		
Use of forceps on seromuscular layer of bowel only, majority of time		
Minimal damage with forceps		
Use of forceps to handle needle		
Inverting sutures		
Suture spacing 3–5 mm		
Equal bites on each side on 80% of bites		
Individual bites on each side on 90% of bites		
Square knots		
Minimal three throws on knots		
Suture cut to appropriate length		
No mucosal pouting		
Apposition of bowel without excessive tension on sutures		

Table 4 Global Rating Scale Used in the OSATS

Competencies	Level of performance							
Respect for tissue	1 Frequently uses unnecessary force on tissue or causes damage by inappropriate use of instruments	2	3 Careful handling of tissue but occasionally causes inadvertent damage	4	5 Consistently handles tissue appropriately with minimal damage
Time and motion	1 Many unnecessary moves	2	3 Efficient time and motion but some unnecessary moves	4	5 Clear economy of movement and maximal efficiency
Instrument handling	1 Repeatedly makes tentative or awkward moves with instruments by their inappropriate use	2	3 Competent use of instruments but occasionally appears stiff or awkward	4	5 Fluid moves with instruments and no awkwardness
Knowledge of instruments	1 Frequently asks for wrong instrument or uses inappropriate instrument	2	3 Knows names of most instruments and uses appropriate instrument	4	5 Obviously familiar with the instruments and their names
Flow of operation and forward planning	1 Frequently stops operating and seems unsure of next move	2	3 Demonstrates some forward planning with reasonable progression of procedure	4	5 Obviously planned course of operation with effortless flow from one move to the next
Use of assistants	1 Consistently places assistants poorly or fails to use assistants	2	3 Appropriate use of assistants most of the time	4	5 Strategically uses assistants to the best advantage at all times
Knowledge of specific procedure	1 Deficient knowledge needing specific instruction at most operative steps	2	3 Knows all important steps of operation	4	5 Demonstrates familiarity with all aspects of operation

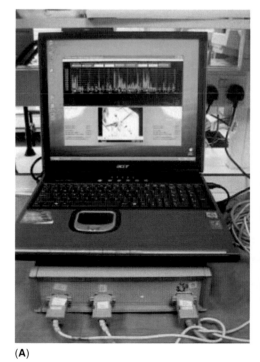

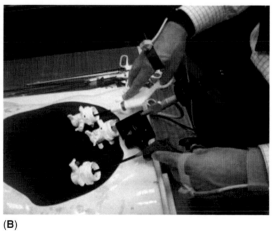

(A) **(B)**

Figure 1 Imperial College Surgical Assessment Device (ICSAD). Raw three-dimensional positional data obtained from the electromagnetic trackers (**A**) are transferred to a computer (**B**) and extrapolated into scores of technical surgical skill. *Source*: Courtesy of Department of Surgical Oncology and Technology, Imperial College, London, UK.

ICSAD evaluates skills, tasks, and procedures. There are now several studies that demonstrate that the ICSAD is a valid and reliable objective method of assessment of technical surgical skill. These have shown that outcome data, such as path length, number and speed of hand movements, and time to completion, are valid indicators of technical surgical skill using standardized surgical tasks. This method of assessment has been validated for minimal access (Taffinder et al. 1999a) and open (Datta et al. 2001) surgical tasks. In laparoscopic surgery, outcome data, such as path length of instrument tips, number of hand movements, and time to completion, are capable of discriminating between different levels of experience, and therefore exhibit construct validity. This is true for simple tasks in a training box (Taffinder et al. 1999b) as well as for complex tasks, such as laparoscopic cholecystectomy on a cadaveric porcine liver model (Smith et al. 1999, 2002). Experienced surgeons tend to use a fewer number of movements (economy of movement) and shorter paths (accuracy in target localization). In open surgery, however, although outcome data, such as number of hand movements and time to completion, are capable of discriminating between different levels of experience, and therefore exhibit construct validity, path length is not.

Virtual Reality Systems

Virtual reality has been described as a collection of technologies that allow people to interact efficiently with three-dimensional computerized databases in real-time using their natural senses and skills (McCloy and Stone 2001). Its strength lies in its ability to allow a surgeon to practice surgical tasks repeatedly, in a short period of time, without the need for a particular clinical situation to arise, and without the pressures of a real-live scenario. It is also preferable for patients that new surgical maneuvers have been practiced outside the operating room before attempts are made during real surgical procedures. The main advantage of virtual reality systems, when compared to motion analysis systems, is that they provide real-time feedback about skill-based errors. Although virtual reality systems are extensively used for training purposes, few have been validated for the assessment of technical surgical skill.

Minimally Invasive Surgical Trainer (MIST)
The Minimally Invasive Surgical Trainer (MIST) is an objective method of assessment of technical surgical skill originally developed in the United Kingdom. It is now commercially available from Mentice AB (Sweden).

The MIST is an example of a low-fidelity virtual reality system, as it attempts to replicate the skills of laparoscopic operating but not the appearance.

The MIST (Fig. 2) consists of a frame holding two standard laparoscopic instruments electronically linked to a computer. The movements of the surgical instruments are viewed in real time on a screen with three-dimensional graphics. Two modules are available: one for core skills and another for suturing. In the core skills module, the user is guided through 12 exercises of progressive complexity that enables the development of essential laparoscopic skills. Each task is based on a key surgical technique employed in laparoscopic cholecystectomy, using simple geometrical shapes rather than tissue, to allow the user to concentrate on the development of key psychomotor skills.

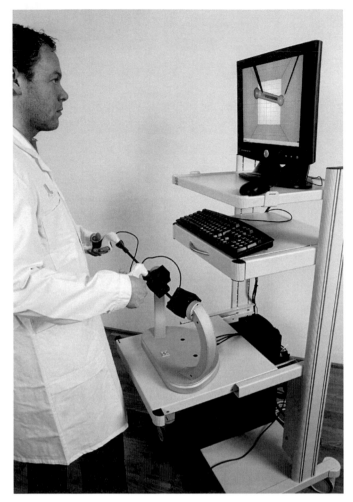

Figure 2 Minimally Invasive Surgical Trainer (MIST). *Source:* Courtesy of Mentice AB, Sweden.

In the suturing module, the user is guided through 12 suturing tasks of progressive complexity, from basic stitching to knot-tying. Right and left repetitions are employed to encourage ambidextrous working. Performance is measured by time, number of errors, and the efficiency with which the exercise is performed.

The MIST evaluates skills (such as transfer/traversal, pegboard, and clamping) and tasks (such as energy use).

There are now several studies that demonstrate that the MIST is a valid and reliable objective method of assessment of technical surgical skill. It is the only virtual reality system that has been extensively validated as a method of assessment of technical skill in minimal access surgery (Taffinder et al. 1998a, Chaudhry et al. 1999). Taffinder et al. (1998a,b) show that the system can distinguish between senior and junior surgeons using outcome data, such as number of movements made, time taken, number of errors made and economy of movement; it therefore exhibits construct validity. Factors that affect surgical performance, such as sleep deprivation, have also been evaluated with the MIST (Taffinder et al. 1998c).

Many improvements may be possible in the future using virtual reality systems. There is much interest in the development of high-fidelity systems, where the appearance, as well as the skills of laparoscopic operating, is replicated.

Other Systems

Advanced Dundee Endoscopic Psychomotor Tester (ADEPT)

The advanced Dundee endoscopic psychomotor tester (ADEPT) is an objective method of assessment of technical surgical skill developed at the University of Dundee (UK).

The ADEPT was originally designed as a tool for the selection of surgeons for laparoscopic surgery, based on the ability of psychomotor tests to predict innate abilities to perform relevant tasks. The ADEPT is a system that uses standardized laboratory-based tasks but real laparoscopic instruments and imaging for the objective assessment of laparoscopic technical surgical skill (Hanna et al. 1997).

The ADEPT consists of an opaque dome that encloses a workspace. The dome has three apertures to reach the workspace: one for a laparoscope, and two for laparoscopic graspers. The apertures for the graspers incorporate hinge mechanisms that have the same degree of freedom as laparoscopic instruments through access ports. A target is situated in the center of the workspace and can be viewed on a standard monitor. The target consists of a rectangular plate mounted on four pins at each corner. If excessive manipulation resulting in contact with the pins occurs, this constitutes a plate error. The target plate has structured tasks involving the manipulation of switches and dials. Between the dome and the target plate there is a transparent spring-mounted sheet with apertures of varying shapes that allow the passage of the manipulating instrument while the sheet is retracted by the assisting instrument. If the assisting instrument establishes contact with the aperture in the sheet, this constitutes a probe error. The system is controlled by a computer. It gives instructions to the user by randomly picking tasks with instructions on the task details. The computer software generates outcome data on performance, such as instrument errors, execution time, and task completion score (involves completing the task within the allocated time and tolerance limit).

The ADEPT evaluates psychomotor abilities (such as tracking, pick and place, translation, aiming, and precision), and skills (such as bimanual dexterity).

There are now several studies that demonstrate that the ADEPT is a valid and reliable objective method of assessment of technical surgical skill. The extent to which the system resembles a situation in real life, and therefore exhibits face validity, includes the use of a real laparoscopic imaging system, and real laparoscopic instruments with the same degree of freedom as real laparoscopic instruments through real access ports. As the performance on the ADEPT is scored by computer software, this eliminates any inter-rater variability. Macmillan and Cuschieri (1999) show that performance on the system correlates well with the independent opinion of senior surgeons regarding the surgical dexterity of more junior surgeons, suggesting that this method of assessment exhibits concurrent validity. The ADEPT evaluates aspects of surgical dexterity that do not improve with practice (innate abilities). Because of this, it could be used to predict future performance, and therefore exhibit predictive validity. Francis et al. (2002) demonstrate that the system can distinguish between senior and junior surgeons, and therefore exhibits construct validity. Senior surgeons tend to incur less instrument errors, with shorter execution times, and higher task completion scores than junior surgeons; the former complete the tasks more accurately without sacrificing execution time.

CONCLUSION

The assessment of surgical competence is certainly a fascinating as well as an important area in our profession that in the last few years has been under the scrutiny of the public, press, and politicians. The development of objective methods of assessment of technical surgical skill was initially seen as the most difficult aspect of assessing surgical competence. Considerable progress has been made in the last decade, and there has been a shift toward using objective rather than subjective systems. The surgical community can now choose from a variety of objective methods of assessment of surgical dexterity. However, as promising as the methods described in this chapter may appear, the objective assessment of technical surgical skill is still in its early stages of development, and some issues are yet to be addressed. These include the further validation of these systems, and the incorporation of these methods for training, evaluation, and potentially for certification and revalidation purposes, proving that once introduced, they do make a difference in outcome. Future research should probably be focused in these directions.

REFERENCES

Bridgewater B, Grayson AD, Jackson M, et al. (2003) Surgeon specific mortality in adult cardiac surgery: comparison between crude and risk stratified data. *BMJ* **327**:13–17.

Chaudhry A, Sutton C, Wood J, et al. (1999) Learning rate for laparoscopic surgical skills on MIST VR, a virtual reality simulator: quality of human–computer interface. *Ann R Coll Surg Engl* **81**.281–6.

Cuschieri A, Francis N, Crosby J, et al. (2001) What do master surgeons think of surgical competence and revalidation? *Am J Surg* **182**:110–16.

Darzi A, Mackay S (2001) Assessment of surgical competence. *Qual Health Care* **10**(Suppl 2):ii64–9.

Datta V, Mackay S, Mandalia M, et al. (2001) The use of electromagnetic motion tracking analysis to objectively measure open surgical skill in the laboratory-based model. *J Am Coll Surg* **193**:479–85.

Faulkner H, Regehr G, Martin J, et al. (1996) Validation of an objective structured assessment of technical skill for surgical residents. *Acad Med* **71**:1363–5.

Francis NK, Hanna GB, Cuschieri A (2002) The performance of master surgeons on the Advanced Dundee Endoscopic Psychomotor Tester: contrast validity study. *Arch Surg* **137**:841–4.

Hanna GB, Drew T, Cuschieri A (1997) Technology for psychomotor skills testing in endoscopic surgery. *Semin Laparosc Surg* **4**:120–4.

Kaufman HH, Wiegand RL, Tunick RH (1987) Teaching surgeons to operate—principles of psychomotor skills training. *Acta Neurochir (Wien)* **87**:1–7.

Kopta JA (1971) An approach to the evaluation of operative skills. *Surgery* **70**:297–303.

Macmillan AI, Cuschieri A (1999) Assessment of innate ability and skills for endoscopic manipulations by the Advanced Dundee Endoscopic Psychomotor Tester: predictive and concurrent validity. *Am J Surg* **177**:274–7.

Martin JA, Regehr G, Reznick R, et al. (1997) Objective structured assessment of technical skill (OSATS) for surgical residents. *Br J Surg* **84**:273–8.

McCloy R, Stone R (2001) Science, medicine, and the future. Virtual reality in surgery. *BMJ* **323**:912–15.

Poloniecki J, Valencia O, Littlejohns P (1998) Cumulative risk adjusted mortality chart for detecting changes in death rate: observational study of heart surgery. *BMJ* **316**:1697–700.

Regehr G, MacRae H, Reznick RK, et al. (1998) Comparing the psychometric properties of checklists and global rating scales for assessing performance on an OSCEformat examination. *Acad Med* **73**:993–7.

Reznick RK (1993) Teaching and testing technical skills. *Am J Surg* **165**:358–61.

Reznick R, Regehr G, MacRae H, et al. (1997) Testing technical skill via an innovative 'bench station' examination. *Am J Surg* **173**:226–30.

Satava RM, Cuschieri A, Hamdorf J (2003) Metrics for objective assessment. *Surg Endosc* **17**:220–6.

Smith SG, Torkington J, Brown TJ, et al. (2002) Motion analysis. *Surg Endosc* **16**:640–5.

Smith SG, Torkington J, Darzi AW (1999) A computerized assessment of surgical dexterity during perfused cadaveric porcine laparoscopic cholecystectomy. *Br J Surg* **86**(Suppl 1):95.

Taffinder N, Smith SG, Huber J, et al. (1999a) The effect of a second-generation 3D endoscope on the laparoscopic precision of novices and experienced surgeons. *Surg Endosc* **13**:1087–92.

Taffinder N, Sutton C, Fishwick RJ, et al. (1998a) Validation of virtual reality to teach and assess psychomotor skills in laparoscopic surgery: results from randomised controlled studies using the MIST VR laparoscopic simulator. *Stud Health Technol Inform* **50**:124–30.

Taffinder NJ, McManus IC, Gul Y, et al. (1998c) Effect of sleep deprivation on surgeons' dexterity on laparoscopy simulator. *Lancet* **352**:1191.

Taffinder NJ, Russell RC, McManus IC, et al. (1998b) An objective assessment of surgeons' psychomotor skills: validation of the MIST-VR laparoscopic simulator. *Br J Surg* **85**(Suppl 1):75.

Taffinder NJ, Smith SG, Mair J, et al. (1999b) Can a computer measure surgical precision? Reliability, validity and feasibility of the ICSAD. *Surg Endosc* **13**(Suppl 1):81.

Valentino J, Donnelly MB, Sloan DA, et al. (1998) The reliability of six faculty members in identifying important OSCE items. *Acad Med* **73**:204–5.

Watts J, Feldman WB (1985) Assessment of technical skills. In: Neufeld VR, Norman GR, eds. *Assessing Clinical Competence*. New York: Springer, pp. 259–74.

Winckel CP, Reznick RK, Cohen R, et al. (1994) Reliability and construct validity of a structured technical skills assessment form. *Am J Surg* **167**:423–7.

34 Meta-analysis of survival data

Srdjan Saso, Jayanta Chatterjee, Ektoras Georgiou, Sadaf Ghaem-Maghami, and Thanos Athanasiou

SURVIVAL DATA IN GYNECOLOGICAL ONCOLOGY

Survival analysis is a valuable statistical tool in medicine as it deals with all possible factors that can lead to death of a biological organism, that is, human. It is a collection of statistical procedures which involve the modeling of time to event data; therefore, the outcome variable of interest is time until an event (*death* being the "event") occurs.

By performing survival analysis in gynecological oncology (GO), the hope is that valuable questions can be answered, thus, allowing us to expand upon the existing knowledge and improve current management protocols for the benefit of patients.

Important questions that one encounters in GO are as follows (Fig. 1):

a. What is the fraction of the GO cancer population which will survive past a certain time?
b. At what rate will the patients die or relapse, if they manage to survive?
c. How does a particular type of surgery/management protocol improve or worsen survival odds?
d. Can multiple causes of death or failure be taken into account?

Time-to-event outcomes help to answer such questions by considering three factors: (1) whether an event takes place; (2) the time at which the event occurs, that is, when the period of observation starts and finishes; and (3) time between response to treatment and recurrence or relapse-free survival time (also called disease-free survival time). However, prior to commencing the analysis, the terms "time" and "event", as well as their relationship to each other must not be left ambiguous. In GO, a cure for ovarian cancer may not be possible, but it is hoped that a new intervention will increase the duration of survival. Therefore, although similar number of deaths may be observed, it is hoped that a new intervention will decrease the rate at which they take place so disease free survival may not be altered but overall survival is prolonged at a given time.

Aims

The aims of this chapter are listed in Box 1.

WHAT IS A META-ANALYSIS?

Historically, clinical decisions in GO were derived from two broad medical areas: gynecology and oncology; these decisions were based on personal experience, unquestioned use of methods suggested by senior colleagues and recommendations from clinical authorities. The progress of absorbing higher forms of evidence into the clinical knowledge base has been slow. This is more evident in surgical practice (which makes up a significant proportion of the practice within GO) where the proportion of systematic reviews and randomized controlled trials (RCTs) in leading surgical journals stands at 5% (Panesar et al. 2006).

Moral–ethical obligations, legal liability, and health economic rationing have heralded the advent of evidence-based healthcare in the last few decades. To ensure the best possible outcomes for patients, clinicians are increasingly required to implement best practices and continuous quality improvement processes within the clinical environment. This inextricably involves the application of the best available knowledge, usually in the form of scientific research, to guide clinical decision making. Hence, the use of clinical research is no longer an option but a necessity. However problems remain for a practicing GO clinician as to what constitutes "best available knowledge" and in particular which type of research should be used (Fig. 2).

Information Overload

With increasing pressures of being a practicing clinician (Royal College of Surgeons of England 2009), two problems remain. One is the ability to synthesize and apply the best evidence to improve patient care, bearing in mind that the average clinician would have to read 19 original articles each day in order to keep up with advances in his chosen field (Davidoff et al. 1995). Furthermore, this problem is compounded by the recent information explosion in the biomedical field within the last quarter century as can be evidenced by the dense cornucopia of articles and journals which are now readily accessible and searchable through a variety of online web-based bibliographic databases like PubMed and EMBASE. In addition to the huge volume of literature, its scattered nature poses further problems. Every time a new article appears, readers must compare new findings with the existing scope of evidence to come to a reframed overall clinical conclusion.

Conflicting Results

The presence of conflicting results among individual research studies does not improve matters. Not only could inconsistent results and conclusions be attributed to the statistical play of chance, but it might also be due to the presence of systematic error from poorly designed study methodology. This would entail the need to critically analyze each individual trial for study quality, adding an extra dimension of burden to the clinician.

Narrative Review and Its Shortcomings

The narrative review partially resolves the problems above by providing a broad, updated and authoritative summary of research and opinion by key leaders in a field. However, this

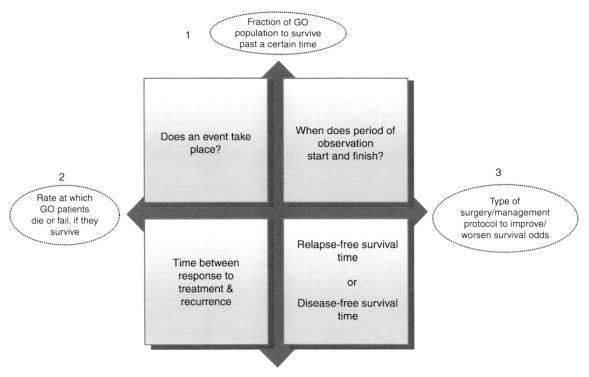

Figure 1 Time-to-event outcomes: how to use them to answer cancer survival related questions?

Box 1

1. Introduce an important branch of statistical analysis to a gynecological oncology surgeon
2. Demonstrate the relevance of meta-analysis to enlarging and improving the management of gyne-oncological practice
3. Focus on survival data (SD) meta-analysis and describe the process required to conduct it thoroughly and precisely
4. Illustrate the drawbacks that can arise when carrying out a SD meta-analysis
5. Discuss alternate meta-analytical methods that can be utilized in the field of gynecological oncology

type of review brings with it its own attendant problems where a number of review authors can provide differing viewpoints and anti-diametric conclusions from the very same source material used. This might be attributed to several factors like the use of an assorted mixture of ambiguous review methodologies, the lack of disclosure and transparency in techniques, the inability to statistically combine results, and the inherent introduction of subjective bias present in the form of "expert" opinion (Williams 1998).

Limitations of RCTs

Furthermore, although RCTs, when conducted properly, offer one of the more objective methods in determining the true relationship between treatment and outcome, the use of this particular type of study design also carries with it a number of limitations.

This includes the need for large numbers of participants in a trial, usually ranging from thousand to tens of thousands of subjects, in order to ensure sufficient statistical power. This is especially so if the treatment effects being studied are small in magnitude but are still deemed clinically useful. It is further compounded by the study of rare diseases of low incidence and prevalence where an RCT might have to be conducted over a prolonged period of time in order to gather sufficient number of required subjects for any statistically significant result to be derived. The presence of a latency period between exposure, treatment, and outcome will also necessitate the need for a longer term follow-up. Hence, although this type of study design is objective and free from bias compared to other study designs, in certain situations it can prove to be costly in terms of time, manpower, and money.

As all groups do not have such resources in excess at their disposal, compromises are reached whereby trials are conducted anyway in smaller discrete populations. These make the results from such smaller studies liable to be statistically insignificant or at best imprecise with larger degrees of uncertainty in result estimates. With that, the overall usefulness of such RCTs is reduced.

Moreover, the design of an RCT mandates that a standardized population demographic be tested in a controlled environment. In comparison with the true multivariate nature of the "real world" clinical setting, the presence of heterogeneity in ethnicity, age, and geography might make any significant result from RCTs inapplicable.

Insufficient High Quality Trial Data (in Surgical Research)

A problem more specific to surgical literature lies in the relatively small proportion of high-quality evidence in most

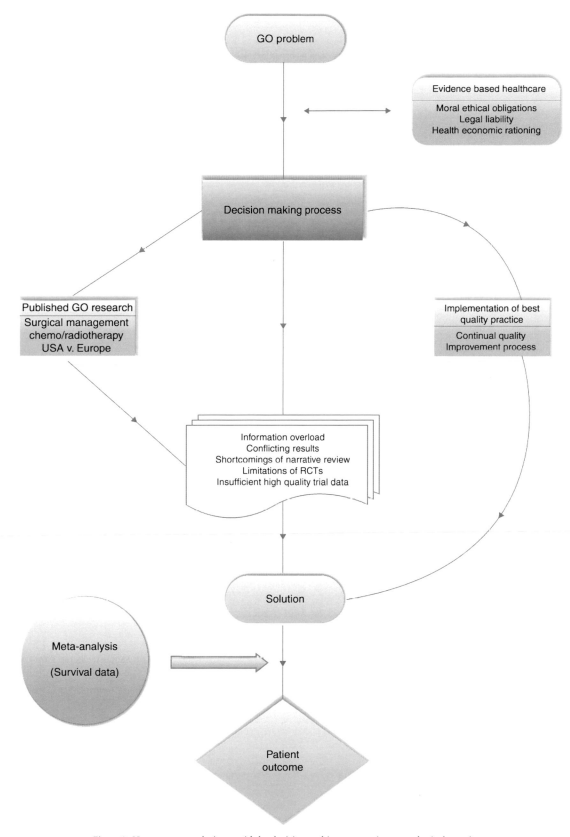

Figure 2 How a meta-analysis can aid the decision making process in gynecological oncology.

surgical journals. The number of surgical RCTs is indeed small and case reports and series still are the predominant publication type. Even then, within surgical studies, there are also heterogeneous differences in study quality, such as insufficient sample size, unclear methodologies, and the use of non-clinical outcomes of interest (Sauerland and Seiler 2005).

The Solution

It is evident that firstly there is a need for a more objective method of summarizing primary research, and secondly it is required to overcome the pitfalls in RCTs. Both these have spurred the development of a formalized set of processes and methodologies in the form of the systematic review and

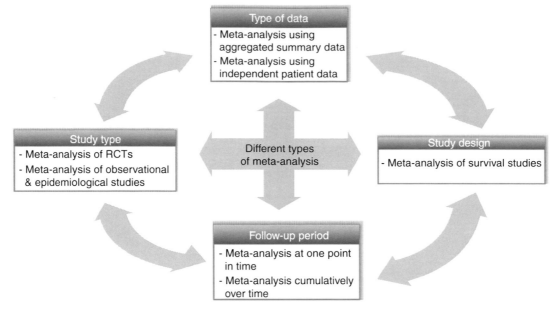

Figure 3 What types of meta-analysis can be used in surgical research?

meta-analysis. In the clinical context, meta-analyses have become an important tool for finding important and valid studies while filtering out the large number of seriously flawed and irrelevant articles. By condensing the results of many trials, they allow the readers to obtain a valid overview on a topic with substantially less effort involved.

Meta-analysis Defined

A systematic review is defined as the objective, transparent and unbiased location and critical appraisal of the complete scope of research in a given topic and the eventual impartial synthesis and, if possible, meta-analysis of individual study findings. Therefore, in order to address a specific research aim, a systematic review collates all evidence that fits pre-specified eligibility criteria.

In a systematic review two types of synthesis can be performed: a qualitative synthesis where primary studies are summarized like in a narrative review and a quantitative synthesis where primary studies are statistically combined. It is this quantitative synthetic component which is termed a meta-analysis: *the statistical quantitative integration of individual study findings to get an overall summary result* (Glass 1976). A common misunderstanding is that a meta-analysis is exactly identical to a systematic review and can be used interchangeably as synonyms. In truth, a meta-analysis is actually a subset component of a systematic review.

A meta-analysis is also not only limited to the summarization of RCT data. Different study designs, data types, and follow-up spans as illustrated in Figure 3 could be also used in a meta-analysis. More details with regard to the usage of meta-analyses most relevant to GO, that is, meta-analysis of SD, together with its attendant pros and cons would be discussed later. For now, emphasis will be given to the aims of meta-analysis in general.

The aims of a meta-analysis are manifold (Box 2).

Each meta-analysis is composed of a discrete number of steps (Box 3).

Box 2

- Critical appraisal of individual studies
- Combination of individual results to create a useful summary statistic
- Analysis for presence of and reasons behind between-study variances
- Exposure of areas of research which might be methodologically inadequate and require further refinement
- Exposure of knowledge gaps and areas of potential future research possibilities

---

Box 3

- Formulation of a specific question to be addressed with a clearly stated set of objectives
- Definition of eligibility (inclusion and exclusion) criteria for primary studies to be included
- Systematic search which identifies and locates all potentially eligible relevant studies whether published or unpublished
- Critical appraisal of each individual study via the use of explicit appraisal criteria
- Performance of a variety of statistical methods to assess for heterogeneity between studies
- Impartial unbiased analysis and assessment of the validity of the results
- Creation of a structured presentation, and synthesis to state and discuss upon findings and characteristics of collected information

---

Furthermore, a meta-analysis can facilitate the synthesis of results for a number of scenarios where the findings of individual studies show: (a) no effect because of a small sample size; (b) varying directions of effect; and (c) effects versus no significant effects.

All these findings can be commonly encountered among surgical topics. A meta-analysis may serve to combine findings from similar studies to help increase the power to detect statistical differences (Ng et al. 2006).

Advantages over Narrative Reviews

From the above, we conclude that the shortcomings of narrative reviews can be readily improved since: (a) presence of explicit inclusion and exclusion criteria ensures the comprehensiveness of the review, while in the process minimizing the inclusion of bias within individual studies; (b) presence of a meta-analysis can provide a quantitative summary of the overall effect estimate; (c) differences between study methodologies which affect results can be explored; and (d) adherence to a strict scientific design with transparent methodology in analysis ensures objectivity and reproducibility of findings.

Narrative reviews by nature also tend to be generically broad and all-encompassing. The systematic review, in contrast, puts forward specific questions to answer which increases the applicability of such reviews in the clinical context.

Advantages over Randomized Controlled Trials

The use of a meta-analysis for the purpose of conducting a systematic review enhances the statistical power of a group of RCTs since the pooling of data from individual studies would increase the study population. With an increase in statistical power comes an increase in the precision of findings and thereby, a reduction in both uncertainty and ambiguity. Systematic reviews can also enhance the applicability of a trial since the pooling and analysis of data from different RCTs with varied patient groups can reveal any heterogeneity or homogeneity of findings.

In conclusion, systematic reviews and meta-analyses have great importance in the summarization and application of scientific surgical research. Their undertaking has become a cornerstone in forming clinical decisions and guidelines, and in the process has given us a better understanding of the areas in need of further research.

Meta-analysis of Survival Data

SD meta-analysis is a particular type of meta-analysis which attempts to qualitatively assess cancer studies by analyzing the main outcome of interest: "time to an event". As explained previously, health care interventions in GO aim to prolong disease-free survival in cancer, thereby affecting the time until an event happens, a possible outcome that can be focused on in studies of GO treatments. However to derive SD, *time to the event* (rather than whether the event happens) becomes the choice outcome of investigation.

"Time" itself in SD meta-analysis means survival time; this can either be time "survived" from complete remission to relapse or progression or time from diagnosis to death. SD analysis offers the best statistical method to analyze "time-to-event" data found in GO research mainly because the "event of interest" does not occur in all individuals during a particular follow-up period. Therefore, SD cannot be analyzed in the same way as continuous data even though time is a continuous variable. This non-observation or non-experience of the "event of interest" by the relevant patients after a period of follow-up is referred to as "censoring", that is, patients' survival times are *censored* and it results in the true "time-to-event" being unknown (Tierney et al. 2007).

SD analysis allows a statistician and in turn a clinician to deal with this particular problem of censoring. It is assumed that the censoring is uninformative; therefore, those patients who are censored, that is, have been lost to follow up, have the same survival prospects as those who continue to be followed up. Two related functions, the survivor function and the hazard function, can be applied to address and model SD, as well as adequately deal with the issue of censoring. The survivor function represents the probability that an individual survives from the time of origin to some time beyond time "t". It directly describes the survival experience of a study cohort, and is usually estimated by the Kaplan–Meier method. More importantly fore the purposes of performing an SD meta-analysis, the hazard function gives the instantaneous potential of having an event at a time, given survival up to that time. It is used primarily as a diagnostic tool or for specifying a mathematical model for survival analysis. Time-to-event outcomes are most appropriately analyzed using hazard ratios (HRs), which take into account of the number and timing of events, and the time until last follow-up for each patient who has been censored. We shall deal with these aspects in greater detail in the next section (Tierney et al. 2007).

Odds ratios (ORs) or relative risks (RRs) are mathematical quantities applied in more generalized forms of meta-analysis. They measure the number of events and are appropriate for measuring dichotomous outcomes, but less suitable for analyzing time-to event outcomes. Dichotomous measures in a meta-analysis of time-to-event outcomes leads to additional problems. For example, the process can involve combining trials reported at different stages of maturity, with variable follow-up, resulting in an unreliable and difficult to interpret type of estimate. Also, if individual trials do not contribute data at each time point, the final estimate can be greatly misleading. Finally, if the time points are subjectively chosen by the systematic reviewer or selectively reported by the trialist, one can see how this could lead to the problem of bias (Tierney et al. 2007).

CONDUCTING A SURVIVAL DATA META-ANALYSIS (FIG. 4)

Importance of Careful Planning

A valid SD meta-analysis requires the same careful planning as any other research study, with particular attention necessary to develop details of design and implementation (Berman and Parker 2002).

Essentially, there are two goals to any type of meta-analysis. One is to summarize the available data and the other is to explain the variability between the studies. Ideally, all studies being meta-analyzed should have similar patient characteristics and similar outcomes of interest. In reality, a certain degree of variability is expected between studies and this is the impetus for performing a meta-analysis (Berman and Parker 2002). Variability is assessed by sub-group analysis, heterogeneity assessment, and sensitivity analysis all of which add "flavor" to the meta-analysis.

The steps involved in a detailed research protocol for an SD meta-analysis are no different to any other type of meta-analysis (Box 4).

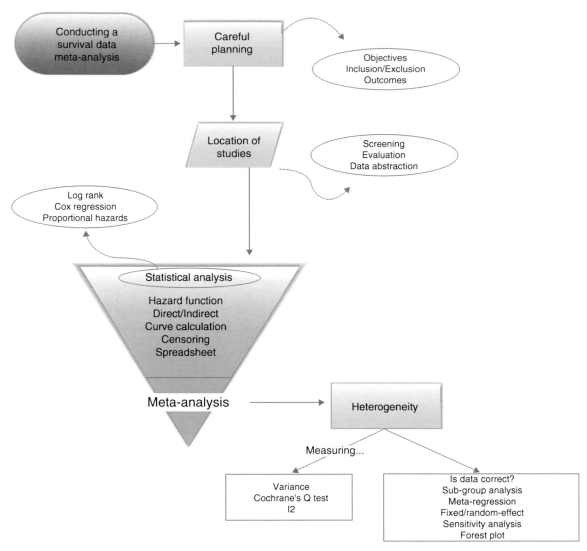

Figure 4 Conducting a survival data meta-analysis.

Defining the Objectives of the Study

The first step is to identify the problem. This includes specifying the oncological disease, condition, management and population of interest, the specific treatments or exposures studied, and the various clinical or biological outcomes investigated.

Defining the Population of Studies to be Included

In order to solve a distinct problem, a discrete and objective statement of inclusion and exclusion criteria for studies can be created. This is crucial in a meta-analysis, helping to eliminate selection bias. These criteria need to be specified in the SD meta-analysis protocol in advance. Any inclusion criteria must include the following:

Study type—It must be decided from the onset whether only RCTs will be included, although there is constant debate and research with regards to this (Stroup et al. 2000, Thompson and Pocock 1991). A hierarchy of evidence has been developed which allows for different types of studies to be included in the analysis. Naturally, the lower the level of evidence of a type of study, the lower the validity of the meta-analysis (Olkin 1995). For more advanced types of meta-analysis, different study designs can also be included. This is termed a "taleo-analysis" which although deemed a best of both worlds has its own limitations and is out of scope for this work.

Patient characteristics—These include age, gender, and ethnicity, presenting condition, co-morbidities, duration of cancer, and method of diagnosis.

Treatment modalities—For the condition in question, the allowable treatment type (surgery, chemotherapy, radiotherapy, novel modalities), dosage, duration, and conversion from one treatment to another should be addressed.

Defining the Outcome Measures

Most studies have multiple outcome measures. The protocol for the SD meta-analysis should specify the outcomes that will be studied (Berman and Parker 2002). There are two schools of thought. The researcher can either focus on one or two primary outcomes or make it a "fishing expedition" and assess as many outcomes as possible.

Locating all Relevant Studies

This is by far the most important, frustrating, and time-consuming part of the meta-analysis. A structured search strategy must be used. This usually involves starting with databases such as NIH Medline, PubMed, EMBASE, CINAHL, and even Google scholar. There are different search strategies for the various databases and effective use must be made of MeSH headings, synonyms, and the "related articles" function in PubMed. It is worth getting a tutorial with a librarian on how to obtain high yield searches that include most of the required (published) studies.

Screening, Evaluation, and Data Abstraction

A rapid review of manuscript abstracts will eliminate those that are fit for exclusion because of inadequate study design, specific population, and duration of treatment or study date. If the published material is just an abstract, there must be sufficient information to evaluate its quality. There must also be summary statistics to put into the meta-analysis, available either from the written material or in writing from the investigator. It is essential that when the available written information is insufficient for the meta-analysis strenuous efforts be made to contact the principal investigator to obtain the information required in order to reduce the effect of publication bias. This becomes even more important for material that has not been formally published and which can only be obtained from the principal investigator (Berman and Parker 2002).

The next step is to collect the full papers. The data will then have to be extracted and added to a pre-designed data extraction form. It is useful if two independent observers extract the data, to avoid errors. Extraction of all patient demographics and baseline characteristics from the included studies and clinical outcomes of interest follows. A table incorporating all the extracted data can then be created which shows all the variables and their values from all the studies included in the meta-analysis. Furthermore, it is essential to ascertain how well matched the studies for various variables are. This is done by scoring them accordingly and noting the overall quality of the studies. No consensus on this issue exists in meta-analysis literature. Quality scores can be used in several ways: as a cut-off, with the meta-analysis including only studies above a pre-determined minimum score; as a weighing value, with studies with higher quality scores being given more weight in the analysis; or as a descriptive characteristic of the study, used in explaining study variability and heterogeneity (Jadad et al. 1996, Moher et al. 1995). Blinding observers to the names of the authors and their institutions, the names of the journals, sources of funding, and acknowledgments can lead to more consistent scores (Jadad et al. 1996).

Statistical Methods for Calculating Overall Effect

SD can be analyzed in several ways, using *log-rank tests*, and *Proportional hazards/Cox regression*, with the obtained results then used for meta-analysis. Once analyzed, data should ideally be combined before commencing with meta-analytical work.

Four methods for combining SD exist: (a) iterative generalized least-squares, (b) meta-analysis of failure-time data with adjustment for covariates, (c) nonlinear regression, and (d) log RR. However, explanation of the above is beyond the scope of this chapter.

Hazard Function and Cumulative Hazard Function

SD meta-analysis can be performed using dichotomous outcomes. They can be created from the data (e.g., death at particular time intervals: three months, one year, three years, five years) and subsequently, analyzed as such. This avoids the problem of censoring and if all the data are collected, the actual analysis is not a burdensome task. However, this approach can only be used when all participants have been followed up to or beyond the time point used for the analysis.

For this reason, SD meta-analysis is most appropriately performed with HRs as the effect measure of choice. Conventionally labeled λ, the hazard function (from which one derives HR) is defined as the event rate at time t conditional on survival until time t or later (i.e., $T \geq t$). The hazard function is always positive, $\lambda(t) \geq 0$, and its integral over must be infinite, thus, allowing the hazard function to increase or decrease. HRs involve the number and timing of events, as well as SD that has been censored. The ratio can be estimated from specific methods that carefully manipulate published or other summary data (Tierney et al. 2007, Parmar et al. 1998, Williamson et al. 2002). This can be done from existing data, which if available to estimate an OR or RR, will also be sufficient to calculate an HR.

Performing a Meta-analysis Based on Hazard Ratios

In order to perform a meta-analysis based on HRs, one must first estimate an HR from each trial, followed by pooling the calculated HRs in an overall meta-analysis. This conveniently follows the approach of more common meta-analyses of other effect measures, such as the RR or OR.

One can use two different methods to arrive at the intended target:

1. A fixed-effect meta-analysis of HRs, can use the following equation derived from Peto's method (Tierney et al. 2007 , Yusuf et al. 1985):

   Pooled log HR

   $$= \frac{\Sigma \text{ log rank observed} - \text{expected events } (O-E)}{\Sigma \text{ log rank variance } (V)}$$

   where Σ denotes "sum of"; the *log rank observed minus expected events* $(O - E)$ and the *log rank variance (V)* are derived from the number of events and the individual times to event on the research arm of each trial.

2. Alternatively, one can use *variance of the log HR* (V^*) and the *log HR* to apply the "inverse variance approach" (Tierney et al. 2007, Parmar et al. 1998):

   $$\text{Pooled log HR} = \frac{\Sigma \text{ log HR}/V^*}{\Sigma 1/V^*}$$

Therefore, if the following measures are presented in a trial report: HR, V, log HR, V^*, O, and/or E, one can employ these statistics to perform a fixed-effect and random-effect meta-analysis. However, if not reported, it would be necessary to estimate the above statistics for each trial, in order to combine them in a meta-analysis.

Calculation of Summary Statistics from Trial Reports
First of all, V and V^* can be derived from each other (Tierney et al. 2007):

$$V^* = 1/V \quad \text{and} \quad V = 1/V^*$$

where V, log rank variance and V^*, variance of the log HR.

Tierney et al. have published a statistical instruction "manual" where the authors describe some of the methods which can be used to calculate an HR by extracting information on the effects of interventions presented in a number of different ways (Tierney et al. 2007). They specifically demonstrate how the summary statistical data presented in trial reports can be used to estimate the $O - E$, V, V^*, HR, and log HR when these values are not listed.

We now list these methods in a hierarchical order, pointing out which summary statistics, when reported, are enough to work out the others as well as the all-important HR, thus permitting a GO clinician to perform an SD meta-analysis. The direct methods are preferable because they make no assumptions.

"Direct" Calculation
1. Trial report presents **O & E** on research and control arm
2. Trial report presents **O & E** on research arm and **log rank V**

"Indirect" Calculation
3. Trial report presents **HR** and **confidence intervals (CIs)**
4. Trial report presents **HR** and **events in each arm** (and the randomization ratio is 1:1)
5. Trial report presents **HR** and **total events** (and the randomization ratio is 1:1)
6. Trial report presents HR, total events, and numbers randomized on each arm
7. Trial report presents *P*-value and **events in each arm** (and the randomization ratio is 1:1)
8. Trial report presents *P*-value and **total events** (and the randomization ratio is 1:1)
9. Trial report presents *P*-value, total events, and numbers randomized on each arm.

"Kaplan–Meier" Curve Calculation
10. Trial report presents Kaplan–Meier curve and information on follow-up
11. Trial report presents Kaplan–Meier curve and numbers at risk.

The issue of "censoring" forces an analysis to undergo a necessary adjustment. This will mean that a clinician performing an SD meta-analysis will have to choose between the two-curve methods, depending on which method is more reliable to address the adjustment issue. If both curve methods are

possible, the following factors can help decide which method to opt for: (a) report/estimation of minimum and maximum follow-up; (b) report of the number at risk at how many time intervals; and (c) event rate between those time points. Further research is required to assess how well all of the methods perform according to variations in trial size, lengths of follow-up, or event rates. Also, in order to optimize the use of available data, a combination of the two-curve methods would be welcome (Tierney et al. 2007).

The resulting summary statistics calculated from the above methods can then be used in the SD meta-analysis procedures found in statistical and meta-analysis software. It is important to state that a number of these methods will be required for most of the trials reported. Thus, more than one method can be adequately used for a particular trial. Importantly, they should be used in preference to using a pooled OR or RR or a series of ORs or RRs at fixed time points, which in turn, improves the interpretation of systematic reviews and "time-to-event outcome" that is, SD meta-analyses.

The formulae employed to perform the above calculations as well as the pros and cons of such methods are explained in further detail in the actual report (Tierney et al. 2007). Appendix A describes a Microsoft Excel spreadsheet developed by *Tierney et al.* which calculates the summary statistics and therefore allows a clinician to avoid the laborious task of performing all the calculations by hand for each and every trial (a potentially error-prone and time-wasting process).

Heterogeneity Between Study Results
Variance between the overall effect sizes in each study might not be due to random sampling variation but instead could be due to the presence of other factors inherent within individual studies. This effect size variation due to slightly different study designs is termed heterogeneity and is defined as the presence of variability among studies included in a meta-analysis. Three different types of heterogeneity exist in literature: (a) clinical heterogeneity (variability in the participants, interventions, and outcomes studied); (b) methodological heterogeneity (variability in study design and risk of bias), and (c) statistical heterogeneity (variability in the intervention effects being evaluated in the different studies), usually a consequence of clinical or methodological diversity, or both, among the studies (The Cochrane Collaboration 2002).

Clinical variation will lead to heterogeneity if the intervention effect is affected by the factors that vary across studies; most obviously, the specific interventions or patient characteristics. In other words, the true intervention effect will be different in different studies. Statistical heterogeneity manifests itself in the observed intervention effects being more different from each other than one would expect due to random error (chance) alone (The Cochrane Collaboration 2002).

Measuring Heterogeneity
There are three ways to measure heterogeneity. First, one can assess the between-studies variance, ^{2}. However, this depends mainly on the particular effect size metric used. The second is Cochrane's Q-test, which follows a chi-square distribution to make inferences about the null hypothesis of homogeneity. The problem with Cochrane's Q-test is that it has poor power

to detect true heterogeneity when the number of studies is small. Because neither of the above-mentioned methods has a standardized scale, they are poorly equipped to make comparisons of the degree of homogeneity across meta-analyses (Huedo-Medina et al. 2006). A third more useful statistic for quantifying inconsistency is I^2 $[= [(Q - df)/Q] \times 100\%]$, where Q is the chi-squared statistic and "df" is its degrees of freedom (Higgins et al. 2003). This statistic is easier to utilize because it defines variability along a scale-free range as a percentage from 0% to 100%. This describes the percentage of the variability in effect estimates that is due to heterogeneity rather than sampling error (chance). Heterogeneity could be considered substantial when this value is >50%. The importance of the observed value of I^2 depends on (i) magnitude and direction of effects and (ii) strength of evidence for heterogeneity (e.g., P value from the chi-squared test, or a CI for I^2). The theory behind the use of I^2 statistic lies in its value of recognizing that statistical heterogeneity is inevitable and therefore moving the focus away from testing whether heterogeneity is present to assessing its impact on the meta-analysis.

Addressing Heterogeneity

A GO clinician performing a SD meta-analysis needs to have several strategies that he/she can use in order to deal with (statistical) heterogeneity identified among a group of studies included in that particular meta-analysis (The Cochrane Collaboration 2002). The description of these strategies, their application and step-by-step guide as to their use in the context of a meta-analysis are beyond the scope of this textbook, but are still listed here in order to act as a guide for the GO surgeon wishing to investigate further.

1. Check that the data inserted is correct
2. Do not perform the meta-analysis
3. Explore heterogeneity (sub-group analysis and metaregression)
4. Fixed-effect/random-effect meta-analysis
5. Sensitivity analysis
6. Graphical display: Forest Plot

Conducting a Meta-analysis in the Surgical Context

The main differences between meta-analysis in surgical fields such as GO and in other fields originate from the reproducibility of treatments and variations in practice that are difficult to compare. The outcomes of a surgical procedure depend on the level of experience of an operating surgeon. This is not the case in other areas of research such as drug trials where the intervention is consistent and the drug acts in a uniform manner. Moreover, standardization and reproducibility in surgical techniques employed by the surgeons is not always consistent. Also, poor outcomes are less likely to be reported which further adds to publication bias (Egger et al. 2001). The experience of a surgeon is one of the key confounders during comparative trials involving interventions. Less experienced surgeons have been reported to have relatively poorer outcomes (Krahn et al. 2006). These issues have the propensity to add to study heterogeneity thus compromising the validity of a meta-analysis of clinical trials in surgery.

Similarly, early meta-analytical assessment of a new procedure or technique may give a misleading picture of its efficacy because issues such as lack of competence of surgeons. Competence is achieved after performing a set of repeated tasks. Factors determining competence include experience, equipment and time. Procedural performance continues to improve until a plateau phase is reached. This constitutes a traditional "learning curve".

The year of publication of a study is a significant determinant of heterogeneity as population characteristics and outcome data may change over time. Also the development in technology and technical expertise may translate into unfavorable outcomes over a defined period. All these factors need to be considered especially in surgical disciplines where new technologies and techniques are continuously developed and the learning-curve is overcome progressively. Increasing accumulation of evidence with time improves the integrity of results reported by a meta-analysis (Lau et al. 1998).

PITFALLS IN CONDUCTING AN SD META-ANALYSIS

Although the aim of a meta-analysis is to reduce uncertainty, there are instances in which the opposite can be true. In the hierarchy of evidence, the systematic review is placed rightly at the top. However, similar systematic reviews with opposite conclusions or those which contradict well-powered high-quality double-blind RCTs are still possible (Petticrew 2003).

Conflicting Results Between Meta-analysis Compared to Large Scale RCTs

Two important questions need to be answered. The first is whether meta-analyses of small trials agree with the results of large trials. No absolute definition exists of what constitutes a large trial, so separating small trials from large trials is not easy. Moreover, when considering the bigger picture, all trials add to the current base of evidence. The extent to which small trials agree or disagree with larger ones is a multifactorial process. Selection bias tends to skew the results. Large trials appearing in high impact journals may have been selected as they provide new insight into the merits and demerits of a particular treatment. Furthermore, there may be less consistency for secondary end points than for primary end points in different trials.

The second important question is whether meta-analyses can in fact validly substitute large trials. It is known that meta-analyses and large trials tend to disagree 10% to 23% of the time, beyond chance. Clinical trials are likely to be heterogeneous, since they address different populations with different protocols. Patients, disease, and treatments are likely to change over time. Future meta-analyses may find an important role in addressing potential sources of heterogeneity rather than always trying to fit a common estimate among diverse studies. With this, meta-analyses and RCTs must be scrutinized in detail for the presence of bias and diversity.

Why Does Bias Exist in Meta-analysis?

Most of the factors responsible for bias are because of assumptions used when combining RCTs. The assumptions are that: (a) results of trials are true approximations to the actual true value of the outcome of study, and are different between trials due to the presence of random chance and not

Box 5

- Publication bias and other forms of reporting bias
- Variable quality of included RCT studies
- Bias and skew due to the presence of small study effects
- Selection bias/personal bias in the selection of studies
- Heterogeneity between individual studies

due to bias; (b) trials selected for combination are representative of all trials possible whether published or unpublished; and (c) studies being combined are sufficiently homogenous in population and methodology such that they are combinable in the first place.

Types of Pitfalls in Conducting an SD Meta-analysis

The statistical methods employed to analyze time-to-event outcomes for individual trials explained in the previous section do not remove the list of problems faced by systematic reviews and SD meta-analyses (Box 5).

IMPACT OF BIAS ON SD META-ANALYSES
Bias

Bias primarily affects internal validity and is defined as *any process at any stage of inference tending to produce results that differ systematically from [their] true values* (Campbell 1957). It refers to "systematic error", the effect of misleading conclusions from multiple replications of the same study. Sampling variation, however, leads to different effect estimates following above replications despite "correct answers" on average. This is known as "random error" and is because of imprecision, a term not to be confused with bias/risk of bias.

Therefore, bias can cause a systematic overestimation or underestimation in outcome which leads to a GIGO effect on meta-analytic results. Hence, in the conduct of a meta-analysis, a key assumption will be that any variability between individual RCTs is due to random variation and not from the presence of bias.

The presence of bias and the extent to which it affects a particular study is usually related to flaws in methodological analysis, conduct, and design of clinical trials. It is more appropriate however to focus on "risk of bias", a more suitable phrase, because results of a study can occasionally be unbiased despite methodological flaws. In addition, variation in the results of included studies can be explained more accurately by differences in risk of bias. These differences will highlight the more rigorous studies with more valid conclusions and will indirectly help us to avoid false-positive/negative conclusions.

Bias is especially of concern within small powered unpublished studies as the methodological quality in smaller trials might not be as vigorous as compared to larger ones where more time, effort, and money might have be involved in the trial design. Moreover, as small studies might not be published, their underlying methodology might not be assessed with as much close scrutiny as during the editorial peer review process in journal publications.

Bias related to methodology design can be of five different kinds: selection, performance, detection, and attrition bias (Fig. 5).

Selection bias: Occurs when candidates in a study are preferentially selected into one group compared to another based on prior knowledge of their pre-existing medical condition.

Performance bias: Occurs if additional treatment interventions are provided preferentially in one treatment group compared to another.

Detection/assessment bias: Arises if the knowledge of patient assignment influences the assessment of outcome. Yet again, blinding of the assessor/observer is the solution.

Attrition bias: Arises where deviations from protocol and loss to follow up lead to the exclusion of patients after they have been allocated to their treatment groups, causing a skew in aggregate treatment effect.

Reporting bias: Occurs when systematic differences between reported and unreported variables are found. Several forms of reporting bias exist and will be dealt with in more detail in subsequent chapters: Publication bias, Time lag bias, English language bias, Citation bias, Duplication bias, and Outcome reporting bias.

Assessing Potential Bias Inherent in RCTs

The use of high-quality trials in a meta-analysis, ideally prospective randomized double blind controlled trials with an intention to treat policy during results reporting, would eliminate many forms of bias.

The solution to selection bias is randomization which will create groups that are equally comparable for any known or unknown potential confounding factors. Adequate *randomization* in the use of pre-generated allocation sequences and concealment of allocation would ensure a standardized group of patients in both treatment and control. Ideally, randomization should be instituted where neither the investigator nor the patient knows the allocation so that they are unable to guide which type of treatment should be used.

Randomization, coupled with *double blinding*, where both patients and investigators are prevented from knowing which group each patient is allocated to, would prevent detection and performance bias. The use of objective compared to subjective measurable outcomes would also further make a trial less prone to assessment bias (Campbell 1957).

To reduce attrition bias, an intention to treat or "per protocol" policy could be used. An intention to treat policy dictates that all randomized patients should be included in the analysis and kept in their original groups, regardless of their adherence or non-compliance to the study protocol or loss to follow up. Conversely, a "per protocol" policy is where only patients who fulfill all protocol directives are included in the analysis.

As a "per protocol", analysis tends to ignore patients who have ceased treatment due to possible adverse outcomes, an intention to treat policy is generally recommended. However, an intention to treat protocol also depends on the use of assumptions to determine the eventual outcome of patients' loss to follow up. It has been recommended that the conduct of both forms of analysis and any underlying comparative differences between them would give the best level of available knowledge (Campbell 1957).

Cochrane Handbook for Systematic Reviews of interventions also describes various methods for assessing bias. It describes a tool titled a "domain-based evaluation", in which critical assessments are made separately for different domains

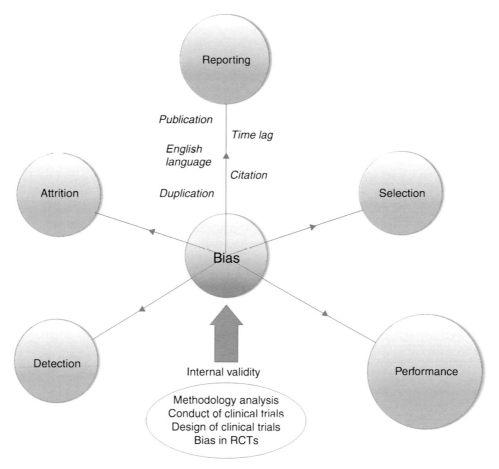

Figure 5 Types of bias encountered in survival data meta-analysis.

(Fig. 6). Each type of domain, described below, assesses a specific type of bias (Higgins 2008).

Sequence generation: A well-designed RCT incorporates and specifies a statistically sound rule for allocating a specific intervention to each patient. This rule has to be based on a chance (random) process (e.g., computer random number generator, coin tossing, shuffling envelopes) and must generate an allocation sequence, thereby allowing an assessment of whether it produces comparable groups. Both this and the next domain could only score positively when assessing RCTs.

Allocation concealment: Method employed to conceal the above allocation sequence in sufficient detail to determine whether allocations could have been predicted in advance, or during, enrolment. For example, using telephone or web-based randomization or sequentially numbered, sealed envelopes.

Blinding of participants, personnel, and outcome assessors: Measures used to remove prior knowledge of which type of intervention a patient received from the patient undergoing the surgery and from the surgeon performing the operation.

Incomplete outcome data: Lack of completeness of outcome data during the follow-up period.

Selective outcome reporting: Study protocol, including the main aims and outcomes of interest, is either incomplete or written with insufficient clarity. Not all of the pre-specified outcomes are reported in the pre-specified way.

Other potential threats to validity that can be considered: Of interest is a detailed description of the surgical methods employed, including whether patients were operated on by one or more surgeons and in one or more hospitals, and the diagnostic methods applied to calculate the necessary outcomes (i.e., techniques and personnel).

Publication Bias

So far, only bias related to actual gathering of data have been considered, that is, methods involved in setting up the trial. Reporting bias is, on the other hand, related to the results' publication process. "Publication bias" is the main subgroup, occurring when the publication of research is reliant upon the nature and direction of results. If the research that appears in the published literature is systematically unrepresentative of the population of completed studies, publication bias occurs. This leads to the preferential publication of certain types of trials compared to others resulting in a fraction of studies being published in an indexed journal, leaving a larger body of research in the form of incomplete draft manuscripts, presentations, and abstracts unpublished. With this, a vast amount of research data could be omitted from indexed bibliographic databases, and thus, becoming difficult to locate. These data eventually are concealed away from systematic reviewers such that not all possible clinical trials could have been included within a meta-analysis of a topic. The end result is a meta-analysis which might not be truly representative

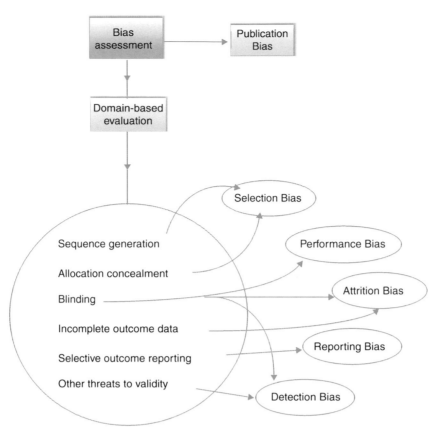

Figure 6 Domain-based evaluations to assess potential bias.

of all valid studies undertaken ending in the development of spuriously precise but inaccurate summary findings (Sterne et al. 2001). Rather frustratingly, wrong conclusions can then be drawn by readers and reviewers with dangerous consequences (e.g., use of falsely deemed safe and effective treatment).

Why Does Publication Bias Exist?

Even though there is no consistent relationship between the publication of a study with study design, methodological quality, study size, or number of study centers, the publication of a trial is more likely when it shows either a statistically significant large effect in the outcome for a new treatment (a positive trial) or when compared to existing treatments (a non-inferiority trial). The publication of a trial is less likely when there are non-significant findings, results with small effect sizes or negative findings (a negative trial) (Sterne et al. 2001).

Reasons for Publication Bias in Negative Trials

Non-significant findings or negative findings are less likely to be published due to (Box 6).

Box 6
• Editorial censorship of uninteresting findings
• Subjective peer review
• Conflicts of interests
• Self censorship dealing with publication bias

BENEFITS OF SD META-ANALYSES (FIG. 7)

A well-conducted systematic review is an invaluable tool for practitioners. A GO specialist can occasionally feel overwhelmed when trying to decide on the best management protocol for a particular cancer, especially if trying to compare between research in the United States and United Kingdom/Europe. The sheer volume of GO literature leads the surgeon to often prefer summaries of information to publications of original investigations. The former type of evidence keeps him/her abreast of the goings-on on a particular GO topic. If deemed to be of high quality, a particular SD meta-analysis can define the boundaries of what is known.

We should also acknowledge that meta-analysis (with all its sub-types) is one of the main pillars of "Evidence-based Health Care" and can be used to make clinical, professional, and policy decisions. First, it can be extremely useful in health technology assessments and cost-effectiveness analysis. Second, meta-analyses identify gaps in GO research and identify beneficial or harmful cancer protocols. Researchers need such meta-analyses to summarize existing data, refine hypotheses, estimate sample sizes, and help define future research agendas. Without these, promising leads may be missed or studies of questions that have been already answered may be embarked on. Industry is particularly interested in meta-analyses as it helps to direct resources to viable and beneficial health interventions.

Administrators and purchasers need integrative publications to help generate clinical policies that optimize clinical outcomes using available resources. For consumers and health policymakers who are interested in the bottom line of evidence,

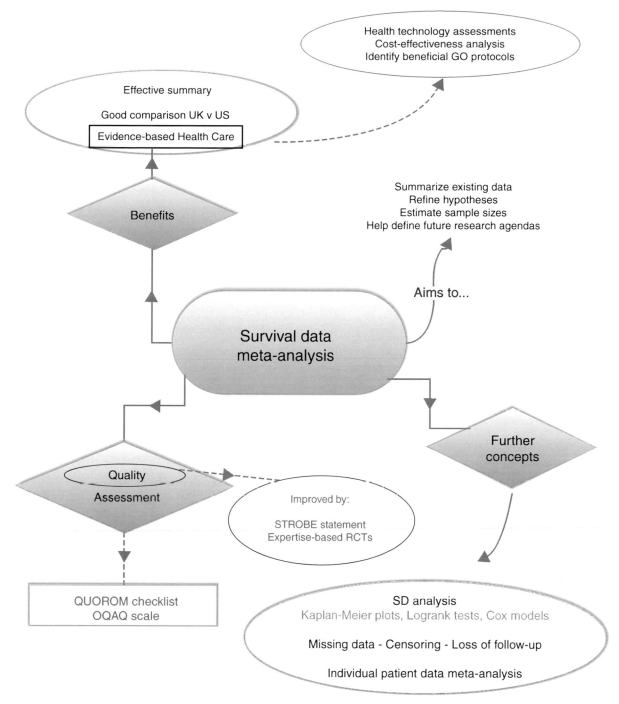

Figure 7 Improvements, benefits, and further concepts of survival data meta-analysis.

systematic reviews and meta-analyses can help harmonize conflicting results of research. They can be used as the basis for other integrative articles produced by policymakers, such as risk assessments, practice guidelines, economic analyses, and decision analyses.

ASSESSING THE QUALITY OF A META-ANALYSIS (FIG. 7)

Two instruments are commonly used to assess the quality of meta-analysis: Quality of Reporting of Meta-analyses (QUOROM) checklist and Overview Quality Assessment Questionnaire (OQAQ) scale (Shea et al. 2001).

The QUOROM statement assesses the quality of reporting. It comprises of a checklist and flow diagram and was developed using a consensus process designed to strengthen the reliability of the estimates it yields when applied by different assessors. It estimates the overall reporting quality of systematic reviews. The checklist asks whether authors have provided readers with information on 18 items, including searches, selection, validity assessment, data abstraction, study characteristics, quantitative data syntheses, and trial flow. It also asks whether authors have included a flow diagram with information about the number of RCTs identified, included and excluded, and the reasons for any exclusions. Individual checklist items included in this instrument are also answered in the following manner: "yes", "no", or "partial/cannot tell" (Moher et al. 1999).

The OQAQ scale has strong face validity, provides data on several essential elements of its development, and has an available published assessment of its construct validity. The OQAQ scale measures across a continuum using nine questions (items 1–9) designed to assess various aspects of the methodological quality of systematic reviews and one overall assessment question (item 10). When the scale is applied to a systematic review, the first nine items are scored by selecting either "yes", "no", or "partial/cannot tell". The tenth item requires assessors to assign an overall quality score on a seven-point scale (Oxman 1994).

IMPROVING THE QUALITY OF GYNECOLOGICAL ONCOLOGY META-ANALYSES (FIG. 7)

The inclusion of RCTs in the process of meta-analysis can be invaluable in improving its quality. The advantages are self-evident; when conducted properly, they offer one of the more objective methods in determining the true relationship between GO treatment and outcome and are free from bias compared to other study designs.

Other benefits are more specific to the surgical practice of GO. "Expertise-based RCT" is a recent technique which offers a solution to overcoming existing biases in surgical trails and can be applied in GO. In this type of trial, a surgeon with expertise in one of the GO procedures being evaluated is paired with a surgeon with expertise in the other procedure who should ideally be from the same institution. Subjects are randomized to treatments and treated by a surgeon who is an "expert" in the procedure. This study overcomes some of the challenges associated with traditional surgical RCTs including the caveat that surgeons who wish to participate in traditional RCTs must be willing to perform both techniques and that a lack of expertise or belief in one of the interventions under evaluation may undermine the validity and applicability of the results (Devereaux et al. 2005). A recent survey of orthopedic surgeons found that most would consider this type of study design as it may decrease the likelihood of procedural cross-overs and enhance validity because unlike the conventional RCT, there is a low likelihood of differential expertise bias (Bednarska 2008).

"Observational studies" make up a significant proportion of the existing GO surgical literature and more specifically meta-analyses. It must be remembered that much of the research into the cause of diseases relies on cohort, case–control, or cross-sectional studies. Also, observational studies can generate significant hypotheses and have a role into delineating the harms and benefits of interventions. To ensure the robustness of reporting observational studies, the STROBE statement was created. It aims to assist authors when writing up analytical observational studies, to support editors and reviewers when considering such articles for publication, and to help readers when critically appraising published articles (von Elm et al. 2007). All these steps will add to the quality of data that is used in future (GO) surgical meta-analyses.

FURTHER CONCEPTS IN SURVIVAL ANALYSIS (FIG. 7)

As already described, most analyses of SD use primarily Kaplan–Meier plots, log rank tests, and Cox models. Prior to proceeding with a meta-analysis of SD manuscripts, it is worth considering limitations that might hinder an accurate portrayal of the final conclusions of each manuscript.

One of the most common problems encountered when developing survival cancer models is missing data. Trial data are reported in such a way that individuals without complete covariate data are usually omitted. This results in a final analysis with reduced power and more importantly, with an unrepresentative subset of patients. Therefore, if substantial missing data are found, methods that could accommodate such a finding should be considered. The most straightforward improvement is a simple recommendation that authors of research papers try to be explicit about the amount of missing data for each variable and indicate how many patients did not have complete data (Clark et al. 2003). More robust is a recent powerful tool which has become increasingly available (Van Buuren et al. 1999). Multiple imputation is a framework method in which missing data are imputed or replaced with a set of plausible values. Several data sets are then constructed, each being analyzed separately, and their results are combined while allowing for the uncertainty introduced in the imputation (Clark et al. 2003).

However, this method must not be looked at as a panacea. The assumption that a model-relating data absence to other measured covariates, as well as survival, exists and can be specified is inherent in the imputation method. Researchers should be aware that such assumptions are not able to be tested, and can apply sensitivity analysis instead to assess the robustness of results (Clark et al. 2003).

Another significant problem that can arise is the extent to which unmeasured factors may affect survival time because of the impossibility of knowing whether all important prognostic factors have been measured (Clark et al. 2003). Such an omission leads to the introduction of bias into the model, reduction of the predictive ability of a model, and exhibition of a large variability in the patients' survival. For example, omissions can occur when some individuals have a shared exposure, such as an environmental factor, which cannot be measured yet ensures that their outcomes cannot be considered independent. Such situations are encountered in multi-center and cluster randomized trials (Yamaguchi et al. 2002) and the variation between and within groups labels them "multi-level". Random-effect models which are widely used in meta-analysis can be applied to allow covariate effects to vary across groups (O'Quigley and Stare 2002). We also note that if a trial does not adjust for an important and omitted prognostic variable, the estimated treatment effect in a randomized trial may be biased even when that variable is balanced between the treatment groups (Clark et al. 2003, Schmoor 1997, Chastang et al. 1988).

Finally, in the authors' opinion, the exploration of cancer relapses may be more informative than focusing only on the time until the first; therefore, analysis of recurrent events can make an important contribution to the understanding of the survival process.

Authors sometimes attempt to explain the above limitations with the following reasons: (a) "keep things simple for the readership" and (b) "lack of computer software with which to perform the statistical tests". However, both types of reasoning are false. The most important factor when conducting a statistical analysis is to ensure that the analysis applied is appropriate for the particular question in mind and that it adequately represents the survival experience of patients in the study. More advanced survival methods may admittedly convey a less straightforward message, but could allow a better understanding of the survival process. Also, recent software packages which are used more by statisticians but less by medical staff are so designed to incorporate complex statistical models personnel.

We would like to point out that prior to conducting a meta-analysis, one must first understand and be able to interpret many and varied methods required to analyze SD. The assumptions made prior to applying the appropriate statistical methods should be clear to the relevant personnel and one must not hesitate to request help from a statistician if more complex methods are required.

META-ANALYSIS AND SOFTWARE (FIG. 7)
The process involved in conducting a meta-analysis, including the benefits and drawbacks (mainly bias and internal and external validity) of the method, has extensively been described in the literature (Athanasiou). Currently, the optimum methodology involves the use of specialized software packages, which have doubled over the last decade. The choice of package is dependent on use requirements. Pre-existing commercial general statistical program suites like SAS, STATA, and SPSS have been enhanced by the provision of add-on third party macro-programs which provide a limited set of basic functions for meta-analysis. Standalone packages are purpose built for meta-analysis and tend to have a greater variety of functions available and have greater methods of input, processing, and output modes. Some software is free such as "RevMan" provided by the Cochrane Centre. Others are commercial.

CONCLUSION
Like primary research, meta-analysis of SD involves a stepwise approach to arrive at statistically justifiable conclusions. It has the potential to provide an accurate, quantitative appraisal of the literature. It may objectively resolve controversies. The greatest challenge in conducting a meta-analysis on a clinical topic is often the lack of available data on the subject, because there are few high-quality, published studies with an acceptable degree of heterogeneity.

With regards to a meta-analysis of SD, the extraction of accurate data in order to derive a log HZR is difficult. This can be explained by the process: (a) estimations via mathematical conversions from the provided summary data of which there might not be enough of sufficient quality in trial reports to derive out HZR; and (b) direct measurements from a Kaplan–Meier survival curve, which can possibly introduce random measurement error and hence reduces the accuracy of results.

If meta-analyses are to continue to have a role in surgical decision making, a key area in GO, clinicians need to be able to perform, assess, compare, and communicate the quality of meta-analyses, particularly in areas where several meta-analyses are available.

APPENDIX A
Instructions on how to apply the calculations spreadsheet in order to facilitate the computational aspects for calculating an HR and/or associated statistics.

Extracted from *Tierney et al.* (2007).

… The user enters all the reported summary statistics and the spreadsheet estimates the HR, 95%CI, lnHR, V, and O-E by all possible methods. The user can also input data extracted from Kaplan–Meier curves and estimate censoring using the minimum and maximum follow-up or the reported numbers at risk, to obtain similar summary statistics. Graphical representations of the input data are produced for comparison with the published curves, to assist with data extraction or to highlight data entry errors. Results from all methods are provided in a single output screen, which facilitates comparison.

REFERENCES
Angelillo IF, Villari P (2003) Meta-analysis of published studies or meta-analysis of individual data? Caesarean section in HIV-positive women as a study case. *Public Health* **117**:323–8.
Saso S, Panesar SS, Siow W, Athanasiou T (2011) Systematic review and meta-analyses in surgery. In: Darzi A, Athanasiou T, eds. *Evidence Synthesis in Healthcare: A practical Handbook for Clinicians.* Springer-Verlag, Berlin Heidelberg.
Bailey KR (1987) Inter-study differences: how should they influence the interpretation and analysis of results? *Stat Med* **6**:351–60.
Bednarska E, Bryant D, Devereaux PJ, et al. (2008) Orthopaedic surgeons prefer to participate in expertise-based randomized trials. *Clin Orthop Relat Res* **466**:1734–44.
Berlin JA, Santanna J, Schmid CH, et al. (2002) Anti-Lymphocyte Antibody Induction Therapy Study Group. Individual patient- versus group-level data meta-regressions for the investigation of treatment effect modifiers: ecological bias rears its ugly head. *Stat Med* **21**:371–87
Berman NG, Parker RA (2002) Meta-analysis: neither quick nor easy. *BMC Med Res Methodol* **9**:10.
Burdett S, Stewart LA (2002) A comparison of the results of checked versus unchecked individual patient data meta-analyses. *Int J Technol Assess Health Care* **18**:619–24.
Campbell DT (1957) Factors relevant to the validity of experiments in social settings. *Psychol Bull* **54**:297–312.
Chalmers I (1993) The Cochrane collaboration: preparing, maintaining, and disseminating systematic reviews of the effects of health care. *Ann NY Acad Sci* **703**:156–63; discussion 163–5.
Chastang C, Byar D, Piantadosi S (1988) A quantitative study of the bias in estimating the treatment effect caused by omitting a balanced covariate in survival models. *Stat Med* **7**:1243–55.
Clark TG, Bradburn MJ, Love SB, et al. (2003) Survival analysis part IV: further concepts and methods in survival analysis. *Br J Cancer* **89**:781–6.
Davidoff F, Haynes B, Sackett D, et al. (1995) Evidence based medicine: a new journal to help doctors identify the information they need. *BMJ* **310**:1085–6.
Devereaux PJ, Bhandari M, Clarke M, et al. (2005) Need for expertise based randomised controlled trials. *BMJ* **330**:88.
Duchateau L, Pignon JP, Bijnens L, et al. (2001) Individual patient-versus literature-based meta-analysis of survival data: time to event and event rate at a particular time can make a difference, an example based on head and neck cancer. *Control Clin Trials* **22**:538–47.
Easterbrook PJ, Berlin JA, Gopalan R, et al. (1991) Publication bias in clinical research. *Lancet* **337**:867–72.
Egger M, Smith GD, Phillips AN (1997) Meta-analysis: principles and procedures. *BMJ* **315**:1533–7.
Egger M, Smith GD, Schneider M (2001) Systematic reviews of observational studies. In: Egger M, Smith GD, Altman D, eds. *Systematic Reviews in Healthcare.* British Medical Association.
Glass GV (1976) Primary, secondary and meta-analysis of research. *Educ Res* **5**:3–8.
Higgins J, Green S (2008) Cochrane handbook for systematic reviews of interventions version 5.0.0 edn. Oxford: The Cochrane Collaboration.
Higgins JP, Thompson SG, Deeks JJ, et al. (2003) Measuring inconsistency in meta-analyses. *BMJ* **327**:557–60.
Huedo-Medina TB, Sanchez-Meca J, Marin-Martinez F, et al. (2006) Assessing heterogeneity in meta-analysis: Q statistic or I2 index? *Psychol Methods* **11**:193–206.

Ioannidis JP, Contopoulos-Ioannidis DG, Lau J (1999) Recursive cumulative meta-analysis: a diagnostic for the evolution of total randomized evidence from group and individual patient data. *J Clin Epidemiol* **52**:281–91.

Jadad AR, Moore RA, Carroll D, et al. (1996) Assessing the quality of reports of randomized clinical trials: is blinding necessary? *Control Clin Trials* **17**:1–12.

Jeng GT, Scott JR, Burmeister LF (1995) A comparison of meta-analytic results using literature vs individual patient data. Paternal cell immunization for recurrent miscarriage. *JAMA* **274**:830–6.

Koopman L, van der Heijden GJ, Hoes AW, et al. (2008) Empirical comparison of subgroup effects in conventional and individual patient data meta-analyses. *Int J Technol Assess Health Care* **24**:358–61.

Krahn J, Sauerland S, Rixen D, et al. (2006) Applying evidence-based surgery in daily clinical routine: a feasibility study. *Arch Orthop Trauma Surg* **126**:88–92.

Lambert PC, Sutton AJ, Abrams KR, et al. (2002) A comparison of summary patient-level covariates in meta-regression with individual patient data meta-analysis. *J Clin Epidemiol* **55**:86–94.

Lau J, Ioannidis JP, Schmid CH (1998) Summing up evidence: one answer is not always enough. *Lancet* **351**:123–7.

Lyman GH, Kuderer NM (2005) The strengths and limitations of meta-analyses based on aggregate data. *BMC Med Res Methodol* **25**:5–14.

Moher D, Cook DJ, Eastwood S, et al. (1999) Improving the quality of reports of meta-analyses of randomised controlled trials: the QUOROM statement. Quality of Reporting of Meta-analyses. *Lancet* **354**:1896–900.

Moher D, Jadad AR, Nichol G, et al. (1995) Assessing the quality of randomized controlled trials: an annotated bibliography of scales and checklists. *Control Clin Trials* **16**:62–73.

Ng TT, McGory ML, Ko CY, et al. (2006) Meta-analysis in surgery: methods and limitations. *Arch Surg* **141**:1125–30.

O'Quigley J, Stare J (2002) Proportional hazards models with frailties and random effects. *Stat Med* **21**:3219–33.

Olkin I, Sampson A (1998) Comparison of meta-analysis versus analysis of variance of individual patient data. *Biometrics* **54**:317–22.

Olkin I (1995) Meta-analysis: reconciling the results of independent studies. *Stat Med* **14**:457–72.

Oxman AD (1994) Checklists for review articles. *BMJ* **309**:648–51.

Panesar SS, Thakrar R, Athanasiou T, et al. (2006) Comparison of reports of RCTs and systematic reviews in surgical journals: literature review. *J R Soc Med* **99**:470–2.

Parmar MKB, Torri V, Stewart L (1998) Extracting summary statistics to perform meta-analyses of the published literature for survival endpoints. *Stat Med* **17**:2815–34.

Petticrew M (2003) Why certain systematic reviews reach uncertain conclusions. *BMJ* **326**:756–8.

Reade MC, Delaney A, Bailey MJ, et al. (2010) Prospective meta-analysis using individual patient data in intensive care medicine. *Intensive Care Med* **36**:11–21.

Royal College of Surgeons of England. Implementing the EWTD: College Response. Available online at http://www.rcseng.ac.uk/publications/docs/ewtd_communicaion.html/attachment_download/pdffile. Last accessed on 1 April 2009.

Sauerland S, Seiler CM (2005) Role of systematic reviews and meta-analysis in evidence-based medicine. *World J Surg* **29**:582–7.

Schmid CH, Stark PC, Berlin JA, et al. (2004) Meta-regression detected associations between heterogeneous treatment effects and study-level, but not patient-level, factors. *J Clin Epidemiol* **57**:683–97.

Schmoor C, Schumacher M (1997) Effects of covariate omission and categorization when analysing randomized trials with the Cox model. *Stat Med* **16**:225–37.

Shea B, Dube C, Moher D (2001) Assessing the quality of reports of systematic reviews: QUOROM statement compared to other tools. In: Egger M, Smith G, Altman D, eds. *Systematic Reviews in Health Care: Meta-analysis in Context.* London: BMJ Publishing, pp. 122–9.

Smith CT, Williamson PR, Marson AG (2005) An overview of methods and empirical comparison of aggregate data and individual patient data results for investigating heterogeneity in meta-analysis of time-to-event outcomes. *J Eval Clin Pract* **11**:468–78.

Sterne JA, Egger M, Smith GD (2001) Systematic reviews in health care: investigating and dealing with publication and other biases in meta-analysis. *BMJ* **323**:101–5.

Stewart LA, Parmar MK (1993) Meta-analysis of the literature or of individual patient data: is there a difference? *Lancet* **341**:418–22.

Stewart LA, Tierney JF (2002) To IPD or not to IPD? Advantages and disadvantages of systematic reviews using individual patient data. *Eval Health Prof* **25**:76–97.

Stroup DF, Berlin JA, Morton SC, et al. (2000) Meta-analysis of observational studies in epidemiology: a proposal for reporting. Meta-analysis of Observational Studies in Epidemiology (MOOSE) group. *JAMA* **283**:2008–12.

Sylvester R, Collette L, Duchateau L (2000) The role of meta-analyses in assessing cancer treatments. *Eur J Cancer* **36**:1351–8.

The Cochrane Collaboration (2002) *Diversity and Heterogeneity:Identifying Statistical Heterogeneity.* The Cochrane Collaboration open learning material 2002 [cited; Available from: http://www.cochrane-net.org/openlearning/HTML/mod13-3.htm.]

Thompson SG, Pocock SJ (1991) Can meta-analyses be trusted? *Lancet* **338**:1127–30.

Thompson SG, Higgins JP (2005) Treating individuals 4: can meta-analysis help target interventions at individuals most likely to benefit? *Lancet* **365**:341–6.

Tierney JF, Stewart LA, Ghersi D, et al. (2007) Practical methods for incorporating summary time-to-event data for meta-analysis. *Trials* **8**:16.

Van Buuren S, Boshuizen HC, Knook DL (1999) Multiple imputation of missing blood pressure covariates in survival analysis. *Stat Med* **18**:681–94.

von Elm E, Altman DG, Egger M, et al. (2007) The Strengthening the Reporting of Observational Studies in Epidemiology (STROBE) statement: guidelines for reporting observational studies. *Lancet* **370**:1453–7.

Williams CJ (1998) The pitfalls of narrative reviews in clinical medicine. *Ann Oncol* **9**:601–5.

Williamson PR, Tudur Smith C, Hutton JL, Marson AG (2002) Aggregate data meta-analysis with time-to-event outcomes. *Stat Med* **21**:3337–51.

Yamaguchi T, Ohashi Y, Matsuyama Y (2002) Proportional hazards models with random effects to examine centre effects in multicentre cancer clinical trials. *Stat Methods Med Res* **11**:221–36.

Yusuf S, Peto R, Lewis JA, et al. (1985) Beta blockade during and after myocardial infarction: an overview of the randomized trials. *Prog Cardiovasc Dis* **27**:335–71.

35 Pain management
Andrew Lawson and Paul Farquhar-Smith

INTRODUCTION

This chapter deals with the management of pain in gynecological malignancy. It does not deal with the management of pain arising from surgical intervention but with pain arising from the effects of the tumor and its treatment (Fig. 1).

Pain from gynecological malignancy is common. For example, over 60% of patients with ovarian cancer experienced pain before diagnosis or recurrence. Furthermore, physical and social function is adversely affected and also pain is associated with higher distress levels.

Pain may be caused by

1. direct effects of the tumor
2. treatment of cancer and cancer symptoms, for example, radiotherapy induced plexopathy, chemotherapy-induced neuropathy, constipation secondary to opioid drug administration
3. secondary problems from malignancy, for example, muscle spasm and musculoskeletal problems after prolonged immobilization.

Patients may therefore complain of different types of pain. These pains can be divided into nociceptive and neuropathic pain. Nociceptive pain (such as caused by tumor erosion or muscle spasm) may be sharp and stabbing, cramping, or throbbing. However, compared to somatic pain, nociceptive pain from the viscera tends to be less localized and can be referred. Neuropathic pain (resulting from a lesion in or damage to the nervous system) is often described as shooting, lancinating, or burning and is often associated with paresthesias and dysesthesias. Local infiltration by tumor into nerves can cause visceral neuropathic pain. Pain generally increases in severity with increasing tumor mass, later in the course of the disease and with metastatic disease. For organs involved in gynecological malignancy, like other viscera, noxious stimuli include distension, smooth muscle contraction, inflammation, and ischemia. Gynecological tumors may become ischemic and necrotic and result in pain associated with infection. Moreover some tumors may release inflammatory mediators as they invade other structures thus increasing the noxious potential. Tumor involvement with a hollow viscus can cause pain from distension and muscle contraction. Bowel obstruction may be associated with ovarian cancer and is an important source of pain.

VISCERAL PAIN PHYSIOLOGY
Anatomy to Explain Clinical Features

Sensory primary afferent neurons that arise in visceral organs are predominantly C and Aδ fibers (somatic sensory primary afferent include Aβ fibers). Furthermore, the total number of primary afferents is only 5% of their somatic counterparts, probably because the visceral system does not require accurate localization. Pelvic visceral also receive dual innervation from the sympathetic and parasympathetic systems. The nociceptive system for the visceral gynecologic organs undergoes primary (in the visceral organ) and secondary (central) sensitization, similar to the somatic system. Inflammation and the release of mediators of the inflammatory soup provides the main impetus that increases activation and sensitization of the nociceptive neurons increasing the afferent input into the spinal cord that drives the development of central sensitization. Visceral central sensitization may be more easily induced than somatic since the N-methyl-D-aspartate (NMDA) receptor is involved in unsensitized spinal transmission and therefore more readily activated by primary sensitization. This process is augmented by recruitment of silent afferents, sensory neurones quiescent (or "silent") in the resting state but activated by inflammation that may account for up to 90% of the total number of visceral primary afferents.

Similar central processes mediate the development of referred pain whereby pain from the viscera is perceived to be in a superficial somatic site. Moreover, pain from one viscus can exacerbate pain from another by a "viscero-visceral sensitization" mechanism. For example, pain from uterine cancer is exacerbated by pain from bowel obstruction.

The consequence of these mechanisms is that pain from gynecological malignancy is poorly localized: pain from a specific lesion may exist in several areas, migrate to different areas, and be referred superficially. Autonomic induced symptoms of sweating and tachycardia may be associated with these pains. Furthermore, distension, ischemia, and tumor-induced inflammation more readily induce the pro-algesic effects of central sensitization potentially increasing the pain burden in these patients.

Pain from Compression of Pelvic Structures

The female pelvic organs are in close proximity to a number of structures within the pelvis, both neurological and vascular. Thus local infiltration by a cervical, endometrial, and/or ovarian tumor may cause pain due to pressure on any of the structures within the pelvis. The pelvis acts as a conduit for the neurovascular supply of the lower limb and consequently nerve involvement may occur at sites of entry and exit from the pelvis as well as within. For example, the sciatic nerve may be affected by malignant infiltration at the point formation at the level of the nerve roots in the sacral plexus. The femoral nerve on the pelvic side wall may be damaged either due to hematoma or malignant infiltration, as may the obturator nerve. Pressure or obliteration of the lymphatic drainage may produce lymphedema of the lower limb. Compression of the venous supply to the lower limb may produce venous edema leading to swelling that may be painful. Although metastatic spread to bone is relatively rare in gynecological malignancy, tumors can invade bone directly.

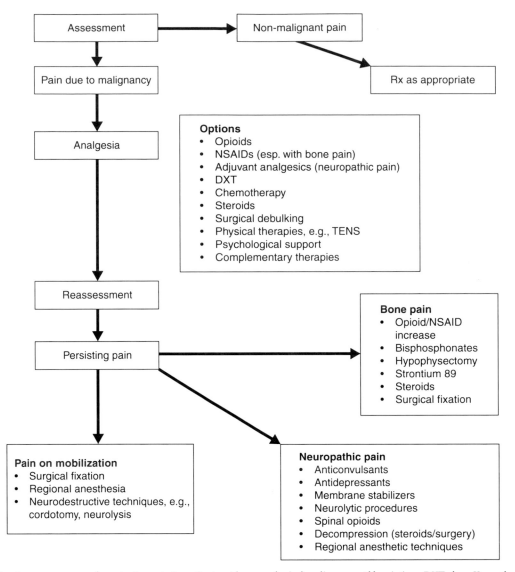

Figure 1 Algorithm for the management of continuing pain in patients with gynecological malignancy. *Abbreviations:* DXT, deep X-ray therapy; NSAID, non-steroidal anti-inflammatory drug; TENS, transcutaneous electrical nerve stimulation.

Initial Management of Pain

In patients with gynecological malignancy who have not had a curative surgical procedure, it is unlikely that simple analgesics alone will provide satisfactory pain relief. In the authors' opinion, patients such as these who have pain should be treated with opioid analgesics from the start. Slow-release morphine preparations and/or regular oral morphine preparations remain the "gold standard" of pain relief in patients with malignant disease. There is no convincing evidence that any of the newer analgesics has significant advantages over morphine. In the United Kingdom and in other parts of the world, diamorphine (diacetylmorphine, heroin) is commonly used as an analgesic agent. Table 1 lists opioid drugs and dosage regimens. Opioids may also be given by the subcutaneous route either intermittently or using a syringe driver. Fortunately, effective management of pain is achievable for the majority of patients with gynecological malignancy who are using opioid-based analgesic drugs in combination with drugs for the treatment of neuropathic pain. For those with pain resistant to standard treatments, perseverance and referral to a specialist at a chronic pain center is likely to result in an improved quality of life.

Table 1 Opioid Drugs in Severe Pain Equianalgesic Dose for 70-kg Adults

Drug	IM (mg)	PO (mg)	Interval (hrs)
Dextromoramide	7.5	10	1.5–3
Diamorphine	5	N/A	2–3
Hydromorphone	1.5	7.5	2–3
Methadone	10	10–15	8–48
Morphine	10	40–60	2–4
Oxycodone	N/A	30	4–6

To optimize analgesia, patients should at the same time be prescribed non-opioid analgesics. Paracetamol (acetaminophen) is widely prescribed in the United Kingdom and overseas and has the advantages of being available without prescription. Patients with bone infiltration may also respond to non-steroidal anti-inflammatory drugs such as diclofenac and ketorolac. Care should be taken in patients with impaired renal, hepatic or cardiovascular function, and in those who have reversible airways obstruction. Steroids may be beneficial in reducing the compressive effects of tumors.

Table 2 Drug Treatment of Neuropathic Pain

Class	Drug	Daily dose (mg)	Route
Tricyclic antidepressants	Amitriptyline	10–150	PO/IM
	Clomipramine	10–150	PO
	Desipramine	10–150	PO
	Doxepin	12.5–150	PO/IM
	Imipramine	12.5–150	PO
Selective serotonin re-uptake inhibitors (SSRIs)	Fluoxetine	20–60	PO
	Parozetine	10–40	PO
Anticonvulsants	Carbamazepine	100–1200	PO
	Clonazepam	2–10	PO
	Gabapentin	300–1200	PO
Membrane stabilizers	Mexiletine	150–1500	PO

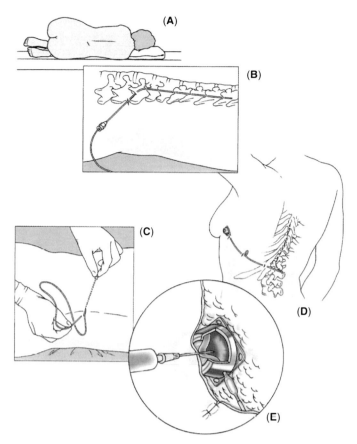

Figure 2 Insertion of tunneled epidural catheter. (**A**) Position of patient: insertion marked at L2. (**B**) Insertion of 16-gauge epidural catheter via a Tuohy needle. (**C**) Second incision over 11th rib allows the catheter to be moved over the anterior chest wall. (**D**) Portal attached to catheter after tensioning loop and second tunnel. (**E**) Injection technique.

Neuropathic Pain

Patients who have nerve involvement may well respond to the usage of antidepressant, anticonvulsant, and membrane-stabilizing agents, all of which have been demonstrated to be efficacious in the treatment of neuropathic pain. Pain due to radiation damage to the sacral plexus is likely to be resistant to standard analgesic techniques and in such circumstances antidepressants and membrane-stabilizing agents may be the first-line drugs of choice (Table 2).

INTERVENTIONAL TECHNIQUES IN GYNECOLOGICAL MALIGNANCY
Epidural and Spinal Opiates

Where standard routes of analgesic administration have failed, the epidural route using a percutaneous epidural catheter can provide optimal analgesia. The benefits of opioid administration by the spinal route have been acknowledged for some time and there is clear evidence that some patients find epidural analgesia of a higher quality with a diminished incidence of unwanted side effects such as nausea, drowsiness, and constipation. Epidural catheters can be inserted percutaneously and brought out through the skin or attached to a number of subcutaneous administration devices (Fig. 2). Subcutaneous pumps have been used to facilitate epidural and spinal analgesia, as have subcutaneous ports through which opiates can be given on a daily or more frequent basis.

All opiates currently on the market have been used in the epidural space. The most commonly used are morphine and (in the United Kingdom) diamorphine. Opiates have been given also in combination with local anesthetic drugs to improve the quality of analgesia. This may be particularly helpful in terminal cases where there is extreme and intractable pelvic and neuropathic pain. Drugs such as clonidine, midazolam, and baclofen have also been given epidurally in such circumstances.

SUPERIOR HYPOGASTRIC PLEXUS BLOCK
The superior hypogastric plexus is formed by the union of the lumbar sympathetic chains in branches of the aortic plexus in combination with the parasympathetic fibers originating in the ventral routes of S2 to S4, which form the pelvic splanchnic nerve, some fibers of which ascend from the inferior

hypogastric plexus to join the superior hypogastric plexus. The superior hypogastric plexus is situated anterior to the lower part of the body of the fifth lumbar vertebra and the upper part of the sacral promontory. It is retroperitoneal and is often called the presacral nerve. The superior hypogastric plexus gives off branches to the ovarian plexuses.

Technique
The patient is placed prone and two 20- or 22-gauge needles are advanced from a point roughly 5 to 7 cm lateral to the L4/L5 interspace to a point just anterior to the L5/S1 interspace. These needles are inserted under fluoroscopic or CT guidance, and injected contrast material demonstrates that the needles are anterior to the vertebral body and not in any of the vascular structures. Following aspiration, neurolytic solution of aqueous phenol 8 to 10 mL is injected, or for local anesthetic blockade, 10 to 20 mL 0.5% bupivacaine (Fig. 3).

Blockade of Ganglion Impar
Ganglion impar block has been described for the treatment of intractable perineal and pelvic pain where the sympathetic input seems to predominate. The ganglion impar is a retroperitoneal structure located at the level of the sacrococcygeal junction. The technique involves placement of a needle through the skin under X-ray control to lie anterior to the coccyx close to the sacrococcygeal junction. Retroperitoneal location of the needle is demonstrated by the injection of contrast

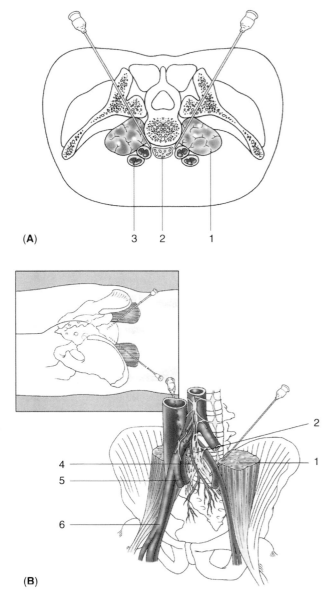

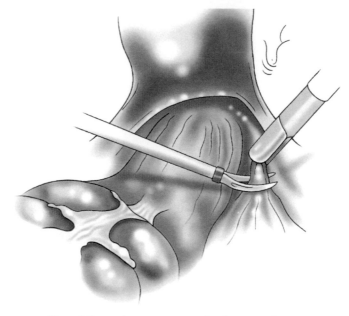

Figure 5 Presacral neurectomy: opening the presacral space.

Figure 3 Superior hypogastric plexus block. (**A**) Sagittal section at L5; (**B**) pelvic anatomy. 1 Psoas major muscle, 2 Superior hypogastric plexus, 3 Bifurcation of iliac vessels, 4 Superior rectal artery, 5 Internal iliac artery and vein, 6 External iliac artery and vein.

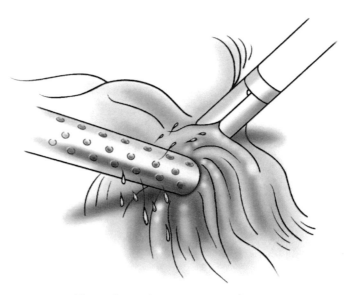

Figure 6 Presacral neurectomy: opened spaces.

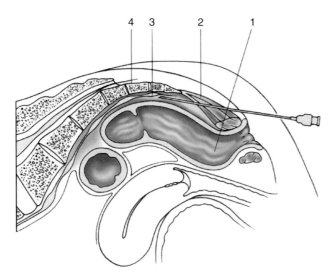

Figure 4 Blockade of ganglion impar. 1 Rectum, 2 Anococcygeal ligament, 3 Ganglion impar, 4 Sacrococcygeal junction.

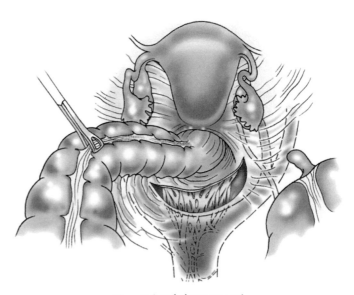

Figure 7 Sacral plexus exposed.

medium. Local anesthetic and/or neurolytic solutions can then be injected. Care must be taken to ensure that puncture of the rectum and accidental trans-bone injection into the epidural space are avoided (Fig. 4).

Presacral Neurectomy

Presacral neurectomy has been used for the control of intractable pelvic pain, whether due to malignancy or chronic pelvic pain syndromes. The technique involves the division of the superior hypogastric plexus at the L5/S1 region as described above. The presacral nerves can be divided as an open procedure or via the laparoscope. Laparoscopic presacral neurectomy is probably the technique of choice (Figs. 5 and 6). Bowel preparation is indicated preoperatively to decompress the bowel. Under direct vision an incision is made in the peritoneum over the lateral sacral promontory and dissecting forceps are used to dissect out the hypogastric plexus. It may then be ligated, cut, or cauterized (Fig. 7).

BIBLIOGRAPHY

Bonica JJ (1990) *The Management of Pain*, 2nd edn. Malvern: Lea & Febiger.

Cervero F, Laird JMA (1999) Visceral pain. *Lancet* **353**:2145–8.

Cousins MJ, Bridenbaugh PO, eds. (1996) *Neural Blockade in Clinical Anaesthesia and the Management of Pain*, 3rd edn. Philadelphia: Lippincott/ Williams & Wilkins.

Doyle D, Hanks GW, MacDonald N, eds. (1997) *The Oxford Textbook of Palliative Medicine*, 2nd edn. Oxford: Oxford University Press.

Farquhar-Smith WP, Jaggar SI (2008) Visceral pain mechanisms. In: Baranowski AP, Fall M, Abrams P, eds. *Urogential Pain in Clinical Practice*. Chapter 6. New York: Informa Healthcare, pp. 61–70.

McMahon SB, Dmitrieva N, Kolzenberg M (1995) Visceral pain. *Br J Anaesth* **75**:132–44.

36 Palliative care

Sarah Cox and Catherine Gillespie

WHAT IS PALLIATIVE CARE?

In 1990 the World Health Organisation defined palliative care as "the active total care of patients whose disease is not responsive to curative treatment. Control of pain, of other symptoms, and of psychological, social and spiritual problems, is paramount. The goal of palliative care is achievement of the best quality of life for patients and their families".

Modern palliative care has evolved from terminal care to a more dynamic multidisciplinary approach which tries to address priorities from an individual patient's perspective. It recognizes that some patients will need palliative care input from diagnosis or soon after. It places emphasis on the need to support the family and carers and to continue that support into bereavement. Above everything is the concept of enabling people to "live well" despite having a life-limiting diagnosis.

Specialist palliative care requires a team approach to identify and address the issues that are having a negative impact on the patient's quality of life. Specialist palliative care teams are now available as a resource to most hospitals, primary care teams and specialist inpatient units or hospices.

The clinical nurse specialist in gyne-oncology complements the palliative care team in the cancer unit or cancer center. They will often have met the patient in the early stages of their disease and will be the key in providing continuity of care as they tend to be the most consistent health professional involved in the patient's management. They will liaise between health professionals and be an important source of information and emotional support to patients throughout their treatment.

Hospices collect together a wide range of disciplines with specialist expertise to provide emotional, practical, and financial help as well as medical and nursing care. Social workers are essential to help with such complex problems as psychosocial counseling, financial and housing issues, immigration, preparing young families for loss, and bereavement support. Occupational therapists help patients cope with sometimes rapidly increasing disability and may enable patients to remain in their own homes for longer. Physiotherapists are essential to maximize mobility, to teach relaxation techniques, and non-pharmacological management of breathlessness. Specialized care may also be available from psychologists, spiritual advisors, art and music therapists, dieticians, pharmacists, and complementary therapists with volunteers to support them all.

Hospices usually have a small number of inpatient beds with a high staff-to-patient ratio. Admissions may be for terminal care but around 40% of patients are discharged back home after a few weeks of symptom control or psychological support. This is an important statistic to emphasis to patients who are may feel referral to hospice is the "first nail in the coffin". Women affected by gynecological malignancy may benefit from the outpatient services available at many hospices which might include day center, complementary therapy such as massage, appointments with dietetics or physiotherapy, or medical outpatients. Hospices may be a useful alternative to consider for women with advanced disease who require medical interventions such as ascitic drainage or blood transfusion (Fig. 1).

Specialist palliative care is also available to patients at home and works alongside the primary care team. Community palliative care teams work across the United Kingdom in a network of interlocking catchment areas. Teams are often based in a hospice and will consist of nurse specialists ("Macmillan nurses" when funded by that charity) with medical, paramedical, and social work input. Nurse specialists in the community complement the input of primary care and social services with specialist advice on symptom control, information, and support. They will communicate closely with other health professionals such as the general practitioner and the hospital gyne-oncology team about the patient's condition. They are also in a position to reflect with the patient issues about their illness and possible treatment options.

WHEN IS PALLIATIVE CARE RELEVANT TO THE WOMAN WITH GYNECOLOGICAL CANCER?

Palliative care is usually considered appropriate when curative treatment is no longer possible. However, there is evidence to suggest that women experience distressing physical and psychological effects during and after successful treatment for gynecological cancer. Persistent difficulties with pain, fatigue, bladder and bowel dysfunction, and sexual problems were reported in a group of disease-free patients. Half were depressed and 39% reported persistent psychosocial difficulties (Steginga and Dunn 1997). Palliative care should therefore be available on the basis of need at all points along the patient pathway. Particularly emotional or symptomatic difficulties may be experienced around the time of diagnosis, during active chemotherapy or radiotherapy, at relapse and in advanced disease.

The U.K. national cancer standards recognize the important role of palliative care in gynecological oncology and expect there to be representation from the specialist palliative care team at the gynecological cancer MDT meeting (Manual of Cancer Standards 2008).

Sexual dysfunction or psychosexual problems can arise either as a direct result of gynecological cancer or as a result of its treatment. Surgery, radiotherapy, and chemotherapy may influence the physical ability to have and gain pleasure from sexual intercourse while altered body image may impact upon a women's ability to enjoy the emotional side of sexual activity. Despite this, the need to feel close to people both physically and emotionally will remain and women will need support in order to come to terms with their altered sexual function.

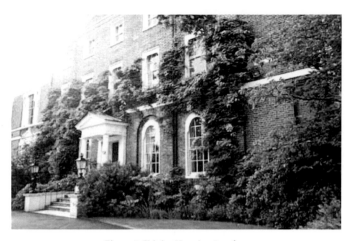

Figure 1 Trinity Hospice, London.

Table 1 Prevalence of Symptoms in Advanced Cancer and Ovarian Cancer

Symptom	Population with advanced cancer (Vainio and Auvinen 1996)	Advanced ovarian cancer (Cox S, unpublished work)
Pain (%)	57	69
Anorexia (%)	30	44
Weakness (%)	51	28
Breathlessness (%)	19	
Confusion (%)	8	
Nausea (%)	21	47
Vomiting (%)		50
Constipation (%)	23	13
Dry mouth (%)		13
Depression (%)		16

Ovarian cancer is often diagnosed at an advanced stage with about 60% of women presenting with stage III or stage IV disease. Other gynecological malignancies usually present earlier but may progress despite treatment. Clinical problems arising commonly in advanced ovarian cancer include malignant bowel obstruction, recurrent ascites, and fistulae. Ureteric obstruction and renal failure are not unusual in end-stage cervical cancer. Decisions around appropriate treatment in these situations will often involve input from the palliative care team. Prognosis depends on patient characteristics and staging of the particular cancer but ovarian cancer represents the fourth commonest cause of cancer death in women. End of life issues may include ethical dilemmas, consideration of place of care, and support for the family into bereavement. Support should be available for staff around the loss of a patient.

GENERAL PRINCIPLES OF PALLIATIVE CARE

A palliative care interview will involve taking a medical history with particular attention to symptoms, insight and understanding, family and social history, and medications—both current and previous. Assessment should also identify psychological and spiritual concerns and anxieties about the present or future. It may be possible to discuss wishes around future care including advanced refusal of treatment, and preferred place of death. The concerns of the family and carers also need to be heard and discussed.

SYMPTOM MANAGEMENT

It is important to determine the likely cause of any symptoms, and to assess their relative significance to the patient in order to plan management. It is common for individuals to have multiple symptoms or problems and a full history should be taken for each. Not all symptoms may be due to the main disease. Symptoms may be caused because of secondary effects of the illness (e.g., weakness or debility), because of side effects of treatment, or because of unrelated, concurrent illness. Symptoms also interact with emotional, social, and spiritual problems, so that pain can be exacerbated by worry, lack of information, fears, anxiety, or any unresolved matters.

Investigations should be considered to aid diagnosis and guide treatment. However if an individual is too frail to receive treatment for a specific problem, invasive tests to diagnose that problem are usually not warranted.

There are many reports of symptom prevalence in mixed populations of cancer patients, but very little published on symptoms associated with advanced gynecological malignancies (Table 1). Symptom surveys vary depending on the stage of disease, but even in cancer center outpatient populations treatable symptoms are very common (Lidstone et al. 2003).

Symptomatic or palliative management embraces an enormous range of interventions from teaching breathing techniques to disease-modifying management like surgery. The common intention with such treatment is not to cure the patient but to make them better, if only for a while. This principle can be applied to every management decision and used to weigh risks against the potential benefit. Treatment decisions need to be individualized and reviewed frequently. It is sensible to minimize the number of medications in order to aid compliance.

Disease-modifying Palliative Treatment

In the treatment of gynecological cancer, surgery, radiotherapy, and chemotherapy are the most commonly used forms of disease-modifying treatment. They may be offered even when cure is not possible to improve quality of life or because they offer the chance of prolonged life.

Non-pharmacological Treatment

Examples of non-pharmacological treatment approaches include the following:

- Breathing control techniques for breathlessness
- Relaxation techniques for anxiety
- Dietary modifications for anorexia
- Provision of a pressure-relieving mattress for debilitated patients
- Acupuncture or TENS for the relief of pain
- Provision of a quiet and supportive environment for agitated or distressed patients

Prescribing for Symptom Control

The aim when prescribing for persistent symptoms is to render the patient symptom-free. Appropriate drugs must therefore be taken regularly rather than on an adhoc basis. Each new drug should be perceived to have benefits which outweigh potential side effects in the context of the patient's condition. It is good practice to avoid polypharmacy; regular review will allow drugs to be stopped that are no longer necessary or helpful. Both patients and carers need clear concise guidelines to ensure maximum cooperation. Drug regimens should ideally be written out in full for patients and families and patient's self-medication charts are a useful adjunct to this. Where patients and families are easily confused by treatment regimens, this should be reviewed to reduce the number of drugs/tablets. Compliance may be further aided by the use of a dossette box, which can be filled by a relative, or pharmacist. Patients and carers also benefit from a clear plan of action should a current management plan not be working and know who to contact and how to contact them. The patient should have an appropriate identified Key Worker at all stages of their cancer journey—this is particularly important in the palliative care setting.

Breathlessness

Breathlessness may become more severe in the last weeks of life, and is often difficult to control. It has many potential causes including pleural effusion, pulmonary embolism, muscle weakness, anemia, pneumonia, chronic heart failure, chronic obstructive pulmonary disease, and/or psychological distress. Consideration should be given to treating reversible causes if the benefit of doing so outweighs the burden to the patient. The goal of symptomatic treatment is to improve the subjective sensation as experienced by the patient, rather than to improve abnormalities in blood gas or pulmonary function. Difficulty breathing is often associated with a high level of anxiety which exacerbates the problem. Patients may need to reduce their expectations and adapt their home environment to make daily activities more manageable. General measures include ensuring that the patient is comfortable, upright positioning, and providing information and reassurance. Teaching breathing exercises can give some feeling of control. Oxygen can be helpful, especially where there is hypoxia, but similar effects can be achieved by a stream of air which produces less practical difficulties. If there is some reversible airways obstruction bronchodilators may be useful. Opioids can improve exercise tolerance in advanced airways limitation and reduce the sensation of breathlessness. Benzodiazepines are central sedatives and can also relieve the unpleasant feeling of dyspnoea. Corticosteroids may be helpful where dyspnoea results from a large tumor mass.

Anorexia

Anorexia is very common in advanced malignancy. It may be associated with considerable weight loss which may be a source of distress to affected women and their relatives. Loss of appetite also results in loss of the social activity of eating with friends and family. Evidence exists to show the ineffectiveness of aggressive nutritional support in very advanced cancer. Women should be advised to try small portions and dietary supplements. Corticosteroids and progestrogens can be used to stimulate appetite where appropriate.

Nausea and Vomiting

Management of nausea and vomiting will be most effective if a cause can be identified and treatment targeted appropriately.

Symptoms may result from gastric irritation or poor gastric emptying because of massive ascites or significant hepatomegaly. Bowel obstruction will often result in vomiting. Raised intracranial pressure should be suspected if there is early morning nausea and vomiting associated with headache and drowsiness or confusion. Since each of these causes has a different mechanism and is mediated by different receptors, specific antiemetics should be chosen. Oral administration may not be effective and parenteral routes (e.g., continuous subcutaneous infusion) should be considered at an early stage.

Constipation

Constipation is a common cause of discomfort in advanced cancer. Causes include inactivity, weakness, dehydration, diminished food intake, low fiber diet, and drugs. In addition, there may be direct or indirect effects of the cancer such as hypercalcemia or bowel obstruction. Patients who are able to should be encouraged to drink plenty of fluids, eat appropriately, and move about. However, in advanced malignancy these measures are usually inadequate by themselves and a laxative such as polyethylene glycol (Movicol) will need to be taken daily. With fecal impaction, rectal intervention will be required as well to initiate bowel movement.

Anxiety and Depression

Anxiety and depression are common in advanced cancer and may be underdiagnosed. Risk factors for the development of depression include previous depressive episodes and uncontrolled pain. Biological symptoms such as loss of appetite and weight, poor sleep, and lethargy are unhelpful in making the diagnosis as they occur with advanced cancer itself. Loss of interest or pleasure and hopelessness may be more discriminating symptoms in this population. Treatment with antidepressants may allow the patient to achieve a better quality for the remainder of her life.

CLINICAL CHALLENGES FOR PALLIATIVE CARE IN GYNECOLOGY ONCOLOGY

Advanced gynecological cancer present a range of clinical challenges for the multiprofessional team. Women with advanced cervical cancer may go into renal failure as a result of bilateral ureteric obstruction. It may be possible to decompress one kidney with a nephrostomy tube and the attempt placement of a J–J stent into the ureter. However, in some cases extrinsic compression makes stenting unsuccessful, or of short-lived benefit. Over-aggressive treatment may result in a woman spending much of her limited time in hospital. The multiprofessional team needs to work closely with the patient and carers and health professionals in the community to make the best decision.

Malignant Bowel Obstruction

Malignant bowel obstruction is a common feature of advanced gynecological malignancy. Retrospective and post-mortem surveys give prevalence rates of 5% to 51% (Ripamionti and Bruera 2002). Malignant bowel obstruction is the most frequent cause of death in ovarian cancer. In these patients, obstruction may be of the small or large bowel, or, most commonly, at multiple sites. The pathophysiology of obstruction is usually by extrinsic compression from mesenteric, omental, and pelvic masses with intra-abdominal adhesions. Contributing factors may include inflammatory edema, fecal impaction, fatigue of intestinal muscles, and constipating effect of drugs.

Clinical presentation may vary depending on the level of the obstruction, but is usually sub-acute with a relapsing and remitting course (Fig. 2).

Surgery should be considered in all patients with malignant bowel obstruction. In advanced malignancy, surgery will be palliative and symptom control may be possible using less invasive means. Most studies of surgery in malignant bowel obstruction have been retrospective and conclusions are difficult to draw. Postoperative morbidity and mortality figures vary widely with reobstruction rates from 10% to 50%. Symptomatic relief is said to be achieved in 42% to over 80% (Feuer et al. 1999). Advanced age, medical frailty, and poor nutritional status may mitigate against operative treatment. The presence of ascites or palpable abdominal masses are poor prognostic signs. Previous abdominal radiotherapy or chemotherapy is associated with poorer outcomes from surgery. Treatment options must be honestly discussed with the patient and their carers in order to come to an appropriate decision.

Symptomatic relief of symptoms can be achieved pharmacologically in a majority of patients. Symptoms are usually a combination of nausea and vomiting, continuous abdominal pain, and/or abdominal colic. Stimulant laxatives should be stopped and prokinetic drugs such as metoclopromide used with caution. Appropriate antiemetics are given parenterally, usually subcutaneously by continuous infusion. To this infusion can be added a strong opioid such as morphine for constant pain and hyoscine butylbromide for intestinal colic.

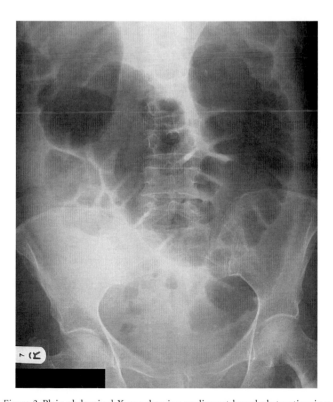

Figure 2 Plain abdominal X-ray showing malignant bowel obstruction in a woman with advanced ovarian cancer.

Patients should be allowed to eat and drink as they choose. Thirst is rarely a problem, but subcutaneous or intravenous fluids can be given if needed. Symptoms can be controlled this way in about 75% of patients with malignant obstruction. In the remainder other measures will be needed which may include the addition of the somatostatin analog, octreotide, corticosteroids, or nasogastric intubation (Mangili et al. 1996). Conservative management with nasogastric intubation and intravenous hydration is appropriate prior to surgery but is not otherwise recommended. A more conservative regime can be managed in the patient's home by the primary care team with specialist palliative care support. Being at home at the end of life is an important goal for many women with cancer and achieving the preferred place of care for a patient is a central priority of the National End of Life Care Strategy 2008.

Recurrent Malignant Ascites

Ovarian cancer is the commonest cause of malignant ascites, occurring in about 30% of patients with ovarian cancer at diagnosis and around 60% at the time of death. In ovarian cancer the ascites is usually associated with peritoneal metastases. Less commonly the fluid may be chylous or can accumulate as a result of portal hypertension in the presence of massive liver metastases. Malignant ascites is not such a poor prognostic sign in a woman with ovarian cancer as in other tumor types because of the potential for response to chemotherapy (Mackey and Venner 1996).

Malignant ascites causes symptoms including anorexia, nausea, abdominal distension and pain, dyspnoea, and fatigue. It can have a negative impact on a woman's body image—she may be treated as if she were pregnant and repeatedly asked "when is the baby due". Knowing her diagnosis these sorts of comments can be devastating (Fig. 3).

Symptoms may be treated empirically as suggested above, but often the best way to gain relief is to drain some of the ascites. Much debate exists over how to make paracentesis most effective. There is an evidence base to guide our practice but it relates largely to cirrhotic ascites. In undiagnosed cases a full history and examination will precede imaging and diagnostic tap of the ascitic fluid (Fig. 4).

In cases of malignant ascites where active treatment is not able to prevent recurrence, the mainstay of treatment is repeated drainage. Symptomatic paracentesis gives good relief of symptoms in 90% of patients. Potential complications include ascitic leaking, infection, and hypovolemia if large volumes are withdrawn. When draining cirrhotic ascites it is usual to provide intravenous fluid replacement with colloids to prevent symptomatic hypovolemia. This is not common practice in the treatment of ascites caused by ovarian cancer. There is no accepted standard rate of drainage or total volume but an average target is 5 L. The drain should be removed as soon as possible to limit the chance of infection and reduce the time spent as an inpatient. Draining to dryness is sometimes advocated although ascitic fluid is likely to recur and the burden of this treatment is greater.

The use of diuretics is also associated with controversy. Small studies have supported the use of a combination of loop diuretics and spironolactone to delay reaccumulation of ascitic fluid. Diuretics appear to be most effective when liver metastases are present.

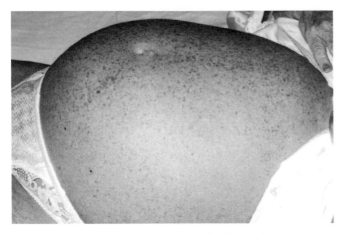

Figure 3 Tense abdominal ascities as a presenting feature of ovarian cancer.

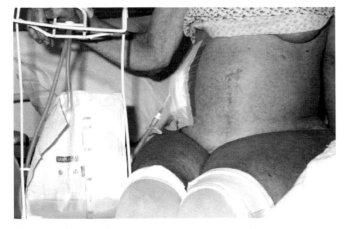

Figure 4 Ascitic drain for symptom relief in a woman with advanced ovarian cancer.

Peritoneovenous shunts may be inserted as an alternative to repeated paracentesis. Originally developed for use in patients with cirrhotic ascites, both Leveen and Denver shunts have been studied in small open trials of recurrent malignant ascites. There is a significant shunt-related operative mortality and morbidity up to 60% in some reports, although others reveal 60% to 80% success rates. Complications include shunt occlusion, coagulopathy, gastrointestinal bleeding, sepsis, and pulmonary edema. Peritoneovenous shunting may be considered for patients who have failed other symptomatic treatments for ascites and who have a prognosis of some months. Tunneled and untunneled percutaneous catheters may represent safer alternatives to peritoneovenous shunts and are increasing in use (Fleming et al 2009).

Intraperitoneal treatments including chemotherapy and monoclonal antibodies have reported some success with the main complication being small bowel adhesions.

COMMUNICATING WITH THE FAMILY AND WITH OTHER PROFESSIONALS

In palliative care, the patient and their family or those important to them are regarded as the unit of care. However, this does not mean that carers should be given information before patients; and professionals need to follow the patient's wishes. The fears, anxieties, and concerns of the carer can to be explored and their more intimate knowledge of the person

drawn out. It may also be helpful to discuss with the family the strain that the situation is placing on them and ways in which services and the professionals may help.

One of the common concerns of patients in hospitals and in the community is that of receiving mixed messages from different professionals. It is important that all of the team involved in the care of the patient, and family are kept fully informed of the important decisions and wishes of the patient and their family or carer. If people are at home and different services are visiting, the carer or patient can sometimes feel that they have a full time job coordinating which services arrive when. It is important in these instances to identify a key worker for that patient and family who helps to take on some of the role of coordination and advocacy, so that the patient and the carer receive the services and benefits to which they are entitled. Similarly, in hospitals patients and carers may ask for information from different nurses and doctors—depending on who is with the patient at one time. There may also be different teams involved. This may be particularly likely with palliative care patients—who may be seeing members of the hospital palliative care team as well as their own doctors. When the circumstances and condition of the patient changes rapidly it is especially important that all the team is kept rapidly informed of relevant changes in the treatment plans or in the person's condition or wishes.

THE DYING PATIENT

The publication in the United Kingdom of the National End of Life Care Strategy (DH 2008) encourages healthcare professionals to work with their patients to discuss and plan for their care toward the end of their life. Most deaths from gynecological cancer can be predicted in advance and therefore planned for and actively managed. Sudden death from associated causes such as pulmonary embolism or sepsis can occur and then the focus is on supporting the relatives.

It can be difficult to recognize that a patient is dying when they have been very slowly deteriorating. It is especially difficult to acknowledge approaching death amongst the team when a relationship has been built up with the woman over a period of time. It may feel like an admission of failure to suggest discussions about preparing for death but there may be important issues which need to be addressed. Integrated care pathways for the care of the dying are increasingly being used in all sites of care to improve recognition and care of the dying patient (Ellershaw and Ward 2003).

Women with advanced disease may ask if they are dying and sensitive honesty is required in answering them. It may be that the medical and nursing team recognize a deterioration and can reflect this to the patient and her family. She can then choose whether to take up an offer of further information. Some women will understand that bad news is available and choose not to pursue it or suggest that their family is told instead.

Information allows patients to plan for their limited future including where they would prefer to die and to deal with "unfinished business". This may include financial plans such as making a will, practical issues such as formalizing a power of attorney and making a living will, or spending precious time with loved ones. Where there are children involved there are particular issues to consider including how to tell them what is happening, how to leave a living written, or video memory, and sometimes who will be their guardian.

Recognition that a woman is entering the terminal phase of her illness is also important for the health care team. Investigations and treatments which had been appropriate may no longer be in the best interests of the patient. A multitude of decisions will need to be made including about continuing chemotherapy, treating new infections, tube feeding, and cardiopulmonary resuscitation. Different patients will want different levels of involvement in such decision making.

As death approaches, patients will become weaker, sleepier, and lose their appetite. They will spend longer periods of time in bed and then longer asleep. They need good nursing care to avoid skin breakdown, and good oral care to prevent mouth discomfort. Blood tests, X-rays, and routine recordings such as blood pressure measurement become unhelpful and should be discontinued. Oral medication becomes more difficult to tolerate and can be cut down and then stopped. Symptomatic drugs must be continued, and may be given by continuous subcutaneous infusion, which is more comfortable than the intravenous route and can be managed by the nursing staff. Pain, nausea, agitation, and bubbly breathing can occur toward the end of life and drugs should be prescribed to be given subcutaneously for each of these symptoms. Fluids are not routinely given at the end of life although this needs to be assessed on an individual basis together with the family.

The health care team should be available regularly to talk with family and friends who often find the bedside vigil emotionally and physically exhausting. They may receive important support from a few minutes conversation a day with one of the teams. They will need an explanation for changes as they happen and in advance if they can be predicted. Enquiries should be made about the patient's spiritual beliefs to allow them and their families to benefit from this support. Support for the family in their bereavement may be available from the palliative care team or locally through the general practitioner or national bereavement agency.

REFERENCES

Department of Health (2008) *End of Life Care Strategy: Promoting High Quality Care for All Adults at the End of Life.* London: Department of Health.

Ellershaw J, Ward C (2003) Care of the dying patient: the last hours or days of life. *BMJ* **326**:30–4.

Feuer D, Broadley K, Shepherd J, et al. (1999) Systematic review of surgery in malignant bowel obstruction in advanced gynecological and gastrointestinal cancer. The Systematic Review Steering Committee. *Gynecol Oncol* **75**(3):313–22.

Fleming N, Alvarez-Secord A, Von Gruenigen V et al. (2009) Indwelling catheters for the management of refractory malignant ascites: a systematic literature overview and retrospective chart review. *J Pain Symptom Manage* **38**(3):341–9.

Lidstone V, Butters E, Seed P, et al. (2003) Symptoms and concerns amongst cancer outpatients: identifying the need for specialist palliative care. *Palliat Med* **17**(7):588–95.

Mackey J, Venner P (1996) Malignant ascites: demographics, therapeutic efficacy and predictors of survival. *Can J Oncol* **6**(2):474–80.

Mangili G, Franchi M, Mariani A, et al. (1996) Octreotide in the management of bowel obstruction in terminal ovarian cancer. *Gynecol Oncol* **61**(3):345–8.

National Cancer Action Team (2008) *National Cancer Peer Review Programme: Manual of Cancer Standards 2008: Gynaecological Cancer Measures.* London: Department of Health.

Ripamionti C, Bruera E (2002) Palliative management of malignant bowel obstruction. *Int J Gynecol Cancer* **12**(2):135–43.

Steginga S, Dunn J (1997) Women's experiences following treatment for gynaecological cancer. *Oncol Nurs Forum* **24**:1403–8.

Vainio A, Auvinen A (1996) Prevalence of symptoms among patients with advanced cancer: an international collaborative study. *J Pain Symptom Manage* **12**:3–10.

37 Doctor–patient communication
J. Richard Smith, Krishen Sieunarine, Mark Bower, Gary Bradley, and Giuseppe Del Priore

INTRODUCTION

Unlike the rest of this book, this final chapter does not concern itself with practical surgical techniques; instead, it looks at the problems of communication between the patient and her gynecologic oncologist. Entire books have been devoted to this subject and it may seem presumptuous even to attempt to address this in a brief chapter. However, we feel that the bare bones of good communication are extremely simple and may be summed up as imparting the truth and nothing but the truth in a compassionate manner.

In gynecologic oncology, patients face a frightening diagnosis and an uncertain future. It is increasingly recognized that patients wish to know their diagnosis and to be kept informed of the progress of treatment. This has resulted in a revolution in the approach to patient–doctor communication. The era of professional paternalism, protecting patients from the diagnosis and remaining unrealistically optimistic to the dying patient, is over. With this change in approach has come a realization that effective communication skills are not innate, but can be taught, learnt, retained, and used to improve patient care. More and more healthcare professionals, including gynecologic oncologists, are receiving training in communication with patients, their families, and other professionals.

This increased communication with cancer patients has costs to healthcare professionals which need to be appreciated and addressed. The improved communication brings healthcare professionals closer to the patient and may increase feelings of inadequacy when faced with insoluble issues and of failure when patients die. Gynecological oncologists dealing with dying patients and their families risk "burn-out"; although the medical profession is notoriously resistant to external help, a team spirit, adequate training through communication workshops, and peer support are important elements in tackling this problem.

Many junior doctors identify breaking bad news as their greatest fear and their top problem in communicating with patients. In many cases, doctors continue to carry this anxiety with them through years of clinical practice. Why do doctors fear breaking bad news? Obviously, the information causes pain and distress to our patients and their relatives, making us feel uncomfortable. We fear being blamed and provoking an emotional reaction. Breaking bad news reminds us of our own mortality and fears of our own death. Finally, we often worry about being unable to answer a patient's difficult questions since we never know what the future holds for either our patients or ourselves. Breaking bad news to patients should not involve protecting them from the truth but rather imparting the information in a sensitive manner at the patient's own pace. The setting for this conversation should be considered carefully. A confidential, quiet, and comfortable location should be used

rather than a busy gynecology ward with neighboring patients eavesdropping. An open-ended interruption-free period of at least 20 to 30 min should be allocated and the patient should be asked if she wishes anyone else to be present. Many patients will already be aware of how serious their condition is and will have guessed the diagnosis. Thus, an initial screening question asking what the patient believes to be the matter may change the interview from breaking to confirming bad news. Subsequently, the conversation may be viewed as a series of cycles repeated for each piece of information imparted. An initial warning shot from the doctor ("I'm afraid that the biopsy result was not normal") should be followed by a pause to enable the patient to respond. Further information can then be given and the patient again asked if she wishes to know any more. In this way it is the patient, not the doctor, who determines the quantity of information delivered and who controls the pace of the conversation without realizing it.

In general, prognostication with respect to "duration of remaining life" and the quoting of five-year mortality statistics is rarely helpful. Few of us are able to explain the implications of skewed distributions, medians, and confidence intervals in a way that is easily understood by patients. Moreover, many of us have enough optimism to believe that we will fall on the lucky side of whatever statistic is quoted and, of course, we might just be right. The last thing that we should do is to destroy all hope. Many patients will ask for predictions as to length of or guarantees of survival, often hoping for reassurance. In these circumstances, it is always easier to give false reassurance but the temptation must be avoided as you will not be doing your patient a favor in the long run. Despite these restrictions, all consultations ideally should end on a positive note, the motto being "never say never". Even in the bleakest of situations, setting short-term achievable goals leaves patients with aims for the future and hope. This maxim applies to both the patient and—where the patient agrees—the next of kin. It is always helpful to leave the patient with a further opportunity for discussion especially about the dozens of questions which arise in the patient's mind and may be generated by her discussions with relatives and friends. We have always given patients' our telephone numbers so that further discussion can be facilitated.

It is desirable to communicate at each stage in a private setting and preferably to the patient and her next of kin at the same time. Failing this, a discussion should take place with the patient and be followed at a future date by a joint consultation between doctor, patient, and her next of kin. It is rarely appropriate to allow relatives to "protect" the patient by withholding information or over-optimistically lying. These issues can become particularly difficult when dealing with cultural differences, particularly if the patient does not speak English.

Table 1 The Four-cusp Approach to Patient Communication

	Cusp 1	Cusp 2	Cusp 3	Cusp 4
Status	Potentially curable	Living with cancer	Pre-terminal	Terminal
Duration	Weeks to years	Months to years	Weeks to months	Days
Treatment	Radical surgery Adjuvant therapy	Palliative chemotherapy or radiotherapy	Supportive care	Terminal care
Aims	Cure Prolong survival	Prolong survival Improve QoL	Improve QoL	Improve QoL End-of-life issues

This act of collusion needs to be explored with relatives, on the basis that the patient needs to understand what is happening to her. With careful negotiation including an acknowledgment of the views of the relatives, access to the patient can usually be secured to determine the patient's own understanding of her illness. It is then common to discover that the patient is well aware of the diagnosis and herself colluding to spare the relatives. In such circumstances honest discussion may reduce anxiety and resolve the relationship difficulties within the family.

In addition to keeping the patient abreast of developments, it is vital to involve the whole multidisciplinary team so that the patient and her relatives hear the same message from all the healthcare professionals. The roles of individuals within the team and their boundaries of care may lead to friction within teams. Philosophical differences in treatment approaches need to be explored. Frequent team meetings and open discussion that avoids a hierarchical structure will enhance team spirit and reduce tensions. Occasionally, an external facilitator may be helpful to coordinate such meetings. The role of the oncology nurse is vital in these circumstances as they are often seen by the patient as accessible and sympathetic, without the formality of the "specialist oncologist".

The following pages set out what could be described as a four-cusp approach which may be useful in discussions on treatment strategies and prognosis (Table 1). We have been surprised at how often patients have taken away the scraps of paper used to demonstrate this four-cusp approach. In addition, we have noticed that our junior staff who frequently lack experience in talking through those difficult issues with patients find this a helpful framework. The cusps are illustrated by case examples. We used to refer to cusps 1, 2, 3, and 4, but a couple of our patients were upset because they confused cusps with "staging" and since then we have referred to four cusps: A, B, C, and D.

THE "FOUR-CUSP" APPROACH
Cusp A: Potentially Curable
The first cusp applies to most patients from the time of the first visit to the clinic when the surgeon imparts the probable diagnosis and discusses with the patient the plan of action to achieve staging and hopefully removal of the tumor. It is rare to feel totally confident that a tumor is incurable before surgery; one may suspect it, but rarely can one know until the histology is confirmed and the staging completed. An honest appraisal of the possibilities is required, coupled with a plan of action. This should include date of surgery, length of time in hospital, and when final and definitive histological and cytological reports will become available. It is almost always possible to achieve these results within 2–4 weeks of the first visit to the clinic. The patients thus know they will have a good idea where they stand by a specific date. The concept of cancer staging should be explained, and that the stage and type of tumor will influence the necessity for further treatment with radiotherapy or chemotherapy. We usually explain that, if we achieve treatment by surgery alone there is a presumption of cure. This, however, can only be confirmed by the passage of time, and the longer all remains well the higher is the likelihood that cure has been achieved. A high level of positivity and a buoyant approach are usually applicable both before and after surgery for those with complete resection of tumor, although the need for careful follow-up and the possibility of relapse should be discussed. This step-by-step approach can be utilized throughout the care of the patient and helps the patient to understand that the whole of care cannot be determined at the first visit. Constant and regular communication is the hallmark of good care.

Case 1
A woman is referred to the gynecological oncology clinic with postcoital bleeding and a suspected cervical cancer. On examination, a small cervical tumor is found which is approximately 2 to 3 cm in diameter. The uterus and cervix are mobile and there are no other detectable abnormalities. A colposcopy and biopsy are performed.

Following the examination, the consultation should continue, usually by asking the patient if she has any idea what she thinks the diagnosis might be. Many patients will state their worst fear, namely cancer; others will say they have no idea. This is generally the point at which to communicate that you also believe the diagnosis to be one of cancer and that the biopsy will confirm or exclude this within the next few days. It is then possible to say that the initial examination suggests that this is an eminently curable cancer, and to outline the plan of action: first, the patient will be admitted on a specific date within the next 1–2 weeks for staging of the tumor and on a subsequent date, probably within the next two weeks, for definitive surgery. Explain that there are four stages of cervical cancer, that stage I is the best and stage IV the worst, but all can be cured. Tell the patient that the first admission will take one day and will deliver an answer which she will probably know later that same day. Explain that you believe the tumor to be stage I and therefore highly curable, probably by surgery alone, but possibly requiring further treatment with chemoradiotherapy. Ask the patient to have her next of kin present at the post-staging ward round if they are not there at the clinic. The patient should be invited to ask any questions and encouraged to write down any questions she thinks of when she is home and to ask them when she is admitted.

It is our practice to copy the letter written to the referring doctor to the patients themselves. We undertook a survey of patient acceptability of this practice, and over 100 patients surveyed all believed it was helpful and none chose not to receive further copies of future letters. This is now a UK-wide policy, although not universally practiced. Carefully organized and coordinated staging protocols allow women rapid access to results, reducing delays, and hence minimizing the anxiety caused by waiting for results. The patient will have the usual prestaging investigations, such as radiographic scans, and will then be admitted for a staging and if for any reason results are delayed this only further increases anxiety.

The operation is then performed, and either the same day or the following day an explanation is given. A few days later the full histological picture is given.

Scenario 1: the histology report shows complete resection of a 2-cm well-differentiated squamous carcinoma with adequate resection margins and negative nodes.

This patient can be told that you believe cure has been achieved, and while long-term follow-up is warranted you expect to see her in the clinic for the next 5 to 10 years (depending on individual protocol) and to discharge her from care at this time "fit and well". At the end of the five years, she enters the cured circle i.e. she is more likely to develop a new cancer than a recurrence of her old one

Scenario 2: the histology report shows complete resection of a moderately differentiated squamous cervical carcinoma with 3 positive metastatic nodes out of 40 removed.

This information is imparted and the patient is told that although there is complete removal of tumor further treatment is required with combination chemoradiotherapy. Such patients can be told that you believe cure is likely and that this is a "belt and braces (suspenders)"approach, but that there is no denying they do have a higher chance of relapse than if their nodes had been negative. The concept of adjuvant therapy following radical surgery may be explained as an "insurance policy" to mop up any tumor cells that could have escaped the surgery. It is always valuable to have the radiotherapeutic member of the MDT to explain the detail of the treatment. She is in cusp B but with a high chance of long-term cure i.e. we are aiming that after 5 years she will return to cusp A, the cured circle. However, psychologically she will be living with her disease.

Case 2

A 55-year-old woman is referred by her general practitioner with abdominal swelling which she has noted in the last few weeks. She has no other symptoms. Abdominal examination reveals fluid in the abdomen on percussion. Vaginal examination is suggestive of a mass arising from the right adnexa, probably ovarian in origin, and nodules are felt in the pouch of Douglas.

The patient is informed that there are findings suggestive of an ovarian mass and that these require urgent investigation. The patient should be told that you suspect cancer and that the investigations you are about to request will go some way to eliciting a diagnosis.

I would do the RMI (risk of malignancy index; see chapter 21, page 156) immediately during the clinic so as to give the patient an early idea of what the likely diagnosis is.

Hematological and biochemical tests are ordered, as are tumor markers, an ultrasound scan with color flow Doppler, and a computed tomography (CT) scan of abdomen and pelvis to detect lymphadenopathy; a magnetic resonance imaging (MRI) of pelvis is also ordered. The patient is reviewed shortly thereafter and the risk of malignancy index is used. The findings are highly suggestive of a stage IC ovarian cancer.

Staging of ovarian cancer is explained to the patient, together with the fact that there are three possible outcomes from the operation which will be communicated to her immediately postoperatively:

- complete macroscopic resection of tumor
- resection of tumor down to nodules less than 1 cm in diameter
- inadequate debulking.

The last two possibilities seem unlikely, bearing in mind the optimistic findings of the investigations. Full staging will be arrived at a few days after surgery when all the cytologic and histologic results will be available. Patient consent is obtained for a total abdominal hysterectomy, bilateral salpingo-oophorectomy, omentectomy, and debulking as required.

Scenario 1: at surgery a smooth-walled cyst is found with some free fluid in the pelvis. There is no evidence of any tumor elsewhere in the abdomen on macroscopic examination.

Postoperatively, the patient can be told that she falls into the first category (fully macroscopically resected tumor) and a few days later the histological report confirms a well-differentiated ovarian epithelial carcinoma, with negative cytology from washings and peritoneum. The patient is informed that she has a stage IA tumor and should have no further problems. She remains at cusp A.

Scenario 2: at surgery the abdomen is opened and 500 ml of straw-colored fluid is aspirated and sent for cytology. Abdominal exploration reveals small studs of tumor on the diaphragm and a small omental deposit. A total hysterectomy, bilateral salpingo-oophorectomy, and omentectomy are performed with minimal residual tumor left at the end of the operation.

The patient is informed postoperatively that she falls into the second category, namely tumor debulked to less than 1 cm, and that she probably has a stage III tumor depending on results and almost certainly will require further treatment. A few days later the histologic and cytologic reports confirm that this clinical impression was correct. The patient is informed and chemotherapy planned. She should be informed that she has now entered the cusp B, "living with cancer", that she may regain cusp A following chemotherapy, this is the goal of the treatment but that only time will tell.

Cusp B: Living with Cancer

Cusp B is for treated patients who are in remission but are less likely to be cured (i.e., "living with cancer") but not terminal. Again a positive approach is appropriate, but the long-term goals are less optimistic. The patient should be informed that it is impossible to determine how long she will remain in remission, that we certainly have many patients who are alive many years after chemotherapy and a few who have returned to cusp A (i.e., presumed cured). Sadly, we also have some who have not survived as long. The golden rule is that the longer one is in complete remission, the better the prospects become. The biggest difficulty is that neither the patient nor the doctor knows which category she is in until time elapses, but it is important that both can see that it is well worth following through with treatment. The patient described in scenario 2 above then undergoes chemotherapy.

Scenario 1: the patient goes into complete remission for five years.

This patient is one of the lucky ones and has returned to cusp A—the cured circle.

Scenario 2: the patient goes into complete remission which lasts for three years and then at the follow-up joint oncology clinic is found to have a raised serum level of CA125 and a palpable nodule in the pouch of Douglas. Staging investigations reveal radiologic evidence of a solitary nodule. She therefore has a second laparotomy: complete excision of the tumor is achieved, followed by a further course of chemotherapy. Again, the patient enters complete remission.

She can be told that she appears to have a relatively non-aggressive tumor and can expect to remain in the second cusp for a good time longer.

Scenario 3: following first-line chemotherapy the patient achieves a partial remission which lasts for five months when she re-presents at follow-up to the joint oncology clinic with a rising serum CA125 level and abdominal swelling. Radiologic investigation suggests that there are widespread metastatic peritoneal nodules.

This patient may be given the choice of whether to be observed until she develops symptoms or to have second-line chemotherapy. The role of chemotherapy is to palliate symptoms rather than prolong survival in this context and the balance between the possible benefits and toxicities of the chemotherapy should be explored with the patient. The patient declines further chemotherapy and then deteriorates over the next few weeks. She needs to be informed that she has moved to cusp C.

Cusp C: Pre-terminal Phase

The third cusp applies to patients with virtually no chance of cure, who have entered the "pre-terminal phase". It is important that the patient is informed and made aware that she has a limited time left to her, and that she is given the opportunity to "put her house in order", see relatives and friends, make a will, etc. No patient should ever be told that there is nothing more than can be done for her. She should be informed that while she has virtually no chance of cure, and aggressive treatments to obtain cure are not appropriate, there are plenty of measures available to ameliorate symptoms, such as pain, nausea or upset bowels. The therapies that are appropriate at this phase of the disease are supportive measures to improve the quality of her life without causing toxicity.

Scenario: a patient with carcinoma of the cervix presents three years after radical radiotherapy for a stage III tumor. She is passing urine permanently from the vagina. On investigation and examination under anesthesia she is found to have extensive recurrence of tumor both in the para-aortic region and on the pelvic side-wall. In addition, she has a large irreparable cysto-vaginal fistula. She also has deteriorating renal function.

The patient is informed that she has recurrent cancer and there are no curative treatments available. She says she had guessed that anyway and is clearly very angry. She is then asked the vital question for cusp C, what in addition to the fact that she is dying is most bothering her? To this she replies that she accepts death as inevitable and this does not make her angry—what makes her angry is her permanent incontinence which is preventing her from going out and seeing family and friends. She is referred to the interventional radiologist and bilateral nephrostomy tubes are inserted, which render her dry. The patient goes home and returns four weeks later, in a terminal condition. She has entered cusp D. She does, however, inform us that she has had a great four weeks, been to the pub every day and seen all her friends. She dies 24 hours later. This decision highlights the importance of not denying patients palliative care even of a complex surgical nature at this time.

An example which could be regarded as non-medical was a patient who was in our ward coming very close to the terminal phase of her disease. She appeared very agitated and when asked "what, apart from cure, she would wish for if she could wave a magic wand?", the answer came back "I have papers at home which I would like to burn and I can't get home". The nurse in charge of her ward was duly informed of this and arranged an ambulance and a nurse to accompany the patient to her house where the papers were retrieved from the loft and burned. The patient returned to hospital much more at peace and was able to move to the terminal phase (cusp D). She died within a few days, mentally at peace.

Cusp D: Terminal Phase

The terminal phase of life lasts from hours to days and all interventions are only designed to "ease the passing". Patients, in general, need no telling that this is where they have arrived, although the relatives may need help in understanding it. Care is focused on emotional support rather than medical intervention, and frequently most of the patient's medication can be stopped apart from analgesia. The death of a patient whose physical symptoms are well controlled and who is spiritually calm is an achievable goal to which we should all strive.

BEREAVEMENT/GRIEF[a]

Bereavement is by definition the process we go through when we suffer loss of something or someone very special to us. In terms of this book it therefore applies to the women diagnosed with cancer who are coping with the loss that this entails and to the relatives of the minority of women who will sadly succumb to their disease.

At the time of diagnosis there is an enormous range of emotions at play. These range from denial, anger, grief, depression, aggression, numbness, etc. There is no doubting that at that first consultation numbness and disbelief will be the strongest emotion, as well as why me? I've done nothing to deserve this, I've eaten healthily, not smoked, not drank, it can't be true. However, over the next few days/weeks when the management plan is clarified, there is the coping with loss of organs if surgery is planned, this may involve loss of fertility, or feelings of loss of womanhood and a true bereavement process unfolds. If this is the first major illness encountered there will also be that loss of invincibility. We all feel invincible, it will never happen to us, until it does—and that is a terrible shock. Anger may center on why me? Why have I been dealt this hand of cards? If one is religious one may wonder why God has allowed this to happen.

---

[a]This section was originally published in Smith JR, Del Priore G, Women's Cancers Pathways to Healing, Springer, London, 2009.

Box 1 Sketch of the "Tapestry of Bereavement/Landscape of Grief"

Denial	D
Anger	A
Bewilderment/Bargaining	B
Depression	D
Acceptance	A
Hope	H

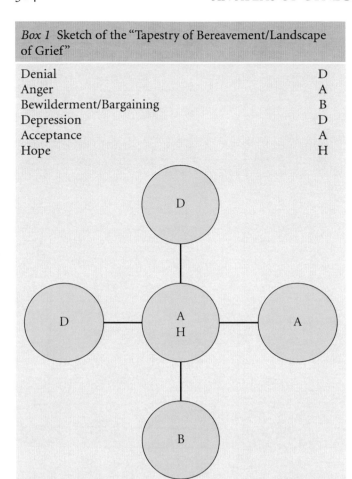

This model is as shown in the sketch with the various emotions cropping up not in any particular order but more randomly, with some predominating at one point and others at another. Hopefully, progress is made to "acceptance and hope". Over time all of the parts of the tapestry fade and whilst they do not disappear the tapestry becomes the new reality.

Traditionally bereavement has been seen in the step-wise progression suggested by Elizabeth Kubla-Ross, from denial to anger to grief to bewilderment to depression to acceptance and hope. Things will never be the same again but life can go on albeit differently. A different model encompassing the same emotions is the "tapestry of bereavement or a landscape of grief" (Box 1). This model was developed by the Rev Gary Bradley, the Founder and Chairman of the Westminster Bereavement Association. The analogy here is with a picture. When one buys a picture there are various features of the picture which one may have noticed, but as the picture hangs on the wall over time one notices different aspects of the picture until after some time one may hardly notice the picture at all, even although it is still there. One may however move the picture and it instantly becomes more visible.

This may all appear somewhat negative but one of the amazing and heartening things which many people say is that their cancer diagnosis finally gave them great inner strength and that they went on to do things that they know they would not otherwise have done—this is the concept of winning through losing—a very difficult place to get to, but something that can be genuinely empowering for the individual.

For those who lose a spouse, relative, or close friend the same range of emotions will occur and the tapestry is similar.

Box 2 Spirituality, Religion, and Psychology

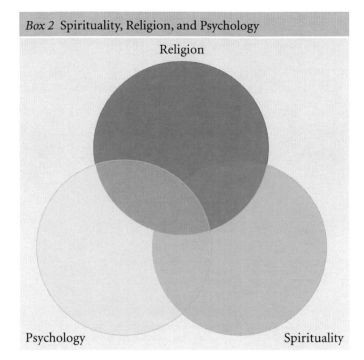

The "tapestry" by its flexibility and its ability to fade and then come back into focus may be a useful model for patients to think about.

This process, particularly when one arrives at hope and acceptance, ties in with the Venn diagram of psychology, spirituality, and religion. These are the areas that most patients will choose to further explore.

SPIRITUALITY, RELIGION, AND PSYCHOLOGY

This is a very difficult area to enter into with one's patients. While it is perfectly acceptable to discuss psychology, the other two namely spirituality and religion are, to a degree, taboo subjects for today's doctors and nurses. However, showing a patient the Venn diagram shown below (Box 2) often allows opening of the conversation. The patient can be invited to say which, if any, or possibly more than one suit her way of thinking. Recently JRS was in a consultation when he asked a patient this question. She said "I have all three covered. My brother is a priest. I see myself as quite a spiritual person and I have already booked up to see a psychologist!" This individual is likely to cope better with her cancer diagnosis than the individual who rejects all three approaches. Allowing the patient to express her views allows suitable onward referral.

BIBLIOGRAPHY

Boyle DCM, Lee M-J (2008) *Fast Facts: Religion and Medicine.* Oxford: Health Press.

Fallowfield LJ (1993) Giving sad and bad news. *Lancet* **341**:476–8.

Maguire P, Faulkner A (1988a) Communication with cancer patients: 1. Handling bad news and difficult questions. *Br Med J* **297**:907–9.

Maguire P, Faulkner A (1988b) Communication with cancer patients: 2. Handling uncertainty, collusion and denial. *Br Med J* **297**:972–3.

Nordin A, ed. (1999) *Gynaecological Cancer. Patient Pictures.* Oxford: Health Press.

Slevin ML (1987) Talking about cancer. How much is too much? *Br J Hosp Med* **38**(1):56–9.

Smith JR, Del Priore G (2009) *Women's Cancers Pathways to Healing.* London: Springer.

Index